PALLIATIVE PRACTICES

An Interdisciplinary Approach

PALLIATIVE PRACTICES

An Interdisciplinary Approach

KIM K. KUEBLER, MN, RN, ANP-CS
Adult Nurse Practitioner
Primary/Oncology/Palliative Care
Private Practice Adjuvant Therapies, Inc.
Atlanta, Georgia

MELLAR P. DAVIS, MD, FCCP
Director of Research
The Harry R. Horvitz Center for Palliative Medicine
Taussig Cancer Center
The Cleveland Clinic Foundation
Cleveland, Ohio

CRYSTAL DEA MOORE, MA, MSW, PhD
Social Work Program Director
Assistant Professor of Social Work
Department of Sociology, Anthropology, and Social Work
Skidmore College
Saratoga Springs, New York

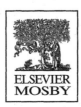

ELSEVIER
MOSBY

ELSEVIER
MOSBY

11830 Westline Industrial Drive
St. Louis, Missouri 63146

PALLIATIVE PRACTICES: AN INTERDISCIPLINARY APPROACH
Copyright © 2005, Mosby, Inc.

NOTICE

Pharmacology is an ever-changing field. Standard safety precautions must be followed, but as new research and clinical experience broaden our knowledge, changes in treatment and drug therapy may become necessary or appropriate. Readers are advised to check the most current product information provided by the manufacturer of each drug to be administered to verify the recommended dose, the method and duration of administration, and contraindications. It is the responsibility of the appropriately licensed health care provider, relying on experience and knowledge of the patient, to determine dosages and the best treatment for each individual patient. Neither the publisher nor the author assumes any liability for any injury and/or damage to persons or property arising from this publication.

The Publisher

ISBN-13: 978-0-323-02821-9
ISBN-10: 0-323-02821-7

Executive Publisher: Barbara Nelson Cullen
Editor: Sandra Clark Brown
Developmental Editor: Sophia Oh Gray
Publishing Services Manager: John Rogers
Senior Project Manager: Cheryl A. Abbott
Design Manager: Bill Drone

Transferred to Digital Printing 2009

To my family
Albert, Carl, and Catherine Kuebler
KK

To my family
Luke, Amanda, Meghan, Jessamyn, Emelyn, and particularly my wife Deborah
MD

To my family
You know who you are
CM

Contributors

Nancy M. Albert, MSN, RN, CCNS, CCRN, CNA
Director, Nursing Research, Division of Nursing
Clinical Nurse Specialist
George M. and Linda H. Kaufman Center for
    Heart Failure
The Cleveland Clinic Foundation
Cleveland, Ohio
6. Cardiovascular

Eduardo Bruera, MD
Professor and Chair
Department of Palliative Care and Rehabilitation
    Medicine
University of Texas M.D. Anderson Cancer Center
Houston, Texas
Foreword

Bushra I. Cheema, MD
Clinical Fellow, Palliative Medicine/
    Hematology-Oncology
The Cleveland Clinic Foundation
Cleveland, Ohio
11. Neurology

Lewis M. Cohen, MD
Associate Professor of Psychiatry
Tufts University School of Medicine
Medford, Massachusetts;
Director, Renal Palliative Care Initiatives
Baystate Medical Center
Springfield, Massachusetts
8. Nephrology

Joshua Cox, PharmD, RPh
Pain Management Consultant
Good Samaritan Hospital
Dayton, Ohio
7. Pulmonary

Mellar P. Davis, MD, FCCP
Director of Research
The Harry R. Horvitz Center for Palliative
    Medicine
Taussig Cancer Center
The Cleveland Clinic Foundation
Cleveland, Ohio
4. Pharmacology
10. Cancer Pain
11. Neurology
Appendixes A and B

Jan L. Frandsen, MSN, CRNP
Nurse Practitioner
The Cleveland Clinic Foundation
Cleveland, Ohio
10. Cancer Pain

Michael Germain, MD, FACD
Assistant Professor of Medicine
Tufts University School of Medicine
Boston, Massachusetts;
Professor of Medicine
Springfield College
Springfield, Massachusetts
8. Nephrology

Mary Magee Gullatte, MN, RN, ANP, AOCN
Adjunct Clinical Faculty
Nell Hodgson Woodruff School of Nursing
Emory University
Atlanta, Georgia;
Director of Nursing, Inpatient Oncology
    and Transplant Services
Emory University Hospitals and Winship Cancer
    Institute of Emory University
Atlanta, Georgia
9. Oncology

Debra E. Heidrich, MSN, RN, CHPN, AOCN
Nursing Consultant, Private Practice
West Chester, Ohio
9. Oncology

Roberta Kaplow, RN, PhD, CCNS, CCRN
Clinical Professor
Nell Hodgson Woodruff School of Nursing
Emory University
Atlanta, Georgia
9. Oncology

Barry M. Kinzbrunner, MD
National Medical Director
Vitas Healthcare Corporation
Miami, Florida
1. Palliative Care Perspectives

Kim K. Kuebler, MN, RN, ANP-CS
Adult Nurse Practitioner
Primary/Oncology/Palliative Care
Private Practice Adjuvant Therapies, Inc.
Atlanta, Georgia
14. The Dying Process
Appendixes A-D

Diane B. Loseth, RN, MSN
Advanced Practice Palliative Care Nurse
Yale-New Haven Hospital
New Haven, Connecticut
13. Cultural and Spiritual Issues

Helen Kathleen Brophy McHale, MSN, RN, FNP, ARNP-BC
Family Nurse Practitioner, Patient Educator
Green Country Free Clinic
Bartlesville, Oklahoma;
Hospice and Palliative Care Primary Nurse
    and Consultant
Jane Phillips Medical Center
Bartlesville, Oklahoma
15. Grief and Bereavement

Crystal Dea Moore, MA, MSW, PhD
Social Work Program Director
Assistant Professor of Social Work
Department of Sociology, Anthropology,
    and Social Work
Skidmore College
Saratoga Springs, New York
2. Advance Care Planning
13. Cultural and Spiritual Issues

John A. Mulder, MD
Clinical Faculty
Vanderbilt University
Nashville, Tennessee;
Chief Medical Officer
Alive Hospital, Inc.
Nashville, Tennessee
13. Cultural and Spiritual Issues

David Oliver, MD, FRCGP
Honorary Senior Lecturer in Palliative Care
Kent Institute of Medicine and Health Science
University of Kent
Kent, United Kingdom;
Consultant Physician in Palliative Medicine
Wisdom Hospice
Rochester, Kent
United Kingdom
11. Neurology

Marilyn O'Mallon, RN, MSN
Assistant Professor, Department of Nursing
Armstrong Atlantic State University
Savannah, Georgia;
Clinical Instructor/ PRN RN
Hospice Savannah, Inc.
Savannah, Georgia
Appendix C

Kathy P. Parker, PhD, APRN, FAAN
Edith F. Honeycutt Professor
Nell Hodgson Woodruff School of Nursing
Emory University
Atlanta, Georgia
5. The Interface of Sleep

Chad S. Peterson, PhD, MD
Resident Physician
University of California at San Francisco
San Francisco, California
13. Cultural and Spiritual Issues

Dana N. Rutledge, RN, PhD
Associate Professor in Nursing
California State University – Fullerton
Fullerton, California
3. Evidence-Based Intervention

Sandra E. Schrader, RN, ADN, BSN
Clinical Manager, Medical Surgical Services
Shands at Alachua General Hospital (AGH)
Gainesville, Florida
14. The Dying Process

Pamela Sue Spencer, B, RN, BSN, FNP
Family Nurse Practitioner
Saginaw Veterans Medical Center
Saginaw, Michigan
11. Neurology

Tom Tomlinson, PhD
Professor
Center for Ethics and Humanities in the Life
  Sciences
Michigan State University
East Lansing, Michigan
12. Ethical Issues

James Varga, RPh, MBA
Palliative Care Consultant
Hospice of the Comforter
Altamonte Springs, Florida
7. Pulmonary
Appendixes A and B

Catherine Vena, RN, PhD(c)
Doctoral Candidate
Nell Hodgson Woodruff School of Nursing
Emory University
Atlanta, Georgia
14. The Dying Process

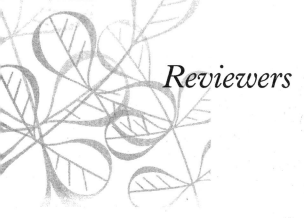

Reviewers

Laurent Adler, MD
Assistant Professor
Department of Internal Medicine, Division
    of Geriatric Medicine and Gerontology
Emory University School of Medicine
Atlanta, Georgia

Donna M. Arena, RN, PhD
Palliative Care Coordinator, Special Projects
    Facilitator Emory Healthcare
Nursing Administration
Emory Healthcare
Emory, Georgia

Eileen R. Chasens, DSN, RN
Assistant Professor
University of Pittsburgh School of Nursing
Pittsburg, Pennsylvania

John W. Finn, MD, FAAHPM
Chief Medical Director
Maggie Allesee Center for Quality of Life
Hospice of Michigan
Detroit, Michigan;
Clinical Assistant Professor
Wayne State University School of Medicine
Detroit, Michigan

Shirley Ann Garick, PhD, MSN, RN
Associate Professor of Nursing
College of Health and Behavioral Sciences
Department of Nursing
Texas A&M University – Texarkana
Texarkana, Texas

Cathy Groeger, MN, RN, NP-C
Associate Professor of Nursing
Our Lady of the Lake College
Baton Rouge, Louisiana

Dianne Husbands, BA, RN, BScN, ENC(c)
Educator, St. Joseph's Healthcare
Hamilton, Ontario, Canada

Maribeth B. Kowalski, PharmD, RPh
Medical Liason
Purdue Pharma LP
Stamford, Connecticut

Lori Ann Ladd, MSN, APRN, BC
Medical Liason, Health Policy
Purdue Pharma
Chesterfield, Missouri

Ronald Allen Mihelic, PharmD
Hematology/Oncology Clinical Pharmacist
Emory University Hospital
Atlanta, Georgia

Nancy K. Nelson, RN, AAS
Advance Illness Care Coordinator,
    Geriatrics/Palliative Care
Stratton VA Medical Center
Albany, New York

Judith L. Reishtein, PhD, RN, CCRN
Post Doctoral Fellow
School of Nursing and Center for Sleep
    and Respiratory Neurobiology
University of Pennsylvania
Philadelphia, Pennsylvania

Paula M. Saunders, MSW
Oncology Social Worker, Social Services
Emory Healthcare
Atlanta, Georgia

Eric Alan Steckelman, MSc, PA-C
Physician Assistant, Anesthesia and Critical
    Medicine
Memorial Sloan Kettering Cancer Center
New York, New York;
Medical Science Liaison
Boehringer Ingelheim
Ridgefield, Connecticut

Connie Henke Yarbro, RN, MS, FAAN
Clinical Associate Professor, Department
    of Medicine;
Clinical Associate Professor, MU Sinclair School
    of Nursing;
Editor, Seminars in Oncology Nursing;
University of Missouri—Columbia
Columbia, Missouri

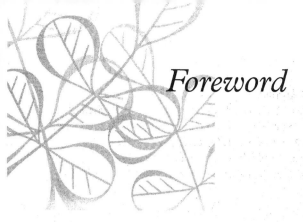

Foreword

Modern palliative care emerged in the United Kingdom during the 1960's as a response to the unmet needs of terminally ill patients and their families. The original palliative care programs were mostly community based and non-academic. The adoption of palliative care in major teaching hospitals, cancer centers, and universities has been very slow, particularly in the United States. The medical and nursing specialty of palliative medicine is already available in the United Kingdom, Canada, and Australia, and it is in an advanced stage of planning in most countries of the European union.

In recent years there has been a major increase in interest in palliative care in North America. However, as compared with other health care disciplines, there are a very limited number of North American books on this subject.

Palliative Practices will help address the educational needs of a large number of North American health care professionals. The editors have produced a book that is eminently practical. The chapters have been authored and edited to continuously address the practical needs of patients and families. The book offers a combination of insights into the palliative care perspective in health care decision making and also very specific chapters addressing issues such as cardiovascular disease and nephrology. This book will be particularly useful to physicians, nurses, and other health care professionals practicing in general hospitals or the community, as well as senior medical students and residents.

I am convinced that this book will have a major impact on the care given to thousands of patients and families in the United States. I strongly recommend it to our colleagues, and I would like to whole-heartedly congratulate the editors and authors for a job well done.

Dr. Eduardo Bruera, Professor and Chair
Department of Palliative Care and Rehabilitation Medicine
University of Texas M.D. Anderson Cancer Center
Houston, Texas

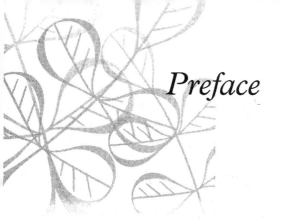

Preface

What do we live for if not to make life less difficult for each other?

—**George Eliot**

The art and science of palliative medicine have gained momentum in the United States and provide clinicians with the framework for improving patient function and quality of life through optimal symptom management including psychoemotional and spiritual support from an interdisciplinary team. This text is written with the intention of providing physicians, advanced practice nurses, physician assistants, and medical social workers with a comprehensive reference and/or a study guide for palliative certification. Palliative practices should be integrated into the traditional management of disease and not reserved for the last weeks and days of life. As Americans age and live longer, the impact on maintaining optimal function will be an ongoing challenge for all clinicians providing care for the adult patient population living and dying from advanced disease.

The editors would like to acknowledge with respect and gratitude the interdisciplinary expertise of our contributors and their commitment to this project. We wish to acknowledge our editors from Elsevier Science, Sandra Brown and Sophia Oh Gray. Becky Phillip from the Cleveland Clinic Foundation is also recognized for her editorial support.

KK, MD, CM

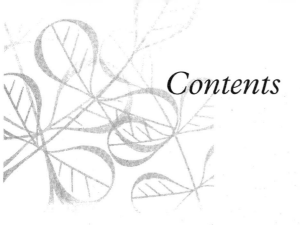

Contents

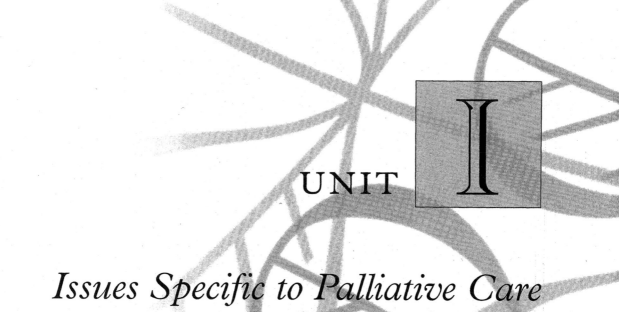

UNIT I

Issues Specific to Palliative Care

CHAPTER 1

Palliative Care Perspectives

Barry M. Kinzbrunner

OBJECTIVES

After the completion of this chapter, the reader should be able to:

1. Describe the various terms used when defining the care provided to patients and families living with advanced disease.
2. Discuss the hospice benefit and role that hospice plays in end-of-life care.
3. Explain the interface between hospice and non-hospice palliative care programs.
4. Demonstrate how to direct patients and families to the appropriate program available that meets individual health care needs.

INTRODUCTION

"The best hospital in the world can't keep you alive forever." This headline appeared in a full-page advertisement in the July 27/Aug. 4, 2003, issue of *U.S. News & World Report*. This ad, sponsored by *Last Acts* and *Partnership for Caring*, two organizations whose missions focus on improving access to end-of-life care for terminally ill patients, goes on to say that "...any hospital has the potential to help those nearing the end of life...(by) offering dying people 'palliative care'—care that addresses the whole person: mind, body, and spirit" (Partnership for Caring & Last Acts, 2003).

Indeed, the American population continues to age and as medical technology continues to advance, providing Americans with the opportunity for longer and healthier lives, it is clear that Americans have become increasingly concerned about how and where they will die. Does death come in a hospital facility, with monitors tracking ebbing vital signs while tubes protrude from every orifice, or does death come at home, in one's own bed surrounded by loved ones? Whatever the circumstances and setting that carry the patient and his or her family to the end of life, the goal should be to provide optimal palliative care.

What about illness prior to death? Is the majority of one's time spent trying every conceivable technologically advanced treatment available, irrespective of its ability to positively affect the trajectory of the illness? Or, even when attempt at cure or remission remains feasible, are significant efforts also focused on relieving the pain and suffering that often accompany the treatments these illnesses may require?

Providing an appropriate answer to these and similar questions is key to the mission of organizations like Partnership for Caring and Last Acts. The answer would appear to be *palliative care*.

DEFINITIONS

Palliative Care Terminology

What exactly is *palliative care*?

The word *palliate* comes from the Latin word *palliare* meaning "to cloak," and according to the Oxford English Dictionary (1975), *palliate* in the context of health care means "to alleviate the symptoms of a disease without curing it." If taken literally, then, *palliative care* could be defined as any care provided to treat the symptoms of any illness without curing that illness, for example, providing a patient with an analgesic medication for the treatment of a painful joint secondary to chronic osteoarthritis. Broadening this further, one could argue that the treatment of diabetes mellitus with exogenous insulin or the treatment of congestive

3

heart failure with digoxin and furosemide is palliative because in both cases symptoms are improved while the underlying pathology remains unchanged. Yet, few would argue that the active treatment of diseases such as diabetes mellitus or congestive heart failure is considered a form of "palliative care" in the context in which it is used today. Therefore it is necessary to better define palliative care in the context in which it is currently understood. To best do that, it is first necessary to define several terms describing care closely associated with palliative care, namely *supportive care, end-of-life care,* and *hospice care.*

Supportive Care

In a number of randomized clinical trials assessing the survival of patients with advanced cancer who were treated with combination chemotherapy, the patients in the control group that did not receive the chemotherapy were treated with what was described as "best supportive care" (Cellerino, Tummarello, Guidi, et al., 1991; Ganz, Figlin, Haskell, et al., 1989). Supportive care in this setting has generally been defined as "the best care available as judged by the attending physician, according to institutional standards for each standard" and is usually believed to include such interventions as antibiotics, analgesics, transfusions, corticosteroids, and/or any other symptomatic therapy including psychosocial therapy when indicated. Although this definition appears to be satisfactory, the reality is that the studies in which "best supportive care" is invoked, such as the ones just cited, do not define the nature of the supportive interventions provided nor do they define how the supportive care is "best," leaving this definition seriously deficient (Klastersky, 1997; Weinreb, 2002).

In the preface to the textbook *Principles and Practice of Palliative Care & Supportive Oncology,* the editors define supportive care in a different fashion (Berger, Portenoy, & Weissman, 2002):

The term supportive oncology refers to those aspects of medical care concerned with the physical, psychosocial, and spiritual issues faced by persons with cancer, their families, their communities, and their health care providers. In this context, supportive oncology describes both those interventions used to support patients who experience adverse effects caused by antineoplastic therapies and those interventions now considered under the broad rubric of palliative care.

This definition better captures the essence of supportive care. It expands supportive care to include the symptomatic treatment of treatment side effects and incorporates the management of other symptoms under the umbrella of palliative care, which is defined in detail later in this chapter. While still leaving the term somewhat open to interpretation, it goes beyond the earlier definition by recognizing that care extends beyond the patient to include the family and the community in which the patient and family live. This also includes the health care workers who provide care for the patient and family. It further acknowledges in more detail that patient and family needs are not only physical but also psychosocial and spiritual.

End-of-Life Care

The definition of end-of-life care on the surface would be self-evident; that is, the care that patients and their families receive when patients are dying or near death—in other words, terminally ill. End-of-life care incorporates multiple forms of care, including supportive care, hospice care, and palliative care, although not all patients who receive supportive or palliative care are actually receiving end-of-life care.

End-of-life care may be provided in any of a number of settings. Obvious settings include patients' homes, adult congregate living facilities (ACLFs), long-term care facilities (LTCFs), and inpatient hospice facilities. However, a significant number of patients are cared for in hospitals, either on the regular hospital unit or in the intensive care unit (ICU) (Fins, Miller, Acres, et al., 1999; Miller & Fins, 1996; Rocker & Curtis, 2003; Sprung, Cohen, Sjokvist, et al., 2003).

With its broad definition, some may think that the term *end-of-life care* is superfluous and that the other terms defined here would be adequate descriptors of the care being provided. However, it is clear, for several reasons, that end-of-life care has become a mainstay in the vocabulary of those who are involved in the care of patients who are terminally ill.

As noted, some patients receiving supportive care and/or palliative care are not at the end of life; this term allows the differentiation between patients receiving supportive and/or palliative care who are *not* terminally ill from those who are. End-of-life care also is a good descriptor for the care that terminal patients receive in less common settings, such as the ICU (Rocker & Curtis, 2003; Sprung et al., 2003). Finally, with increased public awareness of hospice and other available services for people who are terminal, it has become more obvious that describing care as *terminal* or *for the dying* presents negative images. *End-of-life care* on the other hand, although meaning the same thing, has a more positive connotation and many find it to be a more acceptable way to describe the care delivered during this final phase of life.

Hospice Care

The word *hospice* is derived from the Latin term *hospes*, meaning "host" or "guest." Historically and during the hospice movement's modern development in Great Britain, hospices were places where people went to stay and often to die (Kinzbrunner, 2002a). However, as hospice evolved in the United States, it has come to be defined differently.

The National Hospice and Palliative Care Organization (NHPCO) defines hospice as (National Hospice and Palliative Care Organization [NHPCO], 2003a):

…a team-oriented approach to expert medical care, pain management, and emotional and spiritual support expressly tailored to the patient's needs and wishes. Support is provided to the patient's loved ones as well. At the center of hospice care is the belief that each of us has the right to die pain-free and with dignity, and that our families will receive the necessary support to allow us to do so. Hospice focuses on caring, not curing and, in most cases, care is provided in the patient's home. Hospice care also is provided in freestanding hospice centers, hospitals, and nursing homes and other long-term care facilities.

In other words, rather than being a *place*, hospice has evolved in the United States to provide comprehensive care through an interdisciplinary team of health care providers. Care is provided to patients who are near the end of life and their families, preferably in the patient's own home, or in a variety of other settings when necessary, based upon the patient's and/or family's needs (e.g., long-term care).

Hospice in the United States has been further defined by the Medicare Hospice Benefit (MHB), which was enacted by Congress in 1982 (42 Code of Federal Regulations, 1993). (The MHB is discussed in detail later in this chapter.) The MHB, for example, has established that the interdisciplinary team be headed by a registered nurse (RN) and consists of at least a nurse, a physician, a social worker, and a pastoral counselor. The MHB requires that families of patients who have died must receive ongoing bereavement support for at least 1 year following the patient's death. By investing hospice agencies with professional management responsibility and reimbursing hospices a fixed per diem rate, the MHB has further defined hospice care in terms of the therapeutic options that hospice agencies are or are not able to provide and/or cover (the latter especially when the proposed interventions are invasive and/or are prohibitively not cost-effective).

Most important, the MHB has been instrumental in determining which patients receive hospice services by defining patient eligibility for hospice services based on the certification of two physicians that a patient should have "a medical prognosis that his or her life expectancy is 6 months or less if the illness runs its normal course" (42 Code of Federal Regulations, 1993). It is this life expectancy requirement more than any other that has defined hospice care in the United States. And it is this requirement that, in the eyes of many, has severely limited the utilization of hospice services because of the perceived difficulties in predicting prognosis for individual patients, especially those suffering from illnesses other than cancer (Brody & Lynn, 1984; Meier, Morrison, & Cassel, 1997).

Palliative Care

Having examined the definitions of supportive care, end-of-life care, and hospice care, palliative care can now be further defined. In Great Britain, where palliative care has evolved into the specialty of palliative medicine, the latter was defined in 1987 as "the study and management of patients with active, progressive, far-advanced disease for whom the prognosis is limited and the focus is the quality of life" (Doyle, Hanks, & MacDonald, 1998). The addition of care provided by other health care professionals, including nurses, social workers, clergy, and home health aides, as part of an interdisciplinary team expands the definition just mentioned to encompass the more global term *palliative care.*

In 1990 the World Heath Organization (WHO) proposed its own definition of palliative care and most recently expanded and broadened the definition to include all disease entities other than malignancies. Today, it is widely recognized that the principles of palliative care be included as early as possible in the course of chronic illness (Sepuleveda, Marlin, Yoshida, et al., 2002). The new definition includes (World Health Organization, 2002, p. 3):

Palliative care as an approach that improves the quality of life of patients and their families facing the problems associated with life-threatening illness, through the prevention and relief of suffering by means of early identification and impeccable assessment and treatment of pain and other problems, physical, psychosocial and spiritual.

This definition both clarifies and expands on its British predecessor because its focus is on the total patient, inclusive of the patient's family, and on the interdisciplinary nature of the care provided. It includes references to bereavement care and expands palliative care beyond the realm of patients with active, progressive, far-advanced disease by acknowledging the applicability of many of its principles earlier in the course of illness, although it limits this earlier applicability to patients with cancer.

These definitions have sufficed in Great Britain, Canada, and other parts of the world where palliative medicine is a recognized specialty. However, the same has not been true in the United States, where hospice has been the most visible provider of end-of-life care and where palliative medicine is still a fledgling specialty. This prompted the American Academy of Hospice and Palliative Medicine (AAHPM) to weigh in with its own definition of *palliative care* (American Academy of Hospice and Palliative Medicine, 2003):

Palliative care is comprehensive, specialized care provided by an interdisciplinary team to patients and families living with a life-threatening or severe advanced illness expected to progress toward dying and where care is particularly focused on alleviating suffering and promoting quality of life. Major concerns are pain and symptom management, information sharing and advance care planning, psychosocial and spiritual support, and coordination of care.

This definition enhances the WHO's definition by adding to the principles of palliative care the aspects of information sharing, advance care planning, and coordination of care. This definition also has assisted the AAHPM in achieving its goal of fostering better communication between its constituent members who provide palliative care primarily via the hospice model and those who have developed and/or are working to evolve alternative palliative care models in the United States.

These various definitions of palliative care are similar to the definition of hospice care. In recognition of this, NHPCO has incorporated palliative care as an equal partner with hospice care in its definition just quoted and has equated hospice care with palliative care of the dying (NHPCO, 2003a). Also, to address some of the perceived limitations of hospice care around patient eligibility and treatment options as defined by the MHB, NHPCO has added the following to its definition of palliative care (NHPCO, 2003a):

Palliative care extends the principles of hospice care to a broader population that could benefit from receiving this type of care earlier in their illness or disease process. No specific therapy is excluded from consideration. An individual's needs must be continually assessed and treatment options should be explored and evaluated in the context of the individual's values and symptoms. Palliative care, ideally, would segue into hospice care as the illness progresses.

As a final point, it must be noted that all definitions of palliative care presented focus primarily on the patients who have life-limiting illnesses, that is, those who are receiving palliative care as part of their care at the end of life. Although this is the context in which palliative care is often considered, it must be remembered that in actuality palliative care could and should be provided to patients during *all* facets of any illness.

Whether the patient is in the midst of a medical evaluation, newly diagnosed, receiving treatment designed for cure or remission, or receiving disease-directed treatment designed to delay the progress of a chronic, incurable illness, he or she should be provided palliative interventions. Palliative medicine is directed at the myriad physical symptoms accompanying advanced disease and provides the appropriate support for any and all psychosocial and/or spiritual challenges facing the patient and his or her family. What truly defines the unique niche occupied by palliative care is the ability to reach beyond the patient with a life-limiting illness to patients with chronic, long-standing illnesses and even patients with acute, potentially curable illness and provide palliative interventions alongside curative interventions.

HOSPICE CARE AND THE MEDICARE HOSPICE BENEFIT
History

As discussed, the word *hospice* is derived from the Latin term *hospes,* meaning "host" or "guest." Its origins as a way station for travelers between Europe, Africa, and the Middle East can be traced back to the early Middle Ages (Paradis, 1985; Stoddard, 1991). It can be speculated that the association of hospices with the care of the sick and dying may have come from the fact that during the Crusades, wounded soldiers trying to return home would stop at hospices to attempt to recuperate from their injuries, and many would not survive (Kinzbrunner, 2002a).

The modern concept of hospice as an interdisciplinary approach for providing comprehensive care to patients near the end of life had its origins in Great Britain. Calling on the vast health care experience she had gained as a physician, nurse, and social worker, Dame Cicely Saunders established the first hospice facilities in London during the 1960s, initially at St. Joseph's Hospice and then at St. Christopher's Hospice (Corr & Corr, 1983; Saunders, 1983).

The hospice concept found its way across the Atlantic Ocean, in Canada during the 1960s and in the United States during the 1970s. Because of societal differences, the hospice model that developed in the United States did not revolve around providing care in designated inpatient facilities as was the case in Great Britain. Instead, it evolved in a fashion that emphasized the provision of services to patients in the home environment, utilizing inpatient care only when patients had specific needs that could not be managed at home (Lack, 1983; Smith & Granbois, 1992).

Despite mainstream health care showing little interest in hospice, grass roots efforts in many communities led to significant growth of the hospice movement in the United States during the latter half of the 1970s. By 1980, more than 400 hospice agencies were providing care to terminally ill patients, primarily on a voluntary basis because no formal funding was available for these services (Smith & Granbois, 1992). Ultimately, demonstration projects were organized, and the success of these projects led to the establishment of the Medicare Hospice Benefit as part of the Tax Equity and Fiscal Responsibility Act (TEFRA) of 1982 (42 Code of Federal Regulations, 1993; Corless, 1983). The MHB has continued uninterrupted for more than 20 years with only minor modifications. It has served as a model for the provision and reimbursement of end-of-life care services to patients covered by Medicaid, Medicare, and by increasing numbers of managed care and private insurance medical plans.

Hospice Care Under the Medicare Hospice Benefit

Patient Eligibility. The basic features of the Medicare Hospice Benefit are listed in Table 1-1. Patients receiving hospice care under the MHB must be entitled to Medicare Part A benefits and, as discussed, must be certified as terminally ill; this is defined by the Medicare hospice regulations as having "a medical prognosis that his or her life expectancy is 6 months or less if the illness runs its normal course" (Kinzbrunner, 2002a; 42 Code of Federal Regulations, 1993; Rhymes, 1990). Certification that the patient has a prognosis of 6 months or less must be based on the clinical judgment of two physicians—the patient's attending physician and the hospice medical director (or the physician member of the hospice interdisciplinary team) (U.S. Department of Health and Human Services [DHHS], 2001).

Table **1-1**   FEATURES OF THE MEDICARE HOSPICE BENEFIT

Feature	Details of Feature
Patient eligibility	Prognosis of 6 months or less Based on clinical judgment of and certified by two physicians Part A Medicare beneficiary
Benefit periods	Two 90-day periods Unlimited 60-day periods Hospice medical director recertifies 6-month prognosis before each new benefit period
Reimbursement	Per diem rate based on level of care Attending physician professional and care plan oversight services are directly billable under Part B Hospice physician visit services billable outside per diem under Part A
Covered Services	See Box 1-1
Levels of Care	Routine home care Continuous home care General inpatient care Respite inpatient care

Coverage under the MHB is divided into benefit periods. The first 180 days of care are divided into two periods of 90 days each. It is well recognized that predicting patient prognosis is not an exact science; patients who survive longer than 6 months may continue to receive hospice services under the MHB in incremental periods of 60 days each (Palmetto Government Benefits Administrators, 1997). Before the beginning of the second 90-day period within the first 180 days and any subsequent 60-day period, the hospice medical director (or the physician member of the hospice interdisciplinary team) is required to recertify that the patient continues to have a prognosis of 6 months or less (regardless of how long the patient has already been receiving hospice services).

If the hospice medical director determines that a patient no longer has a prognosis of less than 6 months, the patient is discharged from the hospice program with an extended prognosis, in which case all regular Medicare benefits are immediately restored. In this situation, the hospice has the responsibility to ensure continuity of care (which could mean referral to an alternative palliative care program when appropriate). A patient may choose to revoke the hospice benefit and voluntarily leave the hospice program at any time for any reason. Unlike managed care, in which the patient must

wait until the end of the month to have regular Medicare benefits restored (since managed care programs are reimbursed on a fixed monthly basis), patients who revoke the MHB have immediate restoration of all regular Medicare coverage.

Reimbursement. Hospice care provided to patients under the Medicare Hospice Benefit is reimbursed on a per diem basis. Hospice agencies receive a fixed sum per day per patient to provide whatever services are required to care for the patient. The four distinct payment rates are based on the patient's level of care, which are discussed later in this chapter. Hospices can also receive additional reimbursement for patient visits provided by employed or contracted medical directors or hospice physicians and contracted consultant physicians. Administrative and care plan oversight provided by hospice medical directors and physicians are included in the per diem. Attending physician professional services inclusive of visits and care plan oversight are reimbursable as usual under Medicare Part B. All other services provided by the attending physician in his or her office (e.g., diagnostic studies, parenteral medications) that are necessary in the plan of care become the financial responsibility of the hospice.

Covered Services. Under the per diem rate, hospices are responsible for covering all services that are needed to care for "the terminal illness as well as related conditions" (42 Code of Federal Regulations, 1993). These services are delineated in Box 1-1. Hands-on care provided by various members of the hospice interdisciplinary team, including nurses, social workers, pastoral counselors, and home health aides, as well as medical direction and physician care plan oversight, are major components of the services hospices provide. In addition, the hospice program covers all medications, durable medical equipment, and medical supplies that are required by the patient to treat symptoms of the terminal illness, relieving patients and families of significant financial burdens. When patients will benefit nutritionally or functionally, dietary counseling, physical therapy, occupational therapy, and speech therapy are interventions the hospice is required to provide. Diagnostic studies and therapeutic modalities less commonly associated with hospice care, such as chemotherapy, radiation therapy, and transfusion of blood products, should also be paid for by the hospice under the MHB when such interventions are medically indicated for the treatment of symptoms related to the terminal illness.

A unique service offered by hospice programs is bereavement counseling. While it is often said that bereavement counseling actually begins for

Box 1-1 COVERED SERVICES UNDER THE MEDICARE HOSPICE BENEFIT

- Interdisciplinary team care:
  —Nursing services
  —Medical social services
  —Pastoral counseling
  —Medical direction and physician care plan oversight
  —Home health aide and homemaking services
- Bereavement counseling
- Dietary counseling
- Physical therapy, occupational therapy, speech therapy if indicated
- Drugs and biologicals
- Durable medical equipment
- Medical supplies
- Laboratory and diagnostic studies

the patient and family as early as the time that a potentially life-limiting illness is diagnosed, hospices are also required to provide bereavement counseling and support to surviving family members for at least 1 year following the death of the patient (Bozeman, 2002). Hospices must offer this service despite the fact that there is no additional reimbursement for bereavement services after the patient has died.

The care and treatment of conditions "unrelated" to the terminal illness are not included in the per diem reimbursement under the MHB and are not the responsibility of the hospice. In such circumstances, patients have access to regular Medicare Part A and Part B benefits. For example, a patient enrolled in a local hospice program with a diagnosis of congestive heart failure falls at home and fractures his tibia; this requires an emergency department visit, x-ray films, and an orthopedic consultation, all of which is covered under the patient's Medicare plan outside of the MHB.

Levels of Hospice Care. As noted, hospice care in the United States was designed, with intent, to provide care to patients and families in the most familiar and comfortable environment possible—the patient's own home. However, it was recognized that because of chronic care needs, the severity of symptoms, or patient's/family's desire to not have death occur at home, not all patients spend their final days at home. In addition, because the MHB is a Medicare Part A benefit (which covers all inpatient services, as contrasted with Medicare Part B, which covers primarily outpatient and physician services), patients who elect to receive hospice services no longer have hospitalization coverage under Medicare Part A. To address these issues, the MHB defines several "levels of care" (see Table 1-1), reimbursed at different per diem rates that reflect the intensity of services provided by the hospice to meet the needs of the patient and family. The four distinct levels of care are *routine home care, continuous home care, general inpatient care,* and *respite inpatient care* settings.

Routine home care is the basic premise for hospice care provided in the patient's home. It incorporates the services outlined in Box 1-1. For patients who live in an alternative environment, such as an adult congregate living facility (ACLF) or a long-term care facility (LTCF, i.e., a nursing home), the facility is considered their home for the purpose of the MHB and the care received by the patient in the facility is considered routine home care. In such circumstances, the hospice must have a contract in place with the facility while hospice maintains the professional management responsibile for patient care.

Patients may develop acute medical or psychosocial symptoms in the home environment that require more intensive care and support than can be provided under the routine level of home care. Continuous, around-the-clock home care is available if unrelenting symptoms are present such as uncontrolled pain, dyspnea, or severe decubitus ulcers requiring frequent management or if support for a significant breakdown in family dynamics is needed (Kinzbrunner, 2002a; U.S. DHHS, 1992). The requirements for continuous home care are that the care provided to the patient is primarily (more than 50%) nursing and is for a minimum of 8 hours a day (not necessarily consecutively) to a maximum of 24 hours a day. Reimbursement for continuous care is based on a fixed *hourly* rate rather than *per diem*.

When patients are suffering from uncontrolled physical or psychosocial symptoms and they cannot be effectively managed at home, even under a continuous home care level of care, or if such patients do not wish to remain in the home, the MHB requires hospices to provide patients access to general inpatient hospice care. Such care can be provided in a variety of venues. Freestanding hospice inpatient units are dedicated facilities owned and operated by individual hospice programs. Hospice inpatient units may occupy a wing in a hospital or LTCF, usually leased by the host facility to the hospice and operated either by the hospice or jointly by both organizations. (These types of hospice inpatient units may serve as models for, and often double as, palliative care inpatient units, which are discussed in detail later.) Another alternative for providing hospice inpatient care is for hospices to enter into contractual agreements with local hospitals and/or LTCFs to provide inpatient beds on an individual patient basis. In hospitals,

these beds are most commonly located either on the general medical/surgical floor or the oncology floor, whereas in the LTCF, such patients should be cared for on the skilled nursing floor.

The fourth level of care defined by the MHB is respite inpatient care. This level of care is indicated when patients do not have acute symptom management needs that are required to justify a general inpatient level of care but require an inpatient environment to allow caregiver family members needed respite from the day-to-day care they are providing to the patient at home. Respite care is limited to 5 consecutive days at any time.

At the time of hospice admission, patients may be admitted to any of the four levels of care, based upon their needs at the time of initial assessment. Once admitted to the hospice program, patients are actually "transferred" from one level of care to another within the program. For example, if a patient on a routine home care level of care experiences uncontrolled pain requiring more intensive management than can be provided in the home setting, the patient is transferred, rather than admitted, to a general inpatient level of care. Once the pain is brought under control, the patient is transferred, rather than discharged, back to a routine level of home care.

Hospice in the Twenty-First Century

In the twenty-first century, hospice as a provider of comprehensive service to patients near the end of life and their families is thriving. The number of hospice programs has grown from 400 in 1980 to more than 3200 today, serving patients in many settings, including hospitals, long-term care facilities, adult congregate living facilities, free-standing hospices, and, of course, private homes. In 2002, hospice programs served more than 885,000 patients, which is almost 37% of the approximately 2.4 million people who die in the United States each year. This represents a 14% increase in patients served when compared with 775,000 patients in 2001, and a 64% increase over the 540,000 patients in 1998 (NHPCO, 1999; NHPCO, 2003b). As discussed later, during the mid-1990s, hospice median and mean lengths of stay fell from the highs achieved during the late 1980s and early 1990s. This trend has reversed, and for the first time in several years, the amount of time for patients enrolled in hospice programs has increased. Median length of stay in 2002 increased to 26 days, representing a 27% increase from 20.5 days in 2001, while the mean length of stay during the same period rose to 51 days, a 6% increase over the 48-day mean reported the prior year (NHPCO, 2003b).

PALLIATIVE CARE PROGRAMS

While hospice has become the palliative care provider of choice for increasing numbers of terminally ill patients and their families, for others in need of palliative care, hospice remains out of reach. For those patients who have a life expectancy of

6 months or less, this may be the result of the continued barriers mentioned earlier. However, for others, hospice cannot provide the palliative care they require because, although they may be acutely or chronically ill or have a life-limiting illness with uncontrolled symptoms, they have a prognosis in excess of the 6 months required to be eligible (at least under Medicare and Medicaid) for hospice services. For these patients and families, the need to find other ways to deliver the palliative care services that they require has led to the development of palliative care programs and care delivery models throughout the United States. Table 1-2 provides some comparison and contrast between hospice programs and palliative care.

Table **1-2** COMPARISON OF HOSPICE AND PALLIATIVE CARE SERVICES

Characteristic	Hospice	Palliative Care
Eligibility	Prognosis ≤6 months	None required Determined by program
Professional services	Interdisciplinary team: Physician Nurse Social worker Pastoral counselor Certified nursing assistants Others as need	Interdisciplinary or multidisciplinary team: Physician Nurse Social worker Others as needed
Other services	Medications Durable medical equipment (DME) Bereavement care Others (see Box 1-1)	No required services Determined by program
Location of services	Comprehensive: Home care Long-term care facility (LTCF) Inpatient	Based on program: Some comprehensive Some inpatient only Some LTCF-based Some require networking between hospital and hospice or home-based home health programs
Funding	Medicare Hospice Benefit State Medicaid programs Health maintenance organizations (HMOs) and commercial insurers Charity (not-for-profit hospices)	Traditional hospital coverage Traditional home care coverage Support from hospitals and hospice partner organizations Grants Charity

Data from Kinzbrunner, B.M. (2002a). How to help patients access end-of-life care. In B.M. Kinzbrunner, N.J. Weinreb, & J.S. Policzer (Eds.), *Twenty common problems in end-of-life care* (pp. 29-45). New York: McGraw Hill.

Evolution of Palliative Care

Historically, the more broad-based "palliative care movement," similar to its hospice counterpart, had its start in Great Britain. While the hospice movement in England served those patients who were able to access the many hospice inpatient facilities modeled after St. Joseph's and St. Christopher's. Patients in hospitals and at home and not willing or able to relocate to a hospice facility were not receiving the palliative care they needed. This led to the development of hospital-based consult services and by the late 1980s matured to the point where palliative medicine became a recognized specialty, with training programs, research, and inpatient care integrated into the traditional health care system. Care is directed at symptom management and is available to patients irrespective of the severity or prognosis of their illness (Doyle et al., 1998). Hospices continue to provide palliative care services to patients and their families who are terminally ill and, to a lesser degree, work with home care services, which are also integrated into the traditional health care system, to provide palliative care to patients who wish to remain at home (R. Dunlop, personal communication, 1998).

In the United States, despite the successful growth and development of hospice programs through the 1980s and into the early 1990s, approximately 65% of Americans were dying in hospitals, unable to access hospice services at all or at most for only a few days before death (Meier et al., 1997).

This led to significant concerns about how the dying were cared for in the nation's hospitals, resulting in a major multi-institutional research initiative known as the "Study to Understand Prognoses and Preferences for Outcomes and Risks of Treatment." This Robert Wood Johnson funded study is commonly referred to as the SUPPORT study (SUPPORT Principal Investigators, 1995). The objective of the two-phase study was to improve end-of-life decision making and reduce the frequency of a mechanically supported, painful, and often prolonged process of dying.

Phase 1 was designed to identify how seriously ill hospitalized patients who had an estimated 6-month mortality rate of 50% were cared for. This phase demonstrated that serious "shortcomings"

existed in the care provided to these patients in the areas of patient/family communication with physicians, physician knowledge of patients' wishes regarding cardiopulmonary resuscitation (CPR), the number of days spent in an intensive care unit (ICU) before death, and adequate pain control.

With the information obtained from phase I, phase II added specific interventions to the care of a similar group of hospitalized patients, with the hope of improving the outcomes in the areas of communication the need for ICU care and symptom management before patient death. These interventions included patient-specific information supplied to the physician about the probability of patient survival for 6 months, the use of CPR, and the risk of functional disability and were all based from a complex prognostic model (Knaus, Harrell, Lynn, et al., 1995). In addition, a group of nurses were specially trained to serve as conduits to improve communication among patients, families, physicians, and hospital staff members to elicit patient/family preferences, improve the understanding of probable outcomes, improve pain control, and facilitate advance care planning. Regrettably, the interventions were unsuccessful, and the authors concluded that to improve the experience of seriously ill and dying patients, a greater individual and societal commitment and more proactive and forceful measures are needed (SUPPORT Principal Investigators, 1995). In some respects, the SUPPORT study confirmed for academic medicine what those who were working in the field of hospice and end-of-life care already knew—that, perhaps with the exception of the 25% of dying patients who were accessing hospice programs in the United States before death, the care of patients who were near the end of life was severely lacking and needed to be improved.

During this same period and despite the tremendous success and growth of hospice programs during the 1980s and into the early 1990s, hospice utilization in the mid-1990s began to decline, with mean lengths of stay falling from an average of 60 to 45 days and median lengths of stay falling from a little over 1 month to less than 3 weeks (Kinzbrunner, 2002a). Several factors are believed to have played key roles in the underutilization of hospice during this period. Foremost was continued physician discomfort with predicting that a patient has 6 months or less to live, compounded by an increase in regulatory scrutiny regarding the medical necessity of hospice care for individual patients who had been fortunate enough to survive longer than 6 months (Brody & Lynn, 1984; Kinzbrunner, 1997; Kinzbrunner, 2000). Other issues included the lack of open communication among patients, families, and physicians regarding end-of-life care issues (much like the in-hospital experience identified in SUPPORT), the perceived and often real unwillingness of hospices to admit patients receiving certain types of disease-directed or invasive therapies, and the lack of inpatient relationships between hospices and hospitals (Meier et al., 1997).

The results of the SUPPORT study and the decrease in hospice utilization were key elements that spurred into action physicians and others who were committed to providing patients and families with quality end-of-life care. In 1997 the Institute of Medicine (IOM) study on care at the end of life was completed and made several key recommendations focused on improving the end-of-life care in the United States. These recommendations included the need to improve patient access to end-of-life care; improve the education of physicians and other health care providers in end-of-life care; relax regulatory barriers that impede the proper treatment of pain and suffering; create research initiatives in end-of-life care; and elevate palliative care to either a medical specialty or at least a defined area of expertise within the practice of medicine. In parallel, a number of major medical organizations created educational programs for their members with the goal of improving their expertise in palliative and end-of-life care while other initiatives were beginning to incorporate palliative care education and training into undergraduate and graduate medical curricula (Mayer, 1996; Meier et al., 1997; Members of ABIM End-of-Life Patient Care Project, 1996; von Gunten, Neely, & Martinez, 1996; Weissman, 1995).

Hospices motivated by both the apparent decrease in utilization and, perhaps most important, their primary mission of providing access to end-of-life care for all patients and families in need, were considering new and creative ways to provide services to more patients and families. The efforts of both the medical community and the hospice community, have led to the evolution of palliative care in the United States and have given life to a variety of different palliative care program delivery models.

Hospital-Based Palliative Care Programs

Although falling from approximately 65% in the 1990s to 53% at the beginning of the twenty-first century, the majority of patients continue to die in the inpatient hospital setting. These patients are very likely to require pain and symptom management, coordination of care among multiple providers, and assistance in transition between various healthcare settings. The hospital is often the first place where, because of the acuity of illness, patients confront the reality that their illnesses may be terminal. These patients often require a great deal of support to make the appropriate decisions regarding their care. In addition, inpatient costs in the last year of life continue to rise significantly and Medicare costs during the last year of life increased 9.2% in 2001. It is primarily for these reasons that hospital-based palliative care programs have evolved (Center to Advance Palliative Care [CAPC], 2003a).

Hospice programs are limited to admitting patients who have a prognosis of 6 months or less to be eligible for the Medicare Hospice Benefit and 1 year or less for non-Medicare patients in some states. However, hospital-based palliative care programs have no such limitations. Patients cared for by these programs generally either have advanced, life-limiting illnesses or suffer from chronic, incurable, debilitating illnesses, irrespective of predicted life expectancy.

The typical inpatient palliative care team is interdisciplinary. It consists of professionals experienced in palliative care, including, at minimum, physicians, nurses, social workers, and clergy. These team members work in collaboration with the patient's attending physician, physician consultants, and other members of the primary care team (CAPC, 2003a; Health Care Advisory Board, 2003). In academic institutions with teaching programs, palliative medicine fellows, residents from various services such as internal medicine, family practice, and pediatrics, and advanced trainees and students from the other health care disciplines may all participate as members of the palliative care team (Billings, Block, Finn, et al., 2002; von Gunten et al., 1996). Consultants from various ancillary services within the institution can supplement the care provided by the core palliative care team. Services include but are not limited to nutritional support, physical and occupational therapy, pharmacy, and spiritual counseling.

Referral of patients to hospital-based palliative care programs are usually initiated with palliative care consultations, provided by the palliative medicine physician in conjunction with the palliative care nurse and other team members as patients' needs are identified. Patients may be cared for either on the acute care nursing units they occupy at the time of consultation or, when available, in specially designated palliative care units developed by the institution (Santa-Emma, Roach, Gill, et al., 2002).

Patients may come from any service in the hospital. Hospital-based palliative care services were traditionally initiated by existing oncology services with most of the patients suffering from malignancies. However, the myriad of palliative care needs for patients living and dying from advanced non malignant illnesses have been recognized and have led to the development of palliative care services caring for patients with any diagnosis (Santa-Emma et al., 2002; Smith, 2003).

One of the more unique roles identified for hospital-based palliative care services has been their involvement in the care of patients in the ICU setting. ICU patients receiving acute, life-prolonging therapies may, of course, benefit from the aggressive pain and symptom management that palliative care has to offer. Perhaps more important, when withdrawal of life-prolonging measures, such as ventilators, is being contemplated, a palliative care service can play a major role in working with the patient, the family, and the ICU care team to maintain open communication, facilitate the necessary decision making, and provide a smooth transition from the ICU to palliative or hospice care (CAPC, 2003b).

To illustrate the importance of the availability of hospital-based palliative care services to the management of ICU patients, a recent analysis suggested that the ICU was the single largest source for patients admitted or transferred to palliative care units, with 33% of all palliative care unit referrals coming from the ICU (Health Care Advisory Board, 2003).

Not surprising, the greatest challenge facing these new palliative care services is funding. At present, no specific funding exists for an interdisciplinary palliative care service. Palliative care within hospitals is often funded through the regular diagnosis-related group (DRG) reimbursement system (CAPC, 2003a). Physician services are billed using standard current procedural terminology (CPT) visit or consult codes. Because palliative medicine is not yet a recognized subspecialty, denial of payment because of perceived duplication of physician services may be avoided by having the palliative medicine physician use a symptom-based International Classification of Diseases (ICD)-9 diagnosis code (von Gunten, Ferris, Kirschner, et al., 2000). Additional funding for these programs has been provided primarily through grants from organizations such as the Robert Wood Johnson Foundation and the Soros Foundation, which are currently focusing research efforts on increasing the access to and improving the quality of end-of-life care for terminally ill patients and their families.

Several published studies have demonstrated the success of inpatient palliative care units both in terms of quality of care and, at least in part, from a financial perspective. Improvement in the management of symptoms, such as pain and dyspnea, in patients' care on palliative care units have been well chronicled (CAPC, 2003a; Elyasem, Swint, Roach, et al., 2003). Financially, it has been shown that the presence of palliative care units in hospitals can reduce costs significantly, with at least one study showing a greater than 50% reduction in the cost of an inpatient day of care. This is the result of a number of factors, including a decrease in the number of costly ICU days (and substituting much less expensive palliative care inpatient days), reducing the use of unnecessary and expensive futile medical interventions, and, when the inpatient palliative care program is coordinated with a hospice or home palliative care program, a reduction in total inpatient days. However, with the degree of cost savings, the net effect on hospitals' bottom lines appears to be positive (Elyasem et al., 2003; Health Care Advisory Board, 2003; Smith, 2003). The overall success of hospital-based palliative care programs can be further shown by the growing number of hospitals that wish to join the 17% of community hospitals and 20% of academic teaching hospitals that already have such programs in place (CAPC, 2003a).

Hospital/Hospice Partnerships in Hospital-Based Palliative Care

One method that hospitals have used to further improve the cost-effectiveness of palliative care units is to form partnerships with hospices (Kinzbrunner, 2002c; NHPCO & CAPC, 2001). This approach, used by some hospices since the earliest days of the Medicare Hospice Benefit, generally takes the form of a contractual agreement between the hospice and the host hospital, defining the roles of both agencies in the development and day-to-day operation of the unit.

If the hospice is the primary responsible agency, reimbursement to the hospital is usually in the form of rent for space and often coupled with either a discounted fee-for-service or fixed per diem charge for the various ancillary services provided (e.g., food services, laundry services, laboratory services, radiology services, pharmacy). Cost sharing is usually arranged for capital improvements to the space, and the hospice is responsible for providing staffing for the unit. When the hospital requires a palliative care bed for a patient who is not on the hospice program, the two agencies usually have an agreed-upon rate of reimbursement that the hospital provides to the hospice for the inpatient services. If the hospital is the primary responsible agency, the hospital provides the staff and all ancillary services and the hospice will usually pay the hospital an agreed-upon daily rate for each bed that a hospice patient occupies (which is usually at or close to the hospice per diem rate for general inpatient care). The two parties may also agree to have equal

responsibility, in which case responsibility for staffing is often shared (Kinzbrunner, 2002c; NHPCO & CAPC, 2001).

Both the hospital and hospice can benefit from such a partnership. For the hospital, the presence of the hospice interdisciplinary team on a daily basis provides the institution with on-site palliative care expertise. This can assist the hospital in providing its patients with quality pain and symptom management as well as psychosocial and spiritual counseling without drawing from existing staff already stretched thin. The hospice medical director, for example, can serve as the hospital's palliative medicine consultant, extending pain and symptom management expertise to patients outside the hospice arena and increasing hospice access by acquainting patients with the availability of hospice services when appropriate. The medical director and other hospice staff can also provide end-of-life education or opportunities for patient/family and hospital and medical staff education. The inpatient unit's presence in the facility provides the hospital with the added opportunity of demonstrating its commitment to the community by providing end-of-life care as part of its continuum of comprehensive services. The unit can also serve as an anchor for medical student and other health care professional student training in palliative care, as well as a center for palliative care research (Kinzbrunner, 2002c; NHPCO & CAPC, 2001).

For the hospice, a partnership with a hospital provides it with an identity in the community that it is linked to the inpatient facility, increasing the hospice's credibility. The hospice's presence in the hospital facilitates medical and hospital staff education as to the benefits of hospice services, resulting in earlier referral and increased patient utilization of hospice services. The hospice is also afforded the opportunity of being exposed to the broader continuum of palliative care needs that patients not yet ready for hospice services require. Together with the hospital, hospice can provide the impetus for integration of hospice services earlier into the continuum of care (Kinzbrunner, 2002c; NHPCO & CAPC, 2001).

Finally, a distinct advantage is continuity of care. With the presence of a hospice/palliative care inpatient unit in the hospital, patients who require end-of-life care do not need to leave the facility they are in to access the added benefits that a hospice program can provide. This is especially crucial for patients who are being transferred from an ICU setting or who are otherwise too ill to be discharged from the acute care hospital to home or a long-term care facility. Further continuity is provided by the clinicians who can continue to follow and attend to their patients on an active basis. In addition, pain and symptom management, not only for patients referred to the inpatient unit but potentially for all patients at the facility, is positively impacted by the presence of the hospice/hospital palliative care unit (Kinzbrunner, 2002c; NHPCO & CAPC, 2001).

Palliative Care in Long-Term Care

Of the 47% of patients who do not die in the hospital, slightly more than half die in nursing homes (CAPC, 2003a). In addition, studies have demonstrated that, just as in the acute care hospital setting, the undertreatment of pain and poor physician/patient communication regarding end-of-life care planning are significant problems in long-term care facilities (LTCFs) (DeSilva, Dillon, & Teno, 2001; Ferrell, 1995; Teno, 2003; Teno, Weitzen, Wetle, et al., 2001b). Logically, LTCFs would be an ideal place to offer palliative care services.

LTCFs have been partnering with hospices to provide end-of-life care in nursing homes since the middle to late 1980s when the Medicare Hospice Benefit was modified to recognize that the nursing home, for the purposes of the benefit, was to be considered the patient's primary residence (Ersek & Wilson, 2003; Kinzbrunner, 2002a). LTCF residents receiving care under the Medicare Hospice Benefit receive the same comprehensive services had they lived in a private home. Hospice services are reimbursed at the "routine home care" per diem rate. One very important exception is when a patient's custodial nursing home care is covered by Medicaid. In this case the hospice program is reimbursed at a "unified rate," consisting of 95% of the sum of the Medicaid nursing home room-and-board rate and the "routine home care"

per diem rate. Hospice then becomes responsible to pay the LTCF for the patient's room and board (Kinzbrunner, 2002a; Zerzan, Stearns, & Hanson, 2000).

Hospices must have contractual agreements with each LTCF in which they care for patients. The hospice maintains the professional management responsibility for facility patients enrolled on the hospice program. To ensure that patients' needs are appropriately met and are consistent with a palliative plan of care, hospices and LTCFs are mandated to develop "coordinated plans of care" for the patients that are jointly served by the two health care organizations.

In addition to providing "home care" for LTCF residents, LTCF/hospice relationships are evolving to include inpatient relationships as well. It was reported in 1997 that more than 200 nursing homes have dedicated hospice units, and the number of such units is growing, at least in part related to a decrease in the hospital bed availability for hospital-based hospice inpatient units (Castle, Mor, & Banaszak-Holl, 1997).

The hospice experience in serving patients residing in LTCFs has, overall, been a positive one. The additional care provided by the hospice interdisciplinary team is invaluable in supplementing the care provided by the LTCF staff and ensures that patients receive the necessary palliative symptom management, optimal skin care, nutritional assistance, and psychosocial and spiritual support. Hospice social workers and chaplains can also provide support to family members of LTCF patients who may have strong feelings of guilt about having placed a loved one in a LTCF, especially when death is near. This support can be provided either at the facility or off-site, such as in the family member's home (Ersek & Wilson, 2003; Kinzbrunner, 2002a). This augmentation of services that hospice provides to nursing home residents and their families has resulted in an increase in family satisfaction with the end-of-life care provided in the facility setting (Baer & Hanson, 2000).

Another major benefit to the LTCF/hospice partnership is a documented decrease in the hospitalization rates of patients living in nursing homes who are near the end of life. A direct correlation was demonstrated between the utilization of hospice (low, medium, or high, based on the percentage of patients in the facility enrolled in hospice) and the hospitalization rate of the residents. Most interesting, this correlation was not confined to patients who were enrolled in hospice but extended to non-hospice residents in the facility as well (Miller, Gozalo, & Mor, 2001).

As important but probably less-appreciated benefit to the presence of hospice in LTCFs is the support that the hospice program provides to the LTCF staff after the death of the patient. The members of the LTCF staff are considered members of the patient's extended family and often have developed relationships with many of the residents, some of whom have lived in the facility for many years. Just as members of a deceased patient's biologic family have needs, the facility staff needs and greatly benefits from the psychosocial and bereavement support that a hospice program provides (Kinzbrunner, 2002a; Katz, Sidell, & Komaromy, 2001).

However, not all patients residing in LTCFs who require palliative care have the opportunity to receive hospice services. In fact, based on recent studies, only 1% of all facility residents and about 6% of terminally ill residents utilize hospice before death (Miller et al., 2001; Petrisek & Mor, 1999). Some of the reasons for the underutilization of hospice services in LTCFs, such as physician concerns about determining patient prognosis, are the same barriers to hospice access in general (see earlier discussion). However, there are several reasons for poor hospice utilization in LTCFs.

Foremost among these barriers is the relationship between the Medicare Hospice Benefit and the Medicare skilled nursing facility (SNF) benefit. Both benefits are Medicare Part A benefits and are mutually exclusive, meaning a patient who accesses the Medicare SNF benefit cannot use the Hospice Benefit, and vice versa. The implications of this are that patients who require palliative care services and are eligible for the Medicare SNF benefit are not eligible to receive hospice services under the Medicare Hospice Benefit (Kinzbrunner, 2002a).

Another barrier to patient access to hospice unique to LTCF settings is the variable willingness of both hospice and LTCF providers to contract with each other. On the hospice side, programs may selectively choose to work only with facilities who will attempt to maintain a certain average number of patients, allowing the hospice to concentrate staff and resources, thereby increasing the cost-effectiveness of the care. Small hospices may not be able to provide the education and training to the LTCF staff that is necessary to ensure proper hospice utilization. On the flip side, LTCFs may choose not to work with hospices at all or limit the number of providers they work with, potentially reducing the ability of their patients to access such services. LTCF staff members may sometimes perceive the hospice staff presence as intrusive to their already established relationships with facility patients. Finally, both the nursing facility staff and the hospice staff may not be familiar with the rules, regulations, and policies of the respective agencies, creating significant coordination and collaboration challenges (Ersek & Wilson, 2003; Wilson & Daley, 1998).

Not surprising, these challenges and an attempt to meet the palliative care needs of LTCF patients have led investigators to consider alternative models of delivering palliative care in the nursing home environment. One model has developed palliative care units within the LTCF, designed to meet the palliative care needs of patients, irrespective of their potential eligibility for or agreement to hospice services. The prototype project, known as the *hospice households project*, uses case managers selected by the facility and trained in hospice, care planning, assessment techniques, and case management to manage the care of end-stage dementia patients in a specialized setting. The results of this project included decreased physical, psychosocial, and spiritual discomfort of patients, improvement in dementia-related behavioral abnormalities, and increased staff job satisfaction, with little or no additional cost to the facility (Ersek & Wilson, 2003).

The success of this project has led to additional studies comparing the quality and cost of care of a dementia special care unit, which, although not designated as a palliative care unit, was primarily designed for patients with advanced dementia, with the quality and cost of care of a traditional long-term care. Results demonstrated superior quality of care, as measured by less patient discomfort and fewer hospitalizations, and reduced costs in the dementia special care unit (Ersek & Wilson, 2003; Volicer, Collard, Hurley, et al., 1994).

Another method of providing palliative care in the LTCF is through the development of a palliative care consult service. The service can be established by the facility itself, utilizing clinicians already on staff at the facility, or expertise can be sought from outside the facility and is often accompanied by significant education to the LTCF staff by the palliative care consult team. Successful modeling of this approach to palliative care in the LTCF setting can be found in the recently reported Genesis ElderCare, University of Pennsylvania School of Nursing Project. This project evaluated the impact of either a palliative care educational intervention alone or the combination of a palliative care educational intervention plus the establishment of a palliative care consult team on the delivery of palliative care interventions to appropriate LTCF residents. Although measurable outcomes are not yet available, the perceived success of this program can be documented by the fact that the program is being sustained beyond the grant study period by the LTCF organization (Ersek & Wilson, 2003; Tuch, Parrish, & Romer, 2003).

Following this model, a number of other organizations, including medical institutions, ethics consortiums, and bioethics centers, have developed or are developing significant palliative care education programs and palliative care guidelines, as well as providing palliative care and ethics consults geared specifically to LTCFs. Although these programs have been somewhat helpful, they have not yet demonstrated effectiveness at changing LTCF organizational behavior or physician practice patterns to any great degree.

Therefore efforts are ongoing to identify other educational needs to enhance these programs and to produce the desired outcomes (Ersek & Wilson, 2003).

Home-Based Palliative Care

Motivated by the desire to reach patients sooner in the course of terminal illness, some hospice providers have created home-based palliative care programs, often referred to as *pre-hospice* or *bridge* programs (Casarett & Abrahm, 2001). These programs were designed to provide hospice-like services to patients who would benefit from such services but who do not meet hospice eligibility requirements, are not yet ready to accept the implications of hospice regarding their prognosis, and/or are receiving life-prolonging therapy that is not consistent with a hospice plan of care. The bridge program parallels hospice regarding the interdisciplinary approach to care. If the bridge and hospice programs are part of the same agency, continuity of care, at least in theory, may be enhanced as the same team members may care for patients from the time of admission to death, regardless of whether they are on the bridge program or hospice.

Bridge programs are primarily established and reimbursed as home health agencies. Therefore for the services to be reimbursable, the patient must require skilled nursing care and be confined to the home (neither of which are requirements for the Medicare Hospice Benefit). Supplementary funding from outside organizations (e.g., community fund raising, financial gifts, grants) can assist hospice and home health agencies who operate bridge programs to provide uncovered services, such as nursing visits for patients who are not homebound and care from non-nursing disciplines. This is easier to accomplish with larger versus smaller hospice programs.

A study published in 2001 did a comparative analysis of cancer patients cared for by a hospice bridge program and its parent hospice. The bridge program patients qualified for the program by having a prognosis of 1 year or less (as opposed to the 6 months or less required by the Medicare Hospice Benefit) and desired what was described as "life-prolonging" treatment. Demographically, bridge program patients were somewhat younger, married, in a higher income bracket, and less likely to be covered by Medicare or Medicaid. Clinically, the bridge patients had as many symptoms and/or needs of care as the hospice patients, with the bridge patients most notably demonstrating increased needs for pain management (62% vs. 54% for hospice patients) and intravenous (IV) medication management (24% vs. 10%). Survival data demonstrated that bridge patients had longer median survival than hospice patients (52 days vs. 20 days), and a lower percentage of patients lived less than 6 months (87% vs. 94%). Although these differences were statistically significant, one could certainly argue that the bridge patients, as a population, fulfilled the Medicare Hospice Benefit eligibility criterion of having a prognosis of 6 months or less. Yet there was no evidence that hospice was ever offered to this group of patients at the time of bridge program enrollment, nor were there reasons given for why they refused hospice if it was offered. Furthermore, the study does not provide data on how many patients "crossed the bridge" into hospice before death. The lack of this information forces one to raise some significant questions as to whether the bridge program actually accomplished its goal of attracting patients with a longer prognosis (1 year or less vs. 6 months or less) (Casarett & Abrahm, 2001).

Disease-Based Palliative Care

In addition to bridge programs, several plans have been developed to provide palliative care services to patients that are disease-specific. These programs are designed to provide services that assist patients in making end-of-life decisions and provide symptom management while considering the unique needs of patients who suffer from various diseases. For example, a renal palliative care initiative was developed that not only demonstrated improvements in pain and symptom management of patients with advanced end-stage renal disease but also improved the skill and comfort of the physicians and nurses caring for these patients in discussing dialysis withdrawal and advance care planning (Poppel, Cohen, & Germain, 2003).

Efforts to improve the end-of-life care of patients suffering from Alzheimer's disease and other forms of dementia and integrate that care into primary care of these patients has led to creation of the Palliative Excellence in Alzheimer Care Efforts (PEACE) program. This program, developed through the efforts of the primary care geriatrics practice at the University of Chicago, includes patient and caregiver interviews, a post-death

caregiver interview, and a nurse coordinator who, following a review of the interviews, provides the primary care physicians with feedback that enhances patient care. Initial results suggest adequate pain control, patient satisfaction with the quality of care, attention to the patient's wishes, and the occurrence of death in the patient's location of choice. Family satisfaction was also demonstrated to be high regarding quality of care (Shega, Levin, Hougham, et al., 2003).

With the roots of hospice in the field of oncology, partnering with cancer centers and oncologists to reach patients earlier in the course of advanced disease continues to be a major goal. Two models chosen from several that have been developed as part of the Robert Wood Johnson *Promoting Excellence in End of Life Care* project will be reviewed (Beresford, Byock, & Twohig, 2002; Schapiro, Byock, Parker, et al., 2003). The first, called *Project Safe Conduct*, was designed to integrate a team from a community-based hospice. This team consisting of a nurse practitioner, a social worker, and a spiritual counselor integrated into the normal operations of a cancer center. Project Safe Conduct has been shown to reduce unplanned emergency room visits and the number of hospitalizations of patients served by the cancer center while increasing the proportion of patients cared for by hospice from 13% to 80%, median length of hospice stay from 3 days to 30 days, and the mean hospice length of stay from 10 to 43 days (Beresford et al., 2002; Pitorak, Armour, & Sivec, 2003; Schapiro et al., 2003).

The second project created the role of a palliative care coordinator (PCC) to work with a group of cancer patients receiving antineoplastic treatment through an academic comprehensive cancer center in a randomized control study. The study compared these patients with others receiving traditional oncology care from the center without the added benefit of the PCC. The role of the PCC was to facilitate patient/family education regarding the patient's condition, patient/family communication with their oncologists and other health care staff, and ultimately, to ensure that patient/family needs and values were clearly reflected in the treatment decisions that were made. Preliminary results of this study have shown no survival or symptom control differences between the two groups of patients. Patients in the intervention group who worked with the PCC had less reduction in measures of quality of life when compared with the control group. In addition, a statistically significant difference in Medicare costs was reported in favor of the intervention group although the preliminary nature of the results precludes one from concluding whether a true cost savings will be demonstrated (Beresford et al., 2002; Finn, Pienta, Parzuchowski, et al., 2002; Schapiro et al., 2003).

Meeting the palliative care needs of patients with advanced human immunodeficiency virus (HIV) disease and acquired immunodeficiency syndrome (AIDS) has continued to be a challenge, especially as the development and refinement of highly active antiretroviral therapy (HAART) has turned AIDS into more of a chronic disease. Several academic and urban hospital center AIDS palliative care models have evolved, integrating intensive symptom management provided by interdisciplinary palliative care teams with traditional disease management including antiretroviral therapy, opportunistic infection prophylaxis, and treatment of active diseases on both an inpatient and outpatient basis. Although these projects are still too recent to have produced any evidence of improvement in clinical care over traditional services, these projects have served to highlight the many unique challenges of these patients, who generally come from most underserved, resource-poor urban environments (Beresford et al., 2002; O'Neill & Marconi, 2003; Selwyn, Rivard, Kappell, et al., 2003).

Finally, although not truly disease-specific, palliative care initiatives are being undertaken in several special populations. Outreach to minority groups has led hospice and palliative care providers to create end-of-life programs that specifically address the needs and attempt to overcome the inequities and barriers to health care that exist in the African-American community (Barrett & Heller, 2002; Payne, Payne, & Heller, 2002). Other minority groups for whom palliative care models are being explored include Hispanic and Native American communities (DeCourtney, Jones, Merriman, et al., 2003; Policzer, 2002). The special needs of the mentally ill prompted the development of a demonstration project to improve access to advance care planning and end-of-life care in this population (Foti, 2003). Of course, discussion of special populations would be incomplete without discussing the many efforts being made to bring palliative care to children who suffer from advanced illness and whose needs and the needs of their families differ in many significant ways from their adult counterparts (Beresford et al., 2002; Field & Behrman, 2002; Macurda, 2002). One such recently described effort is the Pediatric Palliative Care Project, based at the Seattle Children's Hospital. This project, a collaborative effort throughout the state of Washington to promote family-centered pediatric care, has been able to expand access to home-based palliative care services, including family-centered care planning, in coordination with life-prolonging care across all outpatient and inpatient settings. The success of this project to date has been measured in improved patient/family satisfaction and the quality of medical decision making (Beresford et al., 2002).

Comprehensive Palliative Care Models

As noted, there are myriad ways in which physicians and other providers of health care have been and are continuing to team together to create innovative programs to bring hospice and palliative care services to patients and families in need. However, most efforts are specific to a setting of care or to a disease. The real trick is to integrate these various efforts so that patients and families can receive the services they need irrespective of the disease the patient is living with and dying from or the setting in which the patient requires or chooses to receive the care. Such an effort has taken place in Lexington, Kentucky, where Hospice of the Bluegrass has collaborated with three local hospitals, including an academic medical center, to establish comprehensive palliative care services throughout the community. Components of the program include physician-centered inpatient palliative care consultation services in each hospital (one of which has an existing hospice inpatient unit), the establishment of a hospice liaison nurse in each institution to facilitate continuity of care between the hospital and hospices to which patients are referred, and an outpatient palliative care medical practice. Medical directors from Hospice of the Bluegrass, together with trained nurse practitioners, are primarily responsible for the inpatient and outpatient consultation services.

Since the inception of the program, utilization of the palliative care consult service has continued to increase. For the hospitals, this has resulted in decreased futile care in the ICU, resulting in better ICU bed utilization and reduced costs. For the hospice, the best measurable outcome has been an increase in referrals as a result of patient and physician exposure to palliative medicine earlier in the course of illness (NHPCO & CAPC, 2001; Swinford, 2003).

Another similar model of comprehensive palliative care can be found in Evanston, Illinois. This program, started by Palliative Care and Hospice of the North Shore, integrates their comprehensive hospice program, which includes an inpatient unit, with home health services, a palliative care consult service that provides consults in a variety of settings (inpatient, patient homes, nursing homes), a telephone case management service, and a private duty service that can meet additional patient care needs not provided by hospice or home health care. In addition to the consultation service, either a physician or a nurse practitioner makes follow-up medical home visits to patients. Although those involved in the program report very positive attitudes among patients, families, and physicians who have utilized the service, outcomes data documenting the success of this program have not yet been published (NHPCO & CAPC, 2001; Twaddle, Sheehan, & Romer, 2003).

THE FUTURE

The evolution of end-of-life care in the forms of hospice and palliative care has been a remarkable health care success story. As can be seen from this review, the ability to provide the comprehensive services that patients and families require during the last months or, in some cases, the last years of life has been changed significantly since the seeds from England were planted in the form of hospice and the Medicare Hospice Benefit more than 2 decades ago. True, the introduction of hospice into the health care continuum has not been easy; in its early days it was kept separate and distinct from the traditional health care system and excluded curative or disease-modifying therapy, as illustrated in Figure 1-1.

However, it has been increasingly recognized that patients who require disease-modifying therapy, or sometimes even curative therapy, also need the supportive services that hospice provides. Palliative care programs, including but not limited to the many that were described earlier in the chapter, were introduced. These programs have allowed patients to continue to receive curative or disease-modifying therapy with a gradual increase in the focus on palliation of symptoms occurring as the illness progresses. Although this model, illustrated in Figure 1-2, has been accepted by many as superior to the traditional approach (see Fig. 1-1), it is not a panacea (CAPC, 2003a; Emmanuel, von Gunten, Ferris, et al., 1999). The small amount of palliative care early in the course of illness that is implicit in the placement of the diagonal in Figure 1-2 continues

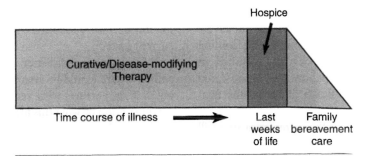

FIGURE 1-1 Traditional model of health care. (Data from Emanuel, L.L., von Gunten, C.F., & Ferris, F.D. [Eds.]. *Plenary 3: Elements and models of end-of-life care.* The Education for Physicians on End-of-life Care [EPEC] Curriculum: ©The EPEC Project, 1999, 2003.)

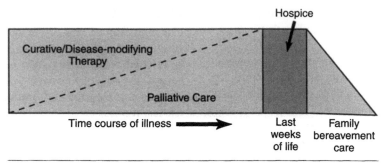

FIGURE **1-2** Integrated palliative care model. (Modified from Emanuel, L.L., von Gunten, C.F., & Ferris, F.D. [Eds.]. *Plenary 3: Elements and models of end-of-life care.* The Education for Physicians on End-of-life Care [EPEC] Curriculum: ©The EPEC Project, 1999, 2003.)

to foster the notion that palliative care's main role is late in the course of illness; this is demonstrated by the fact that most of the palliative care models developed to date are designed for patients with far-advanced disease. As depicted in Figure 1-2, hospice's place is essentially unchanged from that illustrated in Figure 1-1, leaving it as a separate entity outside the mainstream of care, reserved for patients in the last weeks of life.

Moving further into the twenty-first century, the health care needs of our nation will be changing, based on the aging of our society. It is predicted that by 2030, the Medicare population will double from the current 40 million to 80 million. More than 11% (approximately 9 million) of these individuals will be older than 85 years (Lynn & Adamson, 2003). An increase in patient demand for the latest high-technology treatments is already being experienced, especially with increased access to the Internet and consumer-based media advertising, and is sure to rise further in the coming decades. Both of these factors have resulted in significant concerns about how people are cared for when they are chronically ill and in the final stages of life.

However, it is clear that the current measures will be insufficient to meet the needs of the burgeoning population of seniors who will need the kind of services that hospice and palliative care programs currently provide. To meet these needs, an innovative approach has recently been suggested. It is proposed that health care needs be tied to the trajectory of disease, defined as either a short period of decline (typical of cancer), a longer-term period of limitation secondary to disease with intermittent exacerbations and sudden death (typical of organ system failure), and prolonged "dwindling" (typical of dementia, other neurodegenerative diseases, disabling stroke, and frailty). Care would then be tailored to the needs of the patients, based on the predicted trajectory of decline, and would be customized to include appropriate medical treatment, assistance as needed to live as fully as possible, avoidance of gaps in care, proactively anticipating patient needs, and focusing on symptom management. Although this type of proposal sounds very worthwhile and is something to strive for, it would require a major overhaul of the current health care system (Lynn & Adamson, 2003). Therefore although it is something to strive for, it is necessary to create change from within the current system.

It is suggested that better access to hospice and palliative care would be attainable under the existing system, perhaps with very few modifications. An illustration of what this might look like is shown in Figure 1-3. Hospice must be better utilized. Rather than reserve hospice care for the last few weeks of life, as illustrated by both Figures 1-1 and 1-2, patients should be allowed to maximize their ability to access the hospice for the full 6 months to which they are entitled under the Medicare

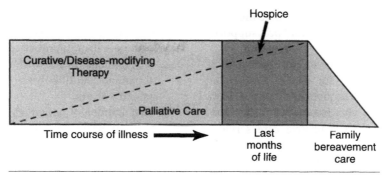

FIGURE 1-3 Proposed model for integrating palliative care and hospice. (Data from Emanuel, L.L., von Gunten, C.F., & Ferris, F.D. [Eds.]. *Plenary 3: Elements and models of end-of-life care.* The Education for Physicians on End-of-life Care [EPEC] Curriculum: ©The EPEC Project, 1999, 2003.)

Hospice Benefit. However, many will continue to cite the barriers of physician inability to predict prognosis and concerns over regulatory scrutiny as reasons why maximizing hospice utilization may be impractical, but the fact is that both of these barriers are more perceived than real.

Based on a 1972 study, repeated and confirmed in 1998, physicians tend to be optimistic when predicting prognosis (Christakis, 1998). Although the SUPPORT investigators reported that physicians were pessimistic, a more thorough analysis of the presented data actually suggests the opposite—that the physicians who participated in the SUPPORT study were quite accurate in predicting prognosis. In a cohort of patients who were predicted by physicians as having an 85% probability of dying in 6 months, 85% of them died (Arkes, Dawson, Speroff, et al., 1995; Kinzbrunner, 2002b; Knaus et al., 1995). In addition, a recent Center for Medicare Services (CMS) memorandum should allay the perceived concerns regarding regulatory scrutiny. The memorandum clearly states that CMS "recognizes that prognoses can be uncertain and may change," and "recognizes that making medical prognostication of life expectancy is not always an exact science. Thus physicians need not be concerned. There is no risk to a physician certifying for hospice care an individual that he or she believes to be terminally ill (U.S. DHHS, 2003)."

Therefore rather than physicians worrying about precisely predicting the prognosis of an individual patient, agonizing over the lack of scientific evidence that established criteria for determining when patients have a prognosis of 6 months or less or about potential regulatory difficulties should the patient live longer than 6 months, a simpler approach is suggested. Perhaps physicians should simply ask themselves the question, "Would I be surprised if this patient were to die of their illness in the next 6 months?" and if the answer is "No," consider utilizing hospice services to provide for the palliative care needs of those patients.

Hospices must adapt as well. As illustrated in Figures 1-1 and 1-2, hospices generally avoid providing any disease-modifying therapy, cited as another barrier to hospice utilization. For patients requesting these types of interventions for whom bridge programs and other models of palliative care have been developed, it appears they are often not given the opportunity to access hospice because of the perceived reluctance of hospices to provide the therapy when medically indicated. As shown in Figure 1-3, hospices must begin to provide patients with disease-modifying interventions such as palliative chemotherapy, radiation therapy, blood transfusions, and minor surgical procedures. These interventions should not be provided haphazardly but should be offered with thoughtful palliative consideration weighing the benefit versus the burden. Hospices also need to find creative ways to serve patients who choose to enroll in phase I clinical trials and to determine how to be included in a clinical trial as the standard for "best supportive care" (Byock & Miles, 2003).

What about patients who do not meet the test "Would I be surprised if the patient died in the next few months?", who do not desire hospice services when offered, or who have non-terminal disease? For these patients, palliative care services should be available throughout the continuum of the illness. These services should be provided by a team of well-trained professionals and may include palliative care consultations in a variety of settings, palliative care units in hospitals and LTCFs, and home visits by members of the palliative care team.

SUMMARY

The practice of palliative care is the primary responsibility of the attending provider. The attending provider is responsible not only for promoting the patient's well-being, diagnosing the patient when ill, and referring to appropriate consultants to treat disease and manage symptoms but also for promoting optimal function and quality of life. Despite the attempts to improve and integrate palliative and hospice care into traditional care settings, it can occur only when the attending physician has recognized the value of these services.

Objective Questions

1. According to the Oxford English Dictionary, palliate in the context of health care means to:

    a. Improve the quality of life of patients.
    b. Alleviate the symptoms of a disease without curing it.
    c. Provide hope to patients who are terminally ill.
    d. Provide interdisciplinary team care to terminally ill patients.

2. The requirement of the Medicare Hospice Benefit that has been most responsible for defining hospice utilization in the United States is:

    a. That the interdisciplinary team is headed by a registered nurse.

    b. The establishment of the nurse, physician, social worker, and pastoral counselor as the four core team members.
    c. The mandate to provide bereavement care to patients' families for 1 year following the patients' death.
    d. The defining of patient eligibility as a 6-month or less prognosis if the illness runs its normal course.

3. Which of the following best describes the group of patients for whom palliative care is best suited?

    a. All patients with life-limiting illnesses with a diagnosis of cancer.
    b. All patients with life-limiting illnesses, irrespective of diagnosis.
    c. All patients, during all phases of illness, with a diagnosis of cancer.
    d. All patients, during all phases of illness, irrespective of diagnosis.

4. Mr. Smith is a 75-year-old Medicare patient with advanced chronic obstructive pulmonary disease (COPD) who is on a local hospice program. He just returned home after visiting his attending physician, reporting increased dyspnea and cough productive of yellow to green sputum. While in the office, his physician took sputum for a culture, obtained a chest x-ray film, and gave the patient a prescription for an antibiotic for what was determined to be an acute bronchitis. Which of the services that Mr. Smith received can be reimbursed under Medicare Part B?

    a. The office visit.
    b. The chest x-ray film.
    c. The sputum culture.
    d. The prescribed antibiotics.

5. The SUPPORT study was conducted in the early 1990s to assess the care that seriously ill and dying patients were receiving in several major academic institutions. Phase I of the study demonstrated deficiencies in patient care in several key areas related to patient/family

communications and advance care planning. To address this, phase II of the study examined the effectiveness of specially trained nurses to serve as liaisons to improve communication among patients, families, physicians, and hospital staff? Phase II of the study showed that the nursing intervention resulted in:

a. An improvement in both the pain control patients received and facilitation of advance care planning.
b. An improvement in the pain control patients received but not in the facilitation of advance care planning.
c. Neither an improvement in the pain control patients received nor in the facilitation of advance care planning.
d. No improvement in the pain control patients received but improvement in facilitation of advance care planning.

6. According to a 2003 Health Care Advisory Board report on hospital-based palliative care programs, what fraction of patients admitted or transferred to palliative care units comes from an ICU setting?

a. One-third.
b. One-fourth.
c. One-sixth.
d. One eighth.

7. Under what circumstances may a patient receive hospice care under the Medicare Hospice Benefit while a resident of a long-term care facility?

a. When the hospice and the LTCF have a contractual relationship and while the patient is receiving skilled nursing home benefits under Medicare Part A.
b. When the hospice and the LTCF have a contractual relationship and the patient is not receiving skilled nursing home benefits under Medicare Part A.
c. When the hospice and the nursing home do not have a contractual relationship and the patient is not receiving skilled nursing home benefits under Medicare Part A.

d. When the hospice and the nursing home do not have a contractual relationship and the patient is receiving skilled nursing home benefits under Medicare Part A.

8. In a 2001 study evaluating the efficacy of a pre-hospice bridge program, the investigators reported which of the following?

a. The majority of patients on the bridge program received care for more than 6 months and had fewer symptoms than hospice patients.
b. The majority of patients on the bridge program received care for less than 6 months and had as many symptoms as hospice patients.
c. The majority of patients on the bridge program received care for more than 6 months and had as many symptoms as hospice patients.
d. The majority of patients on the bridge program received care for less than 6 months and had fewer symptoms than hospice patients.

9. In a study assessing the role of a palliative care coordinator designed to facilitate communication between a group of cancer patients/families and health care providers and to better coordinate care received, the investigators reported which of the following benefits to patients who had the services of the palliative care coordinator as compared with the control group?

a. Improvement in symptom control.
b. Improvement in survival.
c. A true reduction in the costs of care.
d. Less reduction in measures of quality of life.

10. To improve access to end-of-life care over the next decade, which of the following recommendations is most practical?

a. Continue to confine hospice care to the last few weeks of life only while enhancing the development of palliative care.

b. Eliminate the hospice benefit in favor of a more comprehensive palliative care benefit.

c. Maximize utilization of hospice while developing non-hospice palliative care models for patients not desirous of hospice services.

d. Completely redesign the health care system to provide patients with access to all forms of care based on their individual needs.

REFERENCES

American Academy of Hospice and Palliative Medicine. (2003). Position statements: *Definitions of palliative care and palliative medicine.* www.aahpm.org/positions/definition.html.

Arkes, H.R., Dawson, N.V., Speroff, T., et al. (1995). The covariance decomposition of the probability score and its use in evaluating prognostic estimates. *Med Decis Making, 14,* 120.

Baer, W.M., & Hanson, L.C. (2000). Families' perception of the added value of hospice in the nursing home. *J Am Geriatr Soc, 48,* 879-882.

Barrett, D.K., & Heller, K.S. (2002). Death and dying in the black experience. *J Palliat Med, 5*(5), 793-799.

Beresford, L., Byock, I., & Twohig, J.S. (2002). *Financial implications of promoting excellence in end-of-life care.* Missoula, Mont.: Robert Wood Johnson Foundation.

Berger, A.M., Portenoy R.K., & Weissman, D.E. (2002). Preface. In A.M. Berger, R.K. Portenoy, & D.E. Weissman (Eds.), *Principles and practice of palliative care and supportive oncology* (p. xix). Philadelphia: Lippincott Williams & Wilkins.

Billings, J.A., Block, S.D., Finn, J.W., et al. (2002). Initial voluntary program standards for fellowship training in palliative medicine. *J Palliat Med, 5*(1), 23-33.

Bozeman, M. (2002). Bereavement. In B.M. Kinzbrunner, N.J. Weinreb, & J.S. Policzer (Eds.), *Twenty common problems in end-of-life care* (pp. 275-293). New York: McGraw Hill.

Brody H., & Lynn J. (1984). The physician's responsibility under the new Medicare reimbursement for hospice. *N Engl J Med, 310,* 920.

Byock, I., & Miles, S.H. (2003). Hospice benefits and phase I cancer trials. *Ann Int Med, 138,* 335-337.

Casarett, D., & Abrahm, J.L. (2001). Patients with cancer referred to a hospice versus a bridge program: Patient characteristics, needs for care, and survival. *J Clin Oncol, 19,* 2057-2063.

Castle, N.G., Mor, V., & Banaszak-Holl, J. (1997). Special care hospice units in nursing homes. *Hosp J, 12,* 59-69.

Cellerino, R., Tummarello, D., Guidi, F., et al. (1991). A randomized trial of alternating chemotherapy versus best supportive care in advanced non-small cell lung cancer. *J Clin Oncol, 4,* 14.

Center to Advance Palliative Care (CAPC). (2003a). *The case for hospital-based palliative care.* www.capc.org/Files/tmp_133221135.pdf.

Center to Advance Palliative Care (CAPC). (2003b). *Palliative care in the ICU.* www.capc.org/site_root/Documents/documents_251104009.html.

Christakis, N.A. (1998). Predicting patient survival before and after hospice enrollment. *Hosp J, 13,* 71.

42 Code of Federal Regulations, Part 418, Medicare Hospice Regulations, 1993.

Corless, I.B. (1983). The hospice movement in North America. In C.A. Corr & D.M. Coor (Eds.), *Hospice care: Principles and practice* (p. 335). New York: Springer.

Corr, C.A., & Corr, D.M. (1983). Needs and responses: The hospice approach. In C.A. Corr & D.M. Coor (Eds.), *Hospice care: Principles and practice* (p.1). New York: Springer.

DeCourtney, C.A., Jones, K., Merriman, M.P., et al. (2003). Establishing a culturally sensitive palliative care program in rural Alaska Native American communities. *J Palliat Med, 6*(3), 501-510.

DeSilva, D., Dillon J.E., & Teno, J.M. (2001). The quality of care in the last month of life among Rhode Island nursing home residents. *Med Health R I, 84,* 195-198.

Doyle, D., Hanks, G., & MacDonald, N. (1998). Introduction. In D. Doyle, G. Hanks, & N. MacDonald (Eds.), *Oxford textbook of palliative medicine* (2nd ed., p. 3). New York: Oxford University Press.

Dunlop, R. (Nov., 1998). Personal communication.

Elyasem, A.F., Swint, K., Roach, P., et al. (2003). Palliative care inpatient service (PCIS) in a comprehensive cancer center: Clinical and financial outcomes. *Proc Am Soc Clin Oncol, 2099,* 522. Abstract.

Emanuel, L., von Gunten, C.F., Ferris, F.D., et al. (1999). *Education on palliative and end-of-life care (EPEC).* Presentation module 3, Elements and models of end-of-life care.

Ersek, M., & Wilson, S.A. (2003). The challenges and opportunities in providing end-of-life care in nursing homes. *J Palliat Med, 6*(1), 45-57.

Ferrell, B.A. (1995). Pain evaluation and management in the nursing home. *Ann Intern Med, 123,* 681-687.

Field, M.J., & Behrman, R.E. (Eds.) (2002). *When children die: Improving palliative and end-of-life care for children and their families.* Washington: National Academy Press.

Finn, J.W., Pienta, K.J., Parzuchowski, J., et al. (2002). Palliative care project: Bridging active treatment and hospice for terminal cancer patients. *Proc Am Soc Clin Oncol,* 1452.

Fins, J.J., Miller, F.G., Acres, C.A., et al. (1999). End-of-life decision making in the hospital: Current practice and future prospects. *J Pain Symptom Manage, 17,* 6.

Foti, M.E. (2003). "Do it your way": A demonstration project on end-of-life care for persons with serious mental illness. *J Palliat Med, 6*(4), 661-668.

Ganz, P.A., Figlin R.A., Haskell C.M., et al. (1989). Supportive care versus supportive care and combination chemotherapy in metastatic non-small cell lung cancer. Does chemotherapy make a difference? *Cancer, 63,* 1271.

Health Care Advisory Board. (2003). *Best of OI: Success of inpatient palliative care programs.* Washington: The Advisory Board Company. www.advisory.com.

Katz, J.S., Sidell, M., & Komaromy, C. (2001). Dying in long-term care facilities: Support needs of other residents, relatives, and staff. *Am J Hospice Palliat Care, 18*(5), 321-326.

Kinzbrunner, B.M. (1997). FMR: The role of the medical director. *AAHPM Academy Update, 7,* 2.

Kinzbrunner, B.M. (2000). The terminally ill patient. In M.D. Abeloff, J.O. Armitage, A.S. Lichter, et al. (Eds.), *Clinical oncology* (2nd ed., pp. 597-627). London: Churchill Livingstone.

Kinzbrunner, B.M. (2002a). How to help patients access end-of-life care. In B.M. Kinzbrunner, N.J. Weinreb, & J.S. Policzer (Eds.), *Twenty common problems in end-of-life care* (pp. 29-45). New York: McGraw Hill.

Kinzbrunner, B.M. (2002b). Predicting prognosis: How to decide when end-of-life care is needed. In B.M. Kinzbrunner, N.J. Weinreb, & J.S. Policzer (Eds.), *Twenty common problems in end-of-life care* (pp. 3-27). New York: McGraw Hill.

Kinzbrunner, B.M. (2002c). *Providing effective end-of-life care* (pp. 49-50). Hospital Management International.

Klastersky, J. (1997). Supportive care in oncology. *Bull Mem Acad R Med Belg, 152,* 10.

Knaus, W.A., Harrell, F.E. Jr., Lynn, J., et al. (1995). The SUPPORT prognostic model: Objective estimates of survival for seriously ill hospitalized patients. *Ann Int Med, 122,* 191-203.

Lack, S. (1983). The hospice concept: The adult with advanced cancer. In C.A. Corr & D.M. Coor (Eds.), *Hospice care: Principles and practice* (p. 42). New York: Springer.

Lynn, J., & Adamson, D.M. (2003). White paper: *Living well at the end of life. Adapting health care to serious chronic illness in old age.* Rand Health. www.rand.org.

Macurda, J.A. (2002). Care of children at the end of life. In B.M. Kinzbrunner, N.J. Weinreb, & J.S. Policzer (Eds.), *Twenty common problems in end-of-life care* (pp. 399-423). New York: McGraw Hill.

Mayer, R.J. (1996). End-of-life care: It's time to pay attention. *ASCO News, 8,* 1.

Meier D., Morrison S., & Cassel C. (1997). Improving palliative care. *Ann Intern Med, 127,* 225-230.

Members of ABIM End-of-Life Patient Care Project. (1996). *Caring for the dying: Identification and promotion of physician competency.* Philadelphia: American Board of Internal Medicine.

Miller, F.G., & Fins, J.J. (1996). Sounding Board: A proposal to restructure hospital care for dying patients. *N Engl J Med, 334,* 1740.

Miller, S.C., Gozalo, P., & Mor, V. (2001). Hospice enrollment and hospitalization of dying nursing home patients. *Am J Med, 111,* 38-44.

National Hospice and Palliative Care Organization (NHPCO). (1999). *Hospice fact sheet* (updated Spring 1999). www.nhpco.org/facts.html.

National Hospice and Palliative Care Organization (NHPCO). (2003a). *What is hospice and palliative care?* www.nhpco.org/i4a/pages/index.cfm?pageid=3281.

National Hospice and Palliative Care Organization (NHPCO). (2003b). *885,000 Terminally ill Americans served by hospice in 2002.* www.nhpco.org/i4a/pages/index.cfm?pageid=3795&openpage=3795.

National Hospice and Palliative Care Organization (NHPCO), & Center to Advance Palliative Care (CAPC). (2001). *Hospital-hospice partnerships in palliative care: Creating a continuum of service.* www.capc.org/Files/tmp_134090747.pdf.

O'Neill, J., & Marconi, K. (2003). Underserved populations, resource-poor settings, and HIV: Innovative palliative care projects. *J Palliat Med, 6*(3), 457-459.

Oxford English Dictionary (Compact ed.; p. 2059). (1975). New York: Oxford University Press.

Palmetto Government Benefits Administrators. (1997). *Hospice provisions enacted by the Balanced Budget Act (BBA) of 1997.* Medicare Advisory Hospice 97-11, September.

Paradis, L.F. (1985). The development of hospice in America: A social movement organizes. In L.F. Paradis, *Hospice handbook, A guide for managers and planners* (p. 3). Rockville, Md.: Aspen.

Partnership for Caring & Last Acts. (2003, July 27/Aug. 4). Advertisement: The best hospital in the world can't keep you alive forever. *U.S. News & World Report,* p. 67.

Payne, R., Payne, T.R., & Heller, K.S. (2002). The Harlem palliative care experience. *J Palliat Med, 5*(5), 781-792.

Petrisek A.C., & Mor, V. (1999). Hospice in nursing homes: A facility level analysis of the distribution of hospice beneficiaries. *Gerontologist, 39,* 279-290.

Pitorak, E.F., Armour, M.B., & Sivec, H.D. (2003). Project safe conduct integrates palliative care goals into comprehensive cancer care. *J Palliat Med, 6*(4), 645-655.

Policzer, J.S. (2002). Hospice and Hispanics: Strategic issues in providing hospice care to an Hispanic population. *J Palliat Med, 5*(1), 209. AAHPM session abstract.

Poppel, D.M., Cohen, L.M., & Germain, M.J. (2003). The renal palliative care initiative. *J Palliat Med, 6*(2), 321-328.

Rhymes, J. (1990). Hospice care in America. *J Amer Med Assoc, 264,* 369.

Rocker, G.M., & Curtis, J.R. (2003). Caring for the dying in the intensive care unit: In search of clarity. *J Am Med Assoc, 290,* 820-822.

Santa-Emma, P.H., Roach, R., Gill, M.A., et al. (2002). Development and implementation of an inpatient acute palliative care service. *J Palliat Med, 5*(1), 93-100.

Saunders, C.M. (1983). The last stages of life. In C.A. Corr & D.M. Coor (Eds.), *Hospice care: Principles and practice* (p. 5). New York: Springer.

Schapiro, R., Byock, I., Parker, S., et al. (2003). *Living and dying well with cancer: Successfully integrating palliative care into cancer treatment.* Missoula, Mont.: Robert Wood Johnson Foundation.

Selwyn, P.A., Rivard, M., Kappell, D., et al. (2003). Palliative care for AIDS at a large urban teaching hospital: Program description and preliminary outcomes. *J Palliat Med, 6*(3), 461-474.

Sepulveda, C., Marlin, A., Yoshida, T., et al. (2002). Palliative care: The World Health Organization's global perspective. *J Pain Symptom Manage, 24*(2), 91-96.

Shega, J.W., Levin, A., Hougham, G.W., et al. (2003). Palliative excellence in Alzheimer care efforts (PEACE): A program description. *J Palliat Med, 6*(2), 315-320.

Smith, D.H., & Granbois, J.A. (1992). The American way of hospice. *Hastings Cent Rep, 11,* 8.

Smith, T.J. (2003). We can reduce the cost of in-hospital end-of-life care. *Oncology, XXV*(11), 4-6.

Sprung, C.L., Cohen, S.I., Sjokvist P., et al. (2003). End of life practices in European intensive care units: The Ethicus study. *J Am Med Assoc, 290,* 790-797.

Stoddard, S. (1991). *The hospice movement: A better way of caring for the dying* (Revised; pp. 3-28). New York: Vintage.

SUPPORT Principal Investigators. (1995). A controlled trial to improve care for seriously ill hospitalized patients: The study to understand prognoses and preferences for outcomes and risks of treatments (SUPPORT). *J Am Med Assoc, 274,* 1591-1598.

Swinford, S. (2003, Aug. 25). *Successful strategies for hospice-hospital partners in palliative care.* Presented at: Making the most of the Medical Director's position. A conference for Hospice administrators, The Carolina Center for Hospice and End of Life Care.

Teno, J.M. (2003). Now is the time to embrace nursing homes as a place of care for dying patients. *J Palliat Med, 6*(2), 293-296.

Teno, J.M., Weitzen, S., Tennel, M.L., et al. (2001a). Dying trajectory in the last year of life: Does cancer trajectory fit other diseases? *J Palliat Med*, 4(4), 457-464.

Teno, J.M., Weitzen, S., Wetle, T., et al. (2001b). Persistent pain in nursing home residents. *J Am Med Assoc*, 285, 2081.

Tuch, H., Parrish, P., & Romer, A. (2003). Integrating palliative care into nursing homes. *J Palliat Med*, 6(2), 297-309.

Twaddle, M.L., Sheehan, M., & Romer, A.L. (2003). Filling the gaps in service for patients who need supportive care. *J Palliat Med*, 6(1), 117-127.

U.S. Department of Health and Human Services (DHHS). (1992, Dec.). *Medicare hospice manual, section 230.1E* (revised). Springfield, U.S. Department of Commerce.

U.S. Department of Health and Human Services (DHHS), Health Care Financing Administration. (2001, Jan. 24). *Clarification of physician certification requirements for Medicare Hospice.* Program Memorandum. Intermediaries/Carriers. Transmittal AB-01-09.

U.S. Department of Health and Human Services (DHHS), Center for Medicare and Medicaid Services. (2003, March 28). *Hospice care enhances dignity and peace as life nears its end.* Provider education article. Transmittal AB-03-040.

Volicer, L., Collard, A., Hurley, A., et al. (1994). Impact of special care unit for patients with advanced Alzheimer's disease on patients' discomfort and costs. *J Am Geriatr Soc*, 42, 597-603.

von Gunten, C.F., Ferris, F.D., Kirschner, C., et al. (2000). Coding and reimbursement mechanisms for physician services in hospice and palliative care. *J Palliat Med*, 3(2), 157-164.

von Gunten, C.F., Neely, K.J., & Martinez, J. (1996). Hospice and palliative care: Program needs and academic issues. *Oncology*, 10, 1070.

Weinreb, N.J. (2002). Diagnostic tests and invasive procedures. In B.M. Kinzbrunner, N.J. Weinreb, & J.S. Policzer (Eds.). *Twenty common problems in end-of-life care* (pp. 329-364). New York: McGraw Hill.

Weissman, D.E. (1995). Palliative medicine education at the Medical College of Wisconsin. *Wis Med J*, 94, 505.

Wilson, S., & Daley, B. (1998). Attachment/detachment: Forces influencing care of the dying in long-term care. *J Palliat Med*, 1, 21-34.

World Health Organization. (2002). *National cancer control programmes: Policies and managerial guidelines* (2nd ed., p. 2). Geneva: World Health Organization.

Zerzan, J., Stearns, S., & Hanson, L. (2000). Access to palliative care and hospice in nursing homes. *J Amer Med Assoc*, 284, 2489-2494.

CHAPTER 2

Advance Care Planning

Crystal Dea Moore

OBJECTIVES

After the completion of this chapter, the reader should be able to:

1. Discuss the factors that affect communication quality among patients, health care professionals, and families
2. Present nonverbal and verbal strategies to enhance the quality of communication and rapport with patients and families
3. Explicate techniques to facilitate meaningful advance care planning conversations with patients and families
4. Discuss strategies to enhance personal awareness and avoid provider burnout

INTRODUCTION

Effective communication among health care providers, patients, and family members is challenging, particularly when patients are living and dying with advanced illness. Health care professionals' suboptimal communication practices and patterns and how these difficulties can have an impact on the quality of patient care and patients' adjustment to advanced illness are addressed in the literature (e.g., Fallowfield, Jenkins, & Beveridge, 2002; Lee, Back, Block, et al., 2002; Morrison, 1998; Wenrich, Curtis, Shannon, et al., 2001). The purpose of this chapter is to provide practical strategies for palliative care professionals to improve communication effectiveness and advance care planning with patients and families who are coping with myriad challenges that advanced illness presents. Topics include:

- Reasons why advanced illness conversations are so difficult and strategies to initiate and participate effectively in such discussions

- The centrality of the professional-patient relationship to communication effectiveness and the importance of introspection and self-awareness as relationship-building tools
- Effective communication as it relates to advance care planning and the implementation of care plans
- Signs and symptoms of provider burnout and techniques to combat it

ADVANCED ILLNESS CONVERSATIONS

Conversations among health care professionals, patients, and families about advanced illness are often difficult. Clinicians, educated to cure and alleviate patient suffering, may fear causing psychologic and spiritual pain when discussing end-of-life issues or delivering bad news (Morrison, 1998). Health care providers may worry that frank discussions around diagnosis and prognosis will diminish patient and family hope (Steinhauser, Christakis, Clipp, et al., 2001). Clinicians' concern over causing harm, the medical profession's denial of death, and the overall American cultural fear of dying set the stage for clinical avoidance of discussions related to death. On a personal level, professionals may have experienced painful situations related to illness and death and these experiences can have an impact on their willingness and ability to openly confront such topics with their patients (Lee et al., 2002). Most medical professionals have not been properly trained and educated in how to effectively communicate about sensitive issues with patients and families and can overuse professional jargon (Limerick, 2002; Reisfield & Wilson, 2003; The, Hak, Koëter, et al., 2000). On the other hand, medical professionals cannot completely shoulder the blame in the ineffectiveness of patient-provider communication in advanced illness. Patients and families bring their own issues to encounters with providers that can influence communication quality.

The diagnosis of an advanced illness and the concomitant medical decisions that ensue can evoke strong emotions and a psychologic crisis for patients and families (Lee et al., 2002). Depending on personality and previous experiences, patients may react to bad news and the stresses associated with decision making and medical treatments with anger, anxiety, resignation, acceptance, hopefulness, denial, shock, or any combination of these. These emotional reactions influence one's ability to process information and effectively communicate. How a patient and family react to and interact with providers is influenced by their life experiences. These experiences and expectancies emerge during discussions with providers, and how information is exchanged is inextricably linked to the patient's and family's culture; educational level; quality of previous relationships with medical professionals; their understanding of advanced illness, dying, and death; and a host of other factors that makes the patient and family unique. Social and contextual features, such as expected behavior for "good patients," can influence the quality of the communication among providers, patients, and families. Together, these and other variables have an impact on patients' and their loved ones' ability to ask for and process information about diagnosis, prognosis, and treatment options.

Within the context of the "medical (hospital) system culture that values technology over discussion" (Lynn, Arkes, Stevens, et al., 2000), providers' fears of hurting patients or robbing them of hope, along with patients' anxieties, desires to maintain hope, and difficulties in processing medical information, set the stage for problematic communication patterns. The et al. (2000) suggest that patients and physicians "collude" to produce "false optimism about recovery" on the part of the patient through providers' concealment of prognosis, their "medical activism" (i.e., emphasis on treatment), ambiguous communications, and patients' ambivalence about knowing the truth about prognosis to sustain hope about the possibility of cure. This obfuscation may appear to protect patients in the short term but does not shield them from distress or facilitate adjustment to advanced illness over time (Christakis, 1999; Fallowfield et al., 2002). Most research suggests that a vast majority of patients want to be fully informed about their illness and what to expect about their physical condition (Jenkins, Fallowfield, & Saul, 2001; Steinhauser et al., 2001). Clinicians can face the challenge of communicating with patients about their deteriorating condition or providing a less-than-optimistic prognosis by developing caring relationships with their patients, speaking the truth, framing it sensitively, providing emotional support and patient education, and engaging in self-care, which can lead to more effective and humane medical care.

STRATEGIES TO IMPROVE COMMUNICATION QUALITY
Importance of Rapport

The relationship between the health care provider and patient is the vehicle for effective communication. Patients who perceive their provider as caring, emotionally supportive, and empathetic tend to trust and be comfortable with that provider (Friedrichsen, Strang, & Carlsson, 2000), setting the stage for open and genuine dialogue. The health care professional's demonstration of care, concern, and empathy lends itself to the development of rapport with the patient—the foundation for a positive patient-provider relationship and effective communication.

Rapport occurs when the patient feels cared about and is comfortable sharing thoughts and feelings. In developing rapport, the provider conveys warmth and listens to the patient in such a way that he or she feels heard and understood. The health care professional treats the patient as a whole person: an individual with a unique history, a particular set of current circumstances, and a future that is a continuation of the previously lived life. Instead of an assortment of signs and symptoms that present in one's office, the patient is seen as a human being with a full life outside of the medical setting. Rapport can be facilitated through nonverbal and verbal communication strategies.

Nonverbal Communication Strategies

Much information is conveyed through nonverbal behavior. Health care professionals can help establish a productive working relationship and facilitate more effective communication with patients through facilitative nonverbal behaviors that convey compassion, concern, and the desire to listen. The development of self-awareness about one's nonverbal behaviors during patient encounters is the beginning step to making changes that facilitate rapport with patients and families. Much nonverbal behavior is unconscious, and it takes a concerted, long-term individual effort to cultivate self-awareness. Paying conscious attention to one's outward behaviors during patient encounters and asking a trusted colleague who has observed the professional in discussion with patients for feedback are two strategies to develop the needed self-awareness. Larson (1993) describes these nonverbal behaviors through the acronym *SOLVER: s*quarely face the patient, sustain an *o*pen posture, *l*ean forward, *v*erbally follow, maintain good *e*ye contact, and keep one's body *r*elaxed.

Giving a patient one's undivided attention through nonverbal channels, such as squarely facing the patient and being at eye level, sends the message that what the patient has to say is important and that the provider is truly listening. Given the time constraints under which professionals operate, many multitask during patient visits to maximize efficiency. For example, a provider may review the medical chart at the beginning of the visit while the patient is talking or record information into a computer as the patient discusses bothersome symptoms. While multitasking, the provider is listening but the patient may not perceive it that way. When reviewing and recording information during patient visits, providers can develop strategies to minimize the negative impact such activities can have on communication quality. For example, providers may choose to review the patient's record in another setting before the actual appointment or, if that is not possible, ask the patient to wait while the record is reviewed and then begin the discussion with minimal distractions. If information must be recorded during the conversation, the health care professional can explain the necessity of such activity. When the health care professional does focus full attention on the patient and avoid distractions, he or she is communicating a readiness to listen.

Another important nonverbal behavior is maintaining an open posture. A closed posture (e.g., arms folded across the chest or legs tightly crossed) indicates defensiveness and the desire to be cut off from what is being communicated. Slightly leaning forward toward the patient indicates interest and demonstrates that the health care professional is concentrating on the patient's discourse and is engaged and focused on the present moment. Health care professionals may be unaware of their nonverbal behavior when interacting with patients, particularly when conversation topics are difficult or emotionally charged. If providers develop an awareness that their nonverbal behavior does not convey openness or interest, they can ask themselves, "Am I feeling defensive?" "What is impeding my ability to connect with this patient or family?" "What are my fears about addressing this issue with the patient or family?" "How might my attitudes about these topics have an impact on my interactions with the patient and family?" Reflecting on these questions can promote self-awareness about how one's nonverbal behavior is influenced by contextual as well as personal factors.

When patients bring up important issues, providers should allow them to share their concerns in their own words, without cutting them off or steering the discussion in a different direction by asking closed-ended questions or questions not directly related to the patient's presented topic. By giving patients the opportunity to share their unique perceptions of their symptoms, disease, coping methods, and circumstances, providers convey that patient input is key and shared decision making is central to palliative care delivery. They may follow the patient's communication by nodding, saying "yes," "go on," or "tell me more about that." These are ways of minimally influencing topic development while keeping the provider engaged in the listening process.

In the dominant Western culture, eye contact indicates an interpersonal connection between people.

During conversation, it is a way of communicating that one is listening and interested in the topic at hand. Appropriate eye contact, an indicator of emotional connection with another, helps engage individuals in a meaningful discussion. The use of eye contact can vary among cultures, so it is important that providers assess the appropriateness of direct eye contact with patients from diverse backgrounds. For example, certain Native American tribes will avoid making eye contact, especially when discussing serious issues (Ivey, 1988), and averting one's gaze when speaking with those in authority demonstrates respect among some cultural groups (Cournoyer, 2000; Ling, 1997).

Ling (1997) suggests strategies related to nonverbal behavior when interacting with patients and families from diverse ethnic backgrounds. For example, physical closeness and personal space preferences vary among different cultural groups. Health care professionals can show respect for a patient's personal space by initially standing or sitting at arm's length and observing how the family and patient interact and then following their lead for cues about appropriate personal space. In cross-cultural encounters, it is important that providers carefully observe patient behavior and be sensitive to nonverbal nuances. For example, among Asian groups, nodding serves as an acknowledgement, not as an indicator of agreement (Ling, 1997). It is impossible for providers to be fully educated about all cultural practices, but it is important for health care professionals to learn about the beliefs and customs of the groups they will likely encounter in the course of their work.

As discussed, palliative care discussions can be emotionally charged and difficult for providers, patients, and family members alike. When people are uncomfortable, they often engage in nonverbal behaviors that display their emotional state, including shaking their legs, wringing their hands, fidgeting with an object, or other distracting mannerisms. Patients often pick up on these overt manifestations of the provider's emotional state, and this can have an impact on the quality of the communication. Patients may choose to avoid difficult topics in order to be a "good patient" and to protect the provider's feelings. Health care professionals need to become self-aware of how their behavior may foster unintended readings by the patient that can affect the content and quality of palliative care discussions. Appearing distracted, disinterested, or distressed can influence how and what patients reveal.

Building Rapport and Using Active Listening

The advanced illness experience is often frightening and isolating for patients. Their fears and anxieties are numerous: Will my disease get worse? Am I going to suffer? What is going to happen to me? Will I die soon? What will the end be like? What will become of my loved ones? How will they deal with my illness? Patients may choose to bear the burden of their illness in silence to shield their loved ones from psychologic pain, or they may attempt to discuss their concerns with those who are close but find that few can discuss such issues because of their own fears about death and dying (Tobin & Lindsay, 1999). Open-ended questions and empathic listening can reduce patients' sense of isolation and provide an opportunity to explore concerns and hopes. Active listening can be used as a tool to minimize patients' feelings of isolation; to improve diagnostic activities, treatment, and advance care planning; and to promote patient-centered care.

Very few medical care providers are trained psychotherapists. But they do enter into a helping relationship with patients and families that, according to Rogers (1961), encompass those "...in which at least one of the parties has the intent of promoting the growth...improved functioning, improved coping with life of the other." He goes on to say that this "definition covers a wide range of relationships...[and] would include the relationship between the physician and his patient" (Rogers, 1961, p. 40). Central to the helping relationship is the expression of empathy, or the sensitive understanding of the patient's feelings, unique experience with advanced illness, and the meanings assigned to those experiences and circumstances. When a health care provider can effectively communicate that understanding to a patient, empathic understanding is achieved. Empathic listening in and of itself can be therapeutic to palliative care patients and their families (Lo, Quill, & Tulsky, 1999).

Empathic understanding begins with using the nonverbal communication strategies discussed earlier. To *really hear* what a patient or family member is trying to communicate, health care professionals must provide their undivided physical as well as mental attention. Active listening strategies, such as the use of open-ended questions, paraphrases, reflections of feelings, and summarizations, facilitate and demonstrate empathy (Larson, 1993). Active listening promotes issue exploration and patient self-expression. While using such techniques, it is important for providers to remember that silence allows patients to discuss topics at their own pace. Rushing to immediately respond to a patient's communication or countering quickly with a closed-ended question (i.e., a question that has only a limited number of possible responses such as *yes* or *no*) can cut off the exploration process. During patient encounters, there are times when closed-ended questions are appropriate and useful, but an open-ended question followed by a period of silence can be an effective tool in promoting empathy and a deeper understanding of the patient's perspective. Although constraints on medical professionals' time can be a barrier to the full exploration of patient concerns, use of active listening techniques can help providers better understand patient communications and convey to them a sense of being heard and cared about.

Gaining perspective on the patient's unique understanding of his or her diagnosis, treatment options, and prognosis is vital. Patients' perspectives on their advanced illness may be quite different from their providers' or family members' understanding (Norlander & McSteen, 2000). When discussing diagnosis and treatment options, health care professionals' communications may be misheard, not heard, or misconstrued by a patient. What the provider thought was clearly conveyed might not be what the patient actually understood. This misunderstanding could be because of the patient's emotional state during the interaction, the provider's use of medical jargon, or the quality of the patient-provider relationship, among others. In beginning palliative care discussions, assessing

the patient's understanding of the advanced illness and possible treatment options can inform the health care provider about patient goals of care and issues in which the patient needs further education. An effective open-ended question to begin such a discussion is: "What is your understanding of where things stand now with your illness?" (Lo et al., 1999). This question, followed by silence from the provider, can be a powerful tool to gain insight into how the patient views his or her situation.

As the patient discusses his or her perspective, the health care professional can use paraphrases to ensure that the content of the patient's communication is well understood. *Paraphrasing*, communicating back the content of what the patient has said, enhances provider understanding; demonstrates concern, compassion, and empathy; and promotes patient-centered care. Using some of the patient's words in the paraphrasing is helpful, but it is important not to "parrot" what the patient is saying (Larson, 1993). The following is an example of paraphrasing:

Provider: So what do you understand about your illness at this time? (*Pauses.*)

Patient: Well, I know that I have cancer in my lungs and that you people are worried about it spreading to other parts of my body. I think I am supposed to be getting some tests to see if that has happened, but I don't know too much about the tests. I was told that there are some spots or tumors or something on my left lung. I've never smoked so I can't understand why this is happening to me.

Provider: It sounds like you have many unanswered questions. Tests are necessary to determine if the cancer has spread, but you don't have much information about the tests or the cancer itself. Is it fair to say that a lot of this isn't making sense to you at this time?

The provider did not merely repeat back to the patient what was expressed, but used paraphrasing, including some of the patient's own terminology, to demonstrate understanding of and connection with the patient. If the health care professional's paraphrase does not accurately capture the content, the patient has an opportunity to correct any misunderstanding and deepen the provider's understanding of the issue.

Health care professionals in the palliative care setting routinely deal with patients' strong emotions. Patients' displays of anger, fear, hopelessness, or other negative emotions can be difficult to manage. When a patient's strong emotions are unacknowledged in the context of an interaction with a provider, the professional may be perceived as uncaring or distanced, which can hinder further effective communication. Similar to paraphrasing, *reflecting feelings* is a technique that demonstrates empathy and fosters rapport:

> *Patient*: (*Agitated.*) So, now you're telling me the treatment didn't work. You sit there and tell me that I went through all of that for nothing! Don't you know what you are doing? Do you realize how hard this is on my family? You mean I've got to go tell them that the cancer has come back? There has got to be something that you can do!
>
> *Provider*: I can see why you would be angry, given all that you have been through…(*Patient interrupts.*)
>
> *Patient*: Angry?! You're damn right. I'm mad at all you doctors, at God for letting this happen, at myself for not having that pain looked into earlier. Now what's going to happen? This is too much.
>
> *Provider*: You're right, it is overwhelming right now. What can we do right now to help address some of your immediate concerns?

In this example, the provider could have become defensive or began to deliver a detailed medical explanation that the patient might not have been able to process. By listening to the patient's feelings, reflecting and validating them, rapport and trust are facilitated and often the intensity of the situation de-escalated. Using a follow-up open-ended question to probe the patient's concerns and fears can yield valuable information for the patient's care plan and afford the patient the opportunity to explore sensitive issues.

Finally, *summarization* involves recounting the broader themes that occurred over the course of an appointment. A summarization can be helpful at the end of a meeting to recount the important content of the discussion. Summarizations (Larson [1993] refers to them as "big paraphrases") can be used throughout an interaction to ensure that the major topics are being understood and remembered. In the following example, a patient has an appointment with a provider in which the option of hospice care has been discussed:

> *Patient*: OK. This is a lot to think about.
>
> *Provider*: Yes, this is a big decision. As we've been talking, I see that your major concern about receiving hospice care is worry over your family's reaction. You're afraid that they won't understand your decision to stop receiving the chemotherapy. But, as we discussed, your cancer is not responding to the treatment and you say that your quality of life is suffering. As you asked, I will get you a pamphlet on the local hospice program and we will discuss this again over the phone in the next couple of days. If you like, I can meet with you and your family to discuss this.
>
> *Patient*: OK. I'll call you soon.

The provider has reiterated the highlights of the appointment and developed a plan that demonstrates support for the patient and family. These active listening techniques can help health care professionals connect with and emotionally support their patients during difficult times.

Balancing Honesty and Hope

The literature suggests that the balance between provider honesty and the support of patient hope is tenuous (Fallowfield et al., 2002; Morrison, 1998; The et al., 2000). Providers are worried about hurting patients with bad or sad news, but research suggests that a large majority of patients want full disclosure, good or bad, about their disease, prognosis, and treatment options (Fallowfield et al., 2002; Jenkins et al., 2001). Patients and families value provider candor that is tempered with sensitivity, when a realistic picture of diagnosis and prognosis is presented in such a way that hope is not destroyed (Wenrich et al., 2001). In an insightful analysis of the importance of truth in palliative care, Fallowfield et al. (2002, p. 301) indicate, "There is little or no convincing evidence supporting the contention that terminally ill patients who have not been told the truth of their situation die happily in blissful ignorance." Truthful communications, although difficult and anxiety provoking for both patients and providers, can be delivered sensitively and with empathy. When patients are not told the complete truth, they are robbed of the opportunity to make realistic plans about the rest of their lives. They may lose chances to connect with loved ones, take care of unfinished business, or do adequate end-of-life planning. Truth may be difficult in the short term but has the potential to greatly benefit patients and families in the long run (Christakis, 1999).

How can health care professionals better balance hope and truth? In situations where difficult truths must be conveyed, providers can create an appropriate setting in which limited time and distractions (e.g., telephone, staff interruptions) are not a concern. It may also be helpful to assess patients' preferences for receiving information. Providers can ask patients the degree of detail they want when initial diagnostic or prognostic information is relayed. Would a follow-up appointment in the near future be preferable so that the patient can better absorb the information? Some patients may need time to process the basic information about their illness before they are ready to fully explore the details. If the patient desires, having his or her social supports available can be comforting when bad or disappointing news is conveyed. Use of previously discussed nonverbal strategies and active listening techniques can foster rapport and trust, provide a sense of security (Friedrichsen et al., 2000), and demonstrate the professional's empathy and compassion. Reassurance that the patient will not face the situation alone—that the patient's social supports and the medical team will continue to be there as resources—can reduce feelings of isolation. In situations where troubling medical information is discussed, patients' sense of control is diminished and they can feel overwhelmed. Development of a short-term plan that includes setting a time in the near future for follow-up either in person or by telephone can increase patients' sense of control and support their hopes. Referrals to other health care team members may be helpful, including psychiatry, social work, and pastoral care staff.

The delicate balance between hope and truth becomes more complicated when the issue of cultural diversity is considered. Among some cultural groups (e.g., Asian), disclosing the full details of a patient's diagnosis and prognosis directly to the patient is seen as depriving him or her of all hope (Kogan, Blanchette, & Masaki, 2000). Among some Japanese- and Chinese-American families, family members take on the responsibility of protecting an ill member from bad or sad medical news, although some research suggests that many patients belonging to these ethnic groups would want to know the truth about their terminal illness (Yeo & Hikoyeda, 2000). It is inappropriate for health care professionals to make generalizations to individual patients based on broad ethnic group descriptions. To increase cultural competency, providers can ask ethnically diverse patients and families if there are "any cultural traditions that health care workers should keep in mind during the patient's stay" (Yeo & Hikoyeda, 2000, p. 111).

Regardless of one's cultural background, distress, fear, and a sense of helplessness can be common reactions to advanced illness. Providers may be reticent to explore such issues with patients and families because many cannot be solved (Lo et al., 1999), yet the understanding of such fears and concerns are necessary to develop patient-centered care plans. Providers' willingness to enter into such discussions along with their use of open-ended questions and active listening techniques can provide an incredible opportunity for patients and families to explore sensitive and important issues related to the provision of quality palliative care. Lo et al. (1999) provide an example of an exchange between a family member and a provider that demonstrates the effectiveness of exploring fears. Mrs. A., the wife of a cancer patient, is concerned about her husband's bleeding and his discharge plan:

Physician: I would like to know if you have any additional concerns.

Mrs. A.: I am scared that he will bleed uncontrollably at home, and I won't know what to do. I would call 911 if this happens. At least they can help me.

Physician: Yes, bleeding can be frightening, particularly if you're at home with your daughter. Are there other things that are frightening or too much to handle?

Mrs. A.: I know Jim wants to be home, and I want that too. But sometimes it feels that I'm in too far over my head.

As Lo et al. (1999) point out, this exchange gives the physician the opportunity to identify and validate Mrs. A.'s fears. Furthermore, the provider has an opportunity to educate the family member about services, such as hospice or hospital-based palliative care, which addresses her fears about care. Through the use of an open-ended question as an invitation to explore Mrs. A.'s fears, the physician can respond to the issue that is the most troublesome. Avoiding the topic of fears will not make them go away; instead, the patient's and family's isolation may be exacerbated. By bringing fears into the light, the provider has an opportunity to intervene (e.g., patient education, connection with support services).

In discussing fears, health care professionals do not want to rob patients of hope and therefore may be quick to reassure, missing the chance to explore and gain understanding of the patient's concerns. Many patients do rely on hope as a way to cope with advanced illness; however, from the provider's perspective, some patients may have unrealistic hopes. In their discussion of the case of Mr. and Mrs. A., Lo et al. (1999) demonstrate how providers can balance truth and hope. Mr. A., whom the provider believes has a 90% chance of dying within the next 6 months, shares with the physician his hope of being alive for his daughter's next birthday, almost a year away (Lo et al., 1999, p. 747):

The physician might say directly, "I wish I could tell you that you will be here for your daughter's next birthday. It is possible, but unfortunately the odds aren't with you. (*Pause.*) If it doesn't work out that you can be there, are there things that you should consider doing now?" . . .As an alternative, the physician might say, "I know that you're trying very hard to keep your hopes up. Are you sometimes afraid that you won't be there for your family?". . .Statements such as, "I wish that medicine had better answers" may show alliance with the patient's hopes and be more soothing than we expect.

Responses such as these validate patients' desires to maintain hope and do not provide a sense of unrealistic or false optimism.

Palliative care professionals are faced with the challenge of delivering disturbing news to patients and family members over the course of a patient's disease trajectory. Sensitively delivering sad and disappointing news involves more than following a script or recipe for how to deliver such information. The context of the provider-patient relationship, as well as that created within the encounter itself, is central in how patients receive and cope with bad news. Patient-provider relationships characterized by mutual understanding, respect, and empathy promote trust, allowing patients to be comfortable enough to explore concerns, discuss difficult options, and be open to provider expertise and guidance (Friedrichsen et al., 2000).

Use of Medical Terminology

Language is a powerful tool in the decision-making process. Because many health care professionals, patients, and family members do not share the same vocabulary about disease and treatment, ambiguities in language can result in miscommunication (Wenrich et al., 2001). Given the medical terminology that many health care providers employ, what providers mean and what patients understand may be incongruent. Use of technical jargon makes it difficult for patients and families to grasp the medical realities associated with advanced illness and can be used as a tool to obfuscate difficult truths (Reisfield & Wilson, 2003). Providers need to develop self-awareness about their use of medical jargon and be cognizant of how such language affects their interactions with patients. Use of medical vernacular is a technique that may be employed to put the health care professional in a position of distance and power over the patient and often has the outcome of confusing patients and families during a time when a clear understanding of the facts is paramount (Limerick, 2002).

Patients and clinicians may use the same word but give it different meanings. For example, a health care professional may tell a patient that her disease is progressing, wherein the clinical meaning indicates physical deterioration and the lay meaning connotes disease improvement. In referring to biopsy results, a provider may describe the results

Table **2-1** ANTONYMOUS MEANINGS

Term	Clinical Meaning	Lay Meaning
Disease progression	Deterioration	Improvement
Disease regression	Improvement	Deterioration
Advanced	Unfavorable prognosis	Favorable prognosis
Positive (e.g., biopsy)	Presence of disease	Absence of disease
Negative (e.g., biopsy)	Absence of disease	Presence of disease

From Reisfield, G.M., & Wilson, G.R. (2003). Ambiguity in end-of-life communications. *Journal of Terminal Oncology, 2*(2), 62.

as positive, referring to presence of disease, and the patient may understand that the outcome is "good," that is, an absence of disease. See Table 2-1 for several clinical terms that can have the opposite meaning from a lay person's perspective (Reisfield & Wilson, 2003).

In addition to terms with antonymous meanings, the use of euphemisms decreases communication quality. Euphemisms can soften the delivery of bad news, shield patients from psychologic pain, or protect providers from the discomfort of imparting sad information. Reisfield and Wilson (2003, p. 63) indicate, "The more difficult the topic, the more ubiquitous the euphemisms," and those authors provide a series of examples of cancer euphemisms and terms that are routinely used and often misinterpreted. These are shown in Tables 2-2 and 2-3.

Jargon complicates advance care planning discussions as well, when clear communication is vital. Limerick (2002) suggests using "substitutive language" when discussing such medical treatments

Table **2-2** CANCER EUPHEMISMS AND JARGON

Euphemisms	Medical Jargon
• Tumor	• Malignancy
• Growth	• Carcinoma
• Spot	• Metastases
• Lump	
• Mass	

From Reisfield, G.M., & Wilson, G. R. (2003). Ambiguity in end-of-life communications. *Journal of Terminal Oncology, 2*(2), 63.

as artificial nutrition and hydration, cardiopulmonary resuscitation, and other end-of-life treatments. Summaries of Limerick's (2002) suggestions for such language are in Table 2-4. Using medical jargon is second nature to health care professionals given their education and the medical system in which they practice. Becoming aware of how one uses jargon is an important step in making changes in communication patterns with patients and families.

Because each patient and family are unique, providers can use active listening skills and open-ended questions to determine how to best deliver medical information to optimize patient understanding. For example, some patients and families take more time to process information and may have few questions until they can mull over what the provider communicated. For such patients and families, an important strategy could be to schedule a follow-up appointment in the near future, thereby giving them time and "permission" to process and think about the previously shared information. Learning about and accommodating the communication style of patients and families take time and emerges in the context of the ongoing relationship among the patient, family, and health care provider. Table 2-5 summarizes various communication strategies that promote rapport and effective working relationships among patients, families, and health care professionals.

ADVANCE CARE PLANNING

Advance care planning is an important process that emerges in the context of the patient-provider relationship. It involves much more than the completion of formal advance directive documents

Table 2-3 TERMS THAT CAN BE MISINTERPRETED

As "Cure"	As "Curable"
• Response (complete or partial)	• Responsive
• Remission (complete or partial)	• Sensitive
• Control	• Treatable
• Stable disease	• Controllable
• Treated	• Operable
• "Got it all" (surgical)	• Curable (5 years disease-free)
• Clear/clean (x-ray or scan)	
• Cure (!) (5 years disease-free)	

From Reisfield, G.M., & Wilson, G.R. (2003). Ambiguity in end-of-life communications. *Journal of Terminal Oncology, 2*(2), 63.

Table 2-4 SUGGESTED SUBSTITUTIVE LANGUAGE

Technological Terminology	Becomes
What do you want to do?	What is the goal for this patient?
Which treatment do you want us to do/not do?	What is it that you want to have happen for this patient?
Hydration	Artificial water
Nutrition	Artificial food
Ventilation/intubation	Artificial breathing machine/tube
CPR (cardiopulmonary resuscitation)	Artificially providing a heartbeat
Dialysis	Artificial filtration or cleansing of the blood to produce urine
Electrocardioversion	Artificial stimulation or "jump start" of the heart
DNR (do not resuscitate)	AND (allow a natural death)

NOTE: Terms for the living should not be applied to the dying.

From Limerick, M. (2002). Communicating with surrogate decision-makers in end-of-life situations: Substitutive descriptive language for the healthcare provider. *Am J Hospice Palliat Care, 19*(6), 376-380.

Table 2-5 RAPPORT-ENHANCING VERBAL AND NONVERBAL COMMUNICATION STRATEGIES

Verbal Strategies	Nonverbal Strategies
• Use open-ended questions to explore patient concerns.	• Give patient undivided attention.
• Paraphrase the content of the patient's communication using some of the patient's own words.	• Avoid multitasking.
	• Directly face the patient at eye level.
• Validate patients' and family members' feelings.	• Avoid distracting mannerisms.
	• Maintain an open posture.
• Summarize broad themes during the interaction.	• Lean forward.
	• Maintain appropriate eye contact.
• Deliver diagnostic and prognostic information sensitively and with empathy.	• Be sensitive to and aware of cultural differences in nonverbal behavior.
• Assess preferences for receiving medical information.	• Develop self-awareness about one's own nonverbal behaviors and what they communicate to others.
• Avoid the use of medical jargon.	

(e.g., living will, durable power of attorney for health care), although such documents are an integral part of this process. In addition to a thorough discussion of treatment preferences, advance care planning conversations should also address patient values, beliefs, and goals (Norlander & McSteen, 2000). Decisions about treatment preferences are made in the context of a patient's life history, lived experiences, social support systems, cultural norms, and resulting values. Patient values are the foundation for treatment preferences and medical decision making. Instead of focusing only on discrete treatment preferences, learning what matters most to patients can help palliative care providers develop appropriate and meaningful treatment plans in a variety of unforeseen circumstances (Karel, 2000).

Advance care planning done before a crisis and in collaboration with important people in the patient's life can reduce family conflict and burden when decisions must be made on behalf of a loved one (Pearlman, Cole, Patrick, et al., 1995). Advance care planning discussions promote shared decision making among patients and providers, as providers can educate patient and families about viable treatment options and patients can share their values and goals for treatment. Such conversations can be ongoing among the patient, provider, and family over the course of the clinical relationship. Continued discussions about advance care planning issues are particularly important as a patient's medical condition changes. Patient preferences are not static; they can change over time, and providers have an obligation to ensure that patients understand their options as the disease trajectory progresses. Topics to discuss as part of advance care planning include patient goals, values, personal experiences with death, family/social system support of patient goals and values, available resources, and advance directives (Norlander & McSteen, 2000; Quill, 2000; Ratner, Norlander, & McSteen, 2001).

In assessing a patient's goals, the health care provider can determine what the patient wants to accomplish and tailor care to meet those objectives. For example, a patient may want to attend an important family event and therefore choose more aggressive care for a short period to be able to join with loved ones on an important day. Providers can

assess goals by asking open-ended questions such as:
- At this point in your life, what would you like to accomplish?
- As you think about the future, what is most important to you (what matters the most to you)? (Lo et al., 1999)
- What are your hopes for the future?
- What are your fears about the future?
- If you were to die sooner rather than later, what would be left undone? (Quill, 2000)

The identification of patient goals can allow providers to develop patient-centered care plans that consider the patient holistically and not merely a collection of physiologic symptoms to be treated and managed. Values, directly related to patient goals, should also be discussed as part of advance care planning.

In exploring the patient's values, the provider helps the patient elucidate what is truly important and how these personal principles relate to decisions about medical care. Through an understanding of the patient's value structure, medical decisions can be made that are congruent with the patient's life narrative. Patients' values are rooted in their life experiences. Patients, and providers for that matter, cannot adequately anticipate all of the circumstances under which future medical decisions may need to be made on behalf of a patient. Yet through values assessment, providers and families can develop an understanding of patient preferences that can guide decision making in unforeseen circumstances. Providers can utilize completed psychosocial assessments and clinical notes developed by other health care professionals to assist in the assessment of patient values. To explore values with the patient directly, providers may ask questions such as:
- What makes life worth living? (Quill, 2000)
- What would have to happen for your life to be not worth living?
- How do you feel about quality of life versus quantity of life?
- How much input do you want your family/loved ones to have in decisions that are made about your health care?
- What are your thoughts about pain control? Would you want your pain

controlled even if it meant that you might not be as alert?

Ideally such discussion should include the patient's decision-making surrogate so that the responsible decision maker has the same understanding of the patient's values as the provider, thereby decreasing the probability of conflict.

Other fruitful areas for advance care planning discussions include patients' previous experiences with dying and death and their religious beliefs and perspectives on spirituality. If patients have loved ones who experienced a painful, prolonged, and/or frightening death, they can project those fears into their current circumstances. When providers explore such topics with patients, they have the opportunity to further discuss concerns and provide patient education if needed. For many patients, spiritual matters become increasingly important during advanced illness, and addressing such concerns is an integral part of palliative care (Lo et al., 1999). Patients may prefer to discuss spiritual issues with a member of the clergy, but the exploration of these matters by health care professionals can provide substantial insight into a patient's value system and what might be important to this patient over the course of the clinical relationship. For those patients requiring more attention in this realm, health care providers can refer the patient to an appropriate member of the clergy. To begin a conversation about previous experiences with death and dying, health care professionals can ask:

- Has anyone close to you died of an illness? What happened? What was it like for you?
- What other significant losses have you experienced?
- What would you consider a "good death"?

Lo et al. (1999, p. 746) suggest these questions to begin a dialogue about spiritual and existential issues:

- What thoughts have you had about why you got this illness at this time?
- What is your understanding about what happens after you die?
- What legacy do you want to leave your family?
- Is faith (religion, spirituality) important to you in this illness?
- Has faith (religion, spirituality) been important to you at other times in your life?

- Do you have someone to talk to about religious matters? Would you like to explore religious matters with someone?

It is vital that family/support systems be part of advance care planning discussions to decrease the chance for later conflict and regret and to ensure support of and compliance with the patient's stated goals and values. Patients live within the context of social support systems, and these important people are integral to successful patient care and treatment. Providers can encourage patients to discuss advance care planning issues with loved ones at home or during clinical appointments involving the health care provider. Family/social support can be assessed by asking:

- How is your family handling your illness? What are their reactions? (Quill, 2000)
- What kind of conversations have you had with them about care you might need in the future?
- What are your loved ones' fears about your illness? What are their hopes?
- What other types of support might you need?
- What community resources have you utilized?

Providers can assess for additional support that the patient might need, such as pastoral care, home health services, legal services, counseling, hospice, or occupational therapy services.

The written documentation of patient treatment preferences that result from advance care planning discussions take the form of advance directives (legal documents that specify who should make decisions on behalf of a decisionally incapacitated patient [durable power of attorney for health care or health care proxy]) and should list treatment preferences (living will or health care directive). Without an accompanying advance care planning discussion, advance directives may not be very useful in guiding patient care. Without provider input, patients may draft advance directives that are ambiguous, unclear, or so general they cannot be appropriately integrated into the care plan (Teno, Licks, Lynn, et al., 1997). The topic of advance directive completion can be broached by asking patients (Quill, 2000):

- Who would you want to make decisions for you if something happened and you were unable to make decisions about your care? Have you spoken with this person about this? Have you informed other important people in your life that this is your wish?

- How well do you think this person can deal with any disagreements others may have about your wishes? If you anticipate any disagreements, what do you think is the best way to address this?
- What kinds of treatment would you want (and not want) if you become unable to speak for yourself in the future?

If the patient has appointed or wants to appoint a surrogate decision maker in an advance directive, the patient can be encouraged to thoroughly discuss his or her preferences, goals, and values with this person. Too often patients appoint surrogate decision makers and do not directly address with them the very issues that need to be understood for the surrogate to make a substituted judgment that is representative of the patient's values and wishes. Numerous tools exist to structure such conversations among patients and surrogates including *Making Medical Decisions* (AARP, 1996); *Five Wishes* (Commission on Aging with Dignity, 1998); *Talking About Your Choices* (Choice in Dying, 1996); and *Your Life, Your Choices* (Pearlman, Starks, Cain, et al., 2001).

Advance care planning discussions should guide the completion of advance directives, and in terms of specific interventions and goals that should be included in discussions and documents, Quill (2000) suggests those shown in Box 2-1. Patients should be encouraged to place completed advance directives in an accessible place and to give copies of the documents to their surrogate and other physicians involved in their care. Once an advance directive is in place, advance care planning does not stop. Patients need to understand that they can change their advance directive at any time, and health care professionals can ensure that patients' goals, values, and treatment preferences are well represented in advance directive documents by having ongoing discussions with them, particularly if there are changes in the patient's condition or circumstances.

PERSONAL AWARENESS AND SELF-CARE

Working with patients who are living and dying with advanced illness can evoke strong emotions

Box 2-1   WHAT TO INCLUDE IN MOST END-OF-LIFE DISCUSSIONS

GENERAL: GOALS OF TREATMENT
- Relative emphasis on life prolongation
- Relative emphasis on quality of life

SPECIFIC: RANGE OF INTERVENTION
- Advance directives:
  —Living well
  —Health care proxy
- Do not (attempt) resuscitation (DNR) orders
- Other life-sustaining therapies, such as:
  —Mechanical ventilation
  —Feeding tube
  —Antibiotics
  —Hemodialysis
- Palliative care:
  —Management of pain and other symptoms
  —Relief of psychological, social, spiritual, and existential suffering
  —Creating opportunity to address unfinished business

From Quill, T.E. (2000). Initiating end-of-life discussions with seriously ill patients: Addressing the "elephant in the room." *J Amer Med Assoc, 284*(19), 2502-2507.

among and be stressful for professional caregivers. Strong emotions, unchecked and unexamined, can have a negative impact on the quality of patient care and the well-being of the health care professional who experiences them (Meier, Back, & Morrison, 2001; Novack, Suchman, Clark, et al., 1997). Strong reactions in response to patient situations can lead to provider underinvolvement, overinvolvement (Golden & Sonneborn, 1998), or burnout, "a state of emotional exhaustion manifested in low energy, chronic fatigue, and feelings of being emotionally drained, frustrated, and used up" (Larson, 1993, p. 32). Various patients and clinical situations can differentially provoke strong reactions among health care providers, and professionals need to be cognizant of the factors that can "push one's buttons." Increased personal awareness about one's emotional reactions and their triggers can result in a conscious choice to behave or react differently. Personal awareness in the palliative care context can be defined as "insight into how one's life experiences and emotional makeup affects one's interactions with patients, families, and other professionals" (Novack et al., 1997, p. 502). This insight can help providers be aware of the phenomenon of countertransference.

Countertransference, "the conscious or unconscious phenomenon that occurs when the clinician reacts to a [patient] based on the clinician's own past experiences, preferences, preconceptions, fantasies, and fears" (Golden & Sonneborn, 1998, p. 83), can be a source for strong emotions experienced by the provider. Countertransference does not have to have a negative impact on patient care; in fact, it can increase one's compassion and empathy toward the patient (Golden & Sonneborn, 1998). But when the emotions that result from countertransference go unacknowledged and unexplored, patient care could be compromised. Unconsciously acting on one's emotions can be problematic. For example, if a patient reminds a health care professional of a recently deceased uncle and the professional caregiver's behavior is unconsciously and unduly influenced by that perception, patient-centered care could be compromised.

Health care providers may become overengaged or underengaged with patients and families as a result of countertransference phenomena. Providers can overidentify with patients for numerous reasons, including a perception that the patient is similar to one's self or reminds the provider of a family member or someone close (Meier et al., 2001). Countertransference can arise from the provider's own experiences in his or her family of origin. Patterns of behavior and emotion related to conflict, illness, death, caring, intimacy, and communication are learned within one's family, and those lessons can be carried over into interactions health care professionals have with their patients (Novack et al., 1997). Providers' own fears about and experiences with illness, dying, disability, and death can also "leak" into patient interactions if those emotions are not recognized and examined. As Stolick (2003) indicates, fear of death can motivate providers to avoid discussions with patients about dying. To authentically engage with dying patients, self-examination is paramount: "[O]ne must have

considered [death] for oneself" (Stolick, 2003, p. 271).

All professionals overidentify with certain patients, bring their family of origin experiences into patient encounters, and have fears and existential issues around death and dying. These feelings, behaviors, and experiences are what make health care professionals uniquely human, capable of great compassion and empathy. The danger to patients comes when such feelings and experiences are not owned and examined in the context of providing palliative care services. Providers can learn to increase their personal awareness in these areas by reflecting on such questions as:

- What roles did I have in my family? How might I be replicating these roles in my work environment? (Novack et al., 1997)
- If I have a strong, inexplicable emotional reaction to a patient, does he or she remind me of someone close to me? Does the patient's situation resemble my own circumstances? Does the patient remind me of someone I love or a person with whom my relationship is conflicted? How does this influence my caring for this patient?
- What salient personal or professional experiences have I had with illness, death, and dying? How might these experiences color my perceptions of and influence my interactions with patients and families?

Reflecting on questions such as these can lead to a greater awareness of one's own emotional triggers. This awareness can help professionals make conscious behavioral choices that are in the best interest of the patient.

Strong emotional reactions can be provoked not only by issues related to countertransference but also by challenging clinical situations. Providers may characterize some patients and families as "difficult." For example, these patients may come from families with complex dynamics, have psychiatric disorders, exhibit dependent personality traits, or exude anger (Meier et al., 2001; Novack et al., 1997). It is a challenge to develop a relationship with such patients, which complicates communication and medical treatment issues. When faced with a "difficult" patient or family, providers can reflect on what specific behaviors exhibited by the patient are the most troubling. Does the professional possess any personal biases against these behaviors? For example, how does the provider respond to others' anger? Others' dependency? In these situations, it is often helpful for providers to consult with a trusted colleague to gain insight into the situation and identify problem-solving strategies to appropriately treat the patient.

During the illness trajectory, palliative care professionals can develop close relationships with their patients over the course of treatment and are faced with their deaths on a routine basis. Health care professionals must cope with the loss that comes when patients with whom providers have developed attachments die. How professionals deal with their reactions to such losses can have an impact on their level of engagement with living patients (Novack et al., 1997; Wakefield, 2000). Health care professionals are often expected to go on "as usual" after the death of the patient, even if the patient-provider relationship was particularly close (Wakefield, 2000). But grief is a normal response among professional caregivers and should be acknowledged and processed in order to move forward (Radziewicz, 2001). Wakefield (2000) indicates that grief responses among palliative care nurses are repressed because of personal detachment from one's feelings ("intrapsychic disenfranchisement") and societal norms regarding expectations around the professional's grief reactions ("business as usual"). Thus if grief is not openly expressed or publicly acknowledged, "compassion fatigue" or burnout can result.

To facilitate the grieving response, Wakefield (2000) suggests saying goodbye to patients, asking questions about the patient's dying trajectory, expressing feelings through stories, and reflecting on grief. Saying goodbye to a patient who has died could involve viewing the body and saying goodbye before it is removed from the ward or participating in "closure conferences" (Rando, 1984; Wakefield, 2000) with other professional caregivers where feelings about the patient's loss are discussed. Discussing thoughts and questions about the dying trajectory allows professionals to gain greater insight into the dying process and helps professionals

process the clinical facts, avoiding self-blame and guilt. Telling stories about the patient, reminiscing about special experiences, and sharing what the patient meant to the provider on a personal level can also promote closure. Finally, reflecting on grief, allowing one's self to sit with and think about the pain of loss, can help professional caregivers internalize the loss and move through the grieving process. Celebrating and contemplating the memory of patients can be done collectively through periodic memorial services (e.g., every 6 months) held at the health care facility. For those who work with people who are dying, Novack et al. (1997) suggest these reflection questions to increase personal awareness:

- How have my personal experiences with loss and grief affected, enhanced, or limited my abilities to work with dying patients?
- What are my own attitudes and fears of death and vulnerability, and how do they affect my patient care?
- If I were dying, what would I want and need from my physician?

To closely and authentically work with those who are near the end of life, providers must acknowledge, "Death is an essential part of each of our life stories" (Stolick, 2003). Helping others process the feelings and thoughts about their impending death is possible only when one has considered his or her own eventual demise.

Not only can existential and intrapsychic factors have an impact on the quality of providers' interactions with patients and families, systemic forces can influence communication quality. These include time pressures and conflicting or competing interests (e.g., financial concerns, research obligations). Providers practice in settings in which time with patients is limited. Development of a relationship with a patient that is based on trust and mutual respect takes time, and to devote the needed time, competing interests and demands must be juggled. Disagreements about patient management among the health care team can also be a source of stress (Meier et al., 2001). Clarity and quality of communication among the health care team members can affect the primary provider-patient relationship as well. Given the myriad issues with which palliative care professionals must deal, personal awareness and self-care are paramount to avoid burnout and optimize personal well-being as well as patient care.

Meier et al. (2001) discuss burnout from the perspective of the medical model, providing a list of "warning signs and symptoms" that have an impact on the quality of communication and patient care. These signs include various behavioral indicators, such as avoidance of the patient and family, and emotional symptoms including hopelessness, frustration, and anger. Paying attention to the presence of these signs and symptoms can a prompt health care professionals to reflect and identify the etiology of the sign or symptom and promote a healthy response to the patient care situation. For example, health care professionals may avoid "difficult" patients or "dysfunctional" families because of the emotional reactions they experience when interacting with them. As a result, opportunities are lost to fully explore care plans and resolve important issues related to patient care. If providers can acknowledge the difficult emotions they experience and explore possible causes of their reactions, they may be able to develop insight into how their emotional reactions affect patient care and appropriately change their behavior. Under the best of circumstances, providers are not able to "fix" underlying family dynamics or others' troubling personality patterns, but they can employ effective communication skills to provide patient-centered care. Meier et al.'s (2001) listing of warning signs and symptoms that can have a negative impact on patient care is shown in Box 2-2.

When providers become aware of the signs and symptoms of stress and burnout, what can be done to minimize the impact of the experienced emotions on patient care? Meier et al. (2001) suggest these steps: (1) name the feeling; (2) accept the normalcy of the feeling; (3) reflect on the emotion(s) and its possible consequences; and (4) consult a trusted colleague for support and guidance. Identifying and naming the emotional state is the first step in developing personal awareness and making positive behavioral changes. Being able to objectify the feeling can help one gain some conscious control over the emotion, allowing providers to make

Box 2-2   Provider Feelings Influencing Patient Care: Warning Signs and Symptoms

SIGNS (BEHAVIORS)

- Avoiding the patient
- Avoiding the family
- Failing to communicate effectively with other professionals about the patient
- Dismissive or belittling remarks about patient to colleagues
- Failure to attend to details of patient care
- Physical signs of stress or tension when seeing the patient or family
- Contact with the patient more often than medically necessary

SYMPTOMS (EMOTIONS)

- Anger at patient or family
- Feeling imposed upon or harassed by patient or family
- Feeling of contempt for patient or family
- Intrusive thoughts about patient or family
- Sense of failure or self-blame, guilt
- Feeling a personal obligation to save the patient
- Belief that complaints of distress are manipulative efforts to seek attention
- Frequently feeling victimized by the demands of the practice of medicine

From Meier, D.E., Back, A.L., & Morrison, R.S. (2001). The inner life of physicians and care of the seriously ill. *J Amer Med Assoc, 286*(23), 3010.

rational behavioral choices. Acknowledging that strong emotional reactions are normal in the context of providing palliative care to patients is an important step in reducing guilt about one's feelings. Nonjudgmental acceptance of the feeling can give health care professionals permission to explore the consequences of the emotion and how the reaction affects or can affect patient care. This step helps providers perceive the link between their emotional states and behaviors. Finally, it can be valuable to regularly consult trusted colleagues to help health care providers process their emotional reactions, professional behaviors, and patient care options and anticipated outcomes. Group discussions among health care professionals may also be useful to facilitate personal awareness, emotional regulation, and self-monitoring (Novack et al., 1997).

Personal awareness of one's emotions and their precipitants helps facilitate life balance and self-care among palliative care providers. Professional caregivers are often deeply committed to their work, and they face the challenge of balancing their personal and professional lives (Novack et al., 1997). Choices made in one sphere of life, for example, the amount of time dedicated to work, can affect other aspects of life, such as family or leisure time. Novack et al. (1997, p. 505) suggest that providers reflect on the following questions when considering professional and personal choices:

- What would be an ideal distribution of time between work, play, family, and personal growth and development?
- What are the barriers to achieving balance in my life?
- In what ways could my assumptions and beliefs be a barrier to change?
- In what ways is the current imbalance benefiting me, and would I be willing to give that up?

Life balance is a long-term goal that can be promoted with attention to one's assumptions and beliefs about work, relationships, home life, and family. Understanding the link between the content of thoughts and resulting emotional reactions can help health care professionals exert some control over their feelings and behavioral reactions. Self-care also includes attention to the body and spirit, with exercise, diet, and connection to a higher power all contributing to life's balance.

The self is the conduit through which health care professionals communicate and develop relationships with patients and families. Providers' utilization of the previously discussed verbal and nonverbal communication strategies is complemented and enhanced by self-awareness and self-care. Through the practice of communication skills, self-awareness, and self-care, the provider can help patients and families effectively identify and actualize their goals during the patient's final stage of life through shared decision making and advance care planning discussions.

SUMMARY

Palliative care professionals face the challenge of initiating and participating in advanced illness discussions on a regular basis. Effective communication occurs in the context of patient-provider relationships, and the value of building rapport and trust in the context of those relationships cannot be overstated. Communication and relationship skills are affected by one's level of self-awareness and self-care, as providers use the self as the vehicle for sending and receiving communication. Communication skills, self-awareness, and self-care are skills that can be learned and should be practiced to provide effective patient-centered care that holistically addresses patients' needs as they journey to the end of their lives.

Objective Questions

1. Rapport:

   a. Is the foundation for effective communication in the patient-provider relationship.
   b. Is unrelated to provider empathy.
   c. Development is contingent upon nonverbal behavior only.
   d. Is a by-product of effective symptom management.

2. How patients react to "bad news" about diagnosis and prognosis is determined by:

   a. The extent of empathic nonverbal behavior displayed by the clinician in the clinical relationship.
   b. The patient's achieved level of formal education.
   c. Individual, social, and contextual factors inherent in the provider-patient interaction.
   d. The patient's propensity for mental illness.

3. Which of the following acronyms addresses nonverbal attending skills?

   a. SQUARE.
   b. SOLVER.
   c. STRIVE.
   d. SIMPLE.

4. Empathy is:

   a. The sensitive understanding of patients' feelings and their unique experiences with advanced illness.
   b. Facilitated by the provider's sympathy for the patient.
   c. Not central to the development of rapport with the patient.
   d. Demonstrated through "parroting" the patient's words.

5. There is little research evidence to support that:

   a. Patients want providers to shield them from bad news.
   b. Patients seek to hold on to their hopes at the cost of knowing the truth about their prognosis.
   c. Patients who are not told the truth about their prognosis die in blissful ignorance.
   d. Providers are comfortable discussing prognosis with patients.

6. Discussing patient fears directly with them:

   a. Helps patients achieve a sense of control.
   b. Exacerbates patient fears.
   c. Diminishes patient self-efficacy.
   d. Is not good clinical practice.

7. Countertransference:

   a. Does not have an impact on patient care.
   b. Can lead to provider overinvolvement or underinvolvement.
   c. Seldom "leaks" into patient-provider interactions.
   d. Is better left unexamined.

8. To facilitate the grief response among providers who are emotionally affected by their patients' deaths, Wakefield suggests:

   a. Processing one's emotional reactions with a trained professional only.
   b. Asking questions about the patient's dying trajectory.
   c. Writing letters to the surviving family members.

   d. Avoiding rituals concerning the patient's death.

9. Meier (2001) suggests which steps to minimize the impact of experienced emotions on patient care?

   a. Delay acknowledgement of the feeling until the patient is no longer under the provider's direct care.
   b. Name the feeling.
   c. Avoid discussion about the emotional response with colleagues.
   d. Transfer the patient.

10. Advance care planning:

    a. Involves exploring the patient's goals and values.
    b. Stops when an advance directive has been completed.
    c. Typically does not involve family members.
    d. Is best done outside of the provider's office.

REFERENCES

AARP. (1996). *Making medical decisions: Questions and answers about health care powers of attorney and living wills.* Washington, D.C.: AARP.

Choice in Dying. (1996). *Whose death is it anyway: Talking about your choices.* New York: Choices in Dying, Inc.

Christakis, N.A. (1999). *Death foretold.* Chicago: University of Chicago Press.

Commission on Aging with Dignity. (1998). *Five wishes.* Tallahassee, Fla.: Commission on Aging with Dignity.

Cournoyer, B. (2000). *The social work skills workbook.* Belmont, Calif.: Wadsworth.

Fallowfield, L.J., Jenkins, V.A., & Beveridge, H.A. (2002). Truth may hurt but deceit hurts more: Communication in palliative care. *Palliat Med, 16*(4), 297-303.

Friedrichsen, M.J., Strang, P.M., & Carlsson, M.E. (2000). Breaking bad news in the transition from curative to palliative cancer care: Patient's view of the doctor giving the information. *Support Care Cancer, 8*(6), 472-478.

Golden, R., & Sonneborn, S. (1998). Ethics in clinical practice with older adults: Recognizing biases and respecting boundaries. *Generations, 22*(3), 82-86.

Jenkins, V.A., Fallowfield, L.J., & Saul, J. (2001). Information needs of patients with cancer: Results from a large study in UK cancer centres. *Br J Cancer, 84,* 48-51.

Ivey, A.E. (1988). *Intentional interviewing and counseling: Facilitating client development* (2nd ed.). Pacific Grove, Calif.: Brooks/Cole.

Karel, M.J. (2000). The assessment of values in medical decision making. *J Aging Stud, 14*(4), 403-422.

Kogan, S.L., Blanchette, P.L., & Masaki, K. (2000). Talking to patients about death and dying: Improving communication across cultures. In K.L. Braun, J.H. Pietsch, & P.L. Blanchette (Eds.), *Cultural issues in end-of-life decision-making* (pp. 305-325). Thousand Oaks, Calif.: Sage Publications.

Larson, D.G. (1993). *The helper's journey: Working with people facing grief, loss, and life-threatening illness.* Champaign, Ill.: Research Press.

Lee, S.J., Back, A.L., Block, S.D., et al. (2002). Enhancing physician-patient communication. *Hematology,* 464-483.

Limerick, M. (2002). Communicating with surrogate decision-makers in end-of-life situations: Substitutive descriptive language for the healthcare provider. *Am J Hospice Palliat Care, 19*(6), 376-380.

Ling, C.W. (1997). Crossing cultural boundaries. *Nursing, 27*(3), 32d-32f.

Lo, B., Quill, T.E., & Tulsky, J.A. (1999). Discussing palliative care with patients. *Ann Int Med,* 130(9), 744-749.

Lynn, J., Arkes, H.R., Stevens, M., et al. (2000). Rethinking fundamental assumptions: SUPPORTS's implications for future reform. *J Am Geriatr Soc, 48*(5), 214-221.

Meier, D.E., Back, A.L., & Morrison, R.S. (2001). The inner life of physicians and care of the seriously ill. *J Amer Med Assoc, 286*(23), 3007-3014.

Morrison, M.F. (1998). Obstacles to doctor-patient communication at the end of life. In M.D. Steinberg & S.J. Youngner (Eds.), *End-Of-Life decisions: A psychosocial perspective* (1st ed., pp. 109-136). Washington, D.C.: American Psychiatric Press.

Norlander, L., & McSteen, K. (2000). The kitchen table discussion: A creative way to discuss end-of-life issues. *Home Healthc Nurse, 18*(8), 532-539.

Novack, D.H., Suchman, A.L., Clark, W., et al. (1997). Calibrating the physician: Personal awareness and effective patient care. *J Amer Med Assoc, 278*(6), 502-509.

Pearlman, R., Starks, H., Cain, K., et al. (2001). *Your life, your choices,* 2003. From www.va.gov/resdev/programs/hsrd/ylyc.pdf.

Pearlman, R.A., Cole, W.A., Patrick, D.L., et al. (1995). Advance care planning: Eliciting patient preferences for life-sustaining treatment. *Patient Educ Couns, 26*(1-3), 353-361.

Quill, T.E. (2000). Initiating end-of-life discussions with seriously ill patients: Addressing the "elephant in the room." *J Amer Med Assoc, 284*(19), 2502-2507.

Radziewicz, R.M. (2001). Self-care for the caregiver. *Nurs Clin North Am, 36*(4), 855-869.

Rando, T.A. (1984). *Grief, dying, and death: Clinical interventions for caregivers.* Champaign, Ill.: Research Press.

Ratner, E., Norlander, L., & McSteen, K. (2001). Death at home following a targeted advance-care planning process at home: The kitchen table discussion. *J Am Geriatr Soc, 49*(6), 778-781.

Reisfield, G.M., & Wilson, G.R. (2003). Ambiguity in end-of-life communications. *Journal of Terminal Oncology, 2*(2), 61-66.

Rogers, C R. (1961). *On becoming a person: A therapist's view of psychotherapy.* Boston: Houghton Mifflin.

Steinhauser, K.E., Christakis, N.A., Clipp, E.C., et al. (2001). Preparing for the end of life: Preferences of patients, families, physicians, and other care providers. *J Pain Symptom Manage, 22*(3), 727-737.

Stolick, M. (2003). Dying to meet you: Facing mortality and enabling patient styles. *Am J Hospice Palliat Care, 20*(4), 269-273.

Teno, J.M., Licks, S., Lynn, J., et al. (1997). Do advance directives provide instructions that direct care? *J Am Geriatr Soc, 45*(4), 508-512.

The, A., Hak, T., Koëter, G., et al. (2000). Collusion in doctor-patient communication about imminent death: An ethnographic study. *Br Med J,* 321, 1376-1381.

Tobin, D.R., & Lindsay, K. (1999). *Peaceful dying: The step-by-step guide to preserving your dignity, your choice, and your inner peace at the end of life.* Reading, Mass.: Perseus Publishers.

Wakefield, A. (2000). Nurses' responses to death and dying: A need for relentless self-care. *Int J Palliat Nurs, 6*(5), 245-250.

Wenrich, M.D., Curtis, J.R., Shannon, S.E., et al. (2001). Communicating with dying patients within the spectrum of medical care from terminal diagnosis to death. *Arch Intern Med, 161,* 868-874.

Yeo, G., & Hikoyeda, N. (2000). Cultural issues in end-of-life decision making among Asians and Pacific Islanders in the United States. In K.L. Braun, J.H. Pietsch, & P.L. Blanchette (Eds.), *Cultural issues in end-of-life decision-making* (pp. 101-125). Thousand Oaks, Calif.: Sage Publications.

Evidence-Based Interventions

Dana N. Rutledge

OBJECTIVES

After the completion of this chapter, the reader should be able to:

1. Discuss the evolution of evidence-based practice and its terminology.
2. Describe the tools of using evidence in the palliative care setting.
3. Describe factors important to making an evidence-based practice change.

EVOLUTION OF EVIDENCE-BASED PRACTICE

There is a "chasm" between the care that should be delivered in palliative and supportive care and that which exists (Institute of Medicine, 2001). In examining the state of end-of-life health services at the end of the twentieth century, the Institute of Medicine's Committee on Care at the End of Life (Field & Cassell, 1997) reported key threats to effective patient care services, all of which apply to palliative care. The committee identified a lack of evidence-based practice: patients are suffering from errors of *omission*, "when caregivers fail to provide palliative and supportive care known to be effective" (Field & Cassell, 1997, p. 264) and from errors of *commission*, when care providers use ineffective and sometimes harmful interventions. The committee also reported that health care providers, including physicians and nurses, are the products of training and education that often have not prepared them for caring for and communicating with dying patients and their loved ones. Finally, the Institute of Medicine noted an incomplete evidence base framework for providers to determine how best to manage care delivery and symptom management (Field & Cassell, 1997; Johnston & Abraham, 1995). In the meantime, palliative and end-of-life care have emerged as international initiatives and as strategic imperatives for multiple state and organizational settings, with targeted funding dollars from public and private organizations set aside for end-of-life studies and demonstration projects. Examples of these are the Project on Death in America and initiatives from the Robert Wood Johnson Foundation and the Institute of Nursing Research.

Within the past decade, evidence-based practice (EBP) has emerged in international health care as a means to improve the health of individuals and populations of patients for whom care is provided. Practice can be considered evidence-based when it incorporates three core components (Rutledge & Grant, 2002):

- Current best scientific evidence
- Clinical expertise of health care providers, including principles of pathophysiology and psychosociology
- Preferences of patients and family members

First appearing in the medical literature, EBP was seen as an effort to assist in decision making at the level of individual patients (Guyatt, Haynes, Jaeschke, et al., 2000). Its growth was propelled by two simultaneous movements: "(1) the effort to reduce physician practice pattern variation and improve appropriateness of services by using research-based clinical protocols and decision-making algorithms, and (2) an effort to teach medical students critical thinking skills for practice" (Rutledge & Grant, 2002, p.1). Actually, physicians as a professional group have been testing strategies over many years to change practice based upon research (Beck, 2002) and diffusion of research-based evidence has been studied in many disciplines (Berwick, 2003; Estabrooks, 2001; Rogers, 1995). As EBP spread to issues addressing groups of patients, research-based practice guidelines and standards of care became elements of EBP.

EBP is both a process and a product (Rutledge & Bookbinder, 2002). The process of EBP consists of several activities that lead to the product of evidence-based care delivery. These activities can be summarized in three steps: (1) selecting and appraising the evidence to determine a potential practice change; (2) leading a team in planning and implementing a change; and (3) evaluating project outcomes and maintaining the change. In this chapter, each phase of the EBP process is discussed as it relates to palliative care. EBP as an outcome is the translation of evidence into a practice change (Rutledge & Bookbinder, 2002).

In a discussion of evaluating evidence that the National Health Service published in 1972, Cochrane, a British epidemiologist, posited that only interventions and diagnostic tests that had been properly tested and found effective should be provided as national health care. He stressed that evidence from randomized controlled trials (RCT) was much more likely than that from other types of investigations to provide reliable information. Cochrane introduced the idea of levels of evidence: opinion at one end of a continuum with experimental findings at the other (Cochrane, 1999). He also introduced the distinction between effective and efficacious. *Effective* refers to research results from studies with controlled environments with optimal personnel and ideal measures (RCTs), and *efficacious* refers to results in the real world, in routine clinical practice. The distinction between these two cannot be overestimated in importance. This terminology fits well when discussing treatments such as pharmacologic agents and surgical interventions in medicine, and educational interventions and protocols for wound healing in nursing. For example, effective results from studies of congestive heart failure (CHF) have shown improved survival with medical therapy (Quaglietti, Atwood, Ackerman, et al., 2000). However, beneficial effects on quality of life have not been reported consistently and adherence to medical management suffers because of patient quality-of-life issues. Thus efficacious management of CHF may be impaired because patients suffer from quality-of-life issues related to treatment and fail to adhere to recommended treatments.

Evidence-based nursing (EBN) integrates best evidence, nursing expertise, and the values and preferences of the individuals, families, and communities who are served (Sigma Theta Tau International [STTI], 2003) and thus is congruent with EBP. For the remainder of this chapter, EBP assumes to incorporate evidence-based care within medicine and nursing. Both disciplines assume that optimal care is provided when health care providers understand and incorporate findings from a synthesis of current research, value the consensus of expert opinion, and can provide care that takes into account cultural and personal values and preferences. This evidence-based approach ensures that care delivery optimizes the best scientific evidence while ensuring appropriate care of individuals, groups, and populations with varied needs (STTI, 2003).

Evidence

Evidence-based medicine fails to explicitly define evidence, instead describing the process of EBP as "the conscientious, explicit and judicious use of best evidence in making health care decisions" (Sackett, Rosenberg, Gray, et al., 1996, p.71). Initially, proponents equated "evidence" with products of quantitative scientific studies, narrowed even more to the synthesis of randomized controlled trials. However, this has gradually changed to the use of multiple types of evidence in the context of complex clinical decision-making challenges within health care (Forbes & Griffiths, 2002; Radford & Foody, 2001; Rycroft-Malone, Kitson, Harvey, et al., 2002). Non-RCT and qualitative studies can expand the applicability of results to broader populations of patients (Radford & Foody, 2001; Upshur, 2001) and when different types of evidence are needed to answer different clinical questions (Rycroft-Malone et al., 2002). For example, when results of observational studies and randomized trials are congruent with regard to both effect size and direction, the evidence base for an intervention is stronger. When effect sizes are smaller or when an intervention may have risk for harm, observational studies may not concur with trial results (Radford & Foody, 2001), pointing to the need for more tenuous practice recommendations. This is the phenomenon that exists when improved outcomes predicted by randomized studies fail to materialize in less stringent evaluations of an intervention in a real world clinical setting. Synthesizers of evidence must be acutely aware of methodologic limitations of nonrandomized studies (Ioannidis, Haidich, Pappa, et al., 2001) and other types of evidence yet be cautiously open to the use of all potentially relevant observations, facts, or other information that supports or justifies beliefs (Sandelowski & Barroso, 2003; Upshur, 2001).

Qualitative research has begun to be incorporated more formally into thinking about evidence-based practice (Kearney, 2001; Olson, 2001; Sandelowski & Barroso, 2003; Swanson, 2001). Understanding the difference in generalizability between quantitative and qualitative studies assists in seeing how this incorporation can be optimally promoted (Box 3-1)(Olson, 2001). Findings of qualitative studies can "explain processes underpinning the results of quantitative studies, give a voice to the patient, monitor treatment responses, and solve health care delivery problems with respect to organizational behavior and processes, the implementation of change, and the elaboration

of leaders' roles and functions" (Olson, 2001, p. 259). For example, evidence addressing optimal spiritual care for dying patients requires incorporation of qualitative studies that offer explanations of patient needs, belief systems, and acceptable interventions.

Levels of Evidence

Levels or hierarchies of evidence have multiplied as groups attempt to appraise evidence and make sense of findings in terms of strength of sources. These are necessary during the critical appraisal phase of the EBP process. One of the most widely used hierarchies of evidence was created by the Agency for Health Care Policy and Research (AHCPR; now the Agency for Healthcare Research and Quality [AHRQ]) in developing its clinical practice guidelines. Types of evidence are in a hierarchy, with those at the top being the strongest (Box 3-2). Most levels of evidence come from a positivist perspective where meta-analyses or systematic reviews of RCTs are considered the highest level of evidence. A meta-analysis is the statistical analysis of results from several studies in order to integrate the findings (Cooper & Hedges, 1994). It is important to

Box 3-1 GENERALIZABILITY OF QUANTITATIVE AND QUALITATIVE STUDY FINDINGS

QUANTITATIVE STUDIES
- Focus on hypothesis testing
- Data collected through experimentation
- Generalize to groups like the ones studied

QUALITATIVE STUDIES
- Focus on theory development
- Explore detailed description of phenomena and processes
- Generalize to theoretic constructs and the essence of the experience

Box 3-2 TYPE OF EVIDENCE (PER THE AGENCY FOR HEALTHCARE POLICY AND RESEARCH)

Ia. Evidence obtained from meta-analysis of randomized controlled trials.
Ib. Evidence obtained from at least one randomized controlled trial.
IIa. Evidence obtained from at least one other type of well-designed controlled study without randomization.
IIb. Evidence obtained from at least one other type of well-designed quasi-experimental study.
III. Evidence obtained from well-designed nonexperimental studies, such as comparative studies, correlational studies, and case studies.
IV. Evidence obtained from expert committee reports or opinions or clinical experiences of respected authorities.

realize that strict adherence to these hierarchies may lead to good evidence being neglected or judged as unworthy (Gupta, 2003).

Levels of evidence can be more relevant for certain types of research and practice questions than it is for others. For example, when most evidence about an intervention comes from randomized or nonrandomized clinical trials, the AHCPR levels are easy to use. However, when health care providers are trying to determine which patients would benefit most from a clinic for palliative care, clinical trials will not give the answer.

Recently, in a commissioned evaluation of systems of evidence appraisal (Agency for Healthcare Research and Quality [AHRQ], 2002), AHRQ found 40 systems that addressed the strength of a body of evidence (i.e., a synthesis of the available evidence). This is pertinent to health care providers interested in evaluating evidence on palliative care. To determine whether a body of knowledge provides information on which clinicians can base judgments, the quality, quantity, and consistency[1] of the evidence must be evaluated. The AHRQ report concluded

that the systems evaluated varied in their ability to assess each of the three key elements. An important finding from the report was that the dilemma arising from conflicting evidence in a body of literature, particularly between RCT and observational data, may not be resolved using levels or hierarchies of evidence. For example, when RCTs draw conclusions about an intervention from studies with homogeneous populations and when observational studies with diverse multisite samples find other results, grading the strength of the evidence does not tell the health care provider what conclusion to draw about the intervention. The practice context in which a decision is being made may play a key role when deciding to use a specific intervention.

What is important in determining the strength of evidence about any topic is the rigor of the process from which each piece of evidence evolves. Methodologic rigor or quality is "the extent to which a study's design, conduct, and analysis have minimized selection, measurement, and confounding biases" (AHRQ, 2002, Summary p. 1).

In palliative care, a relatively new specialty, evidence to enhance decision making is found from multiple sources. The Cochrane Collaboration Pain, Palliative, and Supportive Care Group outlines the bodies of evidence needed within the specialty (Box 3-3). Much "high level" evidence exists on the effects of pharmacologic agents in managing acute

[1]Definitions used in the AHRQ evaluation. *Quality:* the aggregate of quality ratings for individual studies, predicated on the extent to which bias was minimized; *Quantity:* magnitude of effect, numbers of studies, and sample size or power; *Consistency:* for any given topic, the extent to which similar findings are reported using similar and different study designs.

Box **3-3** COVERAGE BY THE COCHRANE COLLABORATION PAIN, PALLIATIVE, AND SUPPORTIVE CARE GROUP

I. ACUTE PAIN
Treatment of postoperative and post-traumatic pain.

A. Pain Prevention
   • Pharmacologic therapies, e.g., propranolol for migraine prevention
   • Physical therapies, e.g., posture and fluids for preventing post–dural puncture headache
   • Psychological

B. Pain Management
   • Psychological treatments, e.g., distraction therapies
   • Pharmacologic treatments, e.g., aspirin for acute pain
   • Physical treatments, e.g., TENS
   • Complementary treatments, e.g., acupuncture for migraine prevention

Box 3-3   COVERAGE BY THE COCHRANE COLLABORATION PAIN, PALLIATIVE, AND SUPPORTIVE
CARE GROUP—CONT'D

II. CHRONIC PAIN (NON-CANCER)

Includes all chronic non-cancer pain and recurrent acute pain.

A. Pain Prevention

- Psychological therapies, e.g., distraction therapies
- Pharmacologic therapies, e.g., drugs for preventing migraine headaches in children
- Complementary therapies, e.g., feverfew for preventing migraine headaches

B. Pain Management

- Psychological treatments, e.g., coping skills training
- Pharmacologic treatments, e.g., drug treatments for pain in sickle cell disease
- Invasive treatments, e.g., sympathectomy for neuropathic pain
- Physical treatments, e.g., TENS for chronic pain
- Complementary treatments, e.g., acupuncture for idiopathic headache

III. CHRONIC CANCER-RELATED PAIN

A. Pain Management

- Psychological treatments, e.g., coping skills training
- Pharmacologic treatments, e.g., bisphosphonates for relief of pain from bone metastases
- Invasive treatments
- Physical therapies
- Radiotherapy/radioisotopes, e.g., radioisotopes for metastatic bone pain
- Complementary treatments, e.g., aromatherapy and massage for patients with cancer

IV. PALLIATIVE CARE

- Symptom management (physical, pharmacologic, and complementary treatments for anorexia, bowel obstruction, cachexia, constipation, cough, dyspnea, fatigue, hiccup, insomnia, dysphagia, itch, mobility problems, nausea and vomiting, oral health, skin management)
- Communication issues
- Psychological issues
- End-of-life issues
- Organization of support services
- Ethical issues

V. SUPPORTIVE CARE

- Supporting caregivers through the disease process
- Supporting caregivers through bereavement
- Imparting bad news
- Patient and caregiver needs for information about disease and treatment processes
- Nutrition support

TENS, Transcutaneous electrical nerve stimulation.

and chronic pain, whereas less may be available about preventing pain and complementary therapies' effectiveness. Evidence is beginning to be compiled about supporting caregivers through the disease process, whereas less is known about the best ways to impart bad news and specific symptom management related to itch, hiccup, and cough. Although a large-scale trial of palliative home care teams would be ideal (Salisbury & Bosanquet, 2000), such a study would be expensive and difficult. Current providers need to seek evidence from well-conducted observational studies that address pertinent outcomes, physiologic studies, clinical observations, qualitative research, and careful descriptions of processes and context of care delivery (Guyatt & Rennie, 2002). The type of evidence available in palliative care results from the inherent difficulties in doing research with patients who require palliative or supportive care or who are imminently dying (Keeley, 1999; McMillan & Weitzner, 2003).

Best Practices

Best practices were defined by the American Association of Critical Care Nurses (AACN) as fully implemented programs, benchmarked and tested, which meet or set new standards or introduce dramatic innovations in health care delivery (American Association of Critical Care Nurses [AACN], 2003). Based in quality improvement or performance improvement processes, *best practices* is a term used in many industries. It often refers to successful solutions to problems or challenges that are shared by others. It is used in the context of benchmarking, that is, measuring and comparing outcomes among those working toward solutions to a similar problem. In quality improvement, a "best practice" is an outcome to a problem and, although not intrinsically linked to research evidence, may be research-based. Thus a best practice would be the best action, process, or treatment used for individual patients or groups of patients.

Many in quality improvement circles study best practices through a drill-down approach. That is, when a best practice is identified through benchmarking, the search for processes that lead to good results is sought. Then, processes can be linked to

outcomes and others can attempt to improve outcomes by using "tested" processes. The combination of evaluating best practices and benchmarking allows organizations to comprehend how practice changes lead to specific outcomes (Driever, 2002; Goode, 2003). Note that there may not be a link to research evidence through this method.

Others link best practices more to the evidence. According to a group developing European public health policy, best practices are systematic processes that can identify, implement, and monitor the available evidence in health care to achieve improvements (Perleth, Jakubowski, & Reinhard, 2001). This definition clearly goes beyond the issues of quality within one system and is linked more with an evidence-based practice framework. Best practice thus considers the best evidence on (1) effectiveness of health care interventions for a particular clinical condition, (2) ways to disseminate and implement the interventions, and (3) measures useful to monitor the intended effects and other effects of the intervention.

TOOLS OF EVIDENCE-BASED PRACTICE
Guidelines

Clinical practice guidelines (CPGs) or, in some countries, best practice statements are developed by health care professionals and organizations to help support evidence-based clinical decisions in specific contexts. Systematically developed statements aim to guide providers and patients in making decisions related to appropriate care delivery in particular clinical situations (Field & Lohr, 1992). Depending on the rigor of the review methods used by CPG developers, the evidence base varies with the topic and the review process. Particular weaknesses found in some CPGs are that they may come from a weak evidence base, lack input from multidisciplinary expert panels, and poorly report on processes of CPG development.

Users of CPGs are urged to critically appraise how guidelines were developed, seeking those that used the highest quality of primary research available while using a professional consensus methodology. This ensures that the science behind the recommendations is valid and that clinical experts have been part of the recommendation making (Perleth et al., 2001). Users are also urged to evaluate timeliness of CPG recommendations. A recent report commissioned by AHRQ found that of 17 CPGs developed between 1992 and 1998, three quarters were judged to be sufficiently out of date within 3 to 5 years as to need withdrawal from the guidelines database or to require that new evidence be appended to the original guideline (Shekelle, Ortiz, Rhodes, et al., 2001).

Guidelines can be used to direct health care decisions at both the individual patient and the aggregate patient levels. Resources for CPGs are in Box 3-4. CPGs are not intended to mandate care decisions because individual provider and patient preferences need to be part of any decision. To truly optimize care delivery, guidelines must be systematically implemented with strategies that consider barriers and facilitators to practice change.

Reviews

Another important tool for evidence-based practice is synthesized reports of research evidence or systematic reviews (Institute of Medicine, 2001). Few practitioners have the time and energy required to compile comprehensive reviews of evidence. Therefore health care providers must be aware of sources of integrative reviews and knowledgeable about searching primary databases for such reviews. Availability and use of superior reviews in decision making can enhance patient care in palliative care effectiveness.

Internationally, the stimulus for systematic reviews has come from the Cochrane Collaboration, a worldwide group of subject and methodologic specialists who aim to identify and synthesize randomized controlled trials in all aspects of health care. Systematic reviews aim to address a focused area of literature by integrating results of studies on a topic. To be systematic, they require protocols describing how and what literature was searched, read, and evaluated. This contrasts with reviews or overviews that are merely summaries of studies that are available to an author. A meta-analysis is a specific type of systematic review, one that uses a quantitative method of combining the results of independent studies and synthesizing summaries

and conclusions that may be used to evaluate therapeutic effectiveness. Box 3-4 shows select resources available for finding systematic reviews about palliative care topics.

IMPLEMENTING EVIDENCE-BASED PRACTICE

Implementation is translating evidence or information into clinical practice, public health interventions, or policies that effect change (Perleth et al., 2001). In 1998 a conceptual model (Kitson, Harvey, & McCormack, 1998) was developed that has the potential to assist in the implementation of EBP based on collective research experience, practice development, and performance improvement projects (Rycroft-Malone et al., 2002). The main proposition of the model is that successful implementation of evidence-based practices involves the interaction of the "level and nature of the evidence, the context or setting into which the research is to be placed, and the method or way in which the process is facilitated" (Kitson et al., 1998, p.149). In this model, evidence can be a combination of research findings, clinical experience, and patient preferences. Critical elements of context are culture, leadership, measurement, or evaluation, while other factors (e.g., relationships, systems of decision making, innovation potential) also play a part. Facilitation is an appointed role, may be done by an internal or external person or team, and is considered an *enabling* function rather than a *persuasive* one. The model offers a systematic way to approach implementing a practice change.

This EBP model fits with the findings from the science of diffusion of innovation (Berwick, 2003; Rogers, 1995). This science posits that new practices are disseminated or spread according to the influence of the perceptions of the innovation, characteristics of the people who are considering the innovation, and contextual factors such as communication, incentives, leadership, and management. Change agents participate in the diffusion of innovations by influencing decisions to change within the practice setting (Rogers, 1995); thus they may facilitate EBP. The attributes of the innovation include characteristics of the evidence base (e.g., whether based upon randomized trials or

Box 3-4 RESOURCES FOR EVIDENCE-BASED PRACTICE

CLINICAL PRACTICE GUIDELINES

- **"How to Use a Clinical Practice Guideline"** based on the *Users' Guides to Evidence-based Medicine* and reproduced with permission from JAMA. (1995;274[7]:570-574) and (1995;274[20]:1630-1632). Copyright 1995, American Medical Association. www.cche.net/usersguides/guideline.asp
- **Health Services/Technology Assessment Text** (HSTAT) is a searchable collection of large, full-text clinical practice guidelines, technology assessments, and health information. Includes PubMed, Centers for Disease Control and Prevention, and National Guidelines Clearinghouse. hstat.nlm.nih.gov/
- **National Guidelines Clearinghouse (NGC)** is a public resource for evidence-based clinical practice guidelines. NGC is sponsored by the U.S. Agency for Healthcare Research and Quality (formerly the U.S. Agency for Health Care Policy and Research) in partnership with the American Medical Association and the American Association of Health Plans. www.guidelines.gov
- **CMA Infobase** is a repository of guidelines produced or endorsed in Canada by a national, provincial/territorial, or regional medical or health organization, professional society, government agency, or expert panel. mdm.ca/cpgsnew/cpgs/index.asp
- **American College of Physicians' Clinical Practice Guidelines** covers many areas of internal medicine, such as screening for cancer or other major diseases; diagnosis; treatment; and medical technology. www.acponline.org/sci-policy/guidelines/
- **Cancer Care Ontario's Program in Evidence-Based Care** (PEBC) and the **Practice Guidelines Initiative** (PGI) access clinical practice guidelines, evidence-based summaries. www.ccopebc.ca/
- **National Comprehensive Cancer Network Guidelines** access clinical practice guidelines related to patients with cancer (e.g., fatigue, palliative care). www.nccn.org/
- **HIV-AIDS Practice Guidelines**, sponsored by the Infectious Disease Society of America. www.idsociety.org/HIV/CEN/PGindex_HIV.htm
- Kuebler, K.K., Berry, P.H., & Heidrich, D.E. (Eds.) (2001). *End-of-life Care: Clinical Practice Guidelines*, Philadelphia: Saunders.
- Lipman A, Jackson K, & Tyler L. (Eds.) *Evidence Based Symptom Control in Palliative Care: Systematic Reviews and Validated Clinical Practice Guidelines for 15 Common Problems in Patients with Life Limiting Disease.* Pharmaceutical Products PR, 2001.

SYSTEMATIC REVIEWS

- How to search for systematic reviews: www.nlm.nih.gov/bsd/pubmed_subsets/sysreviews_sources.html
- The Cochrane Library consists of a regularly updated collection of evidence-based medicine databases, including The Cochrane Database of Systematic Reviews. www.cochrane.org/
- Evidence-based Practice Centers (EPCs) develop evidence reports and technology assessments on topics relevant to clinical, social science/behavioral, economic, and other health care organization and delivery issues—specifically those that are common, expensive, and/or significant for the Medicare and Medicaid populations. Available reports at www.ahcpr.gov/clinic/epc/#Reports
- Systematic reviews in pain relief: www.jr2.ox.ac.uk/bandolier/painres/srprg.html
- Database of Abstracts of Reviews of Effects (DARE): agatha.york.ac.uk/darehp.htm
- This site lists titles of systematic reviews carried out by members of the Cochrane Pain, Palliative Care and Supportive Care Group, part of the Cochrane Collaboration, and includes links to abstracts where available: www.cochrane.org/cochrane/revabstr/g380index.htm

not, how many studies support) and the characteristics of the clinical problem that provoked the need seeking evidence (Estabrooks, 2001; Rogers, 1995). People considered most likely to accept a new practice may be those who are venturesome or innovative, whereas the next most likely group judiciously accepts changes and has a high degree of opinion leadership; these innovators have strong social connections within their social system and keep abreast of new ideas in their discipline (Rogers, 1995). Other predictors of nurses using research in practice are a positive attitude toward the research process, having attended continuing education programs, and the ability to put aside previous beliefs (Estabrooks, 2001).

A theory that is also useful in understanding how to implement EBP is the social influences model (Zimbrano & Leippe, 1991). Each individual's behavior differentially affects other people's behavior, feelings, or thoughts. This explains how fellow physicians' or nurses' judgments of the importance or value of a practice change can influence its implementation. The social influences model takes into account the importance of habit and custom, values of peers, and social norms on practice behavior (Estabrooks, 2001). Because of these factors, it is quite important to know who the opinion leaders are within an organization before attempting to make a practice change. The influence of these opinion leaders will be critical to the success of a change.

It is important to acknowledge that dissemination of evidence-based information does not ensure its implementation. The processes can overlap, or in some instances, the process never proceeds beyond dissemination. In fact, passive dissemination of information via printed materials, lectures, and conferences has been found to have little or no effect on practice (Beck, 2002; Bero, Grilli, Grimshaw, et al., 1998). Yet these are the most commonly used strategies to circulate information to nurses and physicians. In a survey of research-based practices used by oncology nurses (Rutledge, Greene, Mooney, et al., 1996), 90% of nurses who were aware of 7 of 10 practices used them at least sometimes. This indicates that passive dissemination may work to change awareness and thus is the first step toward implementation. However, it needs to be followed by another type of intervention to ensure that practice change occurs.

Single interventions such as audit and feedback, uses of local opinion leaders, local consensus processes, and patient-mediated interventions have had variable success in changing practice. Better and consistent effects were noted with educational outreach visits (detailing) and reminders (phone, postcard, computer cueing). The most effective way to ensure implementation of a new practice is with multiple methods; in fact, when three or more methods were combined, more than 80% of demonstrations showed positive outcomes (Davis, 1998). The intensity and complexity of interventions may also differentially affect success in bringing forth change.

Newer strategies to bring about practice change are being seen in the United States but are as yet untested. These include action-oriented educational conferences, continuous quality improvement, benchmarking as a strategy to improve use of evidence-based practices, clinical pathways, disease management, financial incentives, and regulatory changes (Beck, 2002; Perleth et al., 2001). Dahl (2002) highlights how regulatory changes across the United States have been necessary to enable implementation of specific elements of evidence-based clinical guidelines related to pain management.

Difficulties in Applying an Evidence-Based Approach

Palliative care has some unique aspects that need to be addressed in developing its evidence base. In many instances, health care providers simply do not know whether a service or treatment is effective (Higginson, 1999). Much available research fails to address desired outcomes in palliative care such as issues of quality of life (e.g., quality of death, best resolution of bereavement). When research outcomes focus only on survival or function, knowledge about other outcomes is absent. As mentioned, studies in palliative care are often full of methodologic limitations such as small or nonrepresentative samples and differential attrition in intervention groups. The very nature of palliative care with its focus on persons with progressive illnesses demands individualization of care, and this is difficult to "standardize" in research interventions. Measuring quality of life among such patients is challenging at best, and evidence for different models of palliative care is limited (Higginson, 1999). The value of desired outcomes is not easy to put into a cost-effectiveness framework. Also, the multiplicity of symptoms addressed by supportive and palliative care makes "showing an effect" difficult across persons with different underlying conditions.

Gaps in Evidence

Some examples of gaps in the palliative care evidence base are:

1. Even though research indicates that where people die is influenced more by where they live than by their preference for location of death (Burge, Lawson, & Johnston, 2003; Gatrell, Harman, Francis, et al., 2003; Pritchard, Fisher, Teno, et al., 1998; Rutledge, Donaldson, & Pravikoff, 2001; Sambamoorthi, Walkup, McSpiritt, et al., 2000), the effects of dying in a non-preferred place on either patient or family members are unknown. Congruence of preference as to place of death and actual site of dying is but one factor that has an impact on satisfaction with decisions related to death (Hays, Galanos, Palmer, et al., 2001; Ringdal, Jordhoy, & Kaasa, 2002; Tiernan, O'Connor, O'Siorain, et al., 2002; Tolle, Rosenfield, Tilden, et al., 1999).

2. Although the analgesic effects of opioids have been documented (Barnett, 2001), lacking is a body of well-designed studies comparing effects of different routes of administration of the same opioid, adverse effects among opioids, and analgesic effects of opioids in treating complex pain. Completely missing is evaluation of the potential beneficial side effects of opioids (e.g., the impact on dyspnea).

3. A recent qualitative systematic review found a lack of scientific basis to support the use of nebulized opioids to treat dyspnea in patients with chronic pulmonary disease including malignancy (Joyce, McSweeney, Carrieri-Kohlman, et al., 2004). This led

authors to recommend further research with random crossover designs involving larger samples that are stratified according to prior opioid use, and consistency of study variables in all future research.

4. A dearth of research and literature exists in the field of pediatric palliative care, complicating the development of clear practice standards and guidelines (Cooley, Adeodu, Aldred, et al., 2000).

5. Other needs are for evidence related to effects of different models of palliative care, the expansion or replication of clinical trials done in persons with cancer to other populations of patients who need palliative services, and extension of work with family-centered care to understand the impact of palliative care services on the family and the effects of family factors on care delivery.

Making an Evidence-Based Practice Change

Below is a discussion of how one group made evidence-based practice changes in palliative care. Table 3-1 shows a summary table analyzing the practice change project. This group (Milligan, McGill, Sweeney, et al., 2001) sought a practical protocol to assist staff in decreasing the prevalence of oral symptoms and problems in hospice patients. Working from this clinical problem, they reviewed and appraised the evidence from the literature and surveyed by telephone other settings similar to their own for extant oral care practices. At this point, they developed a protocol based on the evidence found that met the criteria necessary to make the practice change feasible in the work setting. These criteria were simple, inexpensive, palatable, easily taught, adaptable to different settings, effective, evidence-based, and interdisciplinary. Outlining these criteria before developing the protocol increased the likelihood that those in the setting would accept the practice change, demonstrating the importance of considering factors related to practice context.

Facilitation of the practice change was not well described in the published article, but project leaders developed a written protocol and measured

Table **3-1** SUMMARY TABLE OF PRACTICE CHANGES

Purpose of Project	Practice Change and Setting	Evidence-Based Practice Strategies	Findings	Notes
Implementation of practical oral care for people with advanced cancer	Evidence-based protocol for oral care* in patients admitted to a hospice unit in the United Kingdom	• Literature search • Survey of oral care practices in Scottish hospices and hospice units • Interdisciplinary approach • Implementation with good staff acceptance	• Post-implementation data on 23 patients for days 0 (admission) and 7. • Half or more of patients had multiple oral problems pre-protocol use, including pain and dryness. • On day 7, no patient had a sore mouth, and 30% experienced dryness. On oral assessment, 91% showed improvement.	• No baseline data before protocol implementation. • Authors concluded that this simple protocol enabled changes in oral conditions and quality of life for persons receiving hospice care.

From Milligan, S., McGill, M., Sweeney, M.P., et al. (2001). Oral care for people with advanced cancer: An evidence-based protocol. *Int J Palliat Nurs, 7,* 418-426.
*Protocol includes assessment using the Oral Assessment Guide (Eilers, J., Berger, A.M., & Peterson, M.C. [1988]. Development, testing, and application of the oral assessment guide. Oncol Nurs Forum, 15[3], 325-330.), procedure for offering and giving oral care, and individualized strategies to use with specific groups of patients (e.g., edentulous).

staff use (described as "good"). Outcomes following several months of implementation indicate that oral care conditions of patients within the hospice setting improved after a week of care.

While written as an evidence-based practice project and not as a well-controlled research study, this write-up supports the utility of the conceptual model of EBP (Kitson et al, 1998; Rycroft-Malone et al., 2002). The major proposition of the model as applied to this project is that good evidence supported by a receptive context (work setting) and facilitated by change agents and resources led to a successful practice change.

SUMMARY

Evidence-based practice in palliative care has the potential to enhance patient outcomes by assisting health care practitioners in making sound decisions and implementing optimal systems. Pertinent evidence-based resources are becoming available that can augment other resources in care delivery. Clinician understanding of elements necessary to complete the process of making an evidence-based practice change in palliative care can maximize the chance that such a change will indeed promote optimal clinical outcomes.

Objective Questions

1. In considering the implementation of a practice or intervention, a nurse considers many things. For the practice to be considered evidence-based, there must be:

   a. A scientific basis for the practice.
   b. Best expert opinion for the practice.
   c. Consensus of surrounding work settings on the use of the practice.
   d. Consensus of clinicians in the work setting on the use of the practice.

2. Which best defines effectiveness, as discussed by Cochrane?

   a. A treatment that works most of the time.
   b. A treatment that works in real clinical settings.
   c. A treatment that has been tested in randomized controlled trials.

   d. A treatment that clinicians use consistently, with good results.

3. During the critical appraisal phase of the EBP process, health care providers comparing findings across studies find it useful to use hierarchies or levels of evidence. These systems allow evaluation of the quality, quantity, and consistency of the evidence and are not very useful for evidence that is:

   a. Conflicting.
   b. Done with methodologic rigor.
   c. Needed in palliative care settings.
   d. Based on homogeneous populations.

4. Which of the following best describes a clinical practice guideline?

   a. Standards of care.
   b. Policies and procedures in a work setting.
   c. Local provider-developed statements that describe expected behaviors related to a clinical condition.
   d. Systematically developed statements.

5. For a literature review to be considered "systematic," what information must it include?

   a. The role of expert opinion.
   b. How consensus was achieved.
   c. Which studies were summarized by the author.
   d. The literature search process, and how it was evaluated.

6. Evidence-based practice is most likely to occur when the evidence is robust, the context is ready for change, and facilitation of the change is:

   a. Passively disseminated.
   b. Controlled by administrators.
   c. Done using a single method.
   d. Based on the diffusion of innovation.

7. Evidence in palliative care is spotty across areas of interest because of what factors?

   a. Focus on maladaptation and death.
   b. Minimal research in palliative care.

c. Inappropriate outcomes of research and methodologic limitations.

d. Multiple clinical practice guidelines do not pertain to palliative care.

8. In working toward evidence-based practice, health care professionals who have implemented a change must then:

   a. Select and reappraise the evidence.

   b. Determine a protocol for the practice change.

   c. Lead a team in planning and implementing a change.

   d. Evaluate project outcomes and implement steps to maintain the change.

9. A multidisciplinary team wants to develop a practice protocol related to massage for patients with cancer. In their search for evidence, they want to see if any clinical practice guidelines (CPGs) have been developed already. The best place to find already developed guidelines is:

   a. MEDLINE.

   b. CINAHL Database.

   c. Cochrane Library.

   d. National Guidelines Clearinghouse.

10. The same team also wants to see if there have been any systematic reviews on the topic. The first place to look for a systematic review that would capture randomized clinical trials would be:

    a. MEDLINE.

    b. CINAHL Database.

    c. Cochrane Library.

    d. National Guidelines Clearinghouse.

REFERENCES

Agency for Healthcare Research and Quality (AHRQ). (2002). *Systems to rate the scientific strength of evidence* (Evidence Report/Technology Assessment #47. AHRQ Publication No. 02-E016). Rockville Md: Agency for Healthcare Research and Quality.

American Association of Critical Care Nurses (AACN). (2003). *Best practice network a means to sustainable healthcare improvement.* Retrieved June 8, 2003, from www.aacn.org/AACN/aacnnews.nsf.

Barnett, M. (2001). Alternative opioids to morphine in palliative care: A review of current practice and evidence. *Postgrad Med J, 77*(908), 371-378.

Beck, S.L. (2002). Strategies to translate research into practice. *Semin Oncol Nurs, 18*(1), 11-19.

Bero, L.A., Grilli, R., Grimshaw, J.M., et al. (1998). Closing the gap between research and practice: An overview of systematic reviews of interventions to promote the implementation of research findings. *Br Med J, 317*(7156), 465-468.

Berwick, D.M. (2003). Disseminating innovations in health care. *JAMA, 289*(15), 1969-1975.

Burge, F., Lawson, B., & Johnston, G. (2003). Trends in the place of death of cancer patients, 1992-1997. *Can Med Assoc J, 168*(3), 265-270.

Cochrane, A.L. (1999; original publication 1972). *Effectiveness and efficiency. Random reflections on health services.* Cambridge: University Press.

Cooley, C., Adeodu, S., Aldred, H., et al. (2000). Paediatric palliative care: A lack of research-based evidence. *Int J Palliat Nurs, 6,* 346-351.

Cooper, H., & Hedges, L.V. (Eds.). (1994). *The handbook of research synthesis.* New York: Russell Sage Foundation.

Dahl, J.L. (2002). Working with regulators to improve the standard of care in pain management: The U.S. experience. *J Pain Symptom Manage, 24,* 136-146.

Davis, D. (1998). Does CME work? An analysis of the effect of educational activities on physician performance or health care outcomes. *Int J Psychiatry Med, 28*(1), 21-39.

Driever, M.J. (2002). Are evidence-based practice and best practice the same? *West J Nurs Res, 24*(5), 591-597.

Estabrooks, C. (2001). Research utilization and qualitative research. In J.M. Morse, J.M. Swanson, & A.J. Kuzel (Eds.), *The nature of qualitative evidence.* Thousand Oaks, Calif.: Sage Publications.

Field, M.J., & Cassell, C.K. (Eds.). (1997). *Approaching death: Improving care at the end of life.* Washington D.C.: National Academy Press.

Field, M.J., & Lohr, K.N. (Eds.). (1992). *Guidelines for clinical practice: From development to use. Institute of Medicine.* Washington D.C.: National Academy Press.

Forbes, A., & Griffiths, P. (2002). Methodologic strategies for the identification and synthesis of "evidence" to support decision-making in relation to complex healthcare systems and practices. *Nurs Inq, 9*(3), 141-155.

Gatrell, A.C., Harman, J.C., Francis, B.J., et al. (2003). Place of death: Analysis of cancer deaths in part of North West England. *J Public Health Med, 25*(1), 53-58.

Goode, C.J. (2003). Evidence-based practice. In K.S. Oman, M.E. Krugman, & R.M. Fink (Eds.), *Nursing research secrets* (pp. 7-14). Philadelphia: Hanley & Belfus.

Gupta, M. (2003). A critical appraisal of evidence-based medicine: Some ethical considerations. *J Eval Clin Pract, 9*(2), 111-121.

Guyatt, G.H., Haynes, R.B., Jaeschke, R.Z., et al. (2000). Users' guides to the medical literature. XXV. Evidence-based medicine: Principles for applying the users' guides to patient care. *J Amer Med Assoc, 284*(10), 1290-1296.

Guyatt, G.H., & Rennie, D. (Eds.). (2002). *Users' guides to the medical literature. Essentials of evidence-based clinical practice.* Chicago: AMA Press.

Hays, J.C., Galanos, A.N., Palmer, T.A., et al. (2001). Preference for place of death in a continuing care retirement community. *Gerontologist, 41*(1), 123-128.

Higginson, I.J. (1999). Evidence based palliative care [Editorial]. *Br Med J, 319*, 462-463.

Institute of Medicine. (2001). *Crossing the quality chasm: A new health system for the 21st century.* Washington D.C.: National Academy Press.

Ioannidis, J., Haidich, A.-B., Pappa, M., et al. (2001). Comparison of evidence of treatment effects in randomized and nonrandomized studies. *JAMA, 286*(7), 821-830.

Johnston, G., & Abraham, C. (1995). The WHO objectives for palliative care: To what extent are we achieving them? *Palliat Med, 9*, 123-137.

Joyce, M., McSweeney, M., Carrieri-Kohlman, V., et al. (2004). Evidence synthesis: The use of nebulized opioids in the management of dyspnea. *Oncol Nurs Forum, 31*, 551-561.

Kearney, N. (2001). Levels and applications of qualitative research evidence. *Res Nurs Health, 24*, 145-153.

Keeley, D. (1999). Rigorous assessment of palliative care revisited. *Br Med J, 319*, 1447-1448.

Kitson, A., Harvey, G., & McCormack, B. (1998). Enabling the implementation of evidence based practice: A conceptual framework. *Qual Health Care, 7*, 149-158.

McMillan, S.C., & Weitzner, M.A. (2003). Methodologic issues in collecting data from debilitated patients with cancer near the end of life. *Oncol Nurs Forum, 30*(1), 123-129.

Milligan, S., McGill, M., Sweeney, M.P., et al. (2001). Oral care for people with advanced cancer: An evidence-based protocol. *Int J Palliat Nurs, 7*, 418-426.

Olson, K. (2001). Using qualitative research in clinical practice. In J.M. Morse, J.M. Swanson, & A.J. Kuzel (Eds.), *The nature of qualitative evidence.* Thousand Oaks, Calif.: Sage Publications.

Perleth, M., Jakubowski, E., & Reinhard, B. (2001). What is 'best practice' in health care? State of the art and perspectives in improving the effectiveness and efficiency of the European health care systems. *Health Policy, 56*, 235-250.

Pritchard, R.S., Fisher, E.S., Teno, J.M., et al. (1998). Influence of patient preferences and local health system characteristics on the place of death. *J Amer Geriatr Soc, 46*(10), 1242-1250.

Quaglietti, S.E., Atwood, J.E., Ackerman, L., et al. (2000). Management of the patient with congestive heart failure using outpatient, home, and palliative care. *Prog Cardiovasc Dis, 43*(3), 259-274.

Radford, M.J., & Foody, J.M. (2001). How do observational studies expand the evidence base for therapy? *JAMA, 286*(10), 1228-1230.

Ringdal, G.I., Jordhoy, M.S., & Kaasa, S. (2002). Family satisfaction with end-of-life care for cancer patients in a cluster randomized trial. *J Pain Symptom Manage, 24*(1), 53-63.

Rogers, E.M. (1995). *Diffusion of innovations* (4th ed.). New York: Free Press.

Rutledge, D.N., & Bookbinder, M. (2002). Processes and outcomes of evidence-based practice. *Semin Oncol Nurs, 18*(1), 3-10.

Rutledge, D.N., Donaldson, N.E., & Pravikoff, D.S. (2001). End-of-Life Care Series. Part II. End-of-life care for hospitalized adults in America: Learnings from the SUPPORT and HELP studies. *OJCI, 4*(5), 1-57.

Rutledge, D.N., & Grant, M. (2002). Introduction to evidence-based practice. *Semin Oncol Nurs, 18*(1), 1-2.

Rutledge, D.N., Greene, P., Mooney, K.H., et al. (1996). Use of research-based practices by oncology staff nurses. *Oncol Nurs Forum, 23*(8), 1235-1244.

Rycroft-Malone, J., Kitson, A., Harvey, G., et al. (2002). Ingredients for change: Revisiting a conceptual framework. *Qual Saf Health Care, 11*, 174-180.

Sackett, D.L., Rosenberg, W.M.C., Gray, J.A.M., et al. (1996). Evidence based medicine: What it is and what it isn't. *Br Med J, 312*, 71-72.

Salisbury, C., & Bosanquet, N. (2000). Assessing palliative care is difficult (letter). *Br Med J, 320*, 942.

Sambamoorthi, U., Walkup, J., McSpiritt, E., et al. (2000). Racial differences in end-of-life care for patients with AIDS. *AIDS Public Policy J, 15*(3-4), 136-148.

Sandelowski, M., & Barroso, J. (2003). Creating metasummaries of qualitative findings. *Nurs Res, 52*(4), 226-233.

Shekelle, P.G., Ortiz, E., Rhodes, S., et al. (2001). The validity of the Agency for Healthcare Research and Quality clinical practice guidelines: How quickly do guidelines go out-of-date? *J Amer Med Assoc, 286*, 1461-1467.

Sigma Theta Tau International (STTI). (2003). *STT's position statement on evidence-based nursing.* Retrieved March 1, 2003, from www.nursingsociety.org/research/main.html#ebp.

Swanson, J.M. (2001). The nature of outcomes. In J.M. Morse, J.M. Swanson, & A.J. Kuzel (Eds.), *The nature of qualitative evidence.* Thousand Oaks, Calif.: Sage Publications.

Tiernan, E., O'Connor, M., O'Siorain, L., et al. (2002). A prospective study of preferred versus actual place of death among patients referred to a palliative care home-care service. *Ir Med J, 95*(8), 232-235.

Tolle, S.W., Rosenfield, A.G., Tilden, V.P., et al. (1999). Oregon's low in-hospital death rates: What determines where people die and satisfaction with decisions on place of death? *Ann Int Med, 130*(8), 681-685.

Upshur, R.E.G. (2001). The status of qualitative research as evidence. In J.M. Morse, J.M. Swanson, & A.J. Kuzel (Eds.), *The nature of qualitative evidence.* Thousand Oaks, Calif.: Sage Publications.

Zimbrano, P.G., & Leippe, M.R. (1991). *The psychology of attitude, change and social influence.* Philadelphia: Temple University Press.

Pharmacology

Mellar P. Davis

OBJECTIVES

After the completion of this chapter, the reader should be able to:

1. Discuss the basic principles governing pharmacodynamics and pharmacokinetics.
2. Describe the terms *biophase, EC-50, steep* and *shallow responders, therapeutic index, area under the curve, volume of distribution, half-life* and *clearance.*
3. List the factors associated with non-linear pharmacokinetics.
4. Define the cytochrome P-450 system, glucuronidation, and drug efflux.
5. Examine drug interactions based on metabolism, drug affinity to receptor, and competitive binding.

INTRODUCTION

Many of the illnesses requiring palliation are prevalent in the elderly, in the medically ill, and in patients who require pharmacologic monitoring. The influence of age and disease affects the manner in which drugs are absorbed, distributed, metabolized, and eliminated by the body (pharmacokinetics) and the interaction of the drug at various receptor sites (pharmacodynamics). Wise treatment decisions will balance the relief of disease-related symptoms, prevent adverse drug reactions, minimize drug interactions, and improve patient compliance with drug treatment (Chutka, Evans, Fleming, et al., 1995).

There is a strong association between the age of a patient and the number of medications that he or she receives (Rochon & Gurwitz, 1995). Of Americans older than 65 years, 90% are prescribed

The authors would like to acknowledge the work done by Maribeth B. Kowalski PharmD, RPh, on this chapter.

at least one medication, typically cardiovascular, antihypertensive, analgesic, nonsteroidal antiinflammatory drug (NSAID), sedative, and/or gastrointestinal medications (Chutka et al., 1995). In the long-term care setting it is predicted that more than 60% of patients are taking three or more medications. Medication regimens in the long-term care setting most often include laxatives, analgesics, neuroleptics, and sedatives/hypnotics (Chutka et al., 1995). Patients who are admitted to a palliative unit are generally prescribed 6 or 7 medications at any given time (Bernard & Bruera, 2000). Acute hospitalized patients receive from 7 to 10 medications during their admission (Bernard & Bruera, 2000). These polypharmacy issues contribute to the risk of adverse drug reactions and drug-to-drug interactions. Drug interactions increase proportionately with the number of prescribed drugs at any given time. Patients receiving 1 to 3 medications will have a 3% to 5% incidence of adverse drug interactions, whereas patients on 10 to 20 different medications have a 20% or greater chance of a significant adverse drug-drug event, which can become fatal (Bernard & Bruera, 2000).

Recognizing drug interactions can be difficult because many of the symptoms associated with drug reactions (confusion, nausea, fatigue, constipation) may overlap with common symptoms associated with progressive cancer and debilitating disease (Bernard & Bruera, 2000). Symptomatic patients are at the greatest risk for unrecognized pharmaceutical misadventures because of advanced age, disease, multiple medication use, frequent use of over-the-counter medications, and impaired organ function (influencing drug clearance). As a result, the drug therapeutic index of each individual medication (the serum level or dose that produces toxicity compared with the therapeutic dose) is significantly narrower in these medically ill patients compared with healthy individuals (Bernard & Bruera, 2000). Adverse drug events can be minimized by reducing the number of drugs prescribed and utilizing a dose, interval, and route based on known drug pharmacodynamics and pharmacokinetics (Bernard & Bruera, 2000). Clinicians cannot alter age and frequently cannot modify the course of disease; they can, however, determine the appropriate route, dose, and interval prescribed for each medication. Rote prescribing without an understanding of pharmacology is a recipe for poor outcomes (Rochon & Gurwitz, 1995). Therefore an astute clinician should have the knowledge surrounding pharmacology as a necessity for good palliation. This knowledge contributes to minimal adversity to the patient and enhances his or her quality of life (Fig. 4-1).

PHARMACODYNAMICS

Pharmacodynamics can be described as the interaction of a specific drug at its intended receptor site. *Pharmacokinetics* is defined as the absorption, distribution, metabolism, and excretion of a specific drug. Both of these terms help determine the clinical benefit of specific medications. Pharmacokinetics does not predict a patient's response to medication. An example can be found with opioids because the plasma level of an opioid does not predict the onset or level of analgesia. The measurement and timing of analgesia reflects a minimum drug concentration and activity of an opioid at the opioid receptor site. The intended activation of the receptor by the opioid produces analgesia. The decrease of analgesia over time and a quantifiable duration of analgesic action of an opioid is a surrogate for pharmacokinetics since plasma levels are inaccurate determinants of analgesia (Paalzow, 1982).

A linear relationship exists between the relative degree of analgesia and plasma concentrations for an individual patient, but large individual variations exist in the plasma levels at the onset to pain relief (Paalzow, 1982). Other medications, such as antiseizure and antidepressant agents, have a closer association of receptor sites within tissues (Fig. 4-2).

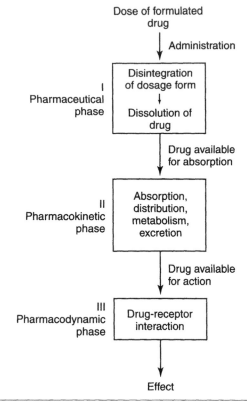

FIGURE **4-1** Three phases to pharmacology before a drug response is seen are the pharmaceutical phase, the pharmacokinetic phase, and the pharmacodynamic phase. The pharmacodynamic phase is dependent upon the previous two phases and has its own individual variations. As a result, the pharmacodynamic phase is subject to the greatest individual variability.

Biophase includes the process of drugs at their receptor site, allowing the drugs to interact in a structural way with their respective receptors by binding with a certain affinity (potency) and activating their specific receptor (intrinsic efficacy), which sometimes changes the shape of the receptor (conformations). Drugs may bind with great affinity but poorly activate the target receptor. A different dose-response relationship can occur with a drug that activates the receptor with greater efficacy yet binds with similar affinity. An example of this is when morphine binds with great affinity

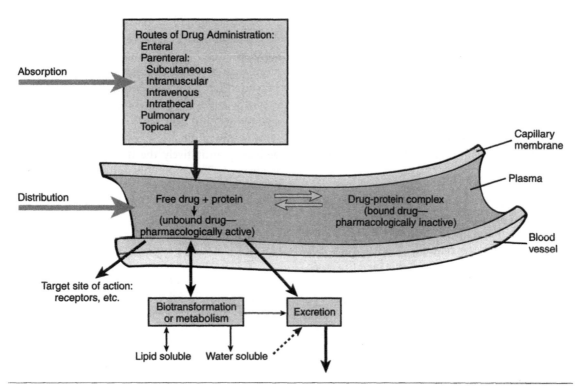

FIGURE 4-2 The schema illustrates the pharmacokinetic phase of drug action. The drug is absorbed, passes through the liver, and circulates in the central compartment. Note that only free drug is capable of being absorbed, distributed to the target site of action, biotransformed, and excreted. The drug-protein complex limits the drug from vascular spaces. As a result of binding to protein, the drug remains in the central compartment and does not reach the biophase (receptor site). (From Principles of drug action. [2003]. In L. McKenry & E. Salerno [Eds.], *Mosby's pharmacology in nursing—Revised & Updated* [Chapter 3, Fig. 3-3]. St. Louis: Mosby.)

to the mu opioid receptors within the central nervous system, but methadone, in contrast, is better at activating the mu receptor than morphine. Morphine needs to bind more opioid receptors to achieve the same degree of pain relief compared with that of methadone. As a result, methadone, at high doses, can produce greater analgesia per dose than morphine (Davis & Walsh, 2001). Because morphine binds to more receptors and induces different receptor conformations than methadone, there is a greater potential for analgesic tolerance and a plateau in pain response at higher doses (Birkett, 2003; Donnelly, Davis, Walsh, et al., 2002).

Once a drug binds to a receptor, a secondary messenger system is frequently involved that activates intracellular processes that clinically create the intended drug response. The secondary messenger becomes responsible for the physiologic drug effect (Birkett, 2003). Most receptors have transmembrane links to guanosine triphosphate binding proteins (G-proteins), which in turn affect other enzymes within the cell. Again, given the example of morphine, G-proteins inhibit adenylyl cyclase but stimulate certain kinases (Birkett, 2003). Activation of the secondary messengers can change with time such that G-proteins become "uncoupled" from the receptor as a negative feedback inhibition or the altered G-proteins stimulate other receptors, which counters the benefits of the drug. This can lead to pharmacologic tolerance, which in the case of morphine may lead to higher dose requirements to maintain optimal pain relief. Opioid receptors activate secondary receptors such as *N*-methyl-D-aspartate receptors and different sodium channels within the cell membrane, which reduces analgesia. This receptor activity is termed *heterologous drug tolerance,* because it involves receptors other than the opioid receptor. Bound receptors may become internalized and may produce analgesic tolerance or resurface on membranes and resensitize the receptor to the drug (Birkett, 2003).

Agonists

Drugs that bind to a receptor and produce a maximum effect are called *agonists.* Partial agonists are those agents that result in a less-than-maximal effect or have a ceiling (maximum dose) to their dose response characteristics. Drugs that bind to a receptor and fail to activate the receptor are *antagonists.* If an antagonist is combined with an agonist, the antagonist could displace the agonist and prevent the receptor from being activated. Generally, antagonists produce an effect only if the agonist is present. For instance, naloxone antagonizes morphine-induced analgesia but alone has very little effect clinically. A partial agonist may also act as an "antagonist," especially when combined with a full agonist, as the partial agonist may prevent favorable receptor conformation.

Efficacy Versus Drug Concentration

The relationship between the drug response and drug concentration is illustrated in Figures 4-3 and 4-4. A specific drug will produce a response that is related to dose and appears as a sigmoid curve. The drug concentration at half maximal effect (e.g., a 50% reduction in pain as in the case of opioids) is called the *EC-50.* The sigmoid appearance of drug response curve illustrates the "ceiling" effect near maximal concentration when receptor reserves are diminished. These dose response sigmoid curves will be different for individual medications within a drug class and among individual patients who are given the same medication. This efficacy versus drug concentration curve resembles a substrate enzyme interaction curve, which is observed with drug metabolism and drug pharmacokinetics. Drug-receptor affinity and activation determine the EC-50 (Birkett, 2003).

The adverse effects of a drug can be graphed in the same way as drug response. Generally, the adverse effects begin at much higher concentrations than the drug concentration for therapeutic benefit. The drug concentrations between drug response and toxicity can be described as the therapeutic window (see Fig. 4-5). The drug concentration ratio of the EC-50 toxicity to EC-50 efficacy defines quantitatively the therapeutic index of a medication. The larger this ratio, the greater is the therapeutic index (Birkett, 2003). The drug response to concentration curves can be replotted using a

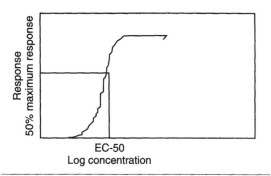

FIGURE **4-3** The EC-50, the dose at which a 50% response is seen, is derived from calculated plasma concentration–response curves. Between 20% and 80% maximal response, there appears to be a linear plasma concentration to response effect. (From Anthony, P. [Ed.]. [2002]. *Pharmacology secrets* [p. 7]. Philadelphia: Hanley & Belfus.)

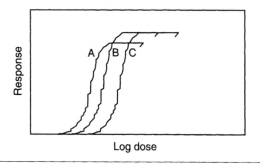

FIGURE **4-4** Drug *A* produces an equivalent response at a lower dose than drug *B* or *C.* The increased biologic effect at lower doses depends on affinity of the drug for receptor (potency) and ability to activate the receptor (intrinsic efficacy). (From Anthony, P. [Ed.]. [2002]. *Pharmacology secrets* [p. 1]. Philadelphia: Hanley & Belfus.)

semi-log graph (Figs. 4-5 and 4-6). This sigmoid curve becomes relatively linear between the EC-20 (the drug concentration at which 20% or the drug response is experienced) and the EC-80 (concentration at which 80% drug response is seen) (see Figs. 4-3 and 4-5).

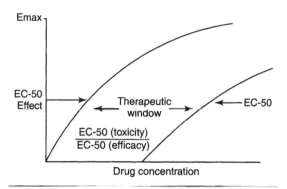

FIGURE 4-5 The drug concentration between efficacy and toxicity is the drug therapeutic window. The therapeutic index is the EC-50 for toxicity over the EC-50 for efficacy (response). The larger the number, the greater is the therapeutic index and the wider is the therapeutic window. Emax is the drug concentration at the maximum drug response.

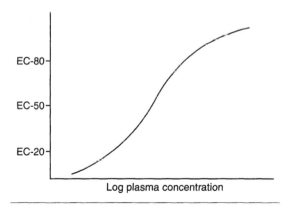

FIGURE 4-6 Responses plotted against log plasma concentrations produce a sigmoid curve. Response per dose diminishes when drug doses are increased beyond EC-80. Between EC-20 (concentrates at which a 20% response is observed) and EC-80 (drug concentrates at 80% response) is a linear response to drug concentration for most drugs and defines the therapeutic drug concentrates.

Another major factor is the slope of the sigmoid curve dose response (Levy, 1998) (see Fig. 4-6). There are shallow responders that have a small incremental response with each dose adjustment (slope of 0.5 gamma) and responders that have a dramatic response per dose increment (gamma >5) (Fig. 4-7). Steep responders have a narrower therapeutic range. Shallow responders will have a wide therapeutic range of EC-20 to EC-80. However, the therapeutic index will be determined largely by the dose at which toxicity occurs. The slope of drug-effect curves is determined by individual rates of drug metabolism and elimination of the drug and the duration and activation of drug receptor interactions.

Though most drugs have a linear dose response between the EC-20 and EC-80, some exceptions do exist. In certain circumstances there is non-linearity in dose efficacy curves, which means that drug response and drug levels assume a more complex relationship (Levy, 1998). If the parent drug is metabolized into an active metabolite, as occurs with morphine to morphine-6-glucuronide and tramadol to O-desmethyl-tramadol, the metabolite will add to the parent drug benefit and alter efficacy curves. If drug binding to circulating protein (albumin or alpha-1 acid glycoprotein) becomes saturated, more drug is proportionately unbound

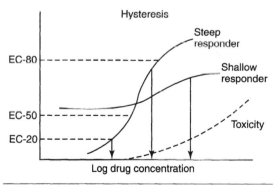

FIGURE 4-7 Patients may have a "steep" response such that profound drug responses are seen with small increment dose but there is a narrow therapeutic window. "Shallow" responders have a gradual response to dose and wider therapeutic window depending on dose toxicity curves.

and available to bind to receptors compared with total circulating drug (as occurs with phenytoin) (Birkett, 2003). Some pharmacologic agents have enantiomers (mirror-image twins), in which one enantiomer is biologically active and has different kinetics and dynamics relative to the non-active enantiomer (as occurs with tramadol and methadone). The active enantiomer will influence dose response curves to a greater extent than the combined active and inactive isomers in the commercially available form (Birkett, 2003).

Two other factors can produce non-linearity between dose response curves. Hysteresis is a delay in drug distribution to the specific receptor, and plasma concentrations can decrease with an increase in drug concentration around the receptor site within extravascular spaces (Fig. 4-8). For instance, the blood-brain barrier delays concentrations of morphine from reaching receptor sites within the brain despite increased concentrations. As the drug concentration in plasma diminishes, the drug effect increases and dose response curves shift to the left (see Fig. 4-7). Morphine, which is hydrophilic, crosses the blood-brain barrier more slowly than lipophilic opioids like fentanyl. Therefore morphine has a delayed onset to action but relative longer dwell time within the central nervous system (Birkett, 2003; Paalzow, 1982).

Analgesic tolerance leads to a "right shift" in the drug concentration-response curve because more drug is needed to produce the same effect (i.e., analgesia) because of changes in receptor, and sensitivity and biophase activity (Birkett, 2003) (Fig. 4-9).

Finally, some medications such as aspirin and warfarin have effects that are not related to the drug per se but are related to the kinetics of the enzyme to which they bind and are not generally related to drug plasma levels. Warfarin, for instance, blocks posttranslational modification of clotting factors to II, VII, IX, and X and the prothrombin time, a measure of warfarin response, is related to clotting factor, enzyme regeneration, and decay rather than warfarin plasma levels (Birkett, 2003).

In summary the following points are important to remember:
- Drug response is proportional to the logarithm of drug concentrations.
- Drug effects decrease in a log linear relationship over time with a single dose.
- Increasing doses above the drug EC-80 increases the duration of drug effects but usually will not improve drug response and can lead to toxicity.
- The therapeutic drug concentrations are characteristically between the EC-20 and EC-80 and secondarily related to minimal adverse effects and the EC-50 toxicity.

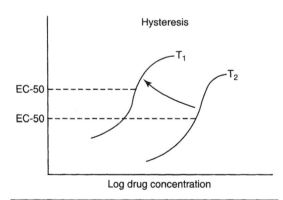

FIGURE 4-8 *Hysteresis* is the apparent increase in response as drug levels decrease in plasma. This leftward shift in dose response is related to the delayed appearance of drug within at the receptor site, delayed clearance from the receptor, and/or prolonged receptor binding.
T_1, Time-1; T_2, Time-2.

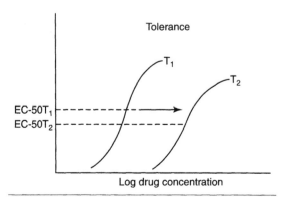

FIGURE 4-9 Tolerance leads to a "right" shift in dose response curves such that higher drug doses are required to maintain the same effect. Tolerance may be caused by changes in drug pharmacokinetics or pharmacodynamics.
T_1, Time-1; T_2, Time-2.

- A number of factors influence drug concentrations: (1) protein binding; (2) active metabolites and enantiomers; (3) receptor modulation; (4) drug targeted enzyme decay and regeneration; and (5) barriers to drug diffusion into receptor sites.

A basic principle difference in pharmacodynamics is much greater between individuals than pharmacokinetics since pharmacodynamics are subject to the kinetic variables influencing drug concentrations at receptor sites and variability in drug receptor interactions (Levy, 1998; Paalzow, 1982) (see Fig. 4-9).

PHARMACOKINETICS

When a drug is introduced into the bloodstream, it is absorbed or diffused out of circulation and binds to tissues. The drug may redistribute back into the bloodstream and be eliminated primarily through the liver or kidneys as unchanged drug and/or metabolites (Paalzow, 1982) (see Fig. 4-2). Plasma concentration curves decline exponentially (logarithmically) as a result of drug diffusion and elimination. Drug concentrations within circulation rapidly decrease with an initial rapid diffusion out of circulation into tissues. Slow diffusion occurs from tissues that are influenced by redistribution from organs that have a higher blood flow to those with lower blood flow (Paalzow, 1982). Tissues with rapid drug distribution (termed the *central compartment*) include heart, lung, liver, and kidney. Poorly perfused tissues are those with a barrier to diffusion and are termed the *peripheral compartment* (which includes bone, fat, muscle, and brain). If the action of a drug is in the peripheral compartment, drug effects will poorly correspond to plasma drug concentrations. A drug with a "two-compartment" model will have two rates of decline in plasma levels: (1) a rapid phase from diffusion; and (2) a slower phase because of redistribution and drug clearance (Fig. 4-10). The slow phase of clearance better reflects the duration of drug action and usually determines dosing intervals. Slow clearance, drug interactions, and organ failure will significantly influence the clearance, thereby influencing drug half-life and dosing intervals.

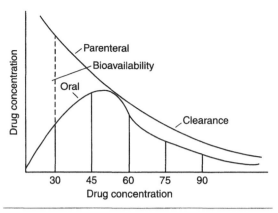

FIGURE **4-10** Route determines bioavailability but plays little role in drug clearance. The latter half of the area under the curve (AUC) of injected and oral medications is super-imposable.

Drugs with a significant redistribution and slow elimination (e.g., methadone) may have biexponential kinetics, which will appear as two peaks in plasma concentration over time. Certain drugs are formulated to have biexponential kinetics (e.g., sustained-release oxycodone) through alterations in the pharmaceutical delivery system. Measuring medication equivalents between drugs with mono-exponential and biexponential kinetics can be inaccurate if done through single-dose studies because of the longer time to steady state concentrations of the biexponential drug. For example, methadone and morphine by single-dose potency studies are said to be equal; however, this is inaccurate and does not reflect equivalence at steady state. At steady state, methadone will have potency at 4 to12 times greater than morphine (Paalzow, 1982).

Drug concentrations over time depend on activity at specific receptor sites, volume of distribution, and liver and/or renal clearance. Other factors contributing to concentration include drug protein binding and drug lipid solubility. These factors indirectly influence the volume of drug distribution (Paalzow, 1982). Diffusion into tissues can be facilitated by an active or passive transport carrier or efflux of drugs from receptor sites by certain membrane pumps (Paalzow, 1982). The volume of distribution depends on how well a drug binds to plasma proteins (either albumin or alpha-1 glycoprotein), which maintains the circulation of the drug relative to the drug's affinity for extravascular tissues. The volume of distribution can greatly exceed normal physiologic volume if it is highly bound to tissue protein (Birkett, 2003; Paalzow, 1982). The "apparent" volume of distribution (which may greatly exceed the body's real volume) reflects the relationship between drug dose and subsequent plasma concentration (Birkett, 2003). Large volumes of drug distribution are caused by tissue binding and help to also determine the loading doses of specific medications. Therefore the greater the volume of distribution, the higher the loading dose will be needed to rapidly achieve therapeutic levels at the specific receptor site (Birkett, 2003).

Drug Half-Life

The volume of distribution and clearance of a drug are the main determinants to a pharmacologic agent's half-life (Urso, Blardi, & Giorgi, 2002). The route of administration plays little role in circulation and elimination. Clearance can be quantified as the volume of blood that is cleared of drug per unit time and similar to the measurement of renal function with creatinine clearance (Birkett, 2003). The total body clearance is the sum of all individual organ clearances of the specific drug. This includes the metabolic conversion of an active drug to active or inactive metabolites produced by liver microsomal enzymes and conjugates, along with the elimination and tubular secretion by the kidney and peripheral non-hepatic drug metabolism (Birkett, 2003) (Figs. 4-11 and 4-12). Components to individual organ clearance can be measured. For instance, liver perfusion is approximately 90 ml per minute, and if at first pass the clearance by the liver is 70% (as occurs with morphine), the hepatic first-pass clearance of morphine is 63 ml per minute. For methadone the first-pass hepatic clearance is 10% to 20% and hepatic first-pass metabolism is 9 to 18 ml per minute (Birkett, 2003). Therefore a proportion of the drug would be eliminated each time it circulates through the liver.

Oral bioavailability is the result of (1) absorption, (2) small bowel metabolism, and (3) first-pass hepatic clearance (Urso et al., 2002). Absorption is influenced by the gut lumen pH and small intestine

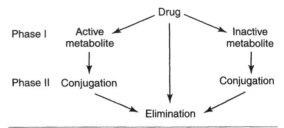

FIGURE 4-11 Drugs that are metabolized by type I enzymes (cytochromes) cause hydroxylation, demethylation, or oxidation of drugs. The second phase of metabolism (phase II) attaches a polar group (glucuronic acid, sulfonyl group, glycine, or glutamate), which renders it soluble for excretion in urine. Drug metabolism may activate or inactivate the parent drug. A conjugated parent drug may also be active. (From Anthony, P. [Ed.]. [2002]. *Pharmacology secrets* [p. 4]. Philadelphia: Hanley & Belfus.)

microvilli, which contain both cytochrome P-450 enzymes (particularly CYP3A4) and glucuronyl transferases and the gut-related efflux protein P-glycoprotein (Schwartz, 2003; Wrighton, Schuetz, Thummel, et al., 2000). Medications that are highly extracted by the liver (and hence have low oral bioavailability) have pharmacokinetics that are highly dependent upon liver blood flow. As liver blood flow diminishes (as in cirrhosis), the oral bioavailability of these highly extracted drugs increases (Birkett, 2003). For example, morphine has oral bioavailability that increases with cirrhosis and worsening portal hypertension (Birkett, 2003; Donnelly et al., 2002). Drugs that are not highly extracted by the liver will have pharmacokinetics that will depend upon the hepatic metabolizing enzyme reserves (cytochrome P-450 and conjugates) and not hepatic blood flow (Birkett, 2003).

Area Under The Curve

One way to determine drug clearance is to measure drug concentrations over time that result in an area under the curve (AUC) graph (Urso et al., 2002) (see Fig. 4-12). Drug concentrations are graphed in relationship to the timing of a dose. Drug clearance is then the dose over the AUC (see Fig. 4-12). The difference in the configuration of the AUC between parenteral and oral dosing is related to the degree

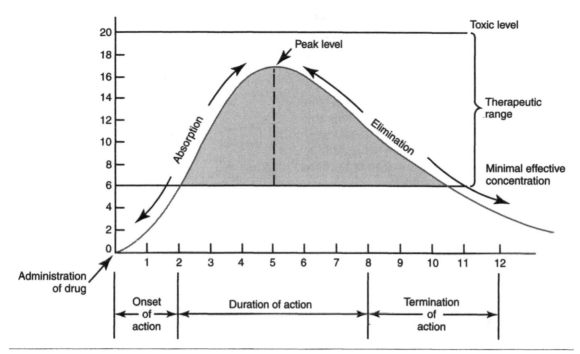

FIGURE 4-12 Plasma profile of a drug consists of absorption, peak levels, and elimination. The time between dose and onset of action is the *hysteresis*. Duration of action and half-life is dependent upon drug elimination. (From Principles of drug action. [2003]. In L. McKenry & E. Salerno [Eds.], *Mosby's pharmacology in nursing—Revised & Updated* [Chapter 3, Fig. 3-7]. St. Louis: Mosby.)

of absorption and hepatic first-pass clearance (Urso et al., 2002). The elimination constant for a particular drug determines clearance (AUC), which is usually a logarithmic process (where a constant proportion of drug is eliminated per unit time).

Elimination

Hepatic Clearance. Hepatic blood flow does not play a major role in overall drug clearance once a medication has reached steady state. When steady-state drug levels are reached, elimination occurs at a constant rate. Elimination will then depend on drug clearance by metabolizing enzymes and renal elimination relative to plasma drug concentrations. Drug clearance is important in that it determines the frequency of maintenance dose administration and influences the dosing interval necessary to maintain therapeutic drug levels and the intended physical responses (whether measured by plasma concentrations as with digoxin or phenytoin or by pharmacodynamic response as with opioids). For a

parenteral infusion rate for a specific drug, the plasma half-life will be shorter if the rate of drug clearance is high with a half-life directly related to the volume of distribution (Birkett, 2003).

In the case of methadone, the volume of distribution is large and the hepatic clearance significantly slower than it is with morphine, thus producing a much longer half-life and as a result extending the dosing interval (Birkett, 2003). Drug half-life will also determine the time to steady state. Generally it takes 3 to 5 drug half-lives to reach steady state. For morphine this is approximately 18 hours, but for methadone it can range from 90 to 120 hours (Birkett, 2003) since the half-life for morphine is 4 hours and the half-life for methadone is 26 hours. It is important for the clinician to appreciate that half-life estimation is an average because there are large differences among individuals. Generally, the appropriate dosing interval for morphine is 4 hours and for methadone it is 8, 12, or 24 hours respectively.

In summary, oral bioavailability is dependent upon absorption and first-pass hepatic excretion. However, at steady state, drug concentrations will depend on the intrinsic clearance of the drug. This will be true whether a drug has a high or a low hepatic first-pass metabolism. At steady state, both high and low hepatic-extracted medications will depend on metabolizing enzymes and renal elimination and not hepatic blood flow. Drug half-life depends on the volume of distribution of the drug and drug clearance (Birkett, 2003).

Renal Clearance and Elimination. The kidneys contain both metabolizing enzymes of the cytochrome P-450 family, efflux protein pumps such as P-glycoprotein, and anion and cation pumps. Renal clearance therefore is the summation of glomerular filtration (of unbound drugs), secretion by anion and cation pumps (in the proximal tubule), and distal tubule reabsorption (Birkett, 2003; Perri, Ito, Rowsell, et al., 2003; Pichette & Leblond, 2003). Competitive drug interactions can occur at the sites of cation or anion pumps both, which are easily saturable at clinically achievable drug concentrations. For example, probenecid prevents the renal secretion of penicillin by competing for the anion pump sites (Birkett, 2003). Passive tubule reabsorption is influenced by (1) urine blood flow, (2) drug lipid solubility, and (3) drug ionization constant (pKa) (Perri et al., 2003). The more un-ionized a drug is, the greater its reabsorption since it will easily pass through lipophilic membranes (Fig. 4-13). As the pH of the urine approximates the pKa, a greater proportion of drug will diffuse back through the tubule membranes. For example, the reabsorption of methadone by the kidney is dramatically increased as urine pH rises above 6 since the pKa of methadone is 9.2 (Birkett, 2003; Davis & Walsh, 2001).

However, if renal excretion accounts for less than 50% of total drug elimination, drug adjustments are usually unnecessary for patients with renal failure unless (1) the drug has a narrow therapeutic index; (2) the parent drug is metabolized to a renally eliminated active metabolite, or (3) uremia reduces hepatic cytochrome enzyme activity (Birkett, 2003). The kidneys contain glucuronyl transferases as well as cytochrome P-450 enzymes, which may play a role

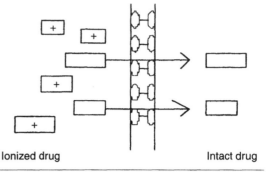

Ionized drug   Intact drug

FIGURE **4-13** pKa is a relationship between ionized and un-ionized drug. It is derived from the Henderson-Hesselbach equation. Un-ionized drug passes freely across membranes. If most of the drug is ionized at physiologic pH, the absorption of the drug will be less. When the pH approximates the pKa, a greater drug effect will occur because of increased absorption. (From Anthony, P. [Ed.]. [2002]. *Pharmacology secrets* [p. 1]. Philadelphia: Hanley & Belfus.)

in drug metabolism. Certain drugs like furosemide are highly eliminated by renal cytochrome metabolism (Pichette & Leblond, 2003).

Protein Binding

Protein binding of a drug within the serum is predominately associated with binding to albumin if the drug is an acidic drug and to alpha-1 acid glycoprotein (AAG) for drugs that are basic (by pKa). Plasma albumin concentrations are much higher than AAG, and albumin holds six separate potential drug-binding sites, which are generally not saturable. AAG has fewer binding sites, but serum levels can increase in the setting of physiologic inflammation. AAG binding is subject to genetic polymorphisms, which can influence drug binding sites (Birkett, 2003). In addition, lipoproteins within red blood cell membranes will non-specifically bind lipophilic medications (Birkett, 2003). Drug protein binding was once thought to be an important determinant to drug interactions and drug kinetics (as a result of competitive binding to albumin or AAG), but more recent studies have determined that this factor may not be clinically relevant (Birkett, 2003; Urso et al., 2002). Unbound drug, a result of competition for binding sites, can lead to increased drug elimination of the unbound portion and increased volume of distribution of the drug. These would pharmacokinetically cancel each other out, thereby reducing efficacy.

Overall, the absolute amount of unbound (biologically active) drug remains unchanged (Birkett, 2003; Urso et al., 2002). As a result, drug monitoring may require the measurement of unbound drug rather than total plasma drug concentration. A clinical example would be monitoring of phenytoin, where therapeutic levels are more accurately reflected by unbound serum concentrations.

Clinical Interactions

P-Glycoprotein. Rifampin reduces morphine's AUC and increases the clearance of morphine-3-glucuronide and morphine-6-glucuronide through stimulation of P-glycoprotein and UGT2B7 (Fromm, Eckhardt, Li, et al., 1997; Venkatesan, 1992).

NON-LINEAR PHARMACOKINETICS

In most instances, increasing drug dosing proportionally increases drug plasma concentrations. If a drug (like alcohol) is given in high doses, the metabolizing enzymes become saturated and further doses increase drug concentrations. As a result, drug kinetics go from first-order (a proportional clearance of drug related to dose) to zero-order kinetics. This means that drug bioavailability is increased because of the saturation of the hepatic first-pass metabolism (Burkitt, 2003). For example, phenytoin is able to saturate its hepatic metabolizing enzyme, leading to an exponential increase in the serum levels in relationship to dose. The overall result of saturation kinetics is that drug half-life is markedly longer at higher doses compared with lower doses (Birkett, 2003).

DOSING REGIMENS IN PHARMACOKINETICS

Continuous drug infusions cause a graded systemic drug accumulation depending upon dose and drug half-life (Birkett, 2003). When doses are given at intervals shorter than the drug half-life, increased serum drug levels can occur. This essentially is similar to increasing a drug dose at half-life intervals while in steady state; drug is eliminated at a rate equal to drug half-life. Dosing interval plasma concentrations can fluctuate twofold if an intermittent bolus is used (Birkett, 2003). Loading doses achieve plasma levels close to steady state quickly but do not achieve steady state more rapidly than non–loading dose regimens (Fig. 4-14). On average, using twice the maintenance dose as a loading dose achieves plasma concentrations close to steady state (the volume of distribution can also influence

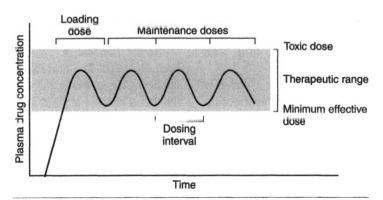

FIGURE 4-14 A loading dose is administered to reach therapeutic drug levels rapidly. Normal loading doses are twice the maintenance doses. Dosing intervals at steady state are usually given at half-life intervals. (From Principles of drug action. [2003]. In L. McKenry & E. Salerno [Eds.], *Mosby's pharmacology in nursing—Revised & Updated* [Chapter 3, Fig. 3-5]. St. Louis: Mosby.)

a loading dose). The greater the volume of the distribution of drug, the greater is the loading dose necessary to fill the volume (Birkett, 2003). Half of the loading dose is eliminated at the drug's half-life and is replaced by the maintenance dose, which should be given at the half-life interval (Birkett, 2003). Problems that can be associated with a loading-dose protocol include the risk of adverse drug effects, particularly if the target organ and receptor site are part of the "central compartment" and flooded with existing drug. Titrating smaller doses at frequent intervals is effective for medications with a low therapeutic index. Medications with a higher therapeutic index may be given at longer than half-life intervals and achieved by using larger doses (Birkett, 2003).

IMPORTANCE OF P-450 ENZYME SYSTEM IN PHARMACEUTICAL MANAGEMENT

Drug metabolism by definition is a chemical modification of a drug within a biologic environment with a primary purpose to increase the drug's solubility (conjugation) to facilitate its excretion. In certain situations, drug metabolism will transform a medication into its active metabolite. This example can be found when codeine is metabolized into morphine and tramadol into desmethyl-tramadol, both of which are the active opioid analgesics of the parent compound. The liver is the primary site of drug metabolism although other major organs and specific extra-hepatic tissues play a role and include kidney, brain, skin, blood, lung, and gastrointestinal tract.

However, most of the metabolizing enzymes (cytochrome and conjugases) are located within the centrilobular region of the liver (Roberts, Magnusson, Burczynski, et al., 2002). The majority of the medications used in palliative medicine are transformed by the type 1 cytochrome P-450 and subsequently conjugated by type 2 conjugase enzymes. The type 1 enzyme is responsible in the conversion of the parent drug either through oxidation, reduction, or hydrolysis into a metabolite that can then be conjugated. The newly formed oxidized or reduced metabolite is then coupled with a glycine, amino acid, or sulfa group such as glucuronic acid, glycine glutamine, sulfate, methyl, or acetate to create a hydrophilic metabolite that is conjugated and prepared for renal excretion.

The rate of drug metabolism is governed by the drug's affinity for a specific enzyme (Km) and the velocity of the enzymatic reaction (Vmax) (Birkett, 2003). The equation for enzyme drug reaction (CLint = Vmax / Km) includes the velocity (Vmax) of the conversion of a drug to the specific metabolite, which depends on the quantity of the enzyme, the enzyme structure, and any potential competing and non-competing drug interactions.

Cytochrome P-450 Enzymes

The cytochrome (CYP) system has been known and studied for more than 20 years and is responsible for the majority of drug metabolism (Meyer, 1996; Oesterheld & Shader, 1998; Pillans, 2001; Tanaka, 1999; Venkatakrishnan, Von Moltke, & Greenblatt, 2001; Why Bother About Cytochrome P-450 Enzymes, 2000). These metabolizing enzymes are located within the endoplasmic reticulum of the cell. The bulk of drug metabolism (and enzyme activity) occurs within the liver although drug metabolizing cytochromes can also be found in the kidney, small bowel, and brain (Bernard & Bruera, 2000; Krishna & Klotz, 1994). A tenfold or greater difference in drug clearance is noted from person to person as a result of genetic polymorphisms of specific enzymes. These polymorphisms govern individualized enzymatic actions on individual drugs (Bertz & Granneman, 1997).

Twenty families of cytochrome enzymes have been identified. The nomenclature for the enzyme family is given an Arabic number as its identifier. The individual enzyme is given an Arabic numeral after the letter, for example, CYP3A4. The most important cytochrome enzymes involved in 90% of drug metabolism are the CYP3A4, CYP2D6, CYP1A2, CYP2C9, and CYP2C19 enzymes (Oesterheld & Shader, 1998; Wrighton et al., 2000). The individual fraction of enzyme to total cytochrome isoforms (based on hepatic mass) are CYP3A4 30%, CYP2C 20%, CYP1A2 13%, and CPY2D 61% to 5% (Bertz & Granneman, 1997). Only a few cytochrome enzymes are involved in the vast majority of medications. These enzymes have wide drug specificity.

Drugs may be rotated within the active enzyme sites and become either oxidized or demethylated into one or several different metabolites by the same enzyme (Wrighton et al., 2000). Alternatively, many drugs are metabolized by more than one cytochrome enzyme. Methadone, for example, is metabolized by the CYP3A4, CYP2D6, CYP1A2, CYP2C9, and CYP2C19 enzymes, with CYP3A4 appearing to be the major enzyme for methadone metabolism. Medications can also activate enzyme production through induction by binding or interacting at the gene promoter sites (Plant & Gibson, 2003). This occurs particularly with CYP3A4 and CYP1A2 enzymes. Enzymes can be inhibited by competitive (reversible) or non-competitive (irreversible) drug binding to the enzyme active site. Non-competitive inhibition will be reversed only by regeneration of a new enzyme. Drug cytochrome interactions are further complicated by the fact that medications (or their metabolites) may simultaneously promote enzyme production and inhibit enzyme activity. Drugs may inhibit cytochromes for which they are not substrate (Inaba, Nebert, Burchell, et al., 1995; Ingelman-Sundberg, 2001; Plant & Gibson, 2003). Several of the cytochromes such as CYP2D6, CYP2C9, and CYP2C19 are subject to structural polymorphisms (structural enzyme mutations occurring in more than 1% of the population), which alter drug clearance and for which frequencies differ among ethnic groups (Bjornsson, Callaghan, Finolf, et al., 2003; Davis & Homsi, 2001; Ingelman-Sundberg, 2001; Jann & Cohen, 2000). Although structural polymorphisms have also been found with CYP3A4, none to date are clinically significant. Polymorphisms are in general a result of deoxyribonucleic acid (DNA) point mutations, ribonucleic acid (RNA) splice site differences, or gene deletions (Bernard & Bruera 2000; Ingelman-Sundberg, 2001).

ETHNICITY AND SPECIAL POPULATIONS

CYP3A4 and CYP1A2 activity does not differ with ethnicity. However, CYP2D6, CYP2C9, and CYP2C19 have distinctly different polymorphisms among Caucasians, Asians, and African-Americans. Poor metabolizers (related to CYP2D6) are found

in 6% to 10% of Caucasians but are rarely found among Asians or African-Americans. Both Asians and Africans have a high frequency of "slow metabolizing" CYP2D6 polymorphisms (Davis & Homsi, 2001). As a result, different ethnic groups may require lower doses of medications that are metabolized through CYP2D6 (such as amitriptyline). Amitriptyline requirements are usually lower for Asians and African-Americans because of the increased frequency of CYP2D6 #10 and CYP2D6 #17, respectively, which slowly metabolize medications relative to usual CYP2D6 isoenzymes (Davis & Homsi, 2001). On the other hand, a reduplication of the CYP2D6 gene occurs in individuals and may lead to ultra-rapid drug clearance. The inheritance of a reduplication (e.g., CYP2D6 #2) leads to a rapid clearance of drugs, and patients with this polymorphism may require higher than "usual" doses to maintain therapeutic levels (Davis & Homsi, 2001). Asians and Pacific Islanders have a different frequency of polymorphisms related to CYP2C9 and CYP2C19, which will influence metabolism of diazepam, phenytoin, and warfarin and thus may influence the frequency of drug interactions (Bjornsson et al., 2003).

P-450 SPECIFIC ENZYMES
CYP3A4

CYP3A4 enzyme levels are variably expressed among individuals and can be as great as tenfold to fortyfold (Bertz & Granneman, 1997). CYP3A4 is subject to enzyme induction by the classic anti-seizure medications (phenobarbital, carbamazepine, phenytoin), as well as dexamethasone and rifampin. CYP3A4 is inhibited by the azole antifungal agents (e.g., ketoconazole and macrolide antibiotics), as well as antidepressants within the selective serotonin reuptake inhibitor (SSRI) family, particularly fluoxamine. Grapefruit juice is an inhibitor of intestinal CYP3A4, which is relevant to first-pass metabolism and absorption in several medications. CYP3A4 has a high capacity to metabolize medications but has a low drug affinity. The CYP3A family of enzymes is found primarily in the kidney, placenta, intestine, lung, and brain (Bertz & Granneman, 1997), and unlike CYP2D6, no structural isoforms produce a clinical difference in pharmacokinetics. CYP3A4 metabolizes a wide range of drugs including alprazolam, triazolam, non-sedating antihistaminics, some calcium channel blockers, fentanyl, methadone, macrolide antibiotics, and several steroids, including corticosteroids such as dexamethasone and methylprednisolone (Bertz & Granneman, 1997).

CYP2D6

CYP2D6 has a significant number of allelic variants or polymorphisms that occur in different frequencies among ethnic groups. Metabolizer status has been determined in several studies by using a "probe" substrate such as dextromethoraphan or debrisoquine (Bertz & Granneman, 1997; Davis & Homsi, 2001; Jann & Cohen, 2000; Kroemer & Eichelbaum, 1995; Wong, Seah, & Lee, 2000). CYP2D6 mutations account for the large individual variation in drug metabolism. CYP2D6 is not inducible, unlike CYP3A4. CYP2D6 metabolizes beta blockers, haloperidol, resperidone, tricyclic antidepressants, fluoxetine, paroxetine, codeine, oxycodone, and tramadol. Major inhibitors of CYP2D6 are paroxetine, fluoxetine, and quinidine (Bertz & Granneman, 1997; Davis & Homsi, 2001; Van der Weide & Steijns, 1999).

Other CYP Isoenzymes

Two important members of the CYP2C family are CYP2C9 and CYP2C19. CYP2C9 metabolizes phenytoin and warfarin. Polymorphisms also exist for the CYP2C9 isoform, and enzyme induction is possible. CYP2C19 is responsible for metabolizing omeprazole, lansoprazole, and diazepam (Bertz & Granneman, 1997). Unlike CYP2D6 where poor metabolizers are found among Caucasians, CYP2C poor metabolizers are frequently found among Asians (Bertz & Granneman, 1997; Van der Weide & Steijns, 1999).

The CYP1A family is expressed in hepatic and extra-hepatic tissues, but the isoform CYP1A2 is found predominantly within the liver (Bertz & Granneman, 1997). CYP1A2 is known to activate carcinogens. CYP1A2 drug substrates include acetaminophen, theophylline, and caffeine. CYP1A2 enzyme expression is also induced by cigarette smoke. Paroxetine is a significant inhibitor (Bertz & Granneman, 1997).

Clinical Interactions

CYP2D6. The SSRIs paroxetine and fluoxetine significantly inhibit CYP2D6, which delays the clearance of tricyclic antidepressants and methadone and prevents the conversion of codeine and tramadol to their active analgesic metabolites (Bernard & Bruera, 2000; Davis & Homsi, 2001). Haloperidol increases plasma levels of tricyclic antidepressants through interactions at CYP2D6 (Tanaka, 1999). Oxycodone is an exception, although converted to oxymorphone by CYP2D6, it has no significant CYP2D6-related drug interactions since the main analgesic constituent is the parent drug (Davis, Varga, Dickerson, et al., 2003).

CYP1A2. Smoking acts like a drug and increases the clearance of methadone by induction of CYP1A2. Fluvoxamine is a strong inhibitor of CYP1A2 and causes methadone to accumulate by prolonging its half-life (Donnelly et al., 2002).

CYP3A4. The classic antiseizure medications induce CYP3A4 and will cause opioid withdrawal symptoms when patients are on stable doses of methadone (Donnelly et al., 2002). Ciprofloxacin and azole antifungals increase methadone levels by delaying clearance through CYP3A4 and CYP1A2. Fentanyl's clearance is delayed by cimetidine and erythromycin, both of which are potent inhibitors of CYP3A4 (Bernard & Bruera, 2000).

CYP2C19. Omeprazole increases phenytoin levels by blocking CYP2C19 (Patsalos, Froscher, Pisani, et al., 2002). Fluconazole inhibits phenytoin metabolism through CYP2C19 and CYP2C9 (Patsalos, Froscher, Pisani, et al., 2002).

CYP2C9. Classic antiseizure medications increase warfarin clearance through the induction of CYP2C9 (Patsalos et al., 2002). Refer to Appendix B for further information on specific medications and their respective metabolism.

METABOLISM THROUGH GLUCURONIDATION

Glucuronidation is another form of drug metabolism. Glucuronidation occurs within the liver and changes hydrophobic compounds into water-soluble metabolites (Tukey & Strassburg, 2000). Biologic substrates are bilirubin, bile acids, steroids, and thyroxine. Medications metabolized via glucuronidation include acetaminophen, morphine, hydromorphone, levorphanol, oxymorphone, codeine, NSAIDs, valproic acid, temazapam, oxapam, and lorazapam (Furlan, Demirdjian, Bourdon, et al., 1999). Certain glucuronidated medications become metabolically active such as what occurs when morphine is metabolized to morphine-6-glucuronide, a strong analgesic metabolite. Like the cytochrome enzymes, glucuronidation subfamilies exist and are indicated by the Arabic numeral (family), letter (subfamily), and Arabic numeral after the letter (individual enzyme) (Liston, Markowitz, & DeVane, 2001). For example, the UGT enzymes responsible for morphine metabolism are UGT2B7 and UGT1A3 (Radominska-Pandya, Czernik, Little, et al., 1999). Genetic polymorphisms for UGTs also exist, but their clinical significance is not well known (unlike the cytochrome system) (Bhasker, McKinnon, Stone, et al., 2000; Holthe, Klepstad, Zahlsen, et al., 2002; Mackenzie, Miners, & McKinnon, 2000). UGT enzymes are located within the luminal space of the endoplasmic reticulum, which functions to limit intracellular drug and glucuronide metabolite diffusion (Gueraud & Paris, 1998; Lin, Lu, Tang, et al., 2001; Radominska-Pandya et al., 1999). UGTs may be induced or inhibited similar to cytochrome enzymes. However, the degree of UGT drug interactions are less than cytochrome-mediated interactions.

Drug metabolism overlaps between the various UGT isoenzymes (Lin et al., 2001). Several isoforms of UGT can be found outside the liver (Straussburg, Kneip, Topp, et al., 2000). Intestinal UGTs (predominantly UGT1A1) play a role in intestinal first-pass metabolism. Intestinal expression of UGTs can vary sevenfold among individuals and can account for variations in UGT drug metabolism (Little, Lester, Kuipers, et al., 1999; Straussburg et al., 2000; Tukey & Strassburg, 2000). Renal UGTs are also capable of metabolizing a diverse number of drugs including furosemide and morphine (Perri et al., 2003; Pichette & Leblond, 2003).

Clinical Interactions

UGT. Morphine is metabolized into morphine-6-glucuronide by UGT2B7 and morphine-3-glucuronide by UGT1A3. However, amitriptyline, nortriptyline, and clomipramine inhibit UGT enzymes and decrease the formation of morphine metabolites and therefore inhibit their analgesic efficacy (Armstrong & Cozza 2003).

MULTIPLE DRUG TRANSPORTERS

Certain carrier proteins located on the plasma membranes efflux will reject certain medications from entering into the cell. These membrane pumps are natural defense barriers against potentially toxic xenobiotic agents (Johnson, 2002; Kruijtzer, Beijnen, & Schellens, 2002). Efflux proteins are adeonosine triposphate (ATP)–dependent and have a wide substrate specificity. The best known efflux pump is P-glycoprotein derived from the MDR_1 gene, but other transporters have also been described (multiple resistant proteins and mitoxantrone resistant protein) (Bodo, Bakos, Szeri, et al., 2003; Johnson, 2002). These carrier proteins are not involved in drug metabolism but limit intracellular concentrations of drugs by extruding them back into interstitial spaces similar to a sump pump. Efflux proteins are located along the blood brain barrier, small bowel, bile canaliculi, and kidney tubules. P-glycoprotein is usually located near CYP3A4 on the intestinal mucosa and has similar substrate specificity as CYP3A4 (Bodo et al., 2002). P-glycoprotein effluxes morphine-6-glucuronide and to a lesser extent methadone and fentanyl and is blocked by certain medications such as verapamil and cyclosporin. P-glycoprotein activity is induced by rifampin. As a result, P-glycoprotein will influence drug delivery to effector sites as well as alter intestinal absorption (bioavailability) (Bodo et al., 2002; Perri et al., 2003; Pichette & Leblond, 2003; Wrighton et al., 2000).

POLYPHARMACY AND DRUG INTERACTIONS

Drug interactions are the result of altered drug kinetics on the initial agent (recipient) by an offending co-medication (precipitant). Drug interactions can occur as a result of interference with absorption, influencing the volume of distribution, altered protein binding, or drug clearance or excretion. Pharmacodynamic interactions are competitive at receptor sites or synergistic because of activation of complementary receptors or through down-regulation of receptors. A precipitant may inhibit the recipient drug receptor, which counters the effect of the recipient drug action. An example is the action of glycopyrrolate, which inhibits the prokinetic activity of metoclopramide through blocking acetylcholine gut receptors. Another example is demonstrated in how ketamine blocks N-methyl-D-aspartate receptor activation that is induced by opioid receptor activation.

Drug interactions that interfere with absorption include drug binding and sequestration (such as occurs with kaolin and morphine) or changes in gut lumen pH (affecting omeprazole and methadone). Altering drug ionization can improve absorption by having the recipient drug in un-ionized form. Blocking P-glycoprotein increases absorption of certain medications, such as that which occurs with grapefruit juice and midazolam. Activation of P-glycoprotein by rifampin reduces morphine levels (through stimulation of P-glycoprotein), as well as morphine-6-glucuronide and morphine-3-glucuronide (through induction of UGT2B7) (Bernard & Bruera, 2000). As mentioned, important interactions at plasma protein binding sites are thought to be rare and are important only if the drug is highly protein bound and has a small volume of distribution and narrow therapeutic index (Bernard & Bruera, 2000).

By far the most common and serious interactions occur during biotransformation of drugs by the cytochrome system. The potential for medication interactions is highest when the recipient shares the same cytochrome isoenzyme or UGTs as the precipitant (Bjornsson et al., 2003). Drug interactions can be inhibitory, which prolongs the clearance of the recipient drug and is either reversible (competitive) or irreversible (non-competitive). Drug interactions may be through the enzyme induction of precipitant binding to gene promoter sites allowing for the transcription of the metabolizing enzyme. As an example, the promoter pregnane x receptor transcript governs CYP3A4 production and is activated by classic antiseizure medications such as carbamazepine, phenobarbital, and phenytoin (Plant & Gibson, 2003). Drug metabolites rather than the parent drug may act as a precipitant as occurs with norfloxentine and the CYP2D6 enzyme (Davis & Homsi, 2001). Drugs can be both an inhibitor and a promoter of the same cytochrome, as commonly seen with antiretrovirals.

If medications have a high presystemic metabolism with significant first-pass clearance and low post-hepatic bioavailability, the precipitant drug could produce a significant increase or decrease in drug effect with the first dose. However if the recipient drug has high oral bioavailability and low first-pass hepatic clearance, accumulation or reduction of recipient drug can be observed with repeated doses. Drug interactions in these circumstances will generally not be observed with initial doses of the precipitant and recipient (Dresser & Bailey, 2002).

Clinical Importance of Polypharmacy

Appropriate medications may be "inappropriate" when given in the wrong way, for a wrong reason, in a wrong dosage, or at inappropriate dosing intervals (Rochon & Gurwitz, 1995). It is easy to misinterpret an adverse drug event or poor drug response as progression of the underlying disease. Poor prescribing adds to the cost of care and increases the patient's symptom burden. It is even worse to prescribe another medication to treat a drug-drug interaction or adverse drug reaction rather than to correct the problem through drug elimination, drug reduction, or drug rotation (Rochon & Gurwitz, 1995). Some of the best prescribing may include drug subtraction through eliminating redundant drugs from the same class or interacting medications. Regular review of drug therapy is mandatory, and a single prescriber is preferred over many as a means to promote safe practice.

PHARMACOKINETICS IN SPECIAL POPULATIONS
Renal Insufficiency

Medications that depend on renal function for elimination will require dose reductions if renal insufficiency is present. Generally, if 50% or more of the drug elimination is related to glomerular filtration, dose reduction will be necessary as kidney function fails. For example, gabapentin is highly dependent upon renal function for elimination and dose schedules need to be adjusted to creatinine clearance (Birkett, 2003). However, medications not normally cleared by the kidneys may also have delayed elimination because of inhibition of liver cytochromes in the presence of uremia. For example, fentanyl clearance is reduced in renal failure despite the fact that it is not cleared by the kidneys because of decreased CYP3A4 activity in the setting of uremia (Dowling, Briglia, Fink, et al., 2003; Koehntop & Rodman, 1997). In addition, there is a down-regulation of certain isoforms of P-glycoprotein and reduction in UGTs with renal failure, which may increase the bioavailability and half-life of certain medications (Pichette & Leblond, 2003). See Chapter 8 for further discussion.

Hepatic Insufficiency

The influence of liver failure on drug metabolism depends on: (1) the dependence of a drug upon hepatic blood flow for first-pass clearance; (2) enzyme reserve (greater for CYP3A4 and UGTs than CYP2D6 and CYP1C9); and (3) extrahepatic enzyme levels (particularly CYP3A4 and UGTs) (Sonne, 1996; Tegeder, Lotsch, & Geisslinger, 1999). Patients with cirrhosis and reduced hepatic blood flow may have increased drug bioavailability with significant first-pass clearance (Birkett, 2003). As cited, morphine's bioavailability increases as liver blood flow diminishes (Donnelly et al., 2002; Tegeder et al., 1999). Protein binding diminishes as the production of albumin is reduced. This can in turn increase unbound drug concentrations, thereby increasing drug elimination and drug action until a new equilibrium is achieved (Birkett, 2003).

Gender

Recent studies have examined the role of gender in pharmacokinetics and drug distribution. Generally, females have more body fat, which can increase the volume of distribution for lipophilic drugs relative to men (Craft, 2003). The bioavailability of drugs dependent upon CYP3A for metabolism is higher in females. The activity of CYP2D6 is diminished in a female, which reduces the clearance of drugs like oxycodone, despiramine, and sertraline (Davis et al., 2003; Schwartz, 2003). Renal function as measured by glomerular filtration and tubular secretion is greater in men than in women when corrected for body size (Schwartz, 2003). Glucuronidation is also diminished in females (Schwartz, 2003). Hence gender-related differences in drug metabolism theoretically may lead to adverse drug reactions and drug-drug interactions. However, confounding factors such as age, disease, and co-medications have a greater influence on pharmacokinetics than differences in gender. In general, drug kinetic differences between genders range between 10% and 30% (AUC) and are unlikely to be clinically relevant (Schwartz, 2003).

SUMMARY

A basic understanding of pharmacology includes pharmacokinetics, pharmacodynamics, and pharmacogenetics. Prescribing without clinical evaluation and regard to polypharmacy guarantees adverse drug events and drug-drug interactions (Box 4-1). Such knowledge will enhance patient care by reducing symptom burden, improve the patient's quality of life, and minimize pharmaceutical risks.

Objective Questions

1. A 56-year-old female with lung cancer is prescribed morphine for metastatic bone pain. She is unable to swallow, and her morphine dose is reduced by 1/3 and given as an intermittent subcutaneous bolus. Regarding the dose intervals:

    a. Intervals by parenteral injection should be shorter because the drug half-life is shorter.
    b. Intervals by parenteral injection should be longer because the drug volume of distribution is larger.
    c. The steady state dose will depend on route of administration.
    d. Drug clearance and volume of distribution determine drug half-life and dosing interval, neither of which are dependent upon route of administration.

Box 4-1   RULES FOR GOOD PRESCRIBING

1. Diagnosis and assessment must precede prescribing.
2. Weigh the risks and benefits of drug therapy.
3. Begin with low doses, particularly for the elderly, for those with organ dysfunction, or with drugs that have a low therapeutic index.
4. Avoid prescribing several medications from the same class.
5. Use one drug for several symptoms if possible.
6. Periodically review medication lists and eliminate redundant or unnecessary medications.
7. Prescribe with the goals of care in mind. Patients who are dying will not benefit from antihypertensives, cardiovascular medications, lipid-lowering agents, or antibiotics.
8. Be aware of drug interactions that adversely affect patients.
9. Simplify the schedule to improve patient compliance.
10. Suspect medications as a cause of cognitive changes in the patient's condition.
11. Prescribe medications with known efficacy, and avoid being "marketed" into using newly released expensive medications unless there is a distinctive advantage over older medications.

2. A 62-year-old female is treated with methadone for cancer-related brachial plexopathy. She is experiencing 80% pain relief (EC-80) with methadone 20 mg every 8 hours. The most appropriate next step would be:

a. Continue to titrate methadone to complete pain relief.
b. Convert to parenteral methadone to improve the therapeutic index.
c. Rotate to alternative opioid because further increases of methadone will lead to toxicity.
d. Review by history her response and satisfaction with her pain response. Review to see if she is having any toxicity. Consider adding a non-interfering co-analgesic.

3. A 46-year-old male with glioblastoma multiforme (high-grade brain tumor) requires dexamethasone 8 mg daily. He develops seizures and is placed on phenytoin. One week later he redevelops neurologic deficits similar to what he had before dexamethasone. The most likely cause for this is:

a. Phenytoin induction of CYP3A4 with increased dexamethasone clearance.
b. Progressive tumor.
c. Radiation recall by phenytoin, leading to increased cerebral edema.
d. Poor absorption of dexamethasone caused by phenytoin.

4. A 32-year-old male has cerebral metastasis and requires phenytoin for seizure control. He is at home with hospice and can no longer swallow. The following medications are good alternatives to give per rectum except:

a. Diazepam.
b. Valproic acid.
c. Carbamazepine.
d. Gabapentin.

5. The most reasonable opioid to use on someone who is a poor metabolizer (homozygote for CYP2D6 mutations) is:

a. Tramadol.
b. Morphine.
c. Codeine.
d. None of the above.

6. A 60-year-old female with kidney cancer and chronic renal failure requiring dialysis requires antiseizure medications and pain control. The combination with the least risk for drug interactions and best safety margin is:

a. Morphine and carbamazepine.
b. Methadone and carbamazepine.
c. Methadone and valproic acid.
d. Morphine and valproic acid.

7. A 55-year-old Asian female is placed on amitriptyline for neuropathic pain related to post-herpetic neuralgia. She develops dry

mouth, urinary retention, and drowsiness with confusion when her dose is increased to 75 mg daily. The most reasonable treatment option is:

a. Add methylphenidate to reduce her drowsiness.
b. Add haloperidol to reduce her confusion.
c. Hold amitriptyline and obtain a blood level.
d. Order urine culture and two blood cultures and start antibiotics.

8. The following is true about morphine in cirrhosis:

a. Morphine protein binding to albumin is significantly impaired by jaundice, and the reduced albumin levels associated with reduced production will significantly alter morphine kinetics.
b. Morphine bioavailability is increased because of reduced hepatic blood flow associated with portal hypertension.
c. Morphine absorption is reduced because of bowel congestion from portal hypertension.
d. Morphine-6-glucuronide accumulates because of reduced bile flow.

9. The volume of distribution:

a. Is an actual volume.
b. Inversely relates to drug clearance.
c. Influences drug half-life.
d. Directly relates to biophase distribution.

10. Morphine kinetics in hepatic failure are altered predominantly because of:

a. Reduced OCI2B7.
b. Loss of total hepatic mass.
c. Reduced hepatic blood flow.
d. Ongoing enterohepatic recirculation.

11. The following is true about CYP2D6 except:

a. There are ethnic differences in CYP2D6 genetics.
b. It has no structural isomers.
c. It is important in morphine metabolism.

d. It can be inhibited by medications such as antidepressants, neuroleptics, and quinine.

12. Reasons for pharmaceutical failure in the management of cancer include:

a. Drug interactions.
b. Drug minimalization.
c. Cost.
d. All of the above.

REFERENCES

Armstrong, S.C., & Cozza, K.L. (2003). Pharmacokinetics drug interactions of morphine, codeine, and their derivatives: Theory and clinical reality, part I. *Psychosomatics, 44,* 167-171.

Bernard, S.A., & Bruera, E. (2000). Drug interactions in palliative care. *J Clin Oncol, 18*(8),1780-1799.

Bertz, R.J., & Granneman, G.R. (1997). Use of in vitro and in vivo data to estimate the likelihood of metabolic pharmacokinetic interactions. *Clin Pharmacokinet, 32*(3), 210-258.

Bhasker, C.R., McKinnon, W., Stone, A., et al. (2000). Genetic polymorphism of UDP-glucuronosyltransferase 2B7 (UGT2B7) at amino acid 268: Ethnic diversity of alleles and potential clinical significance. *Pharmacogenetics, 10*(8), 679-685.

Birkett, D.J. (2003). *Pharmacokinetics made easy.* Australia: McGraw-Hill.

Bjornsson, T.D., Callaghan, J.T., Einolf, H.J., et al. (2003). The conduct of in vitro and in vivo drug drug interaction studies: A PhRMA perspective. *J Clin Pharmacol, 43*(5), 443-469.

Bodo, A., Bakos, E., Szeri, F., et al. (2003). The role of multidrug transporters in drug availability, metabolism and toxicity. *Toxicol Lett, Apr. 11,* 140-141.

Chutka, D.S., Evans, J.M., Fleming, K.C., et al. (1995). Drug prescribing for elderly patients. *Mayo Clin Proc, 70*(7), 685-693.

Craft, R.M. (2003). Sex differences in drug- and non-drug-induced analgesia. *Life Sci, 72,* 2675-2688.

Davis, M.P., & Homsi, J. (2001). The importance of cytochrome P450 monooxygenase CYP2D6 in palliative medicine. *Support Care Cancer, 9,* 442-451.

Davis, M.P., Varga, K., Dickerson, D., et al. (2003). Normal-release and controlled-release oxycodone: Pharmacokinetics, pharmacodynamics, and controversy. *Support Care Cancer, 11,* 74-92.

Davis, M.P., & Walsh, D. (2001). Methadone for relief of cancer pain: A review of pharmacokinetics, pharmacodynamics, drug interactions and protocols of administration. *Support Care Cancer, 9,* 72-83.

Donnelly, S., Davis, M.P., Walsh, D., et al. (2002). Morphine in cancer pain management: A practical guide. *Support Care Cancer, 10,* 13-35.

Dowling, T.C., Briglia, A.E., Fink, J.C., et al. (2003). Characterization of hepatic cytochrome P4503A activity in patients with end-stage renal disease. *Clin Pharmacol Ther, 73,* 427-434.

Dresser, G.K., & Bailey, D.G. (2002). A basic conceptual and practical overview of interactions with highly prescribed drugs. *Can J Clin Pharmacol, 9*(4), 191-198.

Fromm, M.F., Eckhardt, K., Li, S., et al. (1997). Loss of analgesic effect of morphine due to coadministration of rifampin. *Pain, 72*(1-2), 261-267.

Furlan, V., Demirdjian, S., Bourdon, O., et al. (1999). Glucuronidation of drugs by hepatic microsomes derived from healthy and cirrhotic human livers. *J Pharmacol Exp Ther, 289*(2), 1169-1175.

Gueraud, F., & Paris, A. (1998). Glucuronidation: A dual control. *Gen Pharmacol, 31*(5), 683-688.

Holthe, M., Klepstad, P., Zahlsen, K., et al. (2002). Morphine glucuronide-to-morphine plasma ratios are unaffected by the UGT2B7 H268Y and UGT1A1*28 polymorphisms in cancer patients on chronic morphine therapy. *Eur J Clin Pharmacol, 58*, 353-356.

Inaba, T., Nebert, D.W., Burchell, B., et al. (1995). Pharmacogenetics in clinical pharmacology and toxicology. *Can J Physiol Pharmacol, 73*(3), 331-338.

Ingelman-Sundberg, M. (2001). Genetic susceptibility to adverse effects of drugs and environmental toxicants: The role of the CYP family of enzymes. *Mutat Res, 482*, 11-19.

Jann, M.W., & Cohen, L.J. (2000). The influence of ethnicity and antidepressant pharmacogenetics in the treatment of depression. *Drug Metabol Drug Interact, 16*(1), 39-67.

Johnson, W.W. (2002). P-glycoprotein–mediated efflux as a major factor in the variance of absorption and distribution of drugs: Modulation of chemotherapy resistance. *Methods Find Exp Clin Pharmacol, 24*(8), 501-514.

Koehntop, D.E., & Rodman, J.H. (1997). Fentanyl pharmacokinetics in patients undergoing renal transplantation. *Pharmacotherapy, 17*(4), 746-752.

Krishna, D.R., & Klotz, U. (1994). Extrahepatic metabolism of drugs in humans. *Clin Pharmacokinet, 26*(2), 144-160.

Kroemer, H.K., & Eichelbaum, M. (1995). "It's the genes stupid." Molecular bases and clinical consequences of genetic cytochrome P450 2D6 polymorphism. *Life Sci, 56*(36), 2285-2298.

Kruijtzer, C.M.F., Beijnen, J.H., & Schellens, J.H.M. (2002). Improvement of oral drug treatment by temporary inhibition of drug transporters and/or cytochrome P450 in the gastrointestinal tract and liver: An overview. *Oncologist, 7*, 516-530.

Levy, G. (1998). Impact of pharmacodynamic variability on drug delivery. *Adv Drug Deliv Rev, 33*, 201-206.

Lin, Y., Lu, P., Tang, C., et al. (2001). Substrate inhibition kinetics for cytochrome P450-catalyzed reactions. *Drug Metab Dispos, 29*(4 Pt. 1), 368-374.

Liston, H.L., Markowitz, J.S., & DeVane, C.L. (2001). Drug glucuronidation in clinical psychopharmacology. *J Clin Psychopharmacol, 21*(5), 500-515.

Little, J.M., Lester, R., Kuipers, F., et al. (1999). Variability of human hepatic UDP-glucuronosyltransferase activity. *Acta Biochem Pol, 42*(6), 351-363.

Mackenzie, P.I., Miners, J.O., & McKinnon, R.A. (2000). Polymorphisms in UDP glucuronosyltransferase genes: Functional consequences and clinical relevance. *Clin Chem Lab Med, 38*(9), 889-892.

Meyer, U.A. (1996). Overview of enzymes of drug metabolism. *J Pharmacokinet Biopharm, 24*(5), 449-459.

Oesterheld, J.R., & Shader, R.I. (1998). Cytochromes: A primer for child and adolescent psychiatrists. *J Am Acad Child Adolesc Psychiatry, 37*(4), 447-450.

Paalzow, L.K. (1982). Pharmacokinetic aspects of optimal pain treatment. *Acta Anesthesiol Scand Suppl, 74*, 37-43.

Patsalos, P.N., Froscher, W., Pisani, F., et al. (2002). The importance of drug interactions in epilepsy therapy. *Epilepsia, 43*(4), 365-385.

Perri, D., Ito, S., Rowsell, V., et al. (2003). The kidney: The body's playground for drugs: An overview of renal drug handling with selected clinical correlates. *Can J Clin Pharmacol, 10*(1), 17-23.

Pichette, V., & Leblond, F.A. (2003). Drug metabolism in chronic renal failure. *Curr Drug Metab, 4*, 91-103.

Pillans, P.I. (2001). Increasing relevance of pharmacogenetics of drug metabolism in clinical practice. *Intern Med J, 31*(8), 476-478.

Plant, N.J., & Gibson, G.G. (2003). Evaluation of the toxicological relevance of CYP3A4 induction. *Curr Opin Drug Discov Devel, 6*(1), 50-56.

Radominska-Pandya, A., Czernik, P.J., Little, J.M., et al. (1999). Structural and functional studies of UDP-glucuronosyltransferases. *Drug Metab Rev, 31*(4), 817-899.

Roberts, M.S., Magnusson, B.M., Burczynski, F.J., et al (2002). Enterhepatic circulation: Physiological, pharmacokinetic and clinical implications. *Clin Pharmacokinet, 41*(10), 751-790.

Rochon, P.A., & Gurwitz, J.H. (1995). Drug therapy. *Lancet North Am Ed, 346*(8966), 32-36.

Schwartz, J.B. (2003). The influence of sex on pharmacokinetics. *Clin Pharmacokinet, 42*(2), 107-121.

Sonne, J. (1996). Drug metabolism in liver disease: Implications for therapeutic drug monitoring. *Ther Drug Monit, 18*(4), 397-401.

Straussburg, C.P., Kneip, S., Topp, J., et al. (2000). Polymorphic gene regulation and interindividual variation of UDP-glucuronosyltransferase activity in human small intestine. *Biol Chem, 275*(46), 36164-36171.

Tanaka, E. (1999). Update: Genetic polymorphism of drug metabolizing enzymes in humans. *Clin Pharmacol Ther, 24*(5), 323-329.

Tegeder, I., Lotsch, J., & Geisslinger, G. (1999). Pharmacokinetics of opioids in liver disease, *Clin Pharmacokinet, 37*(1), 17-40.

Tukey, R.H., & Strassburg, C.P. (2000). Human UDP-glucuronosyltransferase: Metabolism, expression, and disease. *Annu Rev Pharmacol Toxicol, 40*, 581-616.

Urso, R., Blardi, P., & Giorgi, G. (2002). A short introduction to pharmacokinetics. *Eur Rev Med Pharmacol Sci, 6*, 33-44.

Van der Weide, J., & Steijns, L.S. (1999). Cytochrome P450 enzyme system: Genetic polymorphisms and impact on clinical pharmacology. *Ann Clin Biochem, 36*(Pt. 6), 722-729.

Venkatakrishnan, K., Von Moltke, L.L., & Greenblatt, D.J. (2001). Human drug metabolism and the cytochromes P450: Application and relevance of in vitro models. *J Clin Pharmacol, 41*(11), 1149-1179.

Venkatesan, K. (1992). Pharmacokinetic drug interactions with rifampicin. *Clin Pharmacokinet, 22*(1), 47-65.

Why bother about cytochrome P450 enzymes? (2000). *Drug Ther Bull, 38*(12), 93-95.

Wong, J.Y., Seah, E.S., & Lee, E.J. (2000). Pharmacogenetics: The molecular genetics of CYP2D6 dependent drug metabolism. *Ann Acad Med Singapore, 29*(3), 401-406.

Wrighton, S.A., Schuetz, E.G., Thummel, K.E., et al. (2000). The human CYP3A subfamily: Practical considerations. *Drug Metab Rev, 32*(3-4), 339-361.

CHAPTER 5

The Interface of Sleep

Kathy P. Parker

OBJECTIVES

After the completion of this chapter, the reader should be able to:

1. Discuss normal sleep and common sleep disorders.
2. Describe the sleep of selected clinical populations often seen in the palliative care setting and related factors that have the potential to impair sleep.
3. Identify research-based interventions designed to optimize sleep.

INTRODUCTION

Throughout the millennia, poets, philosophers, scientists, and literary figures have been fascinated by sleep (Thorpy, 1991). Although most recognized it as an essential human need, the phenomenon itself has been poorly understood. Before the twentieth century, many believed that sleep was a simple, passive phenomenon, similar in many aspects to death, and often valued it for its mystical properties (Thorpy, 1991). Today, sleep is described as an active process and one that is regulated by numerous behavioral, neuroendocrine, and central nervous system factors (Carskadan & Dement, 2000). It is also well appreciated that sleep deprivation and/or disruption of sleep can adversely affect important clinical outcomes such as quality of life and functional health status (Newman, Spiekerman, Enright, et al., 2000; Nugent, Gleadhill, McCrum, et al., 2001; Whitney, Enright, Newman, et al., 1998). Yet, in spite of numerous scientific advances recently made in the field, much remains to be discovered about the nature and purposes of sleep.

The goal of palliative care is "to provide symptom control and supportive care for patients and their families when cure is no longer the goal of therapy" (Rozans, Dreisbach, Lertora, et al., 2002, p. 35). Unfortunately, although sleep can play a major role in optimizing these goals, the manner in which sleep interfaces with the palliative care experience has received little, if no, attention. In this setting, numerous factors can have significant detrimental effects on a patient's sleep as well as his or her ability to stay awake and alert during the day. In addition, a patient's sleep problems often affect the sleep of family members and others who provide care—compounding an already difficult situation (Carter, 2002, 2003).

Nurses can play an important role in the development of a plan of care that promotes sleep, optimizes waking, and maximizes life quality for patients and their caregivers. This chapter provides a brief review of normal sleep and sleep disorders, highlights the sleep problems of selected clinical populations often seen in the palliative care setting, and discusses related factors that are associated with impaired sleep. In addition, research-based interventions designed to optimize sleep are presented.

NORMAL SLEEP

Definition

Sleep is defined as "a reversible behavioral state of perceptual disengagement from and unresponsiveness to the environment" (Carskadan & Dement, 2000). Sleep is further defined according to both behavioral and physiologic criteria. Behavioral criteria include the following: closed eyes, decreased response to external stimuli, recumbent position, quiescence, and reversible unconsciousness (Carskadan & Dement, 2000; Chokroverty, 1999; Tobler, 1995). The physiologic criteria are based on polysomnographic recordings

(Table 5-1 and Figure 5-1) (Rechtschaffen & Kales, 1968). Although these definitions and criteria certainly address the phenomenon, they fail to capture the meaning and significance that sleep has within the context of life. Thus subjective measures or descriptions of a person's experience with sleep are also recognized as important in defining the state.

Measurement of Sleep

Subjective measures of sleep can be particularly useful for assessing, screening, and evaluating the effects of treatment (Cohen, 1997). They typically include an individual's assessment of sleep latency (time it takes to fall asleep), number of awakenings, depth and length of sleep, refreshing quality of sleep, satisfaction with sleep, and soundness of sleep (Shaver & Giblin, 1989). This information can be collected through the use of sleep questionnaires (Buysse, Reynolds, Monk, et al., 1989, 1991; Ellis, Johns, Lancaster, et al., 1981), sleep diaries, visual analog scales (Parrott & Hindmarch, 1980), and interviews (Shaver & Giblin, 1989).

Another method sometimes used to measure both sleep and wake patterns is actigraphy (Ancoli-Israel, Cole, Alessi, et al., 2003). Using a wrist-watch-size microprocessor that senses movement, continuous motion recordings can be obtained for long periods. Computer algorithms permit analysis of activity and rest, as well as sleep and wakefulness (Pollak, Tryon, Nagaraja, et al., 2001). Although actigraphy cannot determine sleep stages, information on total sleep time, percent of time spent awake, number of awakenings, time between awakenings, and sleep onset latency can be obtained. Actigraphy data may correlate well with polysomnography (PSG) data, particularly when sleep is normal (Ancoli-Israel et al., 2003; Jean-Louis, von Gizycki, Zizi, et al., 1996).

The gold standard for the measurement of sleep is PSG, a procedure involving the simultaneous recording of the electroencephalograph (EEG), the electromyograph (EMG), and the electrooculograph (EOG). In addition, PSG often includes the measurement of other physiologic parameters, such as respiratory movements of the chest and abdomen, airflow at the nose and mouth, arterial oxygen saturation, electrocardiogram (ECG), and leg movements (anterior tibialis EMG).

PSG has demonstrated that there are two kinds of sleep: non-rapid-eye-movement sleep (NREM; 75% to 80% of sleep period) and rapid-eye-movement sleep (REM; 20% to 25% of sleep period)(see Table 5-1 and Figure 5-1). NREM sleep includes stage 1, stage 2, and stages 3 and 4 collectively referred to as *slow-wave sleep* (*SWS*). Measures typically obtained during PSG include sleep latency (SL) or the time taken to fall asleep, latency to the various sleep stages, the percent of time spent in each of the stages, the distribution of the sleep stages of the total sleep time (TST), sleep efficiency (SE) or the time spent sleeping while in bed, and numbers of brief arousals and awakenings (Carskadon & Rechtschaffen, 2000).

A PSG is scored by examining each recorded page or "epoch" of the recording. At the usual recording speed of 1 centimeter/second (cm/sec), a standard 30-cm page represents a 30-sec epoch. Each epoch is assigned a sleep stage based on changes in EEG frequency (in cycles/sec, or hertz [Hz]) and amplitude (in microvolts [μV]) and the EOG and EMG patterns (Rechtschaffen & Kales, 1968) (see Figure 5-1).

Stages of Sleep

Stage 1 is a transitional phase between wakefulness and sleep and is characterized by low-amplitude, mixed-frequency EEG activity and a level of muscle tone somewhat lower than that of relaxed wakefulness. Some individuals experience myoclonic (hypnic) jerks of the arms, legs, or entire body accompanied by dreamlike mentation (e.g., falling). These jerks are normal but can increase in frequency during stress, opioid toxicities, or in response to a fragmented sleep schedule. During stage 1 sleep, reactivity to outside stimuli is diminished, mental processes change, thoughts begin to drift, thinking is less "reality-oriented," and short dreams often develop. Many people feel that they are awake during this stage because they are easily aroused. In normal sleepers, stage 1 usually represents 2% to 5% of the sleep period.

Table 5-1 A GLOSSARY OF SLEEP-RELATED TERMS

Actigraphy:	A biomedical instrument used to measure body movement.
Apnea:	Cessation of airflow at the nostrils and mouth lasting at least 10 seconds. The three types of apnea are obstructive, central, and mixed. Obstructive apnea is secondary to upper airway obstruction; central apnea is associated with a lack of respiratory effect; mixed apnea has both central and obstructive components. The severity of the apneic condition is typically described in terms of the number of apneic events per hour of sleep, or the respiratory disturbance index (RDI). Five events per hour of sleep (RDI >5) is considered pathologic.
Arousal:	An abrupt change (3-14 sec) from a "deeper" stage of NREM sleep to a "lighter" stage, or from REM sleep to wakefulness.
Circadian rhythm:	An innate daily fluctuation of physiologic or behavior functions, including sleep-wake states, generally tied to the 24-hour daily light-dark cycle. This rhythm sometimes occurs at a measurably different periodicity (e.g., 23 or 25 hrs) when light-dark and other time cues are removed.
Deep sleep:	A common term for NREM stages 3 and 4 (also called *delta* or *slow-wave sleep; SWS*).
Entrainment:	Synchronization of a biologic rhythm by a reinforcing stimulus such as an environmental time cue (zeitgeber) (see below).
Excessive daytime sleepiness:	Difficulty in maintaining the alert, awake state, usually accompanied by a rapid entrance into sleep when the person is sedentary; somnolence, hypersomnia.
Insomnia:	Difficulty in initiating or maintaining sleep, waking up too early in the morning, or feeling unrefreshed after a night's sleep.
NREM sleep:	Non-rapid-eye-movement sleep; divided into four stages, 1 through 4.
Periodic limb movement disorder:	A disorder characterized by periodic episodes of repetitive and highly stereotyped limb movements that occur during sleep. The leg movements are typically 0.5 to 5 seconds in duration and occur approximately every 20 to 40 seconds. The severity of the condition is described in terms of leg movements per hour of sleep (periodic limb movement index, PLMI), and a PLMI ≥5 is considered abnormal.
REM sleep:	Rapid-eye-movement sleep.
Restless legs syndrome:	A disorder characterized by disagreeable leg sensations that usually occur prior to sleep onset and that cause an almost irresistible urge to move the legs. The sensations are typically worse in the evening and are relieved by movement.
Sleep apnea syndrome:	A disorder characterized by repetitive episodes of reduced or absent respiratory airflow that occur during sleep and that are usually associated with a reduction in blood oxygen level.
Sleep architecture:	The NREM-REM sleep-stage and cycles.
Sleep efficiency (SE):	The proportion of sleep in the episode filled by sleep; the ratio of total sleep time (TST) to time in bed.
Sleep hygiene:	The conditions and practices that promote continuous and effective sleep.
Sleep latency (SL):	The time from lights out to onset of sleep defined as the first of three consecutive epochs of stage1sleep or the first epoch of any other stage of sleep.
Total sleep time (TST):	The amount of actual sleep time in a sleep episode; the time is equal to the total sleep episode less the awake time.
Zeitgeber:	An environmental time cue, such as sunlight, noise, social interaction, alarm clocks, that usually helps an individual entrain to the 24-hour day.

Data from American Sleep Disorders Association (ASDA) (1997). *The International Classification of Sleep Disorders.* Rochester, Minn.: Author; Vena, C., Parker, K.P., Cunningham,, M., et al (2004). Sleep-wake disturbances in people with cancer. Part 1: An overview of sleep, sleep regulation, and effects of disease and treatment. *Oncol Nurs Forum,* 31(4):735-746.

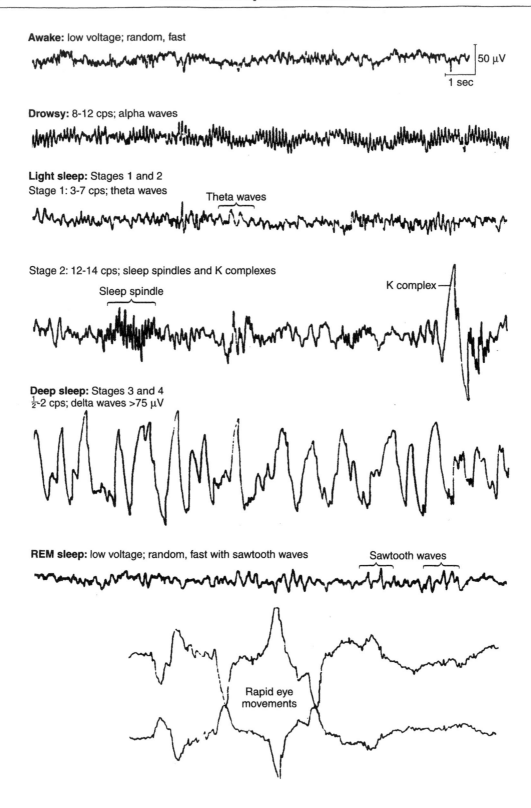

Awake: low voltage; random, fast

50 µV

1 sec

Drowsy: 8-12 cps; alpha waves

Light sleep: Stages 1 and 2
Stage 1: 3-7 cps; theta waves

Theta waves

Stage 2: 12-14 cps; sleep spindles and K complexes

Sleep spindle

K complex

Deep sleep: Stages 3 and 4
$\frac{1}{2}$-2 cps; delta waves >75 µV

REM sleep: low voltage; random, fast with sawtooth waves

Sawtooth waves

Rapid eye
movements

Stage 2 is marked by distinct EEG changes including the appearance of "sleep spindles" (brief bursts of EEG activity), large amounts of theta waves (4 to 7 Hz or cycles/sec), and K complexes (EEG wave forms consisting of a high amplitude, negative sharp wave immediately followed by a positive wave) (see Figure 5-1). Muscle tone is slightly more reduced, eye movements are absent, and mentation consists of short, mundane, and fragmented thoughts. Stage 2 typically makes up 45% to 55% of the sleep period.

Stages 3 and 4 are distinguished by high-amplitude, slow-frequency delta waves (0.5 to 2 Hz or cycles/sec), making up 20% to 50% of the epoch, respectively (see Figure 5-1). Of the NREM stages, SWS is the deepest; random stimuli will usually not arouse the individual. As in stage 2, eye movements are typically absent during stages 3 and 4; EMG activity remains at a decreased level compared with wakefulness. During SWS, the cardiac and respiratory rates, metabolic rate, and blood pressure decrease to basal levels. Growth hormone (GH) is secreted by the anterior pituitary, and levels of other anabolic hormones, such as prolactin and testosterone, are high. Thus NREM sleep may be a time of energy conservation, body renewal, and tissue building.

The EEG pattern of REM sleep resembles that of NREM stage 1 and is characterized by low-amplitude, mixed-frequency EEG activity (see Figure 5-1). However, there are bursts of binocularly symmetric eye movements that give REM sleep its name. The EMG is essentially flat because of hyperpolarization of motor neurons in the brainstem and spinal cord, which causes loss of muscle tone (Siegel, 2000). Blood pressure, heart rate, cardiac output, and respiratory rate become erratic. Oxygen consumption and cerebral blood flow increase. In about 80% of awakenings from REM sleep, people recall dreams, whereas only about 5% of NREM awakenings result in dream reports. Many believe that REM sleep provides psychologic renewal and/or memory consolidation.

Sleep usually progresses through repetitive cycles beginning with NREM stages 1 through 4, back again to stage 2, and subsequently into REM (Figure 5-2). These cycles occur approximately every 70 to 120 minutes in the adult, with four to five cycles normally completed during a sleep period. NREM sleep dominates the first third of the sleep period, whereas REM periods increase in length later in the sleep period. This may explain why morning naps are frequently composed of REM sleep whereas those in the afternoon are more often NREM sleep. After prolonged wakefulness, SWS increases during the first night with recovery of REM sleep postponed to the second or third night.

Sleep in Aging

Age has been shown to be one of the most powerful determinants of sleep patterns (Bliwise, 2000) (Figure 5-3). Children typically have very efficient sleep and have maximal amounts of SWS. SWS decreases markedly during the second decade of life, a decline that continues into old age. REM sleep percentage remains relatively constant across the life span unless a cognitive impairment or medical condition that decreases REM is present. Arousals (see Table 5-1) from sleep markedly increase with age and may contribute to the poor subjective sleep quality often experienced by elders. Physiologic age, however, is not always an accurate reflection of chronologic age, and thus age in years itself may not necessarily predict sleep quality.

FIGURE 5-1 Electroencephalogram patterns in wakefulness and sleep in a young adult. *Awake to Drowsy:* Rhythmic alpha-wave activity at 8 to 10 Hz in relaxed wakefulness with the eyes closed. *Stage 1:* Mixed-frequency, relatively low-amplitude waves with a vertex sharp wave toward the end of the tracing. *Stage 2:* K complex and sleep spindles begin in stage 2. *Stages 3 and 4:* Progressively greater percentages of slow, high-amplitude waves. *REM:* Mixed-frequency, relatively low-amplitude waves in rapid-eye-movement sleep, similar to the pattern in stage 1 appear in REM sleep; rapid eye movements that are characteristic of REM sleep; EMG inhibition characteristic of REM. *cps,* Cycles per second; *μV,* microvolt. (From Lee, K. [1999]. In C. Lindeman & M. McAthie [Eds.]. *Fundamentals of contemporary nursing practice.* Philadelphia: Saunders.)

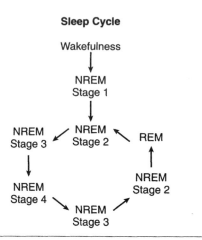

Sleep Cycle

FIGURE 5-2 Sleep cycle. Sleep usually progresses through repetitive cycles beginning with NREM stages 1 through 4, back again to stages 3 and 2, and subsequently into REM. These cycles occur approximately every 70 to 120 minutes in the adult, with four to five cycles normally completed during a sleep period.

Sleep in the elderly, for example, may actually be more adversely affected by co-morbidities and sleep disorders, such as sleep apnea and periodic leg movements (see Table 5-1), which are common in older adults and can cause significant sleep disruption (Ancoli-Israel, 2000; Ancoli-Israel, Kripke, Klauber, et al., 1991b; Ancoli-Israel, Martin, Kripke, et al., 2002; Cohen-Zion, Stepnowsky, Marler, et al., 2001). Other factors contributing to sleep disruption in the elderly may include poor sleep habits, a reduced activity level, psychologic concerns, and medications (Bliwise, 2000). Older people often complain about their sleep and use sleeping pills more often than other age-groups (Wysowski & Baum, 1991). Although women maintain their SWS longer than men, they complain more often of difficulty falling asleep and midsleep awakenings. In contrast, men are more likely to complain of daytime sleepiness (Ancoli-Israel, 2000).

Preferences for the timing of a sleep period within the 24-hour day may also vary with age. Adolescents, for example, often prefer to go to bed later and sleep later, a pattern referred to as *delayed sleep phase syndrome* ("night owls"). Carskadon and Acebo (2002) noted that this is most likely caused by biologic factors (e.g., the timing of melatonin or sex hormone secretion) rather than social factors. The sleep loss that can result (related to the need for early rise times to attend school, etc.) may adversely affect mood, ability to learn, behavior, and the use of drugs and alcohol (Carskadon, 1990). This condition can continue into adulthood and interfere with daytime function. In contrast, older patients often prefer to go to bed and get up earlier (*advanced sleep phase syndrome* ["morning larks"]) and complain of not being able to stay awake long enough in the evening to enjoy family and social activities. By assisting individuals to schedule their sleep period with consideration of possible age-related or developmental preferences can help avoid unrealistic expectations (on the part of the patient as well as the caregivers) regarding sleep and can enhance subjective sleep quality.

The Function of Sleep

Major controversy still exists over the exact function of sleep. Some suggest that it is important for mental and physical restoration (Adam & Oswald, 1984), energy conservation (Zepelin & Rechtschaffen, 1974), memory reinforcement and consolidation (Crick & Mitchison, 1983), and/or the maintenance of synaptic and neuronal network function (Kavanau, 1997, 2000; Krueger & Obal, 2002; Zepelin & Rechtschaffen, 1974). Others propose that, during waking, humoral factors accumulate in the blood that induce tiredness and then are removed by sleep (Jones, 2000). Horne (1988) suggests that sleep is a state of decreased activity and protein conservation caused by the lack of food intake during the night. Some have even wondered if sleep is necessary at all (Baker, 1985). Despite the conflicting reports regarding the function of and need for sleep, it is generally agreed that there is a physiologic imperative to sleep in human beings and that the "drive to sleep can be as strong as the drive to breathe" (Bonnet, 2000, p. 67).

Sleep deprivation studies have been used extensively to help uncover the function of sleep. Early studies suggested that keeping healthy young subjects awake for an entire night made them very sleepy but had almost no effect on their next-day performance (Patrick & Gilbert, 1986). More recent studies have shown that sleep deprivation is associated with fatigue, changes in mood and cognitive

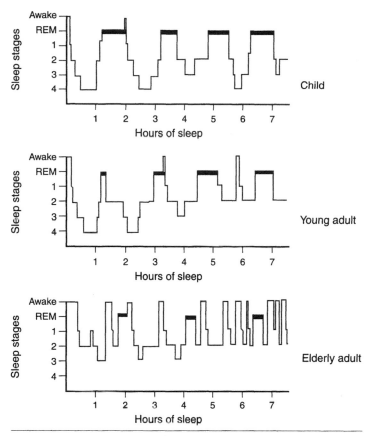

FIGURE 5-3 Sleep across the life span. Normal sleep cycles in children, young adults, and the elderly. Rapid-eye-movement (REM) sleep (*darkened area*) occurs cyclically throughout the night at intervals of approximately 90 minutes in all age-groups and shows little variation in the different age-groups, whereas stage 4 non-REM (NREM) sleep decreases with age. In addition, the elderly have frequent awakenings and a marked increase in total wake. (From Lee, K. [1999]. In C. Lindeman & M. McAthie [Eds.], *Fundamentals of contemporary nursing practice.* Philadelphia: Saunders.)

performance, increased illness, increased sensitivity to pain, restlessness, disorientation, combativeness, delusions, and hallucinations (Adam & Oswald, 1984; Anderson, Getto, Mendoza, et al., 2003; Dinges, Pack, Williams, et al., 1997; Hong & Dimsdale, 2003; Miller, 2003; Nicassio, Moxham, Schuman, et al., 2002). Sleep loss may also affect survival. Kripke (2003) recently demonstrated an increased risk of mortality associated with chronic nocturnal sleep periods of 6 hours or less. In a 10-year follow-up from the National Health and Nutrition Examination Survey (NHANES) I,

Qureshi, Giles, Croft, et al. (1997) also found an increase in stroke in persons who reported more than 8 hours or less than 6 hours of sleep per night. Increased napping has also been associated with increased mortality in the elderly (Bursztyn, Ginsberg, Hammerman-Rozenberg, et al., 1999; Bursztyn, Ginsberg, & Stessman, 2002).

There appears to be an important relationship between sleep and thermoregulation, an observation supported by the finding that SWS at night (a brain and body cooling state) increases after exposure to body warming (Horne & Reid, 1985;

Szymusiak & McGinty, 1990; Szymusiak, Steininger, Alam, et al., 2001). In addition, a decline in core body temperature is typically associated with and may *precede* not only nocturnal sleep onset but also the actual decision to go to bed (Campbell & Broughton, 1994; van den Heuvel, Noone, Lushington, et al., 1998; Van Someren, 2000). Sleep offset and wakefulness are associated with a core body temperature increase (Czeisler, Weitzman, Moore-Ede, et al., 1980; Gillberg & Akerstedt, 1982; Zulley, Wever, & Aschoff, 1981). Body temperature also has prominent effects on sleep architecture as REM sleep is closely linked to the nadir of the body temperature rhythm (Glotzbach & Heller, 2000). The interaction of sleep and temperature appears to be directly related to feedback systems between thermoregulatory and hypnogenic controls located in the preoptic anterior hypothalamus (POAH) and the suprachiasmatic nucleus (SCN) (McGinty & Szymusiak, 1990; Van Someren, 2000).

Sleep may also play an important role in immune function (Benca, Kushida, Everson, et al., 1989; Dinges, Douglas, Hamarman, et al., 1995; Savard, Laroche, Simard, et al., 2003). Many immune factors released during infections, such as interleukin-1, interleukin-2, and tumor necrosis factor-α (TNF-α) (which have both somnogenic and pyrogenic properties), have been shown to promote SWS, possibly because of the associated increased heat production (Krueger & Obal, 2002). This interaction of thermoregulatory and immunologic process may explain why people become sleepy when febrile. Compelling evidence that sleep loss adversely affects immune function comes from a number of animal and human studies. For example, chronically sleep-deprived rats have been shown to spontaneously die in a matter of weeks (Everson, Bergmann, & Rechtschaffen, 1989; Rechtschaffen & Bergmann, 1995; Rechtschaffen, Gilliland, Bergmann, et al., 1983). Septicemia, resulting from a decreased resistance to pathogens, was the suspected cause of death (Everson & Toth, 2000; Rechtschaffen, Bergmann, Everson, et al., 2002). If allowed to sleep normally before death occurred, the rats experienced reversal of most of the sleep deprivation–induced changes and survived. Human studies also suggest that sleep loss compromises host immune

defense responses (Palmblad, Petrini, Wasserman, et al., 1979; Spiegel, Sheridan, & Van Cauter, 2002). Strong correlations between a decrease in sleep, reduced natural killer (NK) cell activity, and an increased susceptibility to viral infections have been reported (Biron, 1997; Biron, Nguyen, Pien, et al., 1999; Biron, Su, & Orange, 1996).

The Regulation of Sleep

According to the Two-Process Model of Sleep Regulation (Borbely & Acherman, 2000), the major mechanisms controlling sleep and waking across time are (1) a *homeostatic process* (process S), determined by prior sleep and waking; and (2) a *circadian process* (process C), which designates periods of high and low sleep propensity. The homeostatic process reflects the physiologic need for sleep, which builds across the day and dissipates throughout the night (Figure 5-4). A key indicator of this process is SWS, which is greatest in amount during the beginning of a sleep episode but declines as the

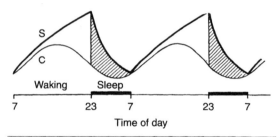

FIGURE 5-4 The Two-Process Model of Sleep Regulation. According to the Two-Process Model of Sleep Regulation, the major mechanisms controlling sleep and waking across time are (1) a homeostatic process (process S) determined by prior sleep and waking; and (2) a circadian process (process C), which designates periods of high and low sleep propensity. The homeostatic process reflects the physiologic need for sleep, which builds across the day and dissipates throughout the night. The circadian process, a sinusoidal rhythm of approximately 24 hours, is controlled by a biologic oscillator (suprachiasmatic nucleus). (From Borbely, A.A., & Acherman, P. [2000]. Sleep homeostasis and models of sleep regulation. In M.H. Kryger, T. Roth, & W.C. Dement [Eds.], *Principles and practice of sleep medicine* [3rd ed., p. 384]. Philadelphia: Saunders.)

night progresses. The circadian process, a sinusoidal rhythm of approximately 24 hours, is controlled by a biologic oscillator (suprachiasmatic nucleus). This process regulates sleep propensity, and its effects are greatest in the early morning hours and to a lesser extent in the late afternoon. The rhythm of core body temperature (which decreases at night), melatonin secretion, and cortisol production are key indicators of the circadian process. External cues (zeitgebers) such as light, activity, and social interactions help keep the circadian rhythm fixed (entrained) within the 24-hour day.

Factors that either oppose or enhance processes S and C can have significant effects on the timing, duration, and structure of sleep and daytime alertness. For example, excessive sleep during the daytime can decrease the drive for sleep and both delay and alter nocturnal sleep depth. Insufficient or poor nocturnal sleep quality can lead to excessive daytime sleep. Displacement of sleep within the 24-hour day, such as in shift work or travel across times zones, can desynchronize internal body rhythms with those of the external environment. Lack of light exposure during the day, inactivity, and infrequent social interactions can also contribute to circadian dysfunction (Van Cauter, Sturis, Byrne, et al., 1993). Thus a stable sleep-wake pattern is achieved by optimizing both homeostatic and circadian factors. Many behavioral interventions designed to improve sleep (discussed later) address these issues.

Sleep Need

Individual sleep need varies significantly and appears to have a strong genetic component (Franken, Chollet, & Tafti, 2001). On an average, people report needing approximately 7 to 8 hours of sleep per night (National Sleep Foundation [NSF], 1995). Some need as little as 5 hours (short sleepers), whereas others report needing 10 or more (long sleepers) (American Sleep Disorders Association [ASDA], 1997). The sleep need is fulfilled when an individual reports feeling refreshed after a nocturnal sleep period and is able to maintain the desired alertness level through the day. In addition to appropriate quantity, the restorative functions of sleep also depend on its quality—not

being interrupted and having limited nighttime awakenings and arousals. Fragmented sleep, whether secondary to a sleep disorder or medical illness, is associated with daytime sleepiness, fatigue, and other functional decrements (Engleman, Kingshott, Martin, et al, 2000; Lee, 2001; Roehrs, Carskadon, Dement, et al., 2000).

IMPAIRED SLEEP AND SLEEP DISORDERS

Impaired Sleep

Impaired sleep can be categorized as either *sleep deprivation* (resulting from inadequate sleep) or *sleep disruption* (resulting from fragmented sleep during the night). Sleep deprivation occurs more often in association with particular lifestyles or stages of development. Sleep disruption, on the other hand, is more often seen in illness and in those with sleep disorders. Both sleep deprivation and sleep disruption result in sleep loss, the primary manifestations of which are insomnia and daytime sleepiness. Possible adverse health outcomes related to impaired sleep include increased pain and fatigue, altered immune function, decrease daytime functioning, altered mood, decreased memory, and impaired social interactions (Lee, 2003).

Sleep Disorders

Primary sleep disorders are specific diagnostic entities and include a wide array of problems characterized by the symptoms of insomnia (difficulty initiating or maintaining sleep or early morning awakening), excessive daytime sleepiness, and/or abnormal movements, behaviors, or sensations during sleep (Table 5-2) (ASDA, 1997). Three primary groups of sleep disorders are outlined in the International Classification of Sleep Disorders (ASDA, 1997). *Dyssomnias* are those disorders that produce difficulty initiating or maintaining sleep or excessive sleepiness. Dyssomnias may be related to intrinsic factors (idiopathic insomnia, obstructive sleep apnea, periodic limb movements), extrinsic factors (medications, environmental conditions), or circadian rhythm factors (shift work, irregular sleep-wake pattern, advanced or delayed sleep phase). *Parasomnias* include abnormal behaviors, movements, or sensations during sleep, such as

Table **5-2**   International Classification of Sleep Disorders

DYSSOMNIAS

Intrinsic Sleep Disorders	Extrinsic Sleep Disorders	Circadian Rhythm Sleep Disorders
Psychophysiologic insomnia	Inadequate sleep hygiene	Time zone change (jet-lag) syndrome
Sleep state misperception	Environmental sleep disorder	Shift-work sleep disorder
Idiopathic insomnia	Altitude insomnia	Irregular sleep-wake pattern
Narcolepsy	Adjustment sleep disorder	Delayed sleep phase syndrome
Recurrent hypersomnia	Insufficient sleep syndrome	Advanced sleep phase syndrome
Idiopathic hypersomnia	Limit-setting sleep disorder	Non–24-hour sleep-wake disorder
Obstructive sleep apnea syndrome	Sleep-onset association disorder	
Central sleep apnea syndrome	Food allergy insomnia	
Central alveolar hypoventilation syndrome	Nocturnal eating (drinking) syndrome	
Periodic limb movement disorder	Hypnotic-dependent sleep	
Restless legs syndrome	Stimulant-dependent sleep disorder	
	Alcohol-dependent sleep disorder	
	Toxin-induced sleep disorder	

PARASOMNIAS

Arousal Disorders	Sleep-wake Transition Disorders	Parasomnias Usually Associated With REM Sleep	Other Parasomnias
Confusional arousals	Rhythmic movement disorder	Nightmares	Sleep bruxism
Sleepwalking	Sleep starts	Sleep paralysis	Sleep enuresis
Sleep terrors	Sleeptalking	Impaired sleep-related penile erections	Sleep-related abnormal swallowing syndrome
	Nocturnal leg cramps	Sleep-related painful erections	Nocturnal paroxysmal dystonia
		REM sleep-related sinus arrest	Sudden unexplained nocturnal death syndrome
		REM sleep behavior disorder	Primary snoring
			Infant sleep apnea
			Congenital central hypoventilation syndrome
			Sudden infant death syndrome
			Benign neonatal sleep myoclonus

Table 5-2   INTERNATIONAL CLASSIFICATION OF SLEEP DISORDERS—CONT'D

SLEEP DISORDERS ASSOCIATED WITH MEDICAL OR PSYCHIATRIC DISORDERS

Associated With Mental Disorders	Associated With Neurological Disorders	Associated With Other Medical Disorders
Psychoses	Cerebral degenerative disorders	Sleeping sickness
Mood disorders	Dementia	Nocturnal cardiac ischemia
Anxiety disorders	Parkinsonism	Chronic obstructive pulmonary disease
Panic disorder	Fatal familial insomnia	Sleep-related asthma
Alcoholism	Sleep-related epilepsy	Sleep-related gastroesophageal reflux
	Electrical status epilepticus of sleep	Peptic ulcer disease
	Sleep-related headaches	

PROPOSED SLEEP DISORDERS

Short sleeper	Menstrual-associated sleep disorder	Terrifying hypnagogic hallucinations
Long sleeper	Pregnancy-associated sleep disorder	Sleep-related neurogenic tachypnea
Subwakefulness syndrome		
Fragmentary myoclonus		
Sleep hyperhidrosis	Sleep choking syndrome	Sleep-related laryngospasm

From American Sleep Disorders Association (ASDA). (1997). *The International Classification of Sleep Disorders*. Rochester, Minn.: Author.

nightmares, sleep walking, sleep terrors, REM behavioral disorder, and bruxism. The third category, *Sleep Disorders Associated with Mental, Neurologic, or Other Medical Disorders*, includes sleep abnormalities associated with conditions such as Parkinson's disease, sleep-related epilepsy, mood disorders, nocturnal cardiac ischemia, sleep-related gastroesophageal reflux, and chronic obstructive pulmonary disease. A final category of *Proposed Sleep Disorders,* for which sufficient information is not available to confirm the unequivocal existence of the disorders (i.e., short sleeper, long sleeper, and sleep choking syndrome), is also included in the taxonomy. Because of their high prevalence in the general population, three primary sleep disorders that may also be seen in patients in the palliative care setting are briefly discussed here, including sleep apnea, restless legs syndrome, and periodic limb movement disorder (see Table 5-1).

Sleep apnea is a syndrome characterized by intermittent episodes of breathing cessation during sleep, either from airway collapse (obstructive sleep apnea [OSA]), cessation of respiratory effort (central sleep apnea [CSA]), or a combination of the two (mixed type). Both conditions are associated with disturbances of sleep initiation and maintenance as well as daytime sleepiness. The prevalence of OSA is approximately 2% to 4% in the general population; risk factors for the condition include obesity, a neck circumference more than 40 cm, nasal obstruction, facial deformities, and macroglossia (Bassiri & Guilleminauolt, 2000). The prevalence of CSA is unknown, but it is believed to be much less common than OSA (ASDA, 1997). CSA is often seen in patients with congestive heart failure, abnormalities of the upper airway, and neurologic lesions of the brainstem areas that regulate respiration (White, 2000). Sleep apnea can be effectively treated with continuous positive airway pressure (CPAP), a device that delivers air under positive pressure through the nose, acting as a splint to maintain an open airway. Dental appliances (that help move the jaw forward) and a variety of surgical procedures are also treatment options (ASDA, 1997; Chesson, Berry, & Pack, 2003; Littner, Hirshkowitz, Davila, et al., 2002). Behavioral interventions such as refraining from alcohol ingestion before bedtime, sleeping in the side position, and elevating the head of the bed may also be helpful.

Restless legs syndrome (RLS) is characterized by disagreeable sensations that usually occur before sleep onset and that cause an almost irresistible urge to move the legs. Symptoms often result in delayed sleep onset and disrupted sleep (ASDA, 1997). RLS can occur in an idiopathic form or secondary to other conditions such as pregnancy, rheumatoid arthritis, uremia, and anemia. Its prevalence is estimated to be between 5% and 15% in the general population. Approximately 80% of patients with RLS also have *periodic limb movement disorder* (PLMD), a condition characterized by episodic limb movements that are associated with nocturnal awakenings and disrupted sleep. PLMD is also a distinct nosologic entity and occurs independent of RLS (ASDA, 1997). PLMD is more common with advancing age and is present in up to 34% of patients older than 60 years (ASDA, 1997).

The pathophysiologic mechanisms involved in RLS and PLMD are unknown (Allen & Earley, 2001; Montplaisir, Nicolas, Godbout, et al., 2000; Winkelmann & Trenkwalder, 2001). Anemia, iron and vitamin deficiencies, disturbances in peripheral and central nervous system functioning, and musculoskeletal abnormalities have all been proposed as contributing factors (ASDA, 1997; Montplaisir et al., 2000; Winkelmann & Trenkwalder, 2001). Abnormalities in dopamine metabolism and endogenous opiate systems likely play an important role (Allen & Earley, 2001; Montplaisir et al., 2000; Winkelmann & Trenkwalder, 2001). Pharmacologic interventions for RLS and PLMD include dopamine agonists, dopamine precursors, benzodiazepines, and opiates. Neuroleptics, such as gabapentin and carbamazepine, are also effective in some patients. Reduction of factors known to exacerbate symptoms, such as high caffeine intake, alcohol, nicotine, and exposure to extreme temperature, may be helpful. Elimination of medications that may precipitate the conditions, such as lithium, tricyclics, selective serotonin reuptake inhibitors, and dopamine antagonists, may be necessary. Careful withdrawal from sedatives, hypnotics, and neuroleptics, if needed, is also recommended

(Chesson, Wise, Davila, et al, 1999). Excellent reviews of the overall management of RLS and PLMD appear elsewhere (Allen & Earley, 2001; Montplaisir et al., 2000; Parker & Rye, 2002).

Symptoms of Impaired Sleep and Sleep Disorders

As previously mentioned, the three symptoms most commonly associated with impaired sleep and/or sleep disorders are insomnia, excessive daytime sleepiness, and abnormal or undesirable nocturnal movements, behaviors, or sensations.

Insomnia. Insomnia is defined as difficulty falling asleep, staying asleep, waking up abnormally early in the morning, or feeling unrefreshed after the major nocturnal sleep period (ASDA, 1997). It is a very common complaint, and studies of large, representative national samples revealed that more than one third had insomnia-related complaints (Balter & Uhlenhuth, 1992; Gallup, 1991, 1995; Mellinger, Balter, & Uhlenhuth, 1985). Factors that appear to predispose an individual to insomnia include female gender, low socioeconomic status, marital status (divorced or widowed as opposed to married), stress, drug/alcohol use, and other health problems (Gallup, 1991, 1995; Mellinger et al., 1985). Triggers of insomnia include stressful events, environmental disturbances, anxiety, depression, pain or discomfort, or medical or surgical conditions—problems that may all stimulate physiologic and cognitive arousal and delay the onset and disrupt the continuity of sleep. Spending too much time in bed, irregular sleep-wake schedules, concern about daytime deficits, too much napping, caffeine consumption, and hypnotic and alcohol ingestion are all factors that may perpetuate the problem (Blais, Morin, Boisclair, et al., 2001; Morin, Daley, & Ouellet, 2001; Morin, Hauri, Espie, et al., 1999). Interventions designed to treat insomnia include a vast array of pharmacologic and behavioral therapies (see "Management of Impaired Sleep," p. 103). Adequate management of the condition is important. Persons with untreated insomnia report significant impairment of their daytime functioning (Morgan, 2003; Riedel & Lichstein, 2000) and may have decreased immune function (Savard, et al., 2003) and increased mortality (Kripke, 2003).

Excessive Daytime Sleepiness. Excessive daytime sleepiness (EDS), the inability to maintain the alert awake state, is the most common consequence of impaired sleep and sleep disorders (D'Alessandro, Rinaldi, Cristina, et al., 1995). Because of its often vague and nonspecific clinical presentation, the condition is frequently unrecognized by health care providers in other clinical settings (ASDA, 1997; El-Ad & Korczyn, 1998). Patients themselves may have very little insight into both the nature and severity of the problem and the negative effects that EDS has on their lives. In its milder forms, EDS may cause only minor, barely perceived decrements in social and occupational functioning (ASDA, 1997). When severe, it can be debilitating, causing a broad range of neuropsychologic deficits affecting both daytime functioning and quality of life (Dinges et al., 1997). EDS can even be life threatening because of associated alterations in alertness and reactivity (Connor, Norton, Ameratunga, et al., 2001; Lloberes, Levy, Descals, et al., 2000; Lyznicki, Doege, Davis, et al., 1998). Behavioral signs of sleepiness include yawning, eyelid ptosis, reduced activity, lapses in attention, and head nodding (Roehrs & Roth, 2000). Daytime sleepiness can be subjectively measured using instruments such as the Epworth Sleepiness Scale (Johns, 1991, 1992, 2000; Roehrs & Roth, 2000). Daytime sleepiness can also be quantified polysomnographically using the Multiple Sleep Latency Test (MSLT) (ASDA, 1986; Carskadon, Dement, Mitler, et al., 1986).

Movements, Behaviors, and/or Sensations. Numerous abnormal or undesirable movements, behaviors, and/or sensations can occur during sleep. For example, sleep starts, sleep talking, body rocking, and leg cramps can occur in otherwise healthy individuals but may lead to discomfort, pain, embarrassment, anxiety, or disturbance of the bed partner's sleep. Abnormal arousals from SWS sleep (e.g., sleep terrors, sleep walking) often occur in young children and disappear by adolescence; in the elderly, in contrast, these behaviors are more commonly associated with pathology. Nightmares, sleep paralysis (feeling unable to move), impaired or painful erections, and periods of dream enactment typically emerge from REM sleep. Bruxism (teeth grinding), enuresis, abnormal swallowing or choking, snoring, dyspnea, chest pain, leg kicking, panic attacks, seizures, and apneic episodes may occur during sleep and be related to one of several sleep disorders or other pathologies (ASDA, 1997).

SLEEP IN THE PALLIATIVE CARE SETTING

Patients with a wide variety of chronic illnesses experience sleep problems. Although the sleep complaints may be relatively similar—such as difficulty initiating or maintaining sleep—exploring how sleep varies according to specific illnesses has the potential to provide unique insights into the assessment and management of these problems. Patients with cancer and human immunodeficiency virus (HIV)/acquired immunodeficiency syndrome (AIDS) are two clinical populations often seen in the palliative care setting. Thus a brief summary of what is known about the sleep of these groups follows. A review of relevant information regarding the sleep of caregivers is also provided. Factors associated with sleep problems in the palliative care setting are discussed in "Factors Associated With Impaired Sleep," p. 98.

Sleep and Cancer

Sleep complaints are common and reported in 30% to 70% of cancer patients surveyed (Davidson, MacLean, Brundage, et al., 2002; Degner & Sloan, 1995; Engstrom, Strohl, Rose, et al., 1999). The variability in prevalence observed likely reflects differences in the way sleep problems were defined and measured and whether they were preexisting conditions (Savard & Morin, 2001). Many patients report that sleep problems occur almost nightly and are moderate to severe in nature (Cleeland, Mendoza, Wang, et al., 2000; Kurtz, Given, Kurtz, et al., 1994; Malone, Harris, & Luscombe, 1994; Portenoy, Thaler, Kornblith, et al., 1994). Unfortunately, the results of a recent study suggest that 85% of cancer patients did not communicate these problems to their physicians—often because they thought nothing could be done (Engstrom et al., 1999). Nonetheless, more than 40% of all prescriptions written for this population are for hypnotics (Derogatis, Feldstein,

Morrow, et al., 1979; Stiefel, Kornblith, & Holland, 1990), an observation that highlights the magnitude of the problem.

Insomnia is a major complaint of cancer patients and includes the classic symptoms of increased sleep latency, poor sleep maintenance, and early morning awakenings (Andersen & Sjogren, 1998; Beszterczey & Lipowski, 1977; Davidson et al., 2002; Engstrom et al., 1999; Owen, Parker, & McGuire, 1999). Many patients also report decreased nocturnal total sleep time. One study found that 45% of a mixed group of cancer patients had a total sleep time of less than 50 hours a week; 23% slept less than 40 hours a week (Beszterczey & Lipowski, 1977). A comparison of cancer patients with those with other medical and surgical patients revealed that cancer patients did sleep less than other patient groups (Kaye, Kaye, & Madow, 1983). Owen et al. (1999) found similar results when comparing sleep quality of cancer patients with normative data. In contrast, other researchers have found no differences in sleep between cancer patients and those with other medical illnesses (Lamb, 1982). Sleep disturbances have also been described in delirium, a cognitive disorder often affecting medically ill patients and that is particularly prevalent among cancer patients (Cole, McCusker, Dendukuri, et al., 2002).

Few polysomnographic studies involving cancer patients have been done. In a study of 14 patients with lung cancer undergoing radiation therapy, 9 of the subjects self-rated their sleep as good and 5 as poor (Silberfarb, Hauri, Oxman, et al., 1985). PSG comparison of the two groups revealed no differences in sleep latency or measures of REM sleep, but poor sleepers had less deep NREM sleep (SWS). Later, the sleep of 17 patients with lung cancer and 15 with breast cancer was studied and compared with 32 healthy insomniacs and 32 normal controls (Silberfarb, Hauri, Oxman, et al., 1993). Patients with breast cancer (50%) were more likely to complain of poor sleep than patients with lung cancer (12%), but they did not have any significant differences in overall sleep measures compared with controls. Although comparable to controls with regard to total bed time, patients with lung cancer had much more disturbed sleep with increased amounts of light NREM sleep, decreased sleep efficiency, and increased awakenings. Both cancer groups showed a greater incidence (47% lung and 60% breast) of PLMs during sleep than either comparison group (20%). In a third study, PSG was used to identify the incidence of sleep apnea in 24 patients who had resection of a head and neck cancer (Friedman, Landsberg, Pryor, et al., 2001); 92% of subjects met the diagnostic criteria for sleep apnea. Of the 22 patients with apnea, 16 had clinical symptoms associated with apnea including restless sleep, loud snoring, and daytime sleepiness.

Although the topic has received much less attention than nocturnal sleep problems, excessive daytime sleepiness has been reported as a significant problem in 30% to 60% of cancer patients (Davidson et al., 2002; Portenoy & Itri, 1999; Sateia & Silberfarb, 1998; Yellen & Dyonzak, 1999). In fact, sleeping more than usual during the day was one of the most troublesome symptoms of patients receiving radiation therapy (Munro, Biruls, Griffin, et al., 1989), although no increase in sleepiness was observed in patients undergoing radiation for prostate cancer (Monga, Kerrigan, Thornby, et al., 1999). Daytime sleepiness and sedation have also been reported in association with opioid analgesics (Hanks, Twycross, & Bliss, 1987; Wilwerding, Loprinzi, Mailliard, et al., 1995).

Numerous factors likely contribute to the poor sleep and daytime sleepiness experienced by these patients, and these are covered in more detail subsequently. However, altered physiology directly related to the cancer may play a prominent role in disrupting sleep and circadian regulatory processes. For example, abnormalities in the circadian production of cortisol have been reported in cancer patients (Mazzoccoli, Carughi, De Cata, et al., 2003; Raida, Kliche, Schwake, et al., 2002). An absent or blunted rhythm of melatonin secretion has also been noted in both lung and colorectal cancer patients (Bartsch & Bartsch, 1999; Khoory & Stemme, 1988; Viviani, Bidoli, Spinazze, et al., 1992). In addition, cancer cells both produce and induce production of cytokines (substances that are sleep promoting) (Ardestani, Inserra, Solkoff, et al., 1999). Further research is needed to more fully understand the extent to which the pathophysiology of cancer itself affects sleep and waking.

Sleep problems are associated with a reduced quality of life (Earlam, Glover, Fordy, et al., 1996; Fortner, Kasprowicz, Wang, et al., 2000; Northouse, Caffey, Deichelbohrer, et al., 1999; Sutherland, Lockwood, & Boyd, 1990) and decreased functional status (Given, Given, Azzouz, et al., 2001) in cancer patients—but the effects may be much more far-reaching. Degner and Sloan reported that insomnia, pain, and fatigue produced the most distress in 434 newly diagnosed patients with cancer; for a subset of 82 patients with lung cancer, symptom distress was predictive of survival time irrespective of age and stage of diagnosis (Degner & Sloan, 1995). Earlam et al. (1996) found that sleep quality was one of six variables that predicted survival in a sample of 50 patients with colorectal cancer and hepatic metastases. Savard, Miller, Mills, et al. (1999) observed that satisfaction with sleep quality was significantly related to levels of T helper and cytotoxic/suppressor cells. Research designed to evaluate the effects of sleep on both the morbidity and mortality in patients with cancer is an important area for future research.

Sleep and HIV/AIDS

HIV infection is often accompanied by sleep disruption. A recent study (Rubinstein & Selwyn, 1998) found that 73% of 115 HIV-positive patients had sleep disturbance, an observation consistent with the results of several additional studies (Cohen, Ferrans, Vizgirda, et al., 1996; Hudson, Lee, & Portillo, 2003). Sleep disturbances appear to develop relatively soon after the initial infection, continue across the disease course, and increase with advancing disease (Moeller, Oechsner, Backmund, et al., 1991; Savard et al., 1999). Sleep problems have also been reported in children with HIV (Franck, Johnson, Lee, et al., 1999)

Difficulties with initiating and maintaining nocturnal sleep and daytime sleepiness are among the most common complaints (Phillips, 1999; Rubinstein & Selwyn, 1998). One study reported that HIV-infected men had more nocturnal wake time when compared with healthy controls (Norman, Chediak, Freeman, et al., 1992). Similar findings have been reported by other researchers (Rubinstein & Selwyn, 1998; Wiegand, Moller,

Schreiber, et al., 1991). Darko, McCutchan, Kripke, et al. (1992) evaluated sleepiness and sleep habits in 62 HIV-positive men and 50 HIV-negative male controls and found that HIV-infected subjects slept more, napped more, had more early morning awakenings, and were less alert in the morning. In a study of 50 men and women with HIV, 43% of the sample had either insomnia (difficulties with sleep onset and reduced total sleep time) or excessive sleepiness (total sleep time more than 10 hours) (Cohen et al., 1996). Seventy percent reported waking more than once per night.

Polysomnographic measures of sleep appear to be affected by the disease. In a sample of asymptomatic HIV-infected males, Norman Resnick, Cohn, et al. (1988, 1990, 1992) found that the patients experienced an increase in SWS, especially in the second half of the night. When compared with normative data, they also found an increase in the number of REM periods, shorter length of the REM periods, and an increase in nocturnal arousals (Norman Chediak, Kiel, et al., 1990). Others reported a high level of daytime sleepiness in HIV-positive subjects, possibly related to the presence of significant obstructive sleep apnea secondary to adenotonsillar hypertrophy (Epstein, Strollo, Donegan, et al., 1995).

Numerous physiologic factors regulating sleep and circadian rhythms may be affected by HIV—central to these are changes in the hypothalamic-pituitary-adrenal axis circadian rhythm. HIV has been associated with decreased production of growth hormone, increased production of corticotrophin-releasing factor and adrenocorticotropin hormone (ACTH), and elevation of cytokines (interleukin-1-β, interleukin-6, and TNF-α) (Kumar, Kumar, Walfrop, et al., 2003; Phillips, 1999). Degeneration of central dopaminergic systems may also play a role in the development of sleep-wake cycle abnormalities (Berger & Arendt, 2000; Koutsilieri, Scheller, ter Meulen, et al., 2005).

The impact that sleep problems have on the clinical outcomes of HIV/AIDS patients remains to be described. However, a recent study of 57 HIV-positive men and women observed that higher levels of distress were significantly related to lower T-cytotoxic/ suppressor (CD3, CD8) cells and that sleep disturbances mediated this relationship

(Cruess, Antoni, Gonzalez, et al., 2003). White Darko, Brown, et al. (1995) observed a correlation between CD4 T cell counts and increased SWS during the last half of the night. These results suggest that interventions designed to enhance sleep may improve immune function in these patients.

Sleep in Family Caregivers

Family caregivers endure a tremendous amount of stress related to providing care for a loved one in the palliative setting. Reactive depression is very prevalent and can interfere with daily functioning, quality of life, and ability to continue to provide care (Jepson, McCorkle, Adler, et al., 1999; Kozachik, Given, Given, et al., 2001; Nijboer, Triemstra, Tempelaar, et al., 1999). Higher rates of depressive symptoms have been consistently described among family caregivers than among their same-age peers not caring for relatives who are ill (Dura, Stukenberg, & Kiecolt-Glaser, 1990; Tennstedt, Cafferata, & Sullivan, 1992). Numerous factors have been associated with caregiver depression including time since diagnosis, type of diagnosis, patient age and functional status, social support, and relationship quality (Douglass, 1997; Given, Given, Stommel, et al., 1999; Knop, Bergman-Evans, & McCabe, 1998; Kurtz et al., 1994; Kurtz, Kurtz, Given, et al., 1995). Only recently has chronic sleep loss related to stress and the 24-hours/day demands of caregiving been described as an important contributing factor (Carter & Chang, 2000).

Family caregivers' sleep may be disrupted in several ways. Problems with insomnia and daytime fatigue related to grief, anxiety, and depression are common (Carter, 2003; Carter & Chang, 2000). In a study examining sleep quality of 47 caregivers, 95% reported moderate to severe problems with regard to sleep latency, sleep quality, sleep duration, sleep efficiency, and sleep disturbances (Carter & Chang, 2000). Male caregivers reported an overall sleep quality that was slightly better than that of the female caregivers (Carter, 2002). Total sleep time may also be significantly compromised; Bramwell and colleagues (1995) reported that a majority of 37 family caregivers of patients with terminal cancer slept less than 4 hours per night, often because they were required to provide 24-hour care to their family member.

Caregivers may also be at risk for sleep problems after the loss of a loved one. Recently, a study was conducted to determine if a cancer patient's unrelieved symptoms during the last 3 months of life increased the risk of long-term psychologic morbidity of the surviving partner. Results revealed that the widow's psychologic morbidity, including difficulty falling asleep at night, waking up at night with anxiety, and the need to take sleeping pills, was associated with the patient's unrelieved mental and physical symptoms. Thus inefficient symptom control during the last months of a cancer patient's life may predispose the surviving partner to long-term sleep problems (Valdimarsdottir, Helgason, Furst, et al., 2002).

As part of a comprehensive palliative care plan, nurses should regularly assess the sleep needs of caregivers and tailor interventions to meet those needs (Steele & Fitch, 1996). Recognizing that wide swings in sleep can occur related to factors such as patient disease status, patient symptoms, and caregiver anxiety underscores the need for continual assessment (Carter, 2003). Helping patients maintain or regain some independence may be helpful (Steele & Fitch, 1996). Adherence to good sleep hygiene practices (discussion follows), scheduling rest/nap periods, appropriate management of depression, and obtaining regular assistance with the provision of care may be indicated. Although studies designed to evaluate the effect of sleep-promoting interventions in caregivers are few in number, McCurry, Gibbons, Logsdon, et al. (2003) found that family members had less depression and improved daytime function after adhering to a program of good sleep hygiene.

FACTORS ASSOCIATED WITH IMPAIRED SLEEP

Numerous factors may contribute to impaired sleep in patients in the palliative care setting. These include:

- Demographic features
- Lifestyle and environmental factors
- Psychologic and cognitive factors

- Responses to illness
- Medications and treatments

Demographic Features

In the general population, older age, female gender, lower socioeconomic status, divorced or widowed status, and the presence of co-morbidities have all been associated with reports of increased sleep problems (Karacan, Thornby, Anch, et al., 1976; NSF, 1995). Age appears to be one of the most important because poor sleep quality in this group has been linked to increased sleep fragmentation, decreased amounts of deep sleep, increased daytime napping caused by nocturia, elevated autonomic activity that results in greater susceptibility to arousal, and decreased strength of the circadian rhythms. As previously mentioned, sleep disorders such as periodic limb movements and sleep apnea are more common in the elderly (Ancoli-Israel, Kripke, Klauber, et al., 1991a; Montplaisir et al., 2000).

Given that many patients with cancer are older, age may predispose these individuals to sleep problems; a weak correlation between sleep disturbance and age in a sample of cancer patients has been described (Engstrom et al., 1999). In contrast, the prevalence of sleep disturbance was recently noted to be slightly higher among younger patients (54% vs. 43% for those older than 65 years), possibly because of higher rates of anxiety and depression in the younger group (Walsh, Donnelly, & Rybicki, 2000). Another study of 982 subjects with a variety of cancer diagnoses found that age was linearly and inversely related to insomnia prevalence (Davidson et al., 2002). Redeker et al. (2000) reported similar results. No significant relationship between sleep quality and age was noted in a study of 58 patients with HIV disease (Nokes & Kendrew, 2001).

The results of studies that examined the effects of gender on sleep disturbances in cancer patients have been equivocal; some report that sleep disturbances are more common in men (Walsh et al., 2000), whereas others report no gender differences (Malone et al., 1994; Redeker, et al., 2000). Several demographic-related factors, such as taking sick leave, unemployment, and widowhood, were all

shown to be independent predictors of insomnia in a sample of 300 women with breast cancer (Savard, Simard, Blanchet, et al., 2001). Davidson and colleagues (2002) found that cancer patients with insomnia identified financial concerns as contributing to their sleep problems; lower income was also found to be a risk factor for insomnia in women with lung cancer (Sarna & Brecht, 1997). In HIV/AIDS patients, sleep problems have been associated with unemployment (Nokes & Kendrew, 2001), female gender, and fewer years of education (Cohen et al., 1996; Lee, Portillo, & Miramontes, 2001). A study of 100 women with HIV/AIDS found greater levels of disrupted sleep (lower sleep efficiency as measured by actigraphy) in women who were unemployed; no relationships were noted between sleep quality and age, having a spouse or partner, number of children, or CD4 count (Lee, Portillo, & Miramontes, 1999).

Lifestyle

Poor sleep hygiene, such as going to bed too late and getting up too early, may interfere with normal sleep regulatory processes and decrease the sleep obtained (Zarcone, 2000). In addition, long naps taken during the daytime hours, especially late in the day, decrease the drive to sleep and often delay sleep onset (Roehrs & Roth, 2000). Use of caffeine in coffee and soft drinks, smoking, and ingestion of alcohol also interfere with sleep by producing arousals. Caffeine disrupts sleep by blocking adenosine, a sleep-promoting factor (Landolt, Dijk, Gaus, et al., 1995; Landolt, Werth, Borbely, et al., 1995); nicotine acts as a central nervous system stimulant (Rieder, Kunze, Groman, et al., 2001). Although alcohol ingestion may speed sleep onset, falling blood alcohol levels produce sympathetic arousal and disturb sleep later in the night (Zarcone, 2000). Few studies have examined the effects of these substances on the sleep of patients in the palliative care setting. However, Dreher (2003) conducted a study that tested whether there were differences in subjective sleep quality and well-being in a group of HIV-positive persons who reduced their caffeine intake from baseline by 90% or more for 30 days versus a group who continued their usual caffeine consumption. Although no improvement in well-being was observed, a significant improvement in sleep quality in the experimental group was demonstrated.

Changes in overall activity/rest schedules may also affect nocturnal sleep. Several studies have described disrupted activity/rest patterns in patients in palliative care (Atkinson, Barsevick, Cella, et al., 2000; Mormont, Waterhouse, Bleuzen, et al., 2000), an observation possibly related to decreased exposure to light and irregular meals, periods of inactivity, and decreased social interactions (Klerman, Rimmer, Dijk, et al., 1998). In a study of 72 women with breast cancer, Berger and Farr (1999) found that those who were less active and slept more during the day had increased nighttime awakenings and greater fatigue. Similar findings have been reported in HIV-positive patients (Darko et al., 1992; Lee et al., 2001; Nokes & Kendrew, 2001). It is of interest to note that, in a qualitative study designed to examine the sleep of six women with HIV, many reported that a good night's sleep was often preceded by a busy day giving them a sense of "physical fullness" that helped ensure sleep (Portillo, Tom, Lee, et al., 2003).

Environmental Factors

Animal and human studies have shown that ambient temperature is an important determinant of both the quality and quantity of sleep. In an environment that is excessively warm, nocturnal sleep periods are characterized by increased wakefulness and by reductions in both REM sleep and NREM sleep (Muzet, Libert, & Candas, 1984). There are marked individual differences in sensitivity to temperature variation and in one's optimal sleeping temperature. Therefore ensuring that the room temperature is comfortable for patients is an important part of an overall sleep-promoting plan of care.

Noise in the environment can also disrupt sleep. According to Lipscomb (1976), an individual's reaction to noise is related to the noxious aspect of the sound source, the relative pleasure or displeasure the person is experiencing at the onset of the noise, the person's basic anxiety level, and the evaluation by the individual of the situation at the time

the noise occurs. The meaning of the noise may also be altered because of the effects of pain, stress, medication, and other physiologic problems (Carter, Henderson, Lal, et al., 2002; Griefahn, 2002; Waye, Clow, Edwards, et al., 2003).

Many stressors cited by patients in a variety of care settings stem from the frequent interventions and interruptions caused by caregiving (Edell-Gustafsson, Gustavsson, & Yngman Uhlin, 2003; Olson, Borel, Laskowitz, et al., 2001; Schnelle, Ouslander, Simmons, et al., 1993). Serious sleep disruption can occur unless caregivers strive to promote an optimal sleep environment and minimize interruptions. In a study of 50 hospitalized cancer patients (all with solid tumors), Sheely (1996) observed that sleep quality (and not perceived length of sleep) was adversely affected by increased nocturnal care–related disturbances, total time spent in a patient's room during the night, and level of care participation required of the patient. In a sample of persons with HIV, subjective sleep quality was better in those having a separate room for sleeping and sleeping alone, whereas sleeping in a noisy bedroom adversely affected sleep (Nokes & Kendrew, 2001).

Psychologic and Cognitive Factors

Sleep problems are a symptom of depression and are characterized by changes in sleep architecture (decreases in slow-wave sleep, short REM latency, increased REM percentage) (Borbely & Acherman, 2000; Holsboer-Trachsler & Seifritz, 2000). Similarly, anxiety can interfere with sleep by increasing psychologic and physiologic arousal causing problems falling asleep, awakenings during the night, and decreasing sleep depth (Reynolds, Willson, & Clark, 1983). Nonetheless, it is not always clear whether depressed and/or anxious individuals are more likely to report sleep problems or whether individuals with more sleep disturbances are more depressed/anxious (Dickens, McGowan, & Dale, 2003; Fishbain, 2002; Harman, Pivik, D'Eon, et al., 2002; Moldofsky, 2001; Nicassio et al., 2002; Sayar, Arikan, & Yontem, 2002; Vines, Gupta, Whiteside, et al., 2003). Both anxiety and depression experienced in response to sleep disruption can provoke substantial autonomic, visceral, and skeletal arousal causing enhanced sleep disruption (Galloway, Bubela, McKibbon, et al., 1995; Menza & Rosen, 1995).

Although anxiety and depression are common in patients with cancer (Breitbart, Bruera, Chochinov, et al., 1995), results of research designed to examine the relationship between these problems and sleep in this group remain equivocal. For example, Lamb (1982) reported that, although depression scores of 15 patients with cancer increased during hospitalization, no changes in sleep were noted. Silberfarb and colleagues (1993) also noted the absence of a relationship between sleep and depression in a sample of patients with lung cancer. In contrast, others have reported positive correlations between sleep problems and both anxiety and/or depression (Beszterczey & Lipowski, 1977; Beszterczey & Lipowski, 1997; Redeker et al., 2000). Depression and anxiety are also common in HIV-infected individuals and likely contribute to the sleep problems experienced by this group (Koutsilieri, Scheller, Sopper, et al., 2002). Depression and anxiety were recently found to be significantly related to sleep quality in a sample of 58 men and women with HIV (Nokes & Kendrew, 2001).

Disorders of cognition, particularly delirium, are also often observed in the palliative care setting (Cole, Dendukuri, McCusker, et al., 2003). The incidence of delirium is high among those in advanced stages of illness and may be an independent marker of mortality (Berger & Arendt, 2000; Koutsilieri et al., 2002; McCusker, Cole, Abrahamowicz, et al., 2002). Sleep-wake disturbances appear to be an important component of the disorder. In a study of factors associated with the development of postoperative delirium in elderly medical patients, an increased likelihood of delirium was noted in those who had greater sleep disturbances in the immediate postoperative period (Kaneko, Takahashi, Naka, et al., 1997). Cole and colleagues (2003) also reported a high prevalence of altered sleep-wake cycle patterns in patients with delirium and sleep-wake cycle disturbances were found to distinguish those with hyperactive, versus hypoactive, delirium (Meagher, O'Hanlon, O'Mahony, et al., 2000). Increased numbers of rapid eye movements both before and during delirium

have been described (Matsushima, Nakajima, Moriya, et al., 1997), suggesting that sleep-wake cycle disturbances in this setting may be related to a disruption of circadian rhythms (Meagher & Trzepacz, 2000). The relationship delirium and other circadian markers such as levels of cortisal, melatonin, and body temperature rhythms has never been studied (Meagher & Trzepacz, 2000). Kaneko and colleagues (1997) reported a good clinical response to light therapy given for 2 hours each morning for postoperative delirium.

Responses to Illness

Pain. Between 30% and 60% of patients in pain complain of sleep difficulties (Dorrepaal, Aaronson, & van Dam, 1989; Ripamonti, Zecca, Brunelli, et al., 2000), and the intensity of pain relates inversely to total sleep time (Tamburini, Selmi, De Conno, et al., 1987). Adequate control of pain often results in a reduction in the occurrence and severity of insomnia (Meuser, Pietruck, Radbruch, et al., 2001). Treatment with opioids, a medication commonly used to manage pain in the palliative care setting, has been shown to adversely affect sleep; high doses disrupt virtually all stages of sleep, decrease or abolish REM, and increase nighttime awakenings (Kay, Eisenstein, & Jasinski, 1969; Knill, Moote, Skinner, et al., 1990). In addition, opioids may disrupt the circadian rhythm by altering episodes of sleep and waking (Byku & Gannon, 2000a, 2000b; Byku, Legutko, & Gannon, 2000; Meijer, Ruijs, Albus, et al., 2000). Nonsteroidal antiinflammatory drugs may also decrease SWS and REM sleep and increase nocturnal awakenings (Horne, Percival, & Traynor, 1980; Landis, Levine, & Robinson, 1989).

Sleep disruption itself appears to increase the perception of pain and may even trigger its development (Moldofsky & Scarisbrick, 1976; Shaver, Lentz, Landis, et al., 1997). It has long been noted that waking each morning feeling unrefreshed, fatigued, and tired is commonly experienced by patients with fibromyalgia, a syndrome characterized by somatic pain (Wolfe, Smythe, Yunus, et al., 1990). Moldofsky and Scarisbrick (1976) were the first to describe a particular sleep EEG abnormality, known as *alpha-delta sleep,* that was associated with this condition. When this phenomenon was stimulated in a group of normal volunteers by selective SWS interruption and deprivation, they developed muscular fatigue and tenderness within a few days (Moldofsky & Scarisbrick, 1976). Restricting sleep to an average of approximately 5 hours a night for 7 consecutive nights also resulted in an increase in somatic complaints including headaches, gastrointestinal problems, and sore joints in a group of normal subjects (Dinges et al., 1997). Similarly, in a study of 12 healthy women, Lentz, Landis, Rothermel, et al. (1999) found that disrupting SWS, without reducing total sleep time or sleep efficiency, for several consecutive nights was associated with decreased pain threshold and increased discomfort. Several pain and sleep experts have suggested that these two symptoms are often interrelated and that pain may interact with sleep disturbances predisposing individuals to even greater morbidity (Lee, 2003; Miaskowski & Lee, 1999). The relationship between pain and impaired sleep is complex, and little is known about treating the two problems when both are present together.

Fatigue. Fatigue is one of the most common symptoms experienced by patients in the palliative care setting (Ancoli-Israel, Moore, & Jones, 2001; Nail, 2002). As many as 61% of cancer patients described their quality of life as being more adversely affected by fatigue than by pain (Vogelzang, Breitbart, Cella, et al., 1997). Most would agree that numerous factors contribute to the development of fatigue (Ancoli-Israel et al., 2001; Lee, 2001). Nonetheless, impaired sleep appears to play a significant etiologic role. For example, a study of women with breast cancer observed that increased fatigue at the midpoint of the cytotoxic drug cycle was associated with decreased daytime activity and increased nighttime awakenings (Berger & Farr, 1999). A subsequent study also found that increased fatigue correlated with increased nighttime awakenings in women with breast cancer receiving cytotoxic drug therapy (Berger & Higginbotham, 2000). Poor sleep efficiency has been associated with decreased activity (lower Karnofsky Performance Status scores) in cancer patients (Miaskowski & Lee, 1999). In a sample of 100 women with HIV/AIDS, Lee and colleagues (2001) found that those with high perceived fatigue had significantly more

difficulty falling sleep, more awakenings from nighttime sleep, poorer daytime functioning, and a higher frequency of depressive symptoms.

Research designed to distinguish the symptom of fatigue from daytime sleepiness associated with impaired nocturnal sleep is ridden with conceptual and methodologic issues (Ancoli-Israel et al., 2001; Lee, 2001). These efforts are compounded by the fact that patients most commonly use the terms "fatigue" and "tiredness" to describe what is, in fact, daytime sleepiness (Chervin, 2000). Excellent reviews on this topic appear elsewhere (Lee, 2001).

Other Symptoms. Patients in the palliative care setting may experience a number of additional symptoms that adversely affect sleep such as dry mouth and thirst, nausea, vomiting, anorexia, constipation, diarrhea, night sweats, cough, and difficulty breathing (Cleeland et al., 2000; Lashely, 1999; Walsh et al., 2000). For example, a recent study noted that patients reporting post-chemotherapy nausea and vomiting also experienced more sleep disturbance, an observation possibly related to the use of antiemetic medications known to disrupt sleep (Cassileth, Lusk, & Torri, 1983; Osoba, Zee, & Warr, 1997). Hot flashes in postmenopausal breast cancer survivors may cause sleep impairment (Carpenter, Johnson, Wagner, et al., 2002; Couzi, Helzlsouer, & Fetting, 1995). Some success in treatment of hot flashes has been achieved following administration of paroxetine (Weitzner, Moncello, Jacobsen, et al., 2002); complementary/alternative therapies may also be an alternative, but research in this area remains to be conducted (Moyad, 2002). More research is needed to explore how and to what extent these and other symptoms often experienced by patients in the palliative setting affect sleep.

Medications and Treatments

Patients in the palliative setting frequently receive analgesics, sedatives, hypnotics, and antidepressants. Each class of these medications can affect sleep in specific ways, and excellent information about these effects can be readily found in the literature (Gursky & Krahn, 2000; Schweitzer, 2000). In brief, benzodiazepines tend to suppress SWS and have variable effects on REM sleep. Barbiturates and opioids decrease REM sleep. Hypnotics have very specific pharmacologic profiles regarding their impact on sleep architecture depending on their rate of absorption, distribution, and metabolism. Particularly significant is the fact that withdrawal from drugs, which selectively suppress a stage of sleep, is frequently associated with a rebound of that sleep stage. Some hypnotics are associated with rebound insomnia, a 1- or 2-night sleep disturbance relative to basal sleep. Thus many of these medications need to be tapered before being discontinued. Several other types of medications alter sleep. For example, lithium suppresses REM sleep and increases SWS. Antidepressants typically suppress REM sleep. Theophylline, which may ease respiration and facilitate sleep, can also increase arousals per sleep hour and decrease total sleep time. Insomnia is a side effect of many drugs used to treat HIV, including nucleoside reverse transcriptase inhibitors, non-nucleoside reverse transcriptase inhibitors, protease inhibitors, and drugs used to treat opportunistic infections (Phillips, 1999; Gallego, Barreiro, Rio Rd, et al., 2004).

Other types of treatments may disrupt sleep because of their emotional impact, their physiologic effects, or their side effects (Savard & Morin, 2001). For example, sleep disturbances and daytime sleepiness have been reported in patients undergoing chemotherapy (Berger & Higginbotham, 2000; Broeckel Jacobsen, Horton, et al., 1998; Redeker et al., 2000) and in response to hormonal therapy (i.e., tamoxifen) (Broeckel et al., 1998; Couzi et al., 1995; Mourits, De Vries, Willemse, et al., 2001; Stein, Jacobsen, Hann, et al., 2000). Problems with nocturnal sleep disturbances and/or daytime sleepiness have also been reported in patients undergoing radiotherapy (Beszterczey & Lipowski, 1977; Faithfull & Brada, 1998; Miaskowski & Lee, 1999). While the mechanisms by which chemotherapy and radiotherapy may interfere with sleep remain to be fully elucidated, some suggest that changes in cytokine expression may play a prominent role (Belka, Budach, Kortman, et al., 2001; Greenberg, Gray, Mannix, et al., 1993). Use of cytokines, especially interferon, interleukin-2, and TNF-α, is associated with a variety of side effects including daytime sleepiness, disturbed sleep, and

depression (Capuron, Ravaud, & Dantzer, 2000; Valentine, Meyers, Kling, et al., 1998). As mentioned, estrogen deficiency resulting from treatment can cause menopausal symptoms that interfere with sleep. Hot flashes and night sweats occur in at least one half of women treated with tamoxifen (Fisher, Costantino, & Redmond, 1989; Love, Cameron, & Connell, 1991) and often occur in men with prostate cancer treated with androgen deprivation therapy (Erlichman & Loprinzi, 1997). Couzi and colleagues (1995) noted a linear association between severity of hot flashes and sleep disturbances in women treated for breast cancer.

MANAGEMENT OF IMPAIRED SLEEP

Sleep Assessment

A sleep assessment (Box 5-1) is a systematic collection of data that includes information about a patient's usual sleep patterns, sleep effectiveness, bedtime routines, and sleep environment. As discussed, a variety of factors related to the patient's underlying disorder, treatments, environment, lifestyle, and responses to illness can be associated with impaired sleep. Objective data from a polysomnographic sleep study may be available for occasional patients, but for most, a sleep history and direct observation are the primary assessment methods. When impaired sleep is a significant ongoing problem, a sleep diary is an excellent way to document frequency and severity of symptoms and their effect on daily activities, evaluate progress of treatment, and promote self-management. Referral to a sleep specialist may also be appropriate if it appears that the patients may have a primary sleep disorder. Sleep clinicians often use the acronym "BEARS" as a format to organize available subjective, behavioral, and objective information in performing a sleep history (Lee, 2003) (Box 5-2) (see the website of the American Academy of Sleep Medicine: www.aasmnet.org).

The clinician should regularly assess both the quality and quantity of the patient's sleep—tasks that can be difficult. In a study of sleep in a surgical intensive care unit, Aurell and Elmqvist (1985) found that nurses often misjudged and consistently overestimated their patients' sleep in comparison

Box 5-1 SLEEP ASSESSMENT

Chief Complaint
- Insomnia
- Excessive daytime sleepiness
- Abnormal movements, behaviors, sensations
- Other symptoms

History of Present Problem
- Onset
- Temporal sequence
- Quality/quantity
- Aggravating factors
- Alleviating factors
- Associated factors
- Contemporaneous medical problems

Sleep History—Nocturnal History
- Time retiring/sleep latency
- Bedtime rituals
- Nocturnal awakenings
- Time awakening/method
- Overall quality of sleep/refreshing quality of sleep
- Average length of sleep episode
- Position
- Comparison of weekdays and weekends
- Dreams/nightmares
- Sleep paralysis
- Nocturnal myoclonus (jerking of the legs)
- Nocturnal behaviors (sleep walking, talking, confusional episodes):
  —Time of night
  —Responsiveness during episode
  —Recollection of episode
- Fitful sleep—condition of bed on awakening
- Snoring
- Waking up gasping for breath
- Waking up with dry mouth
- Symptoms awakening at night—chest pain, pain, reflux, nocturia
- Use of sleeping medications
- Problems in the environment/sleep surface/noise/bedding/temperature/bed partner

Sleep History—Diurnal (Daytime) History
- Morning headaches
- Migraines
- Dizziness
- Problems with memory, concentration, irritability
- Sleepiness during the day—naps
- Falling asleep inappropriately
- Timing and duration of light exposure
- Activity level
- Meal times

Past Medical History

Past Surgical History

Past Psychiatric History
- Anxiety
- Depression
- Drug/alcohol abuse
- Psychotic disorders

Family History (Sleep Disorders)
- Obstructive sleep apnea
- Enuresis
- Sleep terrors
- Sleep walking
- Insomnia

Patient Profile
- Weight change over past year
- Caffeine, ETOH, smoking, drugs, OTC drugs
- Academic functioning
- Occupational functioning
- Marital satisfaction
- Current living status
- Health habits

Current Medications and Treatments

ETOH, Alcohol; *OTC,* over-the-counter.

to parallel polysomnographic recordings. In contrast, another study conducted by Edwards and Schuring (1993) found nurses could reasonably identify sleep and wake states more than 80% of the time based on good correlation with recorded data. This is less likely to occur if careful monitoring of the patient includes watching for potential signs of sleep including closed eyes, lack of movement, and decreased awareness of surroundings. Keeping a systematic sleep record can assist in estimating the amount of sleep a patient is receiving.

Box 5-2   Suggested Questions Following the BEARS Format

B   Bedtime problems—elucidate what happens at sleep onset:
- Do you have any difficulty falling asleep?
- How long does it take you to fall asleep?
- What prevents you from falling asleep?
- How long have you had this problem?
- How much and when have you had alcohol, nicotine, and caffeine today?

E   Excessive daytime sleepiness—determine the extent of excessive daytime sleepiness:
- Do you find yourself falling asleep during the day when you don't want to?
- How likely are you to fall asleep when reading or watching TV, during a conversation, while driving?

A   Awakenings during the night—characterize the extent and content of awakenings:
- Are you having difficulty sleeping through the night?
- What awakens you (pain, shortness of breath, etc.)?
- How often and for how long are you awake?
- What keeps you from falling back asleep?

R   Regularity and duration of sleep—delineate sleep habits:
- What time do you usually go to bed and get up in the morning?
- Do you feel that you usually get enough sleep?

S   Sleep disorders—screen for common sleep disorders:
- Have you or anyone else noticed that you snore loudly?
- Have you or anyone else noticed that you stop breathing in your sleep?
- Have you or anyone else noticed that your legs kick or twitch at night?
- Do you have an irresistible urge to move or other types of sensations in your arms or legs that become worse in the evening and are relieved by movement?

From the American Academy of Sleep Medicine: www.aasmnet.org.

Interventions

The general treatment plan should focus on promoting adequate, restful, and restorative sleep for patients. This can be accomplished by preventing or reducing the factors that are disturbing the patient's sleep or that have potential to do so and by providing bedtime routines, comfort measures, and a setting conducive to sleep (Lee, 2003; Parker, 1995).

Behavioral Interventions. Behavioral interventions are designed to promote practices of daily living that promote good sleep (Zarcone, 2000). These behaviors reinforce the time and place for sleep and control factors that interfere with sleep. They are effective, low-technology approaches that fit with common sense principles of sleep and circadian regulation. They are the foundation of intervention when sleep is disturbed and should be an important component of patient teaching for health maintenance (Lee, 2003). A comprehensive program may contain one or more of the following

strategies:
- Changes in sleep behaviors and environmental factors that interfere with sleep (sleep hygiene)
- Reassociation of both temporal and environmental stimuli with rapid sleep onset (stimulus control therapy)
- Curtailment of time in bed to actual sleep time, thus creating a mild sleep deprivation, which results in more efficient sleep (sleep restriction)
- Changing dysfunctional beliefs that create anxiety and unrealistic sleep expectation (cognitive therapy)

To reinforce the time for sleep, patients should be advised to go to bed and get up at approximately the same times each day, carry out a regular bedtime routine, and limit napping. Although naps and rest period may be necessary, particularly in the palliative care setting, prolonged daytime sleep decreases the drive for sleep and can delay both sleep onset and continuity. Caffeine after 10 AM should be avoided. Limitation of alcohol and nicotine is recommended. Exposure to outdoor morning light helps maintain the setting of the circadian timing system; exposure to bright light in the evening typically delays sleep onset. To the extent possible, patients should have the opportunity to sleep during their accustomed hours and to maintain familiar routines.

The place for sleep should be physically comfortable and psychologically conducive to sleep. When lying in bed does not lead to sleep, the patient should be advised to get up if possible, engage in quiet activity until drowsy, and then return to bed. Trying too hard to sleep is counterproductive; it is better to engage in some distraction and let sleep come naturally. Keeping the clock turned around and away from view during periods of nocturnal waking may help prevent anxiety.

Strenuous physical activity, worry, and anxiety lead to physiologic arousal that interferes with sleep. Moderate exercise usually is perceived as more beneficial to sleep when performed early in the day rather than late in the evening (Young-McCaughan, Mays, Arzola, et al., 2003). If patients tend to dwell on their concerns after going to bed, setting aside planned "worry time" an hour or two before bedtime may be helpful.

The results of two recent meta-analyses suggest that a combination of the interventions just mentioned are effective in treating insomnia (Morin et al., 1999; Murtagh, Culbert, & Schwartz, 1995). Unfortunately, few clinical trials designed to study the efficacy of sleep-promoting interventions in palliative care populations have been conducted (Savard & Morin, 2001). However, some studies show promising results. Davidson, Waisberg, and Brundage (2001) reported improvement in total sleep time and fatigue following a six-session behavioral intervention (stimulus control, relaxation, and sleep hygiene) in a group of 12 patients with cancer. Cannici, Malcom, and Peek (1983) observed that a program of muscle relaxation given to a group of cancer patients over 3 days reduced sleep latency; an effect was sustained at a 3-month follow-up assessment. Stam and Bultz (1986) described the effectiveness (reduced sleep latency and increased total sleep time) of a combination of somatic focusing and imagery training over five

sessions in a 27-year-old man with severe insomnia secondary to cancer and chemotherapy. Most recently, Berger, VonEssen, Kuhn, et al. (2003) evaluated an intervention designed to promote sleep after adjuvant breast cancer chemotherapy. The intervention was an Individualized Sleep Promotion Plan and included components of sleep hygiene, relaxation therapy, stimulus control, and sleep restriction. Sleep was measured subjectively and via actigraphy. Some improvements in sleep latency, sleep efficiency, and total rest time at night were observed (Berger et al., 2003). These results suggest that behavioral interventions hold promise in reducing sleep disturbances in the palliative setting.

Comfort and Relaxation. Patients with pain, other symptoms, or simply wrinkled bedding can find it difficult to sleep or even rest at ease. Analgesics should be administered when indicated to alleviate pain. Careful positioning and dry, wrinkle-free beds enhance patient comfort. Enabling patients to perform their desired bedtime rituals may facilitate sleep onset.

Various kinds of relaxation techniques may be used to produce a calm inner state through reduction of arousal. For example, massage has been shown to be beneficial in reducing anxiety and inducing sleep in some patients (Richards & Bairnsfather, 1988). The relaxing effects of music therapy on both patients (adults and children) and caregivers in the palliative setting have also been demonstrated (Clair, 2002; Hilliard, 2003; Krout, 2003). White noise, such as ocean, rain, and waterfall sounds, may similarly decrease arousal and facilitate sleep onset (Richards, Nagel, Markie, et al., 2003; Spencer, Moran, Lee, et al., 1990; Williamson, 1992). A sleep program that included relaxation training in addition to good sleep hygiene improved sleep at 4 weeks and 8 weeks in a small sample of cancer patients (n = 12) with insomnia (Davidson et al., 2001).

Medications. In general, sleep hygiene and other nonpharmacologic strategies should be used before sleep-promoting medications are considered in managing sleep problems (Chesson, Anderson, Littner, et al., 1999). In the palliative care setting, their use is very common and may be indicated on both an acute and chronic basis (Bruera, Fainsinger, Schoeller, et al., 1996; Derogatis et al., 1979). Benzodiazepines or benzodiazepine-like medications are generally the hypnotics of choice. Short-acting agents such as zaleplon, zopiclone, or zolpidem are generally preferred to avoid a daytime carryover effect (Table 5-3). If daytime sedation is desired, longer-acting agents such as flurazepam, temazepam, or estazolam can be used. When hypnotics are abruptly discontinued, sleep is likely to worsen (rebound insomnia), an effect that can be reduced by tapering the dose (medications with a longer half-life are less likely to cause this problem). Antidepressants with sedative properties may also be used to facilitate sleep onset (Thulasimani & Ramaswamy, 2002). Patients with sleep apnea or heavy snoring are generally not good candidates for hypnotic medications because they may worsen hypoxemia and the related sleep disturbance. Long-term use of hypnotics has been associated with increased risk of mortality in the general population (Kripke, Klauber, Wingard, et al., 1998). Unfortunately, a recent analysis of the literature regarding the use of benzodiazepines and related drugs for insomnia in the palliative care setting revealed no evidence of rigorous randomized controlled studies, suggesting that it is not yet possible to make specific recommendations regarding their use (Hirst & Sloan, 2002).

Excessive daytime sedation from anxiolytics or pain medications can seriously impair a patient's ability to stay awake during the day, lead to excessive napping, and interfere with sleep onset at night. Thus medications with activating properties may be used to increase daytime alertness. Several antidepressants, such as fluoxetine and bupropion, have both activating and antidepressant effects. Methylphenidate, a dopamine reuptake inhibitor, has also been used effectively in cancer patients to decrease daytime sedation and fatigue associated with opioids (Bruera, Driver, Barnes, et al., 2003; Rozans et al., 2002). It has also been used to improve depression; a large study of 30 cancer patients with a wide variety of malignances, including HIV-associated malignancies, observed that more than 75% of subjects treated with methylphenidate had improvement in their depression (Fernandez,

Adams, Holmes, et al.,1987). Modafinil is widely used to treat daytime sleepiness and fatigue in patients with sleep apnea, narcolepsy, and depression (DeBattista, Doghramji, Menza, et al., 2003; Douglas, 2003; Schwartz, Hirshkowitz, Erman, et al., 2003) and has recently been shown to reduce opioid-induced sedation in patients treated for nonmalignant pain (Webster, Andrews, & Stoddard, 2003).

Exogenous melatonin taken before bedtime has been shown to enhance sleep onset—especially in circadian rhythm disorders; its safety and efficacy for treatment of chronic insomnia remains to be demonstrated. Research has not focused on drug interactions with exogenous melatonin, but its effects also depend on the amount and timing of endogenous production, which can be increased by selective serotonin re-uptake inhibitors, antidepressants, and antipsychotic drugs and reduced by beta blockers, benzodiazepines, and nonsteroidal antiinflammatory drugs. Furthermore, because it is not regulated by the Food and Drug Administration, it is currently not recommended for routine use. The results of one study suggested that when melatonin is used in conjunction with chemotherapy, it may improve survival (Lissoni, Chilelli, Villa, et al., 2003), but whether this is related to its sleep/circadian rhythm–promoting properties remains to be determined (Bartsch, Bartsch, & Karasek, 2002; Sainz, Mayo, Rodriguez, et al., 2003).

Body Position. The results of several studies suggest that body position may play an important role in sleep. De Koninck, Lorrain, and Gagnon studied sleep position in 25 normal subjects over five age-groups ranging from 3 to 80 years old (De Koninck et al., 1992). They found that adults and the elderly demonstrated a preference for sided positions, particularly on the right side, as opposed to supine and prone positions in childhood. The supine position seems to elicit snoring and sleep apnea (Berger, Oksenberg, Silverberg, et al., 1997; Cuhadaroglu, Keles, Erdamar, et al., 2003). Therefore assisting the patient to assume a sided position or elevating the head of the bed before sleeping might have a beneficial effect on sleep in some patients and may facilitate optimal breathing.

Table **5-3** Drugs That Affect Sleeping and Waking

Medication	Half-Life (Hr)	Usual Dose (mg)	Side Effects	Effects on Sleep	Clinical Implications
SEDATIVE/ HYPNOTICS—BENZODIAZEPINES					
Quazepam	48 to 120	7.5 to 15	Muscle relaxation, reduced anxiety, anticonvulsant, daytime sedation, hangover, impairment of psychomotor performance, anterograde amnesia, depression, dependency. Longer-acting medications (quazepam and flurazepam) may be associated with drug accumulation, especially in the elderly or those with metabolic abnormalities.	↓Sleep latency and wake time after sleep onset; ↓REM sleep with REM rebound following withdrawal (increased vivid dreams and nightmares). Sleep is usually more consolidated with fewer sleep-stage transitions.	Use with caution in the elderly or in those with liver dysfunction; may worsen obstructive sleep apnea. Use shorter-acting drugs (half-lives ≤8 hr) for hypnotic indication. Use longer-acting drugs (half-lives ≥12 hr) for anxiolytic action. Avoid alcohol/barbiturate intake. Rapid withdrawal may lead to worsening of original symptoms/seizures.
Flurazepam	48 to 120	15 to 30			
Triazolam	2 to 6	0.125 to 0.25			
Estazolam	8 to 24	1 to 2			
Temazepam	8 to 20	15 to 30			
SEDATIVE/HYPNOTICS—NON-BENZODIAZEPINES					
Zolpidem	1.5 to 2.4	5 to 10	Headache, anxiety, depression, anterograde amnesia, residual daytime somnolence.	Little or no effect on sleep architecture in usual doses; may reduce nocturnal arousals.	Tolerance, dependency, and withdrawal symptoms much less of a problem than with benzodiazepines. Rebound insomnia may occur upon abrupt discontinuation. Use with caution in the elderly or those with impaired liver function.
Zaleplon	1	5 to 10			
Zopiclone	5 to 6	7.5 to 10			
STIMULANTS					
Modafinil	10 to 12	100 to 400	Headache, dry mouth, nervousness, irritability, talkativeness, anorexia, insomnia.	Little or no effect on sleep but can lead to insomnia if taken later in the day.	Do not take after 3 PM. Modafinil may cause oral contraceptives to be less effective. Liver function should be monitored regularly.
Methyl-phenidate	2 to 4	10 to 60			

ANTIDEPRESSANTS—TRICYCLICS

Drug	Half-life (h)	Dosage (mg)	Effects on Sleep	Side Effects	Comments
Amitriptyline	10 to 50	75 to 150	Generally ↑total sleep time and ↓wake time. REM suppression, ↑REM latency, ↑stage 2.	Anticholinergic effects—blurred vision, dry mouth, urinary retention, orthostatic hypotension, confusion, daytime sedation, weight gain.	May impair driving ability. Rapid withdrawal may cause REM-sleep rebound, leading to increased dreaming and/or nightmares. Amitriptyline and doxepin are sedating and should be taken at bedtime.
Doxepin	6 to 8	75 to 150			
Nortriptyline	16 to 90	75 to 150			
Desipramine	7 to 90	100 to 200			

ANTIDEPRESSANTS—SELECTIVE SEROTONIN REUPTAKE INHIBITORS

Drug	Half-life (h)	Dosage (mg)	Effects on Sleep	Side Effects	Comments
Fluoxetine	48 to 72	20 to 60	↑total sleep time, ↓sleep latency. REM sleep suppression.	Few anticholinergic effects, priapism (trazodone), nausea, dizziness, dry mouth, sexual dysfunction, insomnia, somnolence.	Fluoxetine, paroxetine, sertraline are more activating—take in morning. Trazodone is sedating—take at bedtime. Rapid withdrawal may cause REM-sleep rebound, leading to increased dreaming and/or nightmares.
Paroxetine	24	20 to 60			
Sertraline	24	50 to 200			
Trazodone	5 to 9	150 to 600	↑total sleep time, ↓sleep latency.		

ANTIDEPRESSANTS—OTHERS

Drug	Half-life (h)	Dosage (mg)	Effects on Sleep	Side Effects	Comments
Bupropion	8 to 24	150 to 300	Insomnia, ↑REM sleep.	GI upset; lowering of seizure threshold.	Activating; take in the morning. Monitor blood pressure.
Venlafaxine	3 to 4	150 to 375	Insomnia, ↑total sleep time.	Anxiety, anorexia, sexual dysfunction, insomnia, somnolence, hypertension.	
Mirtazapine	20 to 40	15 to 45	↑total sleep time, ↓sleep latency.	Increased appetite, weight gain, dizziness, hypertension, sedation.	Sedating—take at bedtime. May cause "hangover"-like symptoms initially, but this typically resolves with continued use.

GI, Gastrointestinal; *REM*, rapid eye movement.
Data from Arcangelo, V.P., & Peterson, A.M. (2001). *Pharmacotherapeutics for advanced practice.* Philadelphia: Lippincott; Benca, R.M. (2000). Mood disorders. In M.H. Kryger, T. Roth, & W.C. Dement (Eds.), *Principles and practice of sleep medicine* (3rd ed., pp. 1140-1157). Philadelphia: Saunders; Mitler, M.M., & Aldrich, M.S. (2000). Stimulants: Efficacy and adverse effects. In M.H. Kryger, T. Roth, & W.C. Dement (Eds.), *Principles and practice of sleep medicine* (3rd ed., pp. 429-440). Philadelphia: Saunders; Roehrs, T., & Roth, T. (2000). Hypnotics: Efficacy and adverse effects. In M.H. Kryger, T. Roth, & W.C. Dement (Eds.), *Principles and practice of sleep medicine* (3rd ed., pp. 414-418). Philadelphia: Saunders.

SUMMARY

Patients in the palliative setting are at high risk for and often have impaired sleep. Despite the widely held belief that sleep promotes well-being, care practices are rarely designed to encourage optimal sleep and promote maximal daytime alertness. Research is needed to clarify the role of both night-time sleep and daytime naps in the palliative setting. Furthermore, additional work is needed to identify clinical interventions that prevent sleep problems and optimize the effectiveness of care.

Objective Questions

1. Sleep is defined according to:

   a. Sleep stages via polysomnography.
   b. Behavioral, physiologic, and subjective criteria.
   c. Subjective reports of quality.
   d. State of quiescence and time of day.

2. The specific functions of sleep are:

   a. Restorative.
   b. Neurologic development/maintenance.
   c. Memory consolidation.
   d. Physical growth and immune function.
   e. Not well understood but likely serve multiple purposes.

3. Daytime sleepiness is best defined as:

   a. Falling asleep after lunch in the afternoon.
   b. Taking a nap.
   c. The tendency to fall asleep during the day.
   d. Fatigue and tiredness.

4. Symptoms often associated with daytime sleepiness include:

   a. Decreased concentration, motivation, memory.
   b. Hyperactivity.
   c. Inability to nap.
   d. Increased illness.

5. Which of the following is true about the sleep of normal young adults:

   a. Sleep is entered through REM.
   b. NREM and REM alternate about every 4 hours.
   c. Slow-wave sleep predominates the last third of the night.
   d. REM predominates the first third of the night.
   e. NREM = 75% to 80% of sleep; REM = 20% to 25% of sleep.

6. Good sleep hygiene includes:

   a. Staying in bed for as long as possible.
   b. Getting sleep any time of the day or night.
   c. Eating a meal before bedtime.
   d. Avoiding working and other stimulating activities right before bedtime.

7. Insomnia can be expressed as:

   a. Difficulty falling asleep.
   b. Difficulty staying asleep.
   c. Difficulty falling asleep, staying asleep, early morning awakenings, and having unrefreshing sleep.
   d. Daytime napping.

8. The most common cause of sleep deprivation is:

   a. Primary sleep disorders.
   b. Circadian rhythm abnormalities.
   c. Chronic illness.
   d. Decreased total sleep time and lifestyle/environment interactions.

9. Poor sleep affects a wide range of physiologic, cognitive/behavioral, psychologic, and social outcomes. Thus helping patients obtain optimal sleep should be an important part of any palliative care plan. Sleep is also important for caregivers; a recent study demonstrated that when caregivers exercise good sleep hygiene, they:

   a. Had more energy.
   b. Were more patient.
   c. Were less depressed and had improved daytime function.
   d. Were able to stay awake for longer periods.

10. Daytime sedation is a common side effect of treatments with anxiolytics or pain medications. Daytime alertness may be enhanced by what pharmacologic agents?

a. Zolpidem.

b. Trazodone.

c. Modafinil and methylphenidate.

d. Temazepam.

REFERENCES

Adam, K., & Oswald, I. (1984). Sleep helps healing. *Br Med J (Clin Res Ed), 289*(6456), 1400-1401.

Allen, R.P., & Earley, C.J. (2001). Restless legs syndrome: A review of clinical and pathophysiologic features. *J Clin Neurophysiol, 18*(2), 128-147.

American Sleep Disorders Association (ASDA). (1986). Guidelines for the Multiple Sleep Latency Test (MSLT): A standard measure of sleepiness. *Sleep, 9*(4), 519-524.

American Sleep Disorders Association (ASDA). (1997). *The International Classification of Sleep Disorders.* Rochester, Minn.: Author.

Ancoli-Israel, S. (2000). Insomnia in the elderly: A review for the primary care practitioner. *Sleep, 23*(Suppl. 1), S23-30; discussion S36-28.

Ancoli-Israel, S., Cole, R., Alessi, C., et al. (2003). The role of actigraphy in the study of sleep and circadian rhythms. *Sleep, 26*(3), 342-392.

Ancoli-Israel, S., Kripke, D.F., Klauber, M.R., et al. (1991a). Periodic limb movements in sleep in community-dwelling elderly. *Sleep, 14*(6), 496-500.

Ancoli-Israel, S., Kripke, D.F., Klauber, M.R., et al. (1991b). Sleep-disordered breathing in community-dwelling elderly. *Sleep, 14*(6), 486-495.

Ancoli-Israel, S., Martin, J.L., Kripke, D.F., et al. (2002). Effect of light treatment on sleep and circadian rhythms in demented nursing home patients. *J Am Geriatr Soc, 50*(2), 282-289.

Ancoli-Israel, S., Moore, P.J., & Jones, V. (2001). The relationship between fatigue and sleep in cancer patients: A review. *Eur J Cancer Care (Engl), 10*(4), 245-255.

Andersen, G., & Sjogren, P. (1998). Epidemiology of cancer pain. *Ugeskr Laeger, 160*(18), 2681-2684.

Anderson, K.O., Getto, C.J., Mendoza, T.R., et al. (2003). Fatigue and sleep disturbance in patients with cancer, patients with clinical depression, and community-dwelling adults. *J Pain Symptom Manage, 25*(4), 307-318.

Arcangelo, V.P., & Peterson, A.M. (2001). *Pharmacotherapeutics for advanced practice.* Philadelphia: Lippincott.

Ardestani, S., Inserra, P., Solkoff, D., et al. (1999). The role of cytokines and chemokines on tumor progression: A review. *Cancer Detect Prev, 23*(3), 215-225.

Atkinson, A., Barsevick, A., Cella, D., et al. (2000). NCCN practice guidelines for cancer-related fatigue. *Oncology, 14*(11A), 151-161.

Aurell, J., & Elmqvist, D. (1985). Sleep in the surgical intensive care unit: Continuous polygraphic recording of sleep in nine patients receiving postoperative care. *Br Med J (Clin Res Ed), 290*(6474), 1029-1032.

Baker, T.L. (1985). Sleep apnea disorders. Introduction to sleep and sleep disorders. *Med Clin North Am, 69*(6), 1123-1152.

Balter, M.B., & Uhlenhuth, E.H. (1992). New epidemiologic findings about insomnia and its treatment. *J Clin Psychiatry, 53*(Suppl.), 34-39; discussion 40-42.

Bartsch, C., & Bartsch, H. (1999). Melatonin in cancer patients and in tumor-bearing animals. *Adv Exp Med Biol, 467,* 247-264.

Bartsch, C., Bartsch, H., & Karasek, M. (2002). Melatonin in clinical oncology. *Neuroendocrinol Lett, 23*(Suppl. 1), 30-38.

Bassiri, A.G., & Guilleminault, C. (2000). Clinical features and evaluation of obstructive sleep apnea-hypopnea syndrome. In M.H. Kryger, T. Roth, & W.C. Dement (Eds.), *Principles and practice of sleep medicine* (pp. 869-878). Philadelphia: Saunders.

Belka, C., Budach, W., Kortman, R.D., et al. (2001). Radiation induced CNS toxicity: Molecular and cellular mechanisms. *Br J Cancer, 85*(9), 1233-1239.

Benca, R.M. (2000). Mood disorders. In M.H. Kryger, T. Roth, & W.C. Dement (Eds.), *Principles and practice of sleep medicine* (3rd ed., pp. 1140-1157). Philadelphia: Saunders.

Benca, R.M., Kushida, C.A., Everson, C.A., et al. (1989). Sleep deprivation in the rat: VII. Immune function. *Sleep, 12*(1), 47-52.

Berger, A.M., & Farr, L. (1999). The influence of daytime inactivity and nighttime restlessness on cancer-related fatigue. *Oncol Nurs Forum, 26*(10), 1663-1671.

Berger, A.M., & Higginbotham, P. (2000). Correlates of fatigue during and following adjuvant breast cancer chemotherapy: A pilot study. *Oncol Nurs Forum, 27*(9), 1443-1448.

Berger, A.M., VonEssen, S., Kuhn, B.R., et al. (2003). Adherence, sleep, and fatigue outcomes after adjuvant breast cancer chemotherapy: Results of a feasibility intervention study. *Oncol Nurs Forum, 30*(3), 513-522.

Berger, J.R., & Arendt, G. (2000). HIV dementia: The role of the basal ganglia and dopaminergic systems. *J Psychopharmacol, 14*(3), 214-221.

Berger, M., Oksenberg, A., Silverberg, D.S., et al. (1997). Avoiding the supine position during sleep lowers 24 h blood pressure in obstructive sleep apnea (OSA) patients. *J Hum Hypertens, 11*(10), 657-664.

Beszterczey, A., & Lipowski, Z.J. (1977). Insomnia in cancer patients. *Can Med Assoc J, 116*(4), 355.

Beszterczey, A., & Lipowski, Z.J. (1997). Insomnia in cancer patients. *Can Med Assoc J, 116*(4), 355.

Biron, C.A. (1997). Activation and function of natural killer cell responses during viral infections. *Curr Opin Immunol, 9*(1), 24-34.

Biron, C.A., Nguyen, K.B., Pien, G.C., et al. (1999). Natural killer cells in antiviral defense: Function and regulation by innate cytokines. *Annu Rev Immunol, 17,* 189-220.

Biron, C.A., Su, H.C., & Orange, J.S. (1996). Function and regulation of natural killer (NK) cells during viral infections: Characterization of responses in vivo. *Methods, 9*(2), 379-393.

Blais, F.C., Morin, C.M., Boisclair, A., et al. (2001). Insomnia: Prevalence and treatment of patients in general practice. *Can Fam Physician, 47,* 759-767.

Bliwise, D.L. (2000). Normal aging. In M.H. Kryger, T. Roth, & W.C. Dement (Eds.), *Principles and practice of sleep medicine* (3rd ed., pp. 26-42). Philadelphia: Saunders.

Bonnet, M.H. (2000). *Sleep deprivation* (3rd ed.). Philadelphia: Saunders.

Borbely, A.A., & Acherman, P. (2000). Sleep homeostasis and models of sleep regulation. In M.H. Kryger, T. Roth, & W.C. Dement (Eds.), *Principles and practice of sleep medicine* (3rd ed., pp. 377-390). Philadelphia: Saunders.

Bramwell, L., MacKenzie, J., Laschinger, H., et al. (1995). Need for overnight respite for primary caregivers of hospice clients. *Cancer Nurs, 18*(5), 337-343.

Breitbart, W., Bruera, E., Chochinov, H., et al. (1995). Neuropsychiatric syndromes and psychological symptoms in patients with advanced cancer. *J Pain Symptom Manage, 10*(2), 131-141.

Broeckel, J.A., Jacobsen, P.B., Horton, J., et al. (1998). Characteristics and correlates of fatigue after adjuvant chemotherapy for breast cancer. *J Clin Oncol, 16*(5), 1689-1696.

Bruera, E., Driver, L., Barnes, E.A., et al. (2003). Patient-controlled methylphenidate for the management of fatigue in patients with advanced cancer: A preliminary report. *J Clin Oncol, 21*(23), 4439-4443.

Bruera, E., Fainsinger, R.L., Schoeller, T., et al. (1996). Rapid discontinuation of hypnotics in terminal cancer patients: A prospective study. *Ann Oncol, 7*(8), 855-856.

Bursztyn, M., Ginsberg, G., Hammerman-Rozenberg, R., et al. (1999). The siesta in the elderly: Risk factor for mortality? *Arch Intern Med, 159*(14), 1582-1586.

Bursztyn, M., Ginsberg, G., & Stessman, J. (2002). The siesta and mortality in the elderly: Effect of rest without sleep and daytime sleep duration. *Sleep, 25*(2), 187-191.

Buysse, D.J., Reynolds, C.F., Monk, T.H., et al. (1989). The Pittsburgh Sleep Quality Index: A new instrument for psychiatric practice and research. *Psychiatry Res, 28*(2), 193-213.

Buysse, D.J., Reynolds, C.F., Monk, T.H., et al. (1991). Quantification of subjective sleep quality in healthy elderly men and women using the Pittsburgh Sleep Quality Index (PSQI) [published erratum appears in *Sleep* 1992 Feb; *15*(1):83]. *Sleep, 14*(4), 331-338.

Byku, M., & Gannon, R.L. (2000a). Opioid induced non-photic phase shifts of hamster circadian activity rhythms. *Brain Res, 873*(2), 189-196.

Byku, M., & Gannon, R.L. (2000b). SNC 80, a delta-opioid agonist, elicits phase advances in hamster circadian activity rhythms. *Neuroreport, 11*(7), 1449-1452.

Byku, M., Legutko, R., & Gannon, R.L. (2000). Distribution of delta opioid receptor immunoreactivity in the hamster suprachiasmatic nucleus and intergeniculate leaflet. *Brain Res, 857*(1-2), 1-7.

Campbell, S.S., & Broughton, R.J. (1994). Rapid decline in body temperature before sleep: Fluffing the physiological pillow? *Chronobiol Int, 11*(2), 126-131.

Cannici, J., Malcom, R., & Peek, L.A. (1983). Treatment of insomnia in cancer patients using muscle relaxation training. *J Behav Ther Exp Psychiatry, 14*(3), 251-256.

Capuron, L., Ravaud, A., & Dantzer, R. (2000). Early depressive symptoms in cancer patients receiving interleukin 2 and/or interferon alfa-2b therapy. *J Clin Oncol, 18*(10), 2143-2151.

Carpenter, J.S., Johnson, D., Wagner, L., et al. (2002). Hot flashes and related outcomes in breast cancer survivors and matched comparison women. *Oncol Nurs Forum, 29*(3), e16-25.

Carskadon, M.A. (1990). Patterns of sleep and sleepiness in adolescents. *Pediatrician, 17*(1), 5-12.

Carskadon, M.A., & Acebo, C. (2002). Regulation of sleepiness in adolescents: Update, insights, and speculation. *Sleep, 25*(6), 606-614.

Carskadan, M.A., & Dement, W. (2000). Normal human sleep: An overview. In M.H. Kruger, T. Roth, & W.C. Dement (Eds.), *Principles and practice of sleep medicine* (3rd ed., pp. 15-25). Philadelphia: Saunders.

Carskadon, M.A., Dement, W.C., Mitler, M.M., et al. (1986). Guidelines for the Multiple Sleep Latency Test (MSLT): A standard measure of sleepiness. *Sleep, 9*(4), 519-524.

Carskadon, M.A., & Rechtschaffen, A. (2000). Monitoring and staging of human sleep. In M.H. Kryger, T. Roth, & W.C. Dement (Ed.), *Principles and practice of sleep medicine* (3rd ed., pp. 1197-1216). Philadelphia: Saunders.

Carter, N., Henderson, R., Lal, S., et al. (2002). Cardiovascular and autonomic response to environmental noise during sleep in night shift workers. *Sleep, 25*(4), 457-464.

Carter, P.A. (2002). Caregivers' descriptions of sleep changes and depressive symptoms. *Oncol Nurs Forum, 29*(9), 1277-1283.

Carter, P.A. (2003). Family caregivers' sleep loss and depression over time. *Cancer Nurs, 26*(4), 253-259.

Carter, P.A., & Chang, B.L. (2000). Sleep and depression in cancer caregivers. *Cancer Nurs, 23*(6), 410-415.

Cassileth, P.A., Lusk, E.J., & Torri, S. (1983). Antiemetic efficacy of dexamethasone therapy in patients receiving cancer chemotherapy. *Arch Intern Med, 143*, 1347-1349.

Chervin, R.D. (2000). Sleepiness, fatigue, tiredness, and lack of energy in obstructive sleep apnea. *Chest, 118*(2), 372-379.

Chesson, A.L. Jr., Anderson, W.M., Littner, M., et al. (1999). Practice parameters for the nonpharmacologic treatment of chronic insomnia: An American Academy of Sleep Medicine report. Standards of Practice Committee of the American Academy of Sleep Medicine. *Sleep, 22*(8), 1128-1133.

Chesson, A.L. Jr., Berry, R.B., & Pack, A. (2003). Practice parameters for the use of portable monitoring devices in the investigation of suspected obstructive sleep apnea in adults. *Sleep, 26*(7), 907-913.

Chesson, A.L. Jr., Wise, M., Davila, D., et al. (1999). Practice parameters for the treatment of restless legs syndrome and periodic limb movement disorder: An American Academy of Sleep Medicine Report. Standards of Practice Committee of the American Academy of Sleep Medicine. *Sleep, 22*(7), 961-968.

Chokroverty, S. (1999). An overview of sleep. In S. Chokroverty (Ed.), *Sleep disorders medicine* (2nd ed., pp. 7-20). Boston: Butterworth Heinemann.

Clair, A.A. (2002). The effects of music therapy on engagement in family caregiver and care receiver couples with dementia. *Am J Alzheimers Dis Other Demen, 17*(5), 286-290.

Cleeland, C.S., Mendoza, T.R., Wang, X.S., et al. (2000). Assessing symptom distress in cancer patients. *Cancer, 89*(7), 1634-1646.

Cohen, F.L. (1997). Measuring sleep. In M. Frank-Stromborg & S.J. Olsen (Eds.), *Instruments for clinical health-care research* (pp. 264-279). Boston: Jones & Bartlett.

Cohen, F.L., Ferrans, C.E., Vizgirda, V., et al. (1996). Sleep in men and women infected with human immunodeficiency virus. *Holist Nurs Pract, 10*(4), 33-43.

Cohen-Zion, M., Stepnowsky, C., Marler, et al. (2001). Changes in cognitive function associated with sleep disordered breathing in older people. *J Am Geriatr Soc, 49*(12), 1622-1627.

Cole, M.G., Dendukuri, N., McCusker, J., et al. (2003). An empirical study of different diagnostic criteria for delirium among elderly medical inpatients. *J Neuropsychiatry Clin Neurosci, 15*(2), 200-207.

Cole, M.G., McCusker, J., Dendukuri, N., et al. (2002). Symptoms of delirium among elderly medical inpatients with or without dementia. *J Neuropsychiatry Clin Neurosci, 14*(2), 167-175.

Connor, J., Norton, R., Ameratunga, S., et al. (2001). Prevalence of driver sleepiness in a random population-based sample of car driving. *Sleep, 24*(6), 688-694.

Couzi, R.J., Helzlsouer, K.J., & Fetting, J.H. (1995). Prevalence of menopausal symptoms among women with a history of breast cancer and attitudes toward estrogen replacement therapy. *J Clin Oncol, 13*(11), 2737-2744.

Crick, F., & Mitchison, G. (1983). The function of dream sleep. *Nature, 304*(5922), 111-114.

Cruess, D.G., Antoni, M.H., Gonzalez, J., et al. (2003). Sleep disturbance mediates the association between psychological distress and immune status among HIV-positive men and women on combination antiretroviral therapy. *J Psychosom Res, 54*(3), 185-189.

Cuhadaroglu, C., Keles, N., Erdamar, B., et al. (2003). Body position and obstructive sleep apnea syndrome. *Pediatr Pulmonol, 36*(4), 335-338.

Czeisler, C.A., Weitzman, E., Moore-Ede, M.C., et al. (1980). Human sleep: Its duration and organization depend on its circadian phase. *Science, 210*(4475), 1264-1267.

D'Alessandro, R., Rinaldi, R., Cristina, E., et al. (1995). Prevalence of excessive daytime sleepiness an open epidemiological problem. *Sleep, 18*(5), 389-391.

Darko, D.F., McCutchan, J.A., Kripke, D.F., et al. (1992). Fatigue, sleep disturbance, disability, and indices of progression of HIV infection. *Am J Psychiatry, 149*(4), 514-520.

Davidson, J.R., MacLean, A.W., Brundage, M.D., et al. (2002). Sleep disturbance in cancer patients. *Soc Sci Med, 54*, 1309-1321.

Davidson, J.R., Waisberg, J.L., Brundage, M.D., et al. (2001). Nonpharmacologic group treatment of insomnia: A preliminary study with cancer survivors. *Psychooncology, 10*(5), 389-397.

DeBattista, C., Doghramji, K., Menza, M.A., et al. (2003). Adjunct modafinil for the short-term treatment of fatigue and sleepiness in patients with major depressive disorder: A preliminary double-blind, placebo-controlled study. *J Clin Psychiatry, 64*(9), 1057-1064.

Degner, L.F., & Sloan, J.A. (1995). Symptom distress in newly diagnosed ambulatory cancer patients and as a predictor of survival in lung cancer. *J Pain Symptom Manage, 10*(6), 423-431.

De Koninck, J., Lorrain, D., & Gagnon, P. (1992). Sleep positions and position shifts in five age groups: An ontogenetic picture. *Sleep, 15*(2), 143-149.

Derogatis, L.R., Feldstein, M., Morrow, G., et al. (1979). A survey of psychotropic drug prescriptions in an oncology population. *Cancer, 44*(5), 1919-1929.

Dickens, C., McGowan, L., & Dale, S. (2003). Impact of depression on experimental pain perception: A systematic review of the literature with meta-analysis. *Psychosom Med, 65*(3), 369-375.

Dinges, D.F., Douglas, S.D., Hamarman, S., et al. (1995). Sleep deprivation and human immune function. *Adv Neuroimmunol, 5*(2), 97-110.

Dinges, D.F., Pack, F., Williams, K., et al. (1997). Cumulative sleepiness, mood disturbance, and psychomotor vigilance performance decrements during a week of sleep restricted to 4-5 hours per night. *Sleep, 20*(4), 267-277.

Dorrepaal, K.L., Aaronson, N.K., & van Dam, F.S. (1989). Pain experience and pain management among hospitalized cancer patients: A clinical study. *Cancer, 63*(3), 593-598.

Douglas, N.J. (2003). Modafinil and sleepiness. *Am J Respir Crit Care Med, 168*(12), 1538; author reply 1538-1539.

Douglass, L.G. (1997). Reciprocal support in the context of cancer: Perspectives of the patient and spouse. *Oncol Nurs Forum, 24*(9), 1529-1536.

Dreher, H.M. (2003). The effect of caffeine reduction on sleep quality and well-being in persons with HIV. *J Psychosom Res, 54*, 191-198.

Dura, J.R., Stukenberg, K.W., & Kiecolt-Glaser, J.K. (1990). Chronic stress and depressive disorders in older adults. *J Abnorm Psychol, 99*(3), 284-290.

Earlam, S., Glover, C., Fordy, C., et al. (1996). Relation between tumor size, quality of life, and survival in patients with colorectal liver metastases. *J Clin Oncol, 14*(1), 171-175.

Edell-Gustafsson, U.M., Gustavsson, G., & Yngman Uhlin, P. (2003). Effects of sleep loss in men and women with insufficient sleep suffering from chronic disease: A model for supportive nursing care. *Int J Nurs Pract, 9*(1), 49-59.

Edwards, G.B., & Schuring, L.M. (1993). Pilot study: Validating staff nurses' observations of sleep and wake states among critically ill patients, using polysomnography. *Am J Crit Care, 2*(2), 125-131.

El-Ad, B., & Korczyn, A.D. (1998). Disorders of excessive daytime sleepiness: An update. *J Neurol Sci, 153*(2), 192-202.

Ellis, B.W., Johns, M.W., Lancaster, R., et al. (1981). The St. Mary's Hospital sleep questionnaire: A study of reliability. *Sleep, 4*(1), 93-97.

Engleman, H.M., Kingshott, R.N., Martin, S.E., et al. (2000). Cognitive function in the sleep apnea/hypopnea syndrome (SAHS) (in process citation). *Sleep, 23*(Suppl. 4), S102-108.

Engstrom, C.A., Strohl, R.A., Rose, L., et al. (1999). Sleep alterations in cancer patients. *Cancer Nurs, 22*(2), 143-148.

Epstein, L.J., Strollo, P.J. Jr., Donegan, R.B., et al. (1995). Obstructive sleep apnea in patients with human immunodeficiency virus (HIV) disease. *Sleep, 18*(5), 368-376.

Erlichman, C., & Loprinzi, C.L. (1997). Hormonal therapies. In V.T. DeVita, S. Hellman, & S.A. Rosenber (Eds.), *Cancer: Principles and practice of oncology* (pp. 395-405). Philadelphia: Lippincott-Raven.

Everson, C.A., Bergmann, B.M., & Rechtschaffen, A. (1989). Sleep deprivation in the rat: III. Total sleep deprivation. *Sleep, 12*(1), 13-21.

Everson, C.A., & Toth, L.A. (2000). Systemic bacterial invasion induced by sleep deprivation. *Am J Physiol Regul Integr Comp Physiol, 278*(4), R905-916.

Faithfull, S., & Brada, M. (1990). Somnolence syndrome in adults following cranial irradiation for primary brain tumours. *Clin Oncol, 10*(4), 250-254.

Fernandez, F., Adams, R., Holmes, V.F., et al. (1987). Methylphenidate for depressive disorders in cancer patients: An alternative to standard antidepressants. *Psychosomatics, 28*(9), 455-461.

Fishbain, D.A. (2002). The pain-depression relationship. *Psychosomatics, 43*(4), 341; author reply 341-342.

Fisher, B., Costantino, J., & Redmond, C. (1989). A randomized clinical trial evaluating tamoxifen in the treatment of patients with node-negative breast cancer who have estrogen-receptor-positive tumors. *N Engl J Med, 320*(8), 479-484.

Fortner, B.V., Kasprowicz, S., Wang, S., et al. (2000). Sleep disturbance and quality of life in cancer patients. *Sleep, 23* (Abstract Suppl. 2), A103-104.

Franck, L.S., Johnson, L.M., Lee, K., et al. (1999). Sleep disturbances in children with human immunodeficiency virus infection. *Pediatrics, 104*(5), e62.

Franken, P., Chollet, D., & Tafti, M. (2001). The homeostatic regulation of sleep need is under genetic control. *J Neurosci, 21*(8), 2610-2621.

Friedman, M., Landsberg, R., Pryor, S., et al. (2001). The occurrence of sleep-disordered breathing among patients with head and neck cancer. *Laryngoscope, 111*(11 Pt. 1), 1917-1919.

Gallego, L., Barreiro, P., Rio Rd, R., et al. (2004). Analyzing sleep abnormalities in HIV-infected patients treated with efavirenz. *Clin Infect Dis, 38*(3), 430-432.

Galloway, S., Bubela, N., McKibbon, A., et al. (1995). Symptom distress, anxiety, depression, and discharge information needs after peripheral arterial bypass. *J Vasc Nurs, 13*(2), 35-40.

Gallup. (1991). *Sleep in America.* Princeton, NJ: Gallup Organization.

Gallup. (1995). *Sleep in America.* Princeton, NJ: Gallup Organization.

Gillberg, M., & Akerstedt, T. (1982). Body temperature and sleep at different times of day. *Sleep, 5*(4), 378-388.

Given, B., Given, C., Azzouz, F., et al. (2001). Physical functioning of elderly cancer patients prior to diagnosis and following initial treatment. *Nurs Res, 50*(4), 222-232.

Given, C.W., Given, B.A., Stommel, M., et al. (1999). The impact of new demands for assistance on caregiver depression: Tests using an inception cohort. *Gerontologist, 39*(1), 76-85.

Glotzbach, S.F., & Heller, H.C. (2000). Thermoregulation. In M.H. Kryger, T.Roth, & W.C. Dement (Eds.), *Principles and practice of sleep medicine* (3rd ed., pp. 289-304). Philadelphia: Saunders.

Greenberg, D.B., Gray, J.L., Mannix, C.M., et al. (1993). Treatment-related fatigue and serum intereukin-1 levels in patients during external beam irradiation for prostate cancer. *J Pain Symptom Manage, 8*(4), 196-200.

Griefahn, B. (2002). Sleep disturbances related to environmental noise. *Noise Health, 4*(15), 57-60.

Gursky, J.T., & Krahn, L.E. (2000). The effects of antidepressants on sleep: A review. *Harv Rev Psychiatry, 8*(6), 298-306.

Hanks, G.W., Twycross, R.G., & Bliss, J.M. (1987). Controlled release morphine tablets: A double-blind trial in patients with advanced cancer. *Anaesthesia, 42*(8), 840-844.

Harman, K., Pivik, R.T., D'Eon, J.L., et al. (2002). Sleep in depressed and nondepressed participants with chronic low back pain: Electroencephalographic and behaviour findings. *Sleep, 25*(7), 775-783.

Hilliard, R.E. (2003). Music therapy in pediatric palliative care: Complementing the interdisciplinary approach. *J Palliat Care, 19*(2), 127-132.

Hirst, A., & Sloan, R. (2002). Benzodiazepines and related drugs for insomnia in palliative care. *Cochrane Database Syst Rev, 4,* CD003346.

Holsboer-Trachsler, E., & Seifritz, E. (2000). Sleep in depression and sleep deprivation: A brief conceptual review. *World J Biol Psychiatry, 1*(4), 180-186.

Hong, S., & Dimsdale, J.E. (2003). Physical activity and perception of energy and fatigue in obstructive sleep apnea. *Med Sci Sports Exerc, 35*(7), 1088-1092.

Horne, J.A. (1988). *Why we sleep.* New York: Oxford University Press.

Horne, J.A., Percival, J.E., & Traynor, J.R. (1980). Aspirin and human sleep. *Electroencephalogr Clin Neurophysiol, 49*(3-4), 409-413.

Horne, J.A., & Reid, A.J. (1985). Night-time sleep EEG changes following body heating in a warm bath. *Electroencephalogr Clin Neurophysiol, 60*(2), 154-157.

Hudson, A.L., Lee, K.A., & Portillo, C.J. (2003). Symptom experience and functional status among HIV-infected women. *AIDS Care, 15*(4), 483-492.

Jean-Louis, G., von Gizycki, H., Zizi, F., et al. (1996). Determination of sleep and wakefulness with the actigraph data analysis software (ADAS). *Sleep, 19*(9), 739-743.

Jepson, C., McCorkle, R., Adler, D., et al. (1999). Effects of home care on caregivers' psychosocial status. *Image J Nurs Sch, 31*(2), 115-120.

Johns, M.W. (1991). A new method for measuring daytime sleepiness: The Epworth Sleepiness Scale. *Sleep, 14*(6), 540-545.

Johns, M.W. (1992). Reliability and factor analysis of the Epworth Sleepiness Scale. *Sleep, 15*(4), 376-381.

Johns, M.W. (2000). Sensitivity and specificity of the Multiple Sleep Latency Test (MSLT), the maintenance of wakefulness test and the Epworth Sleepiness Scale: Failure of the MSLT as a gold standard. *J Sleep Res, 9*(1), 5-11.

Jones, B.E. (2000). Basic mechanisms of sleep-wake states. In M.H. Kryger, T.Roth, & W.C. Dement (Eds.), *Principles and practice of sleep medicine* (3rd ed., pp. 134-154). Phladelphia: Saunders.

Kaneko, T., Takahashi, S., Naka, T., et al. (1997). Postoperative delirium following gastrointestinal surgery in elderly patients. *Surg Today, 27*(2), 107-111.

Karacan, I., Thornby, J.I., Anch, M., et al. (1976). Prevalence of sleep disturbance in a primarily urban Florida County. *Soc Sci Med, 10*(5), 239-244.

Kavanau, J.L. (1997). Memory, sleep and the evolution of mechanisms of synaptic efficacy maintenance. *Neuroscience, 79*(1), 7-44.

Kavanau, J.L. (2000). Sleep, memory maintenance, and mental disorders. *J Neuropsychiatry Clin Neurosci, 12*(2), 199-208.

Kay, D.C., Eisenstein, R.B., & Jasinski, D.R. (1969). Morphine effects on human REM state, waking state and NREM sleep. *Psychopharmacologia, 14*(5), 404-416.

Kaye, J., Kaye, K., & Madow, L. (1983). Sleep patterns in patients with cancer and patients with cardiac disease. *J Psychol, 114*(1st half), 107-113.

Khoory, R., & Stemme, D. (1988). Plasma melatonin levels in patients suffering from colorectal carcinoma. *J Pineal Res, 5*(3), 251-258.

Klerman, E.B., Rimmer, D.W., Dijk, D.J., et al. (1998). Nonphotic entrainment of the human circadian pacemaker. *Am J Physiol, 274*(4 Pt. 2), R991-996.

Knill, R.L., Moote, C.A., Skinner, M.I., et al. (1990). Anesthesia with abdominal surgery leads to intense REM sleep during the first postoperative week. *Anesthesiology, 73*(1), 52-61.

Knop, D.S., Bergman-Evans, B., & McCabe, B.W. (1998). In sickness and in health: An exploration of the perceived quality of the marital relationship, coping, and depression in caregivers of spouses with Alzheimer's disease. *J Psychosoc Nurs Ment Health Serv, 36*(1), 16-21.

Koutsilieri, E., Scheller, C., Sopper, S., et al. (2002). Psychiatric complications in human immunodeficiency virus infection. *J Neurovirol, 8*(Suppl. 2), 129-133.

Koutsilieri, E., Scheller, C., ter Meulen, A., et al. (2004). Monoamine oxidase inhibition and CNS immunodeficiency infection. *Neurotoxicology, 25*(1-2), 267-270.

Kozachik, S.L., Given, C.W., Given, B.A., et al. (2001). Improving depressive symptoms among caregivers of patients with cancer: Results of a randomized clinical trial. *Oncol Nurs Forum, 28*(7), 1149-1157.

Kripke, D.F. (2003). Sleep and mortality. *Psychosom Med, 65*(1), 74.

Kripke, D.F., Klauber, M.R., Wingard, D.L., et al. (1998). Mortality hazard associated with prescription hypnotics. *Biol Psychiatry, 43*(9), 687-693.

Krout, R.E. (2003). Music therapy with imminently dying hospice patients and their families: Facilitating release near the time of death. *Am J Hosp Palliat Care, 20*(2), 129-134.

Krueger, J.M., & Obal, F.J. (2002). Function of sleep. In T. Lee-Chiong, M. Sateia, & M.A. Carskadon (Eds.), *Sleep medicine* (pp. 23-30). Philadelphia: Hanley & Belfus.

Kumar, M., Kumar, A.M., Walfrop, D., et al. (2003). HIV-1 infection and its impact on the HPA axis, cytokines, and cognition. *Stress, 6*(3), 167-172.

Kurtz, M.E., Given, B., Kurtz, J.C., et al. (1994). The interaction of age, symptoms, and survival status on physical and mental health of patients with cancer and their families. *Cancer, 74* (7 Suppl.), 2071-2078.

Kurtz, M.E., Kurtz, J.C., Given, C.W., et al. (1995). Relationship of caregiver reactions and depression to cancer patients' symptoms, functional states and depression: A longitudinal view. *Soc Sci Med, 40*(6), 837-846.

Lamb, M.A. (1982). The sleeping patterns of patients with malignant and nonmalignant diseases. *Cancer Nurs, 5*(5), 389-396.

Landis, C.A., Levine, J.D., & Robinson, C.R. (1989). Decreased slow-wave and paradoxical sleep in a rat chronic pain model. *Sleep, 12*(2), 167-177.

Landolt, H.P., Dijk, D.J., Gaus, S.E., et al. (1995). Caffeine reduces low-frequency delta activity in the human sleep EEG. *Neuropsychopharmacology, 12*(3), 229-238.

Landolt, H.P., Werth, E., Borbely, A.A., et al. (1995). Caffeine intake (200 mg) in the morning affects human sleep and EEG power spectra at night. *Brain Res, 675*(1-2), 67-74.

Lashely, F. (1999). Sleep alterations. In M.E. Ropka & A.B. Willians (Eds.), *HIV nursing and symptom management* (pp. 471-483). Boston: Jones & Bartlett.

Lee, K.A. (2001). Sleep and fatigue. *Annu Rev Nurs Res, 19*, 249-273.

Lee, K.A. (2003). Impaired sleep. In V. Carrieri-Kohlman, A.M. Lindsey, & C.M. West (Eds.), *Pathophysiological phenomena in nursing: Human responses to illness* (pp. 363-385). Philadelphia: Saunders.

Lee, K.A., Portillo, C.J., & Miramontes, H. (1999). The fatigue experience for women with human immunodeficiency virus. *J Obstet Gynecol Neonatal Nurs, 28*(2), 193-200.

Lee, K.A., Portillo, C.J., & Miramontes, H. (2001). The influence of sleep and activity patterns on fatigue in women with HIV/AIDS. *J Assoc Nurses AIDS Care, 12* (Suppl.), 19-27.

Lentz, M.J., Landis, C.A., Rothermel, J., et al. (1999). Effects of selective slow wave sleep disruption on musculoskeletal pain and fatigue in middle-aged women. *J Rheumatol, 26*(7), 1586-1592.

Lipscomb, D. (1976). *Noise: The unwanted sounds.* Chicago: Nelson-Hall.

Lissoni, P., Chilelli, M., Villa, S., et al. (2003). Five years survival in metastatic non-small cell lung cancer patients treated with chemotherapy alone or chemotherapy and melatonin: A randomized trial. *J Pineal Res, 35*(1), 12-15.

Littner, M., Hirshkowitz, M., Davila, D., et al. (2002). Practice parameters for the use of auto-titrating continuous positive airway pressure devices for titrating pressures and treating adult patients with obstructive sleep apnea syndrome. An American Academy of Sleep Medicine report. *Sleep, 25*(2), 143-147.

Lloberes, P., Levy, G., Descals, C., et al. (2000). Self-reported sleepiness while driving as a risk factor for traffic accidents in patients with obstructive sleep apnoea syndrome and in non-apnoeic snorers. *Respir Med, 94*(10), 971-976.

Love, R.R., Cameron, L., & Connell, B.L. (1991). Symptoms associated with tamoxifen treatment in postmenopausal women. *Arch Intern Med, 151*, 1842-1847.

Lyznicki, J.M., Doege, T.C., Davis, R.M., et al. (1998). Sleepiness, driving, and motor vehicle crashes. Council on Scientific Affairs, American Medical Association (see comments). *JAMA, 279*(23), 1908-1913.

Malone, M., Harris, A.L., & Luscombe, D.K. (1994). Assessment of the impact of cancer on work, recreation, home management and sleep using a general health status measure. *J R Soc Med, 87*(7), 386-389.

Matsushima, E., Nakajima, K., Moriya, H., et al. (1997). A psychophysiological study of the development of delirium in coronary care units. *Biol Psychiatry, 41*(12), 1211-1217.

Mazzoccoli, G., Carughi, S., De Cata, A., et al. (2003). Neuroendocrine alterations in lung cancer patients. *Neuroendocrinol Lett, 24*(1-2), 77-82.

McCurry, S.M., Gibbons, L.E., Logsdon, R.G., et al. (2003). Training caregivers to change the sleep hygiene practices of patients with dementia: The NITE-AD project. *J Am Geriatr Soc, 51*(10), 1455-1460.

McCusker, J., Cole, M., Abrahamowicz, M., et al. (2002). Delirium predicts 12-month mortality. *Arch Intern Med, 162*(4), 457-463.

McGinty, D., & Szymusiak, R. (1990). Keeping cool: A hypothesis about the mechanisms and functions of slow-wave sleep. *Trends Neurosci, 13*(12), 480-487.

Meagher, D.J., O'Hanlon, D., O'Mahony, E., et al. (2000). Relationship between symptoms and motoric subtype of delirium. *J Neuropsychiatry Clin Neurosci, 12*(1), 51-56.

Meagher, D.J., & Trzepacz, P.T. (2000). Motoric subtypes of delirium. *Semin Clin Neuropsychiatry, 5*(2), 75-85.

Meijer, J.H., Ruijs, A.C., Albus, H., et al. (2000). Fentanyl, a upsilon-opioid receptor agonist, phase shifts the hamster circadian pacemaker. *Brain Res, 868*(1), 135-140.

Mellinger, G.D., Balter, M.B., & Uhlenhuth, E.H. (1985). Insomnia and its treatment: Prevalence and correlates. *Arch Gen Psychiatry, 42*(3), 225-232.

Menza, M.A., & Rosen, R.C. (1995). Sleep in Parkinson's disease: The role of depression and anxiety. *Psychosomatics, 36*(3), 262-266.

Meuser, T., Pietruck, C., Radbruch, L., et al. (2001). Symptoms during cancer pain treatment following WHO-guidelines: A longitudinal follow-up study of symptom prevalence, severity, and etiology. *Pain, 93*(3), 247-257.

Miaskowski, C., & Lee, K.A. (1999). Pain, fatigue, and sleep disturbances in oncology outpatients receiving radiation therapy for bone metastasis: A pilot study. *J Pain Symptom Manage, 17*(5), 320-332.

Miller, A.H. (2003). Cytokines and sickness behavior: Implications for cancer care and control. *Brain Behav Immun, 17*(Suppl. 1), S132-134.

Mitler, M.M., & Aldrich, M.S. (2000). Stimulants: Efficacy and adverse effects. In M.H. Kryger, T. Roth, & W. Dement (Eds.), *Principles and practice of sleep medicine* (3rd ed., pp. 429-440). Philadelphia: Saunders.

Moeller, A.A., Oechsner, M., Backmund, H.C., et al. (1991). Self-reported sleep quality in HIV infection: Correlation to the stage of infection and zidovudine therapy. *J Acquir Immune Defic Syndr, 4*(10), 1000-1003.

Moldofsky, H. (2001). Sleep and pain. *Sleep Med Rev, 5*(5), 385-396.

Moldofsky, H., & Scarisbrick, P. (1976). Induction of neurasthenic musculoskeletal pain syndrome by selective sleep stage deprivation. *Psychosom Med, 38*(1), 35-44.

Monga, U., Kerrigan, A.J., Thornby, J., et al. (1999). Prospective study of fatigue in localized prostate cancer patients undergoing radiotherapy. *Radiat Oncol Investig, 7*(3), 178-185.

Montplaisir, J., Nicolas, A., Godbout, R., et al. (2000). Restless legs syndrome and periodic limb movement disorder. In M.H. Kryger, T. Roth, & W.C. Dement (Eds.), *Principles and practice of sleep medicine* (3rd ed., pp. 742-752). Philadelphia: Saunders.

Morgan, K. (2003). Daytime activity and risk factors for late-life insomnia. *J Sleep Res, 12*(3), 231-238.

Morin, C.M., Daley, M., & Ouellet, M.C. (2001). Insomnia in adults. *Curr Treat Options Neurol, 3*(1), 9-18.

Morin, C.M., Hauri, P.J., Espie, C.A., et al. (1999). Nonpharmacologic treatment of chronic insomnia. An American Academy of Sleep Medicine review. *Sleep, 22*(8), 1134-1156.

Mormont, M.C., Waterhouse, J., Bleuzen, P., et al. (2000). Marked 24-h rest/activity rhythms are associated with better quality of life, better response, and longer survival in patients with metastatic colorectal cancer and good performance status. *Clin Cancer Res, 6*(8), 3038-3045.

Mourits, M.J., De Vries, E.G., Willemse, P.H., et al. (2001). Tamoxifen treatment and gynecologic side effects: A review. *Obstet Gynecol, 97*(5 Pt. 2), 855-866.

Moyad, M.A. (2002). Complementary/alternative therapies for reducing hot flashes in prostate cancer patients: Reevaluating the existing indirect data from studies of breast cancer and postmenopausal women. *Urology, 59*(4 Suppl. 1), 20-33.

Munro, A.J., Biruls, R., Griffin, A.V., et al. (1989). Distress associated with radiotherapy for malignant disease: A quantitative analysis based on patients perceptions. *Br J Cancer, 60*(3), 370-374.

Murtagh, D.R., Culbert, J.P., & Schwartz, S.M. (1995). Identifying effective psychological treatments for insomnia: A meta-analysis. *J Consult Clin Psychol, 63*, 78-89.

Muzet, A., Libert, J.P., & Candas, V. (1984). Ambient temperature and human sleep. *Experientia, 40*(5), 425-429.

Nail, L.M. (2002). Fatigue in patients with cancer. *Oncol Nurs Forum, 29*(3), 537-546.

National Sleep Foundation (NSF). (1995). *Sleep in America.* Washington, D.C.: Author.

Newman, A.B., Spiekerman, C.F., Enright, P., et al. (2000). Daytime sleepiness predicts mortality and cardiovascular disease in older adults. The Cardiovascular Health Study Research Group. *J Am Geriatr Soc, 48*(2), 115-123.

Nicassio, P.M., Moxham, E.G., Schuman, C.E., et al. (2002). The contribution of pain, reported sleep quality, and depressive symptoms to fatigue in fibromyalgia. *Pain, 100*(3), 271-279.

Nijboer, C., Triemstra, M., Tempelaar, R., et al. (1999). Determinants of caregiving experiences and mental health of partners of cancer patients. *Cancer, 86*(4), 577-588.

Nokes, K.M., & Kendrew, J. (2001). Correlates of sleep quality in persons with HIV disease. *J Assoc Nurses AIDS Care, 12*(1), 17-22.

Norman, S.E., Chediak, A.D., Freeman, C., et al. (1992). Sleep disturbances in men with asymptomatic human immunodeficiency (HIV) infection. *Sleep, 15*(2), 150-155.

Norman, S.E., Chediak, A.D., Kiel, M., et al. (1990). Sleep disturbances in HIV-infected homosexual men. *AIDS, 4*(8), 775-781.

Norman, S.E., Resnick, L., Cohn, M.A., et al. (1988). Sleep disturbances in HIV-seropositive patients. *JAMA, 260*(7), 922.

Northouse, L.L., Caffey, M., Deichelbohrer, L., et al. (1999). The quality of life of African American women with breast cancer. *Res Nurs Health, 22*(6), 449-460.

Nugent, A.M., Gleadhill, I., McCrum, E., et al. (2001). Sleep complaints and risk factors for excessive daytime sleepiness in adult males in Northern Ireland. *J Sleep Res, 10*(1), 69-74.

Olson, D.M., Borel, C.O., Laskowitz, D.T., et al. (2001). Quiet time: A nursing intervention to promote sleep in neurocritical care units. *Am J Crit Care, 10*(2), 74-78.

Osoba, D., Zee, B., & Warr, D. (1997). Effect of postchemotherapy nausea and vomiting on health-related quality of life. *Support Care Cancer, 5*, 307-313.

Owen, D.C., Parker, K.P., & McGuire, D.B. (1999). Comparison of subjective sleep quality in patients with cancer and healthy subjects. *Oncol Nurs Forum, 26*(10), 1649-1651.

Palmblad, J., Petrini, B., Wasserman, J., et al. (1979). Lymphocyte and granulocyte reactions during sleep deprivation. *Psychosom Med, 41*(4), 273-278.

Parker, K.P. (1995). Promoting sleep and rest in critically ill patients. *Crit Care Nurs Clin North Am, 7*(2), 337-349.

Parker, K.P., & Rye, D.B. (2002). Restless legs syndrome and periodic limb movement disorder. *Nurs Clin North Am, 37*(4), 655-673.

Parrott, A.C., & Hindmarch, I. (1980). The Leeds Sleep Evaluation Questionnaire in psychopharmacological investigations: A review. *Psychopharmacology (Berl), 71*(2), 173-179.

Patrick, G.T., & Gilbert, J.A. (1986). On the effects of loss of sleep. *Psychol Rev, 3*, 469.

Phillips, K.D. (1999). Physiological and pharmacological factors of insomnia in HIV disease. *J Assoc Nurses AIDS Care, 10*(5), 93-97.

Pollak, C.P., Tryon, W.W., Nagaraja, H., et al. (2001). How accurately does wrist actigraphy identify the states of sleep and wakefulness? *Sleep, 24*(8), 957-965.

Portenoy, R.K., & Itri, L.M. (1999). Cancer-related fatigue: Guidelines for evaluation and management. *Oncologist, 4*(1), 1-10.

Portenoy, R.K., Thaler, H.T., Kornblith, A.B., et al. (1994). Symptom prevalence, characteristics and distress in a cancer population. *Qual Life Res, 3*(3), 183-189.

Portillo, C.J., Tom, L., Lee, K.A., et al. (2003). Physical and mental fullness as descriptors that influence sleep in women with HIV. *Holist Nurs Pract, 17*(2), 91-98.

Qureshi, A.I., Giles, W.H., Croft, J.B., et al. (1997). Habitual sleep patterns and risk for stroke and coronary heart disease: A 10-year follow-up from NHANES I. *Neurology, 48*(4), 904-911.

Raida, M., Kliche, K.O., Schwake, W., et al. (2002). Circadian variation of dihydropyrimidine deyhdrogenase mRNA expression in leukocytes and serum cortisol levels in patients with advanced gastrointestinal carcinomas compared to healthy controls. *J Cancer Res Clin Oncol, 128*(2), 96-102.

Rechtschaffen, A., & Bergmann, B.M. (1995). Sleep deprivation in the rat by the disk-over-water method. *Behav Brain Res, 69*(1-2), 55-63.

Rechtschaffen, A., Bergmann, B.M., Everson, C.A., et al. (2002). Sleep deprivation in the rat: X. Integration and discussion of the findings. 1989. *Sleep, 25*(1), 68-87.

Rechtschaffen, A., Gilliland, M.A., Bergmann, B.M., et al. (1983). Physiological correlates of prolonged sleep deprivation in rats. *Science, 221*(4606), 182-184.

Rechtschaffen, A., & Kales, A. (1968). *A manual of standard terminology: Techniques and scoring system for sleep stages in human subjects.* (Institute of Health Pub. No. 204). Washington, D.C.: U.S. Government Printing Office.

Redeker, N.S., Lev, E.L., & Ruggiero, J. (2000). Insomnia, fatigue, anxiety, depression, and quality of life of cancer patients undergoing chemotherapy. *Sch Inq Nurs Pract, 14*(4), 275-290; discussion 291-278.

Reynolds, C.R., Willson, V.I., & Clark, P.L. (1983). A four-test short form of the WAIS-R for clinical screening. *Clin Neuropsychol, 3,* 111-116.

Richards, K., Nagel, C., Markie, M., et al. (2003). Use of complementary and alternative therapies to promote sleep in critically ill patients. *Crit Care Nurs Clin North Am, 15*(3), 329-340.

Richards, K.C., & Bairnsfather, L. (1988). A description of night sleep patterns in the critical care unit. *Heart Lung, 17*(1), 35-42.

Riedel, B.W., & Lichstein, K.L. (2000). Insomnia and daytime functioning. *Sleep Med Rev, 4*(3), 277-298.

Rieder, A., Kunze, U., Groman, E., et al. (2001). Nocturnal sleep-disturbing nicotine craving: A newly described symptom of extreme nicotine dependence. *Acta Med Austriaca, 28*(1), 21-22.

Ripamonti, C., Zecca, E., Brunelli, C., et al. (2000). Pain experienced by patients hospitalized at the National Cancer Institute of Milan: Research project "towards a pain-free hospital." *Tumori, 86*(5), 412-418.

Roehrs, T., Carskadon, M.A., Dement, W.C., et al. (2000). Daytime sleepiness and alertness. In M.H. Kryger, T. Roth, & W.C. Dement (Eds.), *Principles and practice of sleep medicine* (3rd ed., pp. 43-52). Philadelphia: Saunders.

Roehrs, T., & Roth, T. (2000). Hypnotics: Efficacy and adverse effects. In M.H. Kryger, T. Roth, & W. Dement (Eds.), *Principles and practice of sleep medicine* (3rd ed., pp. 414-418). Philadelphia: Saunders.

Rozans, M., Dreisbach, A., Lertora, J.J. et al. (2002). Palliative uses of methylphenidate in patients with cancer: A review. *J Clin Oncol, 20*(1), 335-339.

Rubinstein, M.L., & Selwyn, P.A. (1998). High prevalence of insomnia in an outpatient population with HIV infection. *J Acquir Immune Defic Syndr Hum Retrovirol, 19*(3), 260-265.

Sainz, R.M., Mayo, J.C., Rodriguez, C., et al. (2003). Melatonin and cell death: Differential actions on apoptosis in normal and cancer cells. *Cell Mol Life Sci, 60*(7), 1407-1426.

Sarna, L., & Brecht, M.L. (1997). Dimensions of symptom distress in women with advanced lung cancer: A factor analysis. *Heart Lung, 26*(1), 23-30.

Sateia, M.J., & Silberfarb, P.M. (1998). Sleep in palliative care. In D. Doyle, G.W. Hanks & N. MacDonald (Eds.), *Oxford textbook of palliative medicine* (2nd ed., pp. 472-486). New York: Oxford University Press.

Savard, J., Laroche, L., Simard, S., et al. (2003). Chronic insomnia and immune functioning. *Psychosom Med, 65*(2), 211-221.

Savard, J., Miller, S.M., Mills, M., et al. (1999). Association between subjective sleep quality and depression on immunocompetence in low-income women at risk for cervical cancer. *Psychosom Med, 61*(4), 496-507.

Savard, J., & Morin, C.M. (2001). Insomnia in the context of cancer: A review of a neglected problem. *J Clin Oncol, 19*(3), 895-908.

Savard, J., Simard, S., Blanchet, J., et al. (2001). Prevalence, clinical characteristics, and risk factors for insomnia in the context of breast cancer. *Sleep, 24*(5), 583-590.

Sayar, K., Arikan, M., & Yontem, T. (2002). Sleep quality in chronic pain patients. *Can J Psychiatry, 47*(9), 844-848.

Schnelle, J.F., Ouslander, J.G., Simmons, S.F., et al. (1993). The nighttime environment, incontinence care, and sleep disruption in nursing homes. *J Am Geriatr Soc, 41*(9), 910-914.

Schwartz, J.R., Hirshkowitz, M., Erman, M.K., et al. (2003). Modafinil as adjunct therapy for daytime sleepiness in obstructive sleep apnea: A 12-week, open-label study. *Chest, 124*(6), 2192-2199.

Schweitzer, P.K. (2000). Drugs that disturb sleep and wakefulness. In M.H. Kryger, T. Roth, & W.C. Dement (Eds.), *Principles and practice of sleep medicine* (3rd ed., pp. 441-461). Philadelphia: Saunders.

Shaver, J.L., & Giblin, E.C. (1989). Sleep. *Annu Rev Nurs Res, 7,* 71-93.

Shaver, J.L., Lentz, M., Landis, C.A., et al. (1997). Sleep, psychological distress, and stress arousal in women with fibromyalgia. *Res Nurs Health, 20*(3), 247-257.

Sheely, L.C. (1996). Sleep disturbances in hospitalized patients with cancer. *Oncol Nurs Forum, 23*(1), 109-111.

Siegel, J.M. (2000). Brain mechanisms generating REM sleep. In M.H. Kryger, T. Roth, & W. Dement (Eds.), *Principles and practice of sleep medicine* (3rd ed., pp. 112-133). Philadelphia: Saunders.

Silberfarb, P.M., Hauri, P.J., Oxman, T.E., et al. (1985). Insomnia in cancer patients. *Soc Sci Med, 20*(8), 849-850.

Silberfarb, P.M., Hauri, P.J., Oxman, T.E., et al. (1993). Assessment of sleep in patients with lung cancer and breast cancer. *J Clin Oncol, 11*(5), 997-1004.

Spencer, J.A., Moran, D.J., Lee, A., et al. (1990). White noise and sleep induction. *Arch Dis Child, 65*(1), 135-137.

Spiegel, K., Sheridan, J.F., & Van Cauter, E. (2002). Effect of sleep deprivation on response to immunization. *JAMA, 288*(12), 1471-1472.

Stam, H.J., & Bultz, B.D. (1986). The treatment of severe insomnia in a cancer patient. *J Behav Ther Exp Psychiatry, 17*(1), 33-37.

Steele, R.G., & Fitch, M.I. (1996). Needs of family caregivers of patients receiving home hospice care for cancer. *Oncol Nurs Forum, 23*(5), 823-828.

Stein, K.D., Jacobsen, P.B., Hann, D.M., et al. (2000). Impact of hot flashes on quality of life among postmenopausal women being treated for breast cancer. *J Pain Symptom Manage, 19*(6), 436-445.

Stiefel, F.C., Kornblith, A.B., & Holland, J.C. (1990). Changes in the prescription patterns of psychotropic drugs for cancer patients during a 10-year period. *Cancer, 65*(4), 1048-1053.

Sutherland, H.J., Lockwood, A., & Boyd, N.F. (1990). Ratings of the importance of quality of life variables: Therapeutic implications for patients with metastatic breast cancer. *J Clin Epidemiol, 43*(7), 661-666.

Szymusiak, R., & McGinty, D. (1990). Control of slow wave sleep by thermoregulatory mechanisms. *Prog Clin Biol Res, 345,* 53-64; discussion 65-66.

Szymusiak, R., Steininger, T., Alam, N., et al. (2001). Preoptic area sleep-regulating mechanisms. *Arch Ital Biol, 139*(1-2), 77-92.

Tamburini, M., Selmi, S., De Conno, F., et al. (1987). Semantic descriptors of pain. *Pain, 29*(2), 187-193.

Tennstedt, S., Cafferata, G.L., & Sullivan, L. (1992). Depression among caregivers of impaired elders. *J Aging Health, 4*(1), 58-76.

Thorpy, M.J. (1991). History of sleep and man. In M.J. Thorpy & J. Yager (Eds.), *The encyclopedia of sleep and sleep disorders* (pp. ix - xxxiii). New York: Oxford.

Thulasimani, M., & Ramaswamy, S. (2002). The role of tricyclic antidepressants and tramadol in palliative care. *Postgrad Med J, 78*(916), 124.

Tobler, I. (1995). Is sleep fundamentally different between mammalian species? *Behav Brain Res, 69*(1-2), 35-41.

Valdimarsdottir, U., Helgason, A.R., Furst, C.J., et al. (2002). The unrecognised cost of cancer patients' unrelieved symptoms: A nationwide follow-up of their surviving partners. *Br J Cancer, 86*(10), 1540-1545.

Valentine, A.D., Meyers, C.A., Kling, M.A., et al. (1998). Mood and cognitive side effects of interferon-alpha therapy. *Semin Oncol, 25*(1 Suppl. 1), 39-47.

Van Cauter, E., Sturis, J., Byrne, M.M., et al. (1993). Preliminary studies on the immediate phase-shifting effects of light and exercise on the human circadian clock. *J Biol Rhythms, 8*(Suppl.), S99-108.

van den Heuvel, C.J., Noone, J.T., Lushington, K., et al. (1998). Changes in sleepiness and body temperature precede nocturnal sleep onset: Evidence from a polysomnographic study in young men. *J Sleep Res, 7*(3), 159-166.

Van Someren, E.J. (2000). More than a marker: Interaction between the circadian regulation of temperature and sleep, age-related changes, and treatment possibilities. *Chronobiol Int, 17*(3), 313-354.

Vena, C., Parker, K.P., Cunninghan, M., et al. (2004). Sleep-wake disturbances in people with cancer. Part 1: An overview of sleep, sleep regulation, and effects of disease and treatment. *Oncol Nurs Forum, 31*(4), 735-746.

Vines, S.W., Gupta, S., Whiteside, T., et al. (2003). The relationship between chronic pain, immune function, depression, and health behaviors. *Biol Res Nurs, 5*(1), 18-29.

Viviani, S., Bidoli, P., Spinazze, S., et al. (1992). Normalization of the light/dark rhythm of melatonin after prolonged subcutaneous administration of interleukin-2 in advanced small cell lung cancer patients. *J Pineal Res, 12*(3), 114-117.

Vogelzang, N.J., Breitbart, W., Cella, D., et al. (1997). Patient, caregiver, and oncologist perceptions of cancer-related fatigue: Results of a tripart assessment survey. The Fatigue Coalition. *Semin Hematol, 34*(3 Suppl. 2), 4-12.

Walsh, D., Donnelly, S., & Rybicki, L. (2000). The symptoms of advanced cancer: Relationship to age, gender, and performance status in 1,000 patients. *Support Care Cancer, 8*(3), 175-179.

Waye, K.P., Clow, A., Edwards, S., et al. (2003). Effects of nighttime low frequency noise on the cortisol response to awakening and subjective sleep quality. *Life Sci, 72*(8), 863-875.

Webster, L., Andrews, M., & Stoddard, G. (2003). Modafinil treatment of opioid-induced sedation. *Pain Med, 4*(2), 135-140.

Weitzner, M.A., Moncello, J., Jacobsen, P.B., et al. (2002). A pilot trial of paroxetine for the treatment of hot flashes and associated symptoms in women with breast cancer. *J Pain Symptom Manage, 23*(4), 337-345.

White, D.P. (2000). Central sleep apnea. In M.H. Kryger, T. Roth, & W.C. Dement (Eds.), *Principles and practice of sleep medicine* (3rd ed., pp. 827-839). Philadelphia: Saunders.

White, J.L., Darko, D.F., Brown, S.J., et al. (1995). Early central nervous system response to HIV infection: Sleep distortion and cognitive-motor decrements. *AIDS, 9*, 1043-1050.

Whitney, C.W., Enright, P.L., Newman, A.B., et al. (1998). Correlates of daytime sleepiness in 4578 elderly persons: The Cardiovascular Health Study. *Sleep, 21*(1), 27-36.

Wiegand, M., Moller, A.A., Schreiber, W., et al. (1991). Alterations of nocturnal sleep in patients with HIV infection. *Acta Neurol Scand, 83*(2), 141-142.

Williamson, J.W. (1992). The effects of ocean sounds on sleep after coronary artery bypass graft surgery. *Am J Crit Care, 1*(1), 91-97.

Wilwerding, M.B., Loprinzi, C.L., Mailliard, J.A., et al. (1995). A randomized, crossover evaluation of methylphenidate in cancer patients receiving strong narcotics. *Support Care Cancer, 3*(2), 135-138.

Winkelmann, J., & Trenkwalder, C. (2001). Pathophysiology of restless-legs syndrome. Review of current research. *Nervenarzt, 72*(2), 100-107.

Wolfe, F., Smythe, H.A., Yunus, M.B., et al. (1990). The American College of Rheumatology 1990 Criteria for the Classification of Fibromyalgia. Report of the Multicenter Criteria Committee. *Arthritis Rheum, 33*(2), 160-172.

Wysowski, D.K., & Baum, C. (1991). Outpatient use of prescription sedative-hypnotic drugs in the United States, 1970 through 1989. *Arch Intern Med, 151*(9), 1779-1783.

Yellen, S.B., & Dyonzak, J.V. (1999). Sleep disturbances. In C.H. Yarbro, M.H. Frogge, & M. Goodman (Eds.), *Cancer symptom management* (2nd ed., pp. 161-180). Sudburry, Mass.: Jones & Bartlett.

Young-McCaughan, S., Mays, M.Z., Arzola, S.M., et al. (2003). Research and commentary: Change in exercise tolerance, activity and sleep patterns, and quality of life in patients with cancer participating in a structured exercise program. *Oncol Nurs Forum, 30*(3), 441-454; discussion 441-454.

Zarcone, V.P. (2000). Sleep hygiene. In M.H. Kryger, T. Roth, & W.C. Dement (Eds.), *Principles and practice of sleep medicine* (3rd ed., pp. 657-661). Philadelphia: Saunders.

Zepelin, H., & Rechtschaffen, A. (1974). Mammalian sleep, longevity, and energy metabolism. *Brain Behav Evol, 10*(6), 425-470.

Zulley, J., Wever, R., & Aschoff, J. (1981). The dependence of onset and duration of sleep on the circadian rhythm of rectal temperature. *Pflugers Arch, 391*(4), 314-318.

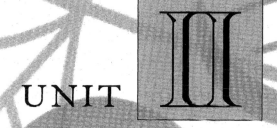

UNIT III

*Specific Disease States
and Symptom Management*

6 *Cardiovascular*

Nancy M. Albert

OBJECTIVES

After the completion of this chapter, the reader should be able to:

1. Describe three main processes involved in the pathophysiology of systolic left ventricular dysfunction.
2. Discuss two issues with current prognostic markers used in heart failure today.
3. State five core drug classes used in the management of advanced systolic heart failure.
4. Describe five lifestyle changes that are essential to optimized systolic heart failure management.
5. Discuss treatment strategies for heart failure exacerbation involving congestion and systemic hypoperfusion.

CARDIOVASCULAR DISEASE

The term *cardiovascular disease* is not equivalent to the term *heart disease*; rather, it is broad in scope and represents diseases of the heart *and* circulatory system. Hypertension is the most prevalent cardiovascular disease and affects about 50 million Americans (American Heart Association [AHA], 2002). Other highly prevalent cardiovascular conditions are coronary heart disease, which includes myocardial infarction and angina pectoris (12.9 million), congestive heart failure (4.9 million), stroke (4.7 million), and congenital cardiovascular defects (1 million). One in five people has a chronic cardiovascular condition. As Americans age, it is expected that the incidence of common chronic cardiovascular diseases, especially coronary heart disease, congestive heart failure, and stroke, will increase as a result of age related diseases. (AHA, 2002).

In 2000, 39.4% of all deaths, equivalent to one of every 2.5 deaths, were caused by cardiovascular disease (AHA, 2002), making it the number-one killer in the United States. Cardiovascular disease claims more lives than the next five leading causes of death combined (cancer, chronic lower respiratory diseases, accidents, diabetes mellitus, and influenza/pneumonia). Of cardiovascular deaths in the year 2000, more women than men died (53.5% vs. 46.5%, respectively) and 32% of all deaths occurred in people younger than 75 years—a reminder that cardiovascular disease is an equal opportunity killer and leads to premature deaths. When cardiovascular deaths were calculated as percentages, 75% were caused by diseases of the heart, with coronary heart disease (54%) and congestive heart failure (5%) the leading causes. In the 10-year period between 1990 and 2000, cardiovascular death rates declined by 17%; however, actual (absolute) cardiovascular deaths increased by 2.5%. The decrease in cardiovascular death rates is largely because of an increasing life expectancy among Americans, which can be attributed to newer and more effective medical treatments for myocardial infarction and stroke with emphasis on risk factor modification and prevention (AHA, 2002).

Today there is a general understanding that cardiovascular disease is a progressive disease. When addressing specific sequelae of cardiovascular disease, some are considered singular events, such as a stroke, chest pain, or myocardial infarction, that require acute intervention and regular, intermittent medical oversight and management to prevent another event and death. However, heart failure is not a singular event but, instead a sequelae that are chronic and may range from subclinical to extremely debilitating. Unlike cardiovascular events, the chronic sequelae require continuous medical oversight, management, and follow-up, even when patients are symptom-free. In both the singular event and sequelae, modification of risk factors is promoted. Because the focus of this book is on palliative practice for advanced illness and because heart failure is a condition whose etiology is most often caused by cardiovascular diseases, such as coronary heart disease, hypertension, valve diseases, congenital disease, and diabetes mellitus, the focus of this chapter is on management of heart failure.

Heart Failure Definition, Nomenclature, and Incidence

Heart failure is a broad term that can have many meanings, depending on the context in which it is discussed. It is defined as a clinical syndrome characterized by specific symptoms (dyspnea and fatigue) and signs (fluid retention) that arise from a structural or functional disorder of the heart and cause a pathophysiologic state in which the heart does not pump enough oxygenated blood to meet the needs of the tissues (ACC/AHA, 2001; Felker, Adams, Konstam, et al., 2003). The two basic hemodynamic derangements in all types of heart failure are high ventricular filling pressures and decreased cardiac output. Heart failure can be the result of right or left ventricular dysfunction. It can be an acute condition that develops shortly after myocardial injury (myocarditis or papillary muscle rupture) or infarction and causes cardiogenic shock, or it may be a chronic condition with ventricular dysfunction that is mild to severe with symptoms that are absent (compensated) to functionally limiting (decompensated). It can be labeled as *systolic* (structural heart disease with depressed ventricular ejection fraction of 40% or less) or *diastolic* (impaired ventricular relaxation or abnormal ventricular stiffness) dysfunction.

Heart failure with chronic left ventricular systolic dysfunction is associated with significant morbidity, mortality, and health care expenditure (AHA, 2002). It is the most frequently sited Medicare hospital discharge diagnosis-related group (DRG), and

more Medicare dollars are spent on heart failure assessment and treatment than on any other diagnosis (ACC/AHA, 2001). Thus the term *heart failure* (*HF*) and the advanced pathophysiology described in this chapter are limited to HF from chronic left ventricular systolic dysfunction. Though diastolic heart failure is often recognized, treatment algorithms are not fully developed. It is likely that palliative care teams will be involved in the care of patients with severe systolic dysfunction and rarely with diastolic ventricular dysfunction. In the past, the term *congestive HF* or the abbreviation *CHF* was used as substitute phrasing for chronic left ventricular systolic dysfunction because congestion was a prominent feature of the patient's clinical picture. In this chapter, the term *CHF* is used only when it applies to describe a congestive or a fluid-overloaded state causing dyspnea and fatigue and is not used as a general term for HF. HF can occur and worsen silently and may not be associated with congestion.

Heart failure is a chronic, progressive, costly, and fatal condition that warrants strategies to improve the quality of life for patients and their families, including expert management at the end of life. About 550,000 new cases occur each year. In the year 2000, approximately 262,300 deaths occurred, increasing by 148% from 1979 (AHA, 2002). In the United States, 999,000 hospital discharges from the year 2000 were assigned a primary diagnosis of HF and hospitalizations increased by 165% relative to 1979 (AHA, 2002). These hospitalizations in 2000 cost Medicare beneficiaries 3.6 billion dollars (AHA, 2002). Research from large multicenter clinical trials showed that the majority of patients died within 8 years of diagnosis (AHA, 2001) and that the elderly population (older than 65 years) were more likely to die, with only 25% of patients living beyond 5 years. In fact, HF was found to be more deadly than all cancers with the exception of lung cancer (Stewart, MacIntyre, Hole, et al., 2001). Survival over a 10-year period in 66,547 consecutive patients was a median of 1.47 years for men and 1.39 years for women after diagnosis (MacIntyre, Capewell, Stewart, et al., 2000). Patients who survived the first 30 days post index hospitalization improved their survival to 2.47 years for men and

2.36 years for women (MacIntyre et al., 2000). Other studies have revealed the bleak survival of heart failure. Investigators have concluded that prognosis has not improved for the past 40 years (Khand, Gemmel, Clark, et al., 2000).

Heart failure is also a symptomatically burdensome, debilitating condition associated with poor quality of life. Murray, Boyd, Kendall, et al. (2002) used a qualitative study method to provide insight into the experience of dying for patients with HF and cancer. Four critical themes emerged:

1. The illness trajectory of HF is unpredictable and non-linear.
2. Patients are less informed with a limited understanding about the course of HF and its prognosis and are less involved in clinical decision making compared with cancer patients.
3. Patients experience frustration, progressive losses, social and emotional isolation, and the stresses of balancing a complex HF medical regimen with normal existence.
4. Health and social services (palliation) are not readily available, do not provide a financial benefit to the patient, and are often poorly coordinated.

These data highlight the need for care that is not limited to pharmacologic and general medical therapies but more comprehensive to include palliation and a focus on improvements at the end of life.

PATHOPHYSIOLOGY OF ADVANCED HEART FAILURE

Many cardiac and non-cardiac conditions can cause impairment of left ventricular systolic function. Coronary artery disease causes heart failure in 59% to 70% of patients. This is also known as ischemic cardiomyopathy (Gheorghiade & Bonow, 1998). Structural cardiac disorders of non-ischemic origin, also known as *non-ischemic cardiomyopathy*, (i.e., valvular disease, hypertension, atrial fibrillation, congenital abnormalities, myocarditis) are identifiable causes. Heart failure can arise from identifiable non-cardiovascular causes such as obesity, alcohol, illicit drug use, cardiotoxic medications, diabetes, sleep apnea, and anemia or have no known etiology, also known as *idiopathic dilated cardiomyopathy*.

The pathophysiology of HF is complex; however, three general processes occur in response to myocardial injury or stress: ventricular remodeling, neuroendocrine activation, and immune system up-regulation. These three processes are generated to promote stroke volume and increase cardiac output when the injured myocardium cannot contract with enough force to maintain organ perfusion. Unfortunately, these adaptive processes become maladaptive and ultimately worsen HF by sustaining and accelerating ventricular remodeling. This in turn further activates and up-regulates neurohormones and cytokines to adversely affect cardiac structure and function. This vicious cycle activates neurohormones and up-regulates cytokines to adversely contribute to morbidity, further stress on the myocardium, further depression of mechanical performance, and eventual morbidity (Fig. 6-1).

Ventricular Remodeling

Ventricular remodeling is the complex cellular interstitial and molecular changes that occur in cardiomyocytes, leading to abnormalities in cardiac geometry, structure, and left ventricular function (Cohn, Ferrari, & Sharpe, 2000). An initial response to injury is myocyte hypertrophy, which increases cardiac mass/wall thickness compared with ventricular internal cavity dimensions (also known as *concentric remodeling*) in an attempt to maintain myocyte wall stress at normal levels and thereby preserve stroke volume and pump function to compensate for ventricular injury and decreased cardiac outputs (Albert, 1999; Peterson, 2002). Concentric hypertrophy will initially increase cardiac output but at the cost of further increasing wall stress, thus continuing the remodeling process.

Myocytes elongate, which causes the left ventricle to dilate and form a spherical or globular (U) shape (eccentric hypertrophy), which differs from the usual elliptical shape. As myocyte mass increases, contractility and stroke volume are initially maintained, but this adaption also increases the strength, number, and distribution of *non*-contractile protein (nonmyocytes) structural components within cardiomyocytes in an attempt

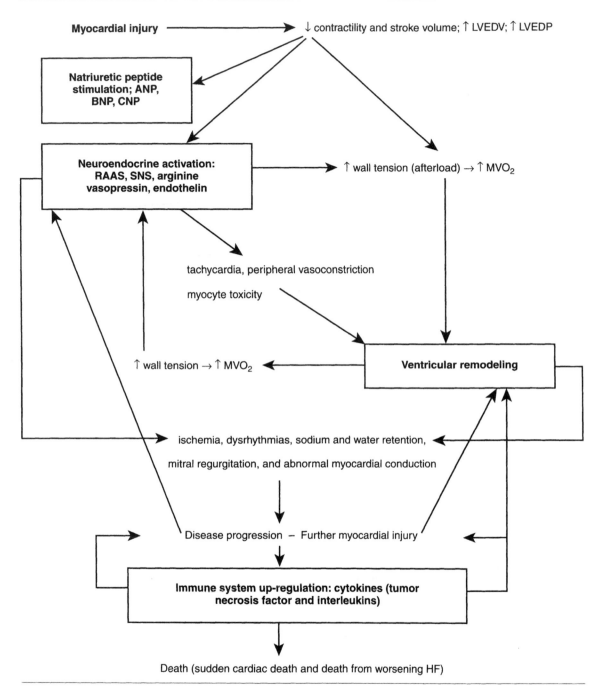

FIGURE **6-1** The pathophysiologic process of advanced systolic left ventricular dysfunction. *ANP*, Atrial natriuretic peptide; *BNP*, brain natriuretic peptide; *CNP*, C-type natriuretic peptide; *LVEDV*, left ventricular end-diastolic volume; *LVEDP*, left ventricular end-diastolic pressure; *RAAS*, renin-angiotensin-aldosterone system; *SNS*, sympathetic nervous system; MVO_2, myocardial oxygen consumption.

to maintain structural integrity (Albert, 1999; Cohn et al., 2000; Zile, 2002). Ultimately, fibroblasts and other non-myocytes proliferate and influence the production and degradation of the collagen network of the extracellular matrix that surrounds and interconnects the cardiomyocytes, myofibrils, muscle fibers, and coronary microcirculation; provides external stimulation by both mechanical and chemical signals; and maintains muscle fiber and cardiac myocyte alignment. The collagen network disruption caused by HF leads to loss of collagen struts that attach myocytes to myocytes and myocytes to capillaries. Changes in the extracellular matrix are believed to impair cardiomyocyte contraction and further depress left ventricular performance (Anand, 2002) leading to cardiac dilatation (Cleutjens & Creemers, 2002; Goldsmith & Borg, 2002).

In post–myocardial infarction HF, remodeling occurs in two phases. Within hours of injury, the inflammatory response becomes localized at the infarct zone and the infarct will extend. Within 72 hours after injury, the remodeling process is already active and includes aneurismal dilation or wall thinning from elevation in systolic and diastolic wall stress (Sutton & Sharpe, 2000). Beyond 72 hours, late remodeling occurs and includes global ventricular dilation and up to 70% increase in cell volume. This phase distributes the increased wall stresses evenly as extracellular matrix forms a collagen-based scar, stabilizing the distending forces. However, the remodeling process fails to normalize increased wall stress and ultimately leads to progressive dilation and worsening contractile function (Jessup & Brozena, 2003; Sutton & Sharpe, 2000).

Myocyte loss occurs through both necrosis and apoptosis (programmed cell death). Apoptosis occurs not only at the site of myocardial injury but also at remote sites from injury in non-infarcted or non-injured myocardium and is believed to accelerate wall thinning and left ventricular dilation, both of which will increase wall stress and enhance further left ventricular dysfunction (Abbate, Biondi-Zoccai, Bussani, et al., 2003; Anand, 2002). Increased interstitial fibrosis with increased interstitial collagen deposition occurs in areas of myocyte apoptosis, causing abnormal fiber shortening, uncoordinated ventricular contraction, and reduction in ejection fraction (Cohn et al., 2000).

With hypertrophy and other systolic dysfunction changes, often there is accompanying diastolic dysfunction. Diastolic ventricular stiffness increases as the left ventricular wall thickens. This is thought to be the result of three factors:
1. Ventricular wall hypertrophy.
2. Interstitial fibrosis.
3. Physiologic abnormalities of hypertrophied myocytes cause impairment of the sarcoplasmic reticulum to handle the flux of calcium across these membranes.

Overall, ventricular remodeling increases intraventricular volume, which helps increase stroke volume through Starling's principles but also increases ventricular filling pressure and wall stress. Therefore while these responses are initially adaptive, ventricular remodeling becomes maladaptive because it leads to worsening ejection fraction and ventricular contractility, mitral regurgitation, exercise intolerance, myocardial ischemia, atrial and ventricular dysrhythmias, and diastolic dysfunction (Cohn et al., 2000). Ventricular remodeling changes occur silently and are initiated early in HF, usually before symptoms appear. Over time, the remodeling process contributes to worsening of symptoms (ACC/AHA, 2001). Reversal of this process is possible, even in advanced HF, and may lead to alleviation or diminishing of symptoms and improvement in functional abnormalities (mitral regurgitation, myocardial ischemia, and atrial and ventricular dysrhythmias) (Jessup & Brozena, 2003).

Neuroendocrine Activation

Myocardial injury reduces mitochondria calcium transport and uptake within cardiomyocytes, leading to depressed myofibril contractility and an overall reduction in left ventricular ejection fraction (Smith & Levine, 1999). By ultrasound, stroke volume decreases and left ventricular diastolic volume increases.

Several compensatory mechanisms are initiated in an attempt to maintain cardiac output. Activation of the sympathetic nervous system increases plasma norepinephrine and epinephrine, which causes vasoconstriction and increased heart rate. These changes will improve cardiac output but also will increase myocardial oxygen demand and wall stress (afterload). In addition, myocardial norepinephrine concentrations fall, which causes cardiac beta-1 receptors to be down-regulated and cardiac beta-2 and alpha receptors to be up-regulated (Dorn, 2002). Beta-1 receptor down-regulation leads to reduced contractility and promotes ventricular remodeling (Adams, Mathur, & Gheorghiade, 2003; Schrier & Abraham, 1999). Beta-2 receptor overexpression leads to depressed systolic function, and alpha-receptor overexpression causes myocyte hypertrophy and ventricular remodeling (Dorn, 2002; Schrier & Abraham, 1999). In addition to sympathetic nervous system stimulation, central mechanoreceptors within the right atrium and arteries trigger release of arginine vasopressin from the posterior pituitary gland to increase systemic blood pressure (through vasoconstriction at the V_1 receptor level) and increase intravascular volume (through water retention at the V_2 receptor level within the kidney) to support cerebral perfusion (Schrier & Abraham, 1999).

Decreased blood flow to the kidney stimulates the renal arteriolar baroreceptors and up-regulation of the renin-angiotensin-aldosterone system (Unger, 2000). The renin-angiotensin-aldosterone system plays an integral role in cardiovascular homeostasis through effects on vascular tone and blood volume. Angiotensin II is a potent vasoconstrictor and also stimulates cardiac myocardium growth and interstitium deposition to promote ventricular hypertrophy and remodeling (Schrier & Abraham, 1999; Unger, 2000). Angiotensin II fosters the sympathetic nervous system to stimulate the presynaptic release of norepinephrine from sympathetic nerve endings, leading to further vasoconstriction. Angiotensin II vasoconstricts both afferent and efferent renal arterioles to maintain the glomerular filtration rate. Angiotensin II stimulates aldosterone synthesis and release from the adrenal cortex, which in turn promotes sodium reabsorption at the distal renal tubules (Schrier & Abraham, 1999). Ultimately the up-regulation of the renin-angiotensin-aldosterone system in HF increases preload and afterload in an attempt to increase stroke volume.

Angiotensin-converting enzyme inhibitors do not diminish the local production of angiotensin II in the heart by the chymase pathway. (Kokkonen, Lindstedt, & Kovanen, 2003; Unger, 2000). Chymase is stored within mast cells and released upon cell activation. In advanced HF, cardiac mast cell density markedly increases and angiotensin II enzymatic activity becomes activated from local chymase, the angiotensin-converting enzyme–independent pathway (Matsumoto, Wada, Tsutamoto, et al., 2003). Recent research has shown that the chymase pathway can be critical to cardiac fibrosis and not only because of angiotensin II production but also because chymase activates transforming growth factor-beta from the mast cells, which in turn increases collagen production and promotes differentiation of fibroblasts to myofibroblasts, leading to ventricular wall stiffness and diastolic dysfunction (Matsumoto et al., 2003). These findings suggest that chymase-mediated tissue fibrosis is not solely responsible for angiotensin II but also other profibrotic molecules that will require further investigation.

Endothelial cells exert an important vasoregulatory function by releasing relaxing and constricting factors. Endothelial peptides are synthesized by endothelial and smooth muscle cells, as well as by cardiomyocytes and neural, renal, pulmonary, and inflammatory cells (Spieker, Noll, Ruschitzka, et al., 2001). Vasodilatory peptides in normal endothelium dominate and allow for increase in blood flow, when appropriate (Elkayam, Khan, Mehboob, et al., 2002). Endothelin-1 is synthesized to endothelin-1, a potent systemic and pulmonary vasoconstrictor peptide that elicits a response from veins to a greater extent than from arteries. Its effects are mediated by activation of two cell-surface receptor subtypes: (1) endothelin-$_A$, which is a selective receptor present mainly in vascular smooth muscle, has high affinity for endothelin-1, and exerts vasoconstriction and proliferation; and (2) endothelin-$_B$, a nonselective receptor found in nonvascular tissues, has affinity for endothelin-1 as well as other endothelins and causes vasodilation by releasing nitric oxide and prostacyclin (Spieker et al., 2001; Suresh, Lamba, & Abraham, 2000). Endothelin-1's vasoconstrictor potency is 10 times that of angiotensin II in vitro and is therefore an important regulator of vascular structure and tone. Many factors and substances will stimulate release of endothelin-1, such as shear-stress, pulsatile stretch, arterial pH, hypoxia, circulating thrombin, angiotensin II, vasopressin, transforming growth factor-beta, endotoxin, and cytokines (Lüscher & Barton, 2000; Suresh et al., 2000). In addition, exercise up-regulates myocardial expression of endothelin-1, suggesting that this peptide has a role in maintaining cardiac function (Lüscher & Barton, 2000).

Endothelin-1 is present in both healthy and failing myocardium and induces contraction and positive inotropic action. However, elevated plasma endothelin-1 is a characteristic of severe HF and not of asymptomatic or mild HF. In addition to controlling vascular tone and cardiac myocyte contraction, it modulates growth properties of vascular smooth muscle and hypertrophy of cardiomyocytes (Suresh et al., 2000). Endothelin-1 is released in response to low cardiac output (similarly to norepinephrine) to maintain blood pressure and increase contractility. However similar to norepinephrine and angiotensin II, endothelin-1 will exert a deleterious action related to vascular and myocardial remodeling (Lüscher & Barton, 2000; Suresh et al., 2000).

In summary, neuroendocrine up-regulation and endothelial cell activation cause increased heart rate, fluid retention, and peripheral vasoconstriction to maintain arterial pressure and perfusion of the cerebral and coronary arteries, which provides an adaptive benefit early after myocardial injury (Zucker & Pliquett, 2002). However, prolonged neuroendocrine and endothelial activation leads to the dire consequences of excessive tachycardia, dysrhythmias, myocardial ischemia, excessive peripheral and renal vasoconstriction, volume overload, hyponatremia, vascular fibrosis, endothelial dysfunction, and worsening ventricular remodeling (myocardial hypertrophy, apoptosis, and fibrosis) (Suresh et al., 2000). The progressive release and elevation of neurohormones and

endothelin-1 results in a vicious feedback cycle of major adverse effects, which exacerbates circulatory congestion, clinical deterioration and death.

Natriuretic Peptide Stimulation. Natriuretic peptide is released from the myocardium early in HF so as to counteract the effects of up-regulation of the sympathetic, and the renin-angiotensin-aldosterone system. Atrial natriuretic peptide (ANP) is secreted primarily from the atria in response to atrial wall stretch. B-type natriuretic peptide (BNP) is secreted by atrial and ventricular myocytes. In HF, the predominant source of BNP is the ventricular myocardium as a response to pressure and volume overload (Chen & Burnett, 1999). At the cellular level, ANP and BNP promote natriuresis (sodium loss); diuresis; arterial and venous dilation and coronary artery flow; renin inhibition (leading to decreased neuroendocrine activation of norepinephrine, aldosterone, and endothelin-1); and lusitropy (ventricular relaxation). In addition, ANP and BNP have an antifibrotic and myocyte anti-proliferative effect, that helps retard ventricular remodeling (Adams et al., 2003; Chen & Burnett, 1999). C-type natriuretic peptide is expressed in the vascular endothelium and also acts to vasodilate and inhibit myocyte hypertrophy in HF (Adams et al., 2003; Chen & Burnett, 1999).

In advanced HF, the generation of endogenous ANP, BNP, and CNP is inadequate to maintain a clinically compensated state (Adams et al., 2003). Even though natriuretic peptide plasma levels are elevated, the reactive vasoconstricting, sodium-retaining, and water-retaining hormones dominate the clinical picture so that the overall net balance is toxic to the heart. Unfortunately, natriuretic receptor activity is down-regulated, which blunts the benefits of elevated circulating endogenous BNP (Adams et al., 2003).

IMMUNE SYSTEM UP-REGULATION

In addition to neurohormones and natriuretic peptides, another group of peptides, the proinflammatory cytokines, are up-regulated in patients with HF. Tumor necrosis factor and interleukin-6 are two cytokines that are thought to play a central role. Other cytokines, such as interleukin-1, interleukin-2, interferon-γ (a.k.a. interleukin-18;

Yamaoka-Tojo, Tojo, Inomata, et al., 2002), are also implicated but to a lesser extent (Murray & Freeman, 2003).

Because HF is a state of progressive cardiac muscle injury and causes stressful stimuli and signals, it should be no surprise that myocardial immune system activation occurs. Cardiomyocytes and other cells in the myocardium synthesize tumor necrosis factor in response to stress; that is, stress from myocardial infarction, left ventricular pressure overload, or left ventricular volume overload (Murray & Freeman, 2003). In humans, tumor necrosis factor was uniformly expressed in the failing heart but not so in the normal heart (Murray & Freeman, 2003). Cytokine serum levels are higher in patients with cardiac cachexia and in those with more advanced, edematous, decompensated HF (Sharma, Al-Nasser, & Anker, 2001). Interleukin-6 is a multifunctional vasodepressor cytokine produced by vascular tissue in patients with HF. It mediates both immune and inflammatory responses, which causes myocardial dysfunction, muscle wasting, and abnormal endothelin-dependent vasodilation (Tsutamoto, Hisanago, Wada, et al., 1998). High plasma levels of interleukin-6 were also associated with vascular resistance and increased vascular permeability (Tsutamoto et al., 1998).

Inflammatory cytokines contribute to ventricular remodeling, peripheral manifestations of HF, and progressive deterioration in functional class (Murray & Freeman, 2003). Tumor necrosis factor provokes myocyte hypertrophy; degrades the extracellular matrix, which is replaced by fibrosis; triggers apoptosis and necrosis; promotes fetal gene expression; blunts adrenergic myocyte responsiveness; and impairs cardiac contractile function (Mann, 2002; Murray & Freeman, 2003). Tumor necrosis factor induces left ventricular dilation by increasing myocardial matrix metalloproteinases (proteolytic enzyme system that degrades the extracellular myocardial matrix) and by decreasing tissue inhibitors of myocardial matrix metalloproteinase (the endogenous system that regulates local matrix metalloproteinase activity) (Wilson, Gunasinghe, Coker, et al., 2002). Tumor necrosis factor, interleukin-6, and other proinflammatory cytokine levels are associated with high levels of

norepinephrine, epinephrine (Tsutamoto et al., 1998), ANP, and BNP (Yamaoka-Tojo et al., 2002) and are positively correlated with insulin resistance (Sharma et al., 2001).

The hallmark pathophysiologic mechanisms discussed initiate the syndrome of HF, which also involves a complex blend of structural, functional, and biologic maladaptive alterations (Box 6-1) (Jessup & Brozena, 2003). Pathophysiologic mechanisms listed in Box 6-1 play a role in initiating and/or aggravating HF and may be important processes in the clinical cascade already discussed.

MANAGEMENT OF HF SYMPTOMS
Common Symptoms
Congestion (fluid overload) is the prevailing problem that links patients to their health care providers. Evidence of congestion includes the *signs* of neck vein distention, elevated right internal jugular venous pressure, positive abdominal-jugular neck vein reflex, edema, ascites, S_3 gallop, and pulmonary crackles. HF *symptoms* are dyspnea, orthopnea, paroxysmal nocturnal dyspnea, exercise intolerance, and fatigue. Patients with HF may experience leg weakness, asthenia, lack of energy, reduced endurance, and a general feeling of malaise.

As HF progresses and organs receive less oxygenated blood, patients will experience the signs and symptoms associated with inadequate systemic perfusion: mental obtundation, orthostatic hypotension, narrow pulse pressure, pulsus alternans, cool forearms and legs (not just hands and feet), worsening renal function (oliguria), hyponatremia (from increased vasopressin and water retention), and nausea/anorexia/early satiety (from reduced gut perfusion). Reduced effective circulating volume produces a racing heart (caused by tachycardia or dysrhythmias) and symptomatic hypotension from angiotensin-converting enzyme (ACE)-inhibitors. Patients with right ventricular dysfunction will have additional signs and symptoms: liver congestion, hepatomegaly, hepatojugular reflux, anasarca, and pitting peripheral edema.

There are many nonspecific signs and symptoms of HF that are frequently seen in patients even with a mild to advanced condition (Box 6-2).

Box 6-1   Other Pathophysiologic Mechanisms in Heart Failure, Cardiac Dysfunction

FUNCTIONAL ABNORMALITIES
- Mitral regurgitation, aortic stenosis, or other primary valvular disease
- Triple-vessel coronary artery disease and hibernating myocardium
- Wide QRS, left bundle branch block, left ventricular septal-to-posterior wall motion delay, and abnormal heart rate variability
- Atrial fibrillation
- Premature ventricular contraction

STRUCTURAL ABNORMALITIES
- Coronary artery occlusion
- Changes in calcium influx/abnormal excitation-contraction coupling
- Necrosis

CIRCULATING AND TISSUE SUBSTANCES
- Impaired endothelium-mediated vasodilation (nitric oxide, prostacyclin, adrenomedullin, and endothelium-derived hyperpolarizing relaxing factor)
- Alterations in peripheral sensory mechanoreceptor transduction, changes in production of central neurotransmitters, and alterations in the synthesis of excitatory and inhibitory substances within the central nervous system

OTHER FACTORS
- Advanced age
- Genetic predisposition, including effects of sex and ethnicity
- Coexisting non-cardiac conditions:
  —Severe hypertension
  —Obesity
  —Diabetes mellitus
  —Renal disease (insufficiency and failure)
  —Anemia
  —Sleep apnea
  —Depression
  —Secondary pulmonary hypertension from pulmonary embolus or chronic pulmonary obstructive disease
  —Primary pulmonary hypertension
  —Thyroid disease (thyroid toxicosis) or hypothyroidism
- Alcohol, tobacco, and toxic drug exposure
- Other environmental factors:
  —Social isolation
  —Medication adherence
  —Lifestyle: activity, diet, recognition of signs and symptoms

These signs and symptoms may be caused by several factors including worsening HF (congestion and inadequate systemic perfusion), medication and dietary indiscretion, coronary artery ischemia, co-morbidity (hypertension, renal disease, valvular heart disease, atrial fibrillation, stroke, anemia, sleep apnea, thyroid disease), medication side effects, acute non-cardiac events (pulmonary embolus, bleeding, systemic infection), and acute cardiac events (myocardial infarction, papillary muscle rupture, conduction abnormalities and dysrhythmias, especially when ventricular response

Box 6-2   Universal Signs/Symptoms Associated With but Not Specific to Heart Failure

- Lightheadedness
- Dizziness
- Confusion
- Fainting
- Wheezing
- Severe cough
- Slow heart rate
- Irregular pulse
- Low blood pressure
- High blood pressure
- Vomiting
- Diarrhea
- Mottled skin
- Weight loss

is markedly slow or fast) (Jain, Massie, Gattis, et al., 2003).

During acute decompensation, patients with HF often experience dyspnea with exertion (90%), dyspnea at rest (36%), peripheral edema (67%), fatigue (34%), and crackles (69%) (Scios, Inc., 2003). These patients may be described in terms such as "wet." The Acute Decompensated Heart Failure National Registry (ADHERE™; Scios, Inc., 2003) found that only 3% of patients admitted with HF had a systolic blood pressure of less than 90 mm Hg. In fact, 47% of patients had a systolic pressure between 90 and 140 mm Hg and 50% had a systolic blood pressure greater than 140 mm Hg. Therefore the majority of patients have elevated ventricular filling pressures but adequate systemic perfusion and would be described as "wet and warm." When patients have inadequate systemic perfusion caused by decreased cardiac output and marked vasoconstriction, they are described as "cold" (Jain et al., 2003.). In recent years, clinicians have created an overall approach to managing exacerbations of HF by developing guidelines for care after assessing to see if their classification is "wet and warm," "wet and cold," or "cold and dry." The fourth grouping, "warm and dry," does not warrant acute therapies and has the best outlook (Jain et al., 2003; Nohria, Lewis, & Stevenson, 2002).

Care Strategies for Chronic Advanced HF With Acute Exacerbation

In advanced HF, patients may no longer respond to standard pharmacologic therapies and the benefits that were realized early may diminish over time. In an acute decompensated state, the immediate goals are to alleviate symptoms and improve the hemodynamics; however, the overriding goal of management is the same as of chronic management: promote reversal or prevent progression of ventricular remodeling. Therefore once the patient is stabilized with intravenous diuretic, vasodilator, and inotropics (as needed), standard pharmacologic and nonpharmacologic management strategies are instituted before discharge and are maintained in the outpatient setting. Figure 6-2 provides an overview of acute management approaches based on the patient's clinical classification (Jain et al., 2003; Loh, 2000; Nohria et al., 2002). These profiles do *not* include treatment for cardiogenic shock; rather, the focus is on treatment of an acute exacerbation of chronic advanced HF. Patients with advanced HF can have an acute event (myocardial infarction), which superimposes acute heart failure upon chronic HF. This is not the norm and is not discussed in this chapter.

During acute exacerbations of HF, patients can benefit from hemodynamic monitoring with a pulmonary artery catheter. In this way, hemodynamic function is easily monitored and improvements in dynamic pressures correlated with improvement in symptoms. There are no randomized trials in the literature, however, to prove that hemodynamic monitoring is efficacious in HF relapse (Loh, 2000). Pulmonary crackles are absent in 80% of patients with chronically elevated ventricular filling pressures. This is because of compensatory accelerated pulmonary lymphatic drainage. Peripheral edema is insensitive to increased pulmonary filling pressures. Patients may have a diastolic gallop (S_3) chronically because of profound mitral regurgitation. As a result, hemodynamic monitoring provides a more accurate assessment of volume status and can monitor therapy more accurately (Nohria et al., 2002). Persistently high left ventricular filling pressures (pulmonary artery wedge pressure ≥16 mm Hg) and signs of volume

CONGESTION

Warm and Dry
- Ideal classification.
- Maintain current core pharmacologic and nonpharmacologic therapies to maintain stable volume status and prevent HF progression.
- Monitor for changes in status.

Warm and Wet (most common, 67%)
- Represents volume overload: need increased diuretics (can be done in hospital, OPD, home care, palliative– or hospice–home care using physician-initiated, nurse-mediated algorithms)
  - IV loop diuretics (bolus or infusions) ‡
  - Supplement with metolazone
- Maintain ACE-I
- Use IV NTG, nesiritide or NTP to relieve congestion, as needed †
- Avoid IV inotropic agents (dobutamine, milrinone)*

Cold and Dry (less common, 5%)
- May need diuresis; however, focus is on improving perfusion, and, generally, patient is vasoconstricted.
- May need IV fluids if *hypo*volemic.
- Continue oral core HF Tx; may need vasodilators (NTP, NTG, nesiritide) if systolic blood pressure is >90 mm hg and no signs of severe hypoperfusion (drug choice based on other presenting signs/symptoms).†
- Oxygen.
- IV inotropic agent if unstable.*
- Initiate BB Tx gradually

Cold and Wet (28% of decompensation)
- If symptomatic hypotension: may need to withdraw ACE-I and BB until stabilized; then restart.
- IV vasodilator Tx alone will improve cardiac output (cold state): NTP, NTG, nesiritide; titrate to optimize hemodynamic profile.†
- Avoid IV inotropic agents.*
- Once stabilized on IV vasodilator Tx, use ACE-I, nitrates, and hydralazine while weaning IV agent.
- IV diuretic Tx:‡
  - —IV loop diuretics (bolus or infusions).
  - —Supplement with metolazone.

SYSTEM PERFUSION (vertical label on left axis)

ACE-I, Angiotensin-converting enzyme inhibitors; BB, beta-blockers; BNP, b-type natriuretic peptide; BP, blood pressure; HF, heart failure; IV, intravenous; NTG, nitroglycerin; NTP, nitroprusside; OPD, outpatient department; PAC, pulmonary artery catheter; RAS, renin angiotensin system; Tx, therapy; PAWP, pulmonary artery wedge pressure

*IV inotropic infusion notes:
A: Dobutamine and milrinone: Associated with increased risk for ischemic events and tachydysrhythmias. These agents increase heart rate and myocardial oxygen consumption and can induce ischemia and damage hibernating (viable) myocardium (especially dobutamine). When used in "cold and dry" class, can lead to dependence and tachyphylaxis.
B: In the "warm and wet" class:
  (1) Appropriate to initiate IV inotropic agents temporarily to provide stability when hemodynamic status is initially unclear and patients have *severe* symptoms of systemic hypoperfusion (i.e., low systolic blood pressure causes lightheadedness and dizziness when resting supine in bed; oliguric; resting heart rate is >120 beats per minute when in normal sinus rhythm) and when IV diuretics + metolazone fail to prompt diuresis in patients with a high baseline blood urea nitrogen.
  (2) Increases complexity when adjusting oral Tx as inotropic agent is weaned. Physiologic effects of agents might mask inadequacy of diuretic regimen and intolerance to vasodilator Tx or high vasodilator doses leading to potential hospital readmission in near future.

†IV vasodilator notes:
NTG. At low doses, induces venous vasodilation. As dose increased, arterial dilation and dilation of coronary arteries occur; initial dose is 5 mcg/minute and can be titrated every 3-5 minutes. Adverse effects: nitrate tolerance, significant hypotension and reflex tachycardia. About 20% of patients are resistant to any form of NTG; if dose is >200 mcg/minute, patient is not likely to respond to higher doses. Use with caution if significant aortic stenosis or an acute right ventricular wall myocardial infarction.

NTP. A balanced, direct, arterial and venous vasodilator. Especially useful in reducing high afterload, high BP, and severe valve regurgitation. Potent vasodilating effects; suggest continuous BP monitoring and PAC monitoring. Start at 0.1 to 0.2 mcg/kg/minute and titrate every 5 minutes to achieve desired hemodynamic response. Also, dilates pulmonary arteries and reduces right ventricular afterload. Can cause coronary steal syndrome in patients with acute MI without HF (prefer NTG over NTP if patient having HF exacerbation and acute ischemic event). Adverse effects: thiocyanide and cyanide toxicity.

Nesiritide. Recombinant human BNP; vasodilates arteries, veins, and coronary arteries. Produces vasodilation, diuresis (mild), and natriuresis (mild). Will decrease PAWP more effectively than IV diuretics alone or NTG. No tolerance (as seen with NTG); therefore no need to up-titrate infusion; does not require PAC or continuous BP monitoring (as seen with NTP), no cyanide toxicity (as seen with NTP); therefore may be used safely on non–critical care nursing units. May produce significant hypotension that lasts longer than NTG and NTP (because of longer half-life of 19 minutes), but the incidence of hypotension is similar to that of NTG. Start dose: bolus of 2 mcg/kg followed by a 0.01 mcg/kg/minute infusion.

‡IV diuretic agent notes:
A: To ensure diuresis and natriuresis, the dose of loop diuretic must be high enough to exceed the threshold drug concentration within the renal tubular lumen. Generally achieved by (1) doubling the IV bolus dose (q 3-4 hr) until an adequate response is achieved or (2) initiating a continuous furosemide infusion.
B: Continuous infusion is associated with smoother and more predictable response and less prerenal azotemia.
C: Excessive diuresis can cause electrolyte abnormalities, worsening renal function, RAS activation (thus worsening HF), and can trigger hypotensive effects of ACE-I.
D: Concomitant vasodilator therapy can counteract the increase in systemic vascular resistance associated with RAS activation to reduce afterload and increase perfusion.

FIGURE **6-2** Acute management approaches for chronic advanced heart failure with acute exacerbation based on the patient's clinical classification.

overload at the time of discharge correlate with post-discharge survival (Fonarow, 2001; Lucas, Johnson, Hamilton, et al., 2000). Therefore an important goal of treatment is to decrease cardiac preload and afterload, decreasing ventricular remodeling and neuroendocrine activation.

PROGNOSTIC INDICATORS FOR PALLIATIVE INTERVENTIONS

Reports in the literature enumerate prognostic markers and risks for hospitalization in HF (Table 6-1). Although each factor independently predicts an

important outcome (mortality and hospital readmission), the routine use of prognostic factors for risk stratification in clinical practice has limitations. First, many markers of these outcomes have been studied in isolation without additional factors taken into account. There is a lack of direct comparative data regarding which markers are better predictors of risk. It is impossible to tell which markers are redundant and which ones offer independent significance in predicting outcomes. If comparative data involve many markers that are statistically significant, then there also must be details regarding

Table **6-1**   PROGNOSTIC TABLE

Markers of Survival in Heart Failure

Clinically Significant Test(s)/Marker(s)	Comments and Hazard Ratio (HR) When Available	Reference
Cardiac norepinephrine spillover rate	More powerful prognosticator than PAWP, mean PAP, and serum sodium level	8
Low SDNN RR intervals	All-cause death (HR 1.05) and HF death (HR 1.07)	9
Low serum sodium level	All-cause death (HR 1.14) and HF death (HR 1.23)	9
High creatinine level	All-cause death (HR 1.09) and HF death (HR 1.13)	9
Higher cardiothoracic ratio	All-cause death (HR 1.23)	9
	All deaths and cardiac deaths	5
Non-sustained VT	All-cause death (HR 1.57)	9
High LVESD	All-cause death (HR 1.23)	9
High LVEDVI	1-year death (HR 1.6)	10
Increasing age (per decade)	All-cause death (HR 1.19)	9
	1-year death (HR 2.3)	10
LV hypertrophy	All-cause death (HR 1.54)	9
MRT >50 seconds	Most powerful predictor of cardiac death and need for Tx (HR 4.44)	15
Predicted VO$_2$ max <50%	Cardiac death (HR 3.50) and need for Tx	15
Resting systolic BP <105 mm Hg	Cardiac death (HR 2.49) and need for Tx	15
ET-1 level >5 pg/ml	Best predictor of cardiac mortality when compared with BNP, LVEF, NYHA class, age, and sex (accounted for 53.4% of variance in multivariate analysis)	16
N-proANF >1000 pg/mL	Cardiac death; accounted for 12.8% of variance in multivariate analysis	16
IVCD	Cardiac death HR 1.84 (many predictors on multivariate analysis but this and ICM [below] were only factors with HR >1.02)	1
ICM	Death HR 2.00 (other significant predictors: resting heart rate, LVEF, mean BP, peak VO$_2$, serum sodium)	1
	5-year mortality (compared with non-ICM)	3
Baseline 6-minute walk <218 meters	Death HR 4.6. Also predicted death or hospitalization; better predictor than age, ICM, LVEF, or sex	17

Table **6-1** Prognostic Table—cont'd

Clinically Significant Test(s)/Marker(s)	Comments and Hazard Ratio (HR) When Available	Reference
LVEF	Cardiac failure and SCD	5
Peak VO$_2$	All deaths and cardiac deaths	5
BNP	Functional status deterioration	11
	BNP was significantly correlated with peak exercise VO$_2$	12
	SCD: only independent predictor on univariate and multivariate analysis; NYHA, HR, history of HTN, CAD, DM, drug history, systolic BP, and LVEF did not predict SCD	4
	Cardiac death; superior to IL-6 but both were significantly elevated	14
Left bundle branch block	All-cause death (HR 1.70) and SCD (HR 1.58). Effects are independent of age, HF severity, and ACE-I and beta-blocker prescriptions	2
	All-cause death (HR 1.07) but not SCD	6
QRS prolongation	All-cause death (HR 1.46) and SCD	6
≥120 milliseconds	All-cause mortality; effect was greater in patients	18
≥110 milliseconds	>65 years old	
Absence of emotional support before hospitalization	Cardiac death and nonfatal cardiovascular events *in women*	13
Depression	Combination of either functional decline or death as severity of depressive symptoms worsened at 6 months	19
	Increased death and rehospitalization at 3 months and 1 year If major depression; independent of age, NYHA class, ejection fraction, and ischemic etiology of HF	7

ACE-I, Angiotensin-converting enzyme inhibitors; *BP*, blood pressure; *BNP*, B-type natriuretic peptide; *CAD*, coronary artery disease; *DM*, diabetes mellitus; *ET-1*, endothelin; *HF*, heart failure; *HTN*, hypertension; *ICM*, ischemic cardiomyopathy; *IL-6*, interleukin-6; *IVCD*, intraventricular conduction delay; *LV*, left ventricular; *LVEF*, left ventricular ejection fraction; *LVEDVI*, left ventricular end-diastolic volume index; *LVESD*, left ventricular end-systolic diameter; *MRT*, mean response time (equals oxygen deficit divided by change in oxygen update during treadmill exercise testing); *N proANF*, N-terminal proatrial natriuretic factor; *NYHA*, New York Heart Association; *SCD*, sudden cardiac death; *SDNN*, standard deviation of normal-to-normal; *Tx*, cardiac transplantation; *VO$_2$ max*, maximum oxygen uptake; *VT*, ventricular tachycardia.

1. Aaronson, K.D., Schwartz, S., Chen, T., et al. (1997). Development and prospective validation of a clinical index to predict survival in ambulatory patients referred for cardiac transplant evaluation. *Circulation, 95*, 2660-2667.
2. Baldasseroni, S., Opasich, C., Gorini, M., et al. (2002). Left bundle branch block is associated with increased 1-year sudden and total mortality rate in 5517 outpatients with congestive heart failure: A report from the Italian Network on Congestive Heart Failure. *Am Heart J, 143*, 398-405.
3. Bart, B.A., Shaw, L.K., McCants, C.B., et al. (1997). Clinical determinants of mortality with angiographically diagnosed ischemic or nonischemic cardiomyopathy. *J Am Coll Cardiol, 30*, 1002-1008.
4. Berger, R., Huelsman, M., Strecker, K., et al. (2002). B-type natriuretic peptide predicts sudden death in patients with chronic heart failure. *Circulation, 105*, 2392-2397.
5. Goldman, S., Johnson, G., Cohn, J.N., et al. (1993). Mechanisms of death in heart failure. The vasodilator-heart failure trials. *Circulation, 87* [Suppl. VI], VI-24–VI-31.
6. Iuliano, S., Fisher, S.G., Karasik, P E., et al. (2002). QRS duration and mortality in patients with congestive heart failure. *Am Heart J, 143*, 1085-1091.
7. Jiang, W., Alexander, J., Christopher, E., et al. (2001). Relationship of depression to increased risk of mortality and rehospitalization in patients with congestive heart failure. *Arch Intern Med, 161*, 1849-1856.
8. Kaye, D.M., Lefkovits, J., Jennings, G.L., et al. (1995). Adverse consequences of high sympathetic nervous activity in the failing human heart. *J Am Coll Cardiol, 26*, 1257-1263.

Continued

Table **6-1**   PROGNOSTIC TABLE—CONT'D

9. Kearney, M.T., Fox, K.A., Lee, A., et al. (2002). Predicting death due to progressive heart failure in patients with mild-to-moderate chronic heart failure. *J Am Coll Cardiol, 40*, 1801-1808.

10. Koelling, T.M., Semigran, M.J., Mijller-Ehmsen, J., et al. (1998). Left ventricular end-diastolic volume index, age, maximal heart rate at peak exercise predict survival in patients referred for heart transplantation. *J Heart Lung Transplant, 17,* 278-287.

11. Koglin, J., Pehlivanli S., Schwaiblmair, M., et al. (2001). Role of brain natriuretic peptide in risk stratification of patients with congestive heart failure. *J Am Coll Cardiol, 38*, 1934-1941.

12. Krüger, S., Graf, J., Kunz, D., et al. (2002). Brain natriuretic peptide levels predict functional capacity in patients with chronic heart failure. *J Am Coll Cardiol, 40*, 718-722.

13. Krumholz, H.M., Butler, J., Miller, J., et al. (1998). Prognostic importance of emotional support for elderly patients hospitalized with heart failure. *Circulation, 97*, 958-964.

14. Maeda K., Tsutamoto, T., Wada, A., et al. (2000). High levels of plasma brain natriuretic peptide and interleukin-6 after optimized treatment for heart failure are independent risk factors for morbidity and mortality in patients with congestive heart failure. *J Am Coll Cardiol, 36*, 1587-1593.

15. Rickli, H., Kiowski, W., Brehm, M., et al. (2003). Combining low-intensity and maximal exercise test results improves prognostic prediction in chronic heart failure. *J Am Coll Cardiol, 42,* 116-122.

16. Selvais, P.L., Robert, A., Ahn, S., et al. (2000). Direct comparison between endothelin-1, N terminal proatrial natriuretic factor, and brain natriuretic peptide as prognostic markers of survival in congestive heart failure. *J Card Fail, 6*, 201-207.

17. Shah, M.R., Hasselblad, V., Gheorghiade, M., et al. (2001). Prognostic usefulness of the six-minute walk in patients with advanced congestive heart failure secondary to ischemic or nonischemic cardiomyopathy. *Am J Cardiol, 88*, 987-993.

18. Silvet, H., Amin, J., Padmanabhan, S., et al. (2001). Prognostic implications of increased QRS duration in patients with moderate and severe left ventricular systolic dysfunction. *Am J Cardiol, 88*, 182-185.

19. Vaccarino, V., Kasl, S.V., Abramson, J., et al. (2001). Depressive symptoms and risk of functional decline and death in patients with heart failure. *J Am Coll Cardiol, 38*, 199-205.

the specific patient population in HF to which these factors apply (i.e., ischemic vs. dilated cardiomyopathy or young vs. elderly patients) and which group would benefit the most from each cluster or groups of markers. Second, many markers are time-consuming to obtain, costly, and lack sensitivity, specificity, or reliability in particular situations (e.g., serum neurohormonal samples should not be obtained until the patient has been resting in a supine position for 20+ min). The marker must be standardized so that it is used properly for comparison and so that the results are meaningful (valid). Because of debility, some patients may not tolerate certain tests (e.g., metabolic stress test). Other markers will need to be repeated over time before results provide reliable prognostic information (e.g., an isolated echocardiogram or serum BNP level may provide risk-stratification but should be repeated after therapeutic interventions are completed in order to determine prognostic information). Finally, identification of a marker for survival or high risk for decompensation should prompt treatment interventions that possibly modify risk. Elevated serum cytokine and endothelin-1 levels are predictors of a failing heart; however, few treatment options are available today (most remain at clinical trial stage or have not exhibited benefit in clinical trials) that target cytokines or endothelin-1 directly. There is a need to develop an algorithm for risk stratification that can be generalized to most patients with HF.

In lieu of using an individual or groups of specific indicators to determine prognosis when a patient qualifies for palliative medicine, investigators have developed clinical classification schemes to determine hospice eligibility and to promote palliation in patients who would truly benefit from these services. Fox, Landrum-McNiff, Zhong, et al. (1999) evaluated the National Hospice Organization criteria specific to HF to determine if factors are appropriate as prognostic criteria. Hospitalized patients with documented progression of HF and an ejection fraction of less than or equal to 20% and/or supraventricular or ventricular dysrhythmias qualified for services. However, at 6 months, 73% with ejection fraction criteria and 75% with dysrhythmia criteria were still alive after hospital discharge. In addition, the 6-month mean survival time greatly exceeded criteria-predicted survival; 38% of patients with a predicted survival of less than or equal to 10% and 53% of patients with a predicted survival of less than or equal to 50% were alive at 6 months (Fox et al., 1999).

Alla, Briancon, Juillière, et al. (2000) developed a prognostic rating system that identified patients with severe HF (hospitalization for New York Heart Association [NYHA] functional class III/IV dyspnea, edema, or hypertension; an ejection fraction ≤30%; and a cardiothoracic index ≥60%) and studied specific demographic, functional, co-morbid conditions, and laboratory characteristics. Once prognostic factors were identified, a prognostic score was developed to identify patients at low, intermediate, and high risk for mortality. Ischemic and dilated cardiomyopathy patients had a separate scoring scheme, and in each, 1-year survival in those in the high mortality class was 25.7% and 24.1%, respectively. Box 6-3 lists specific characteristics that predicted low survival, based on HF etiology (Alla et al., 2000) and other criteria (Albert, Davis, & Young, 2002). The main advantages to this type of scoring system are that it does not rely on expensive, burdensome, or time-intensive testing and is easily repeated on a routine basis. The main disadvantage to these criteria is that there is no assurance patients are treated optimally based on ACC/AHA evidence-based consensus guidelines (2001). Refer to Table 6-2 for optimal core pharmacologic management.

In an effort to combine evidence-based practices and a simple scoring system, Albert et al. (2002) published a scoring system that included initial screening criteria that is consistent with the current ACC/AHA guidelines and also criteria from Alla et al.'s high mortality class (2000). In this way, optimal medical management is required as part of initial screening criteria before specific patient characteristics were considered high-risk for end of life. Although this algorithm eliminated a major disadvantage to the previous work, the 25% 1-year survival rate might be considered problematic for health care providers who do not wish to prematurely promote palliation alone when they believe aggressive therapies might effectively improve patient outcomes (survival).

The major drawback to determining palliation and hospice readiness is that the clinical course of heart failure is, relative to cancer, unpredictable (O'Connell, 2000) and sudden cardiac death adds to this unpredictability. In acutely ill patients with HF, predictions are inaccurate. Physicians have great difficulty predicting survival and are more likely to underestimate both 90-day and 1-year survival (Poses, Smith, McClish, et al., 1997). Adequate risk stratification tools in the future will contribute to patient care by providing guidance for palliation referral. Until definitive guidelines are developed or until reimbursement for end-of-life care in the United States changes, the burden of triaging patients with poor survival into palliative or hospice care rests with health care providers who might be fearful of relinquishing aggressive care. However, patients who remain highly symptomatic after optimized medical therapies, especially those with poor prognostic signs (listed in Table 6-1 and Box 6-3) ought to be referred to a HF specialty team to initiate palliative measures. In this way, patients and families are supported and appropriate conversations about death and dying initiated while the patient has a substantial chance of surviving the index episode of symptomatic progression that raised the awareness of prognosis. Palliative care is not an alternative to aggressive cardiac care but should be complementary. It is clear that HF is a uniformly terminal condition. Advance directives and goals of care need to be addressed early in the course of disease and re-addressed as the patient's clinical status fails. This issue was addressed in the old Agency for Health Care Policy and Research (AHCPR) guidelines, but it is still important to practice today.

INTERVENTIONS BEFORE PALLIATION

Core Pharmacologic Management

The ACC/AHA (2001) uses a stepped approach to manage chronic HF. Patients at high risk for developing HF (stage A HF) are initiated on pharmacologic therapies known to reverse ventricular remodeling and improve morbidity and survival. This specifically includes ACE inhibitors or, if severe cough, angioedema, or symptomatic hypotension

Box 6-3   CHARACTERISTICS THAT PREDICT LOW SURVIVAL IN ADVANCED HEART FAILURE

ISCHEMIC CARDIOMYOPATHY

A combination of three or four factors increases the prognostic risk.
- Resting heart rate >100 beats per minute
- Serum creatinine >2.2 mg/dl (180 μmol/L)
- Serum sodium <134 mg/dl after treatment for dehydration or volume overload
- History of prior decompensation requiring hospitalization
- Age >70 years

DILATED CARDIOMYOPATHY

A combination of four or more factors increases prognostic risk.
- History of serious co-morbidity: cancer, liver failure, chronic pulmonary condition, cerebral vascular disease, or arterial artery disease
- Patient dependent upon others for activities of daily living or is institutionalized
- History of heart failure >3 months prior to the index hospitalization for decompensation
- Resting heart rate >100 beats per minute
- Serum creatinine >2.2 mg/dl (180 μmol/L)
- Serum sodium <134 mg/dl after treatment for dehydration or volume overload
- Age >70 years

OTHER CRITERIA

Assumes patient is in advanced functional class and on core medical therapies with medications administered at recommended dosages.
- Dependent upon a continuous intravenous dobutamine or milrinone infusion, decompensation with inotrope withdrawal, *or* unable to be weaned from intravenous inotropic infusions
- Decompensation despite cardiac resynchronization device implantation *not* caused by suboptimal lead placement or device settings
- Frequent firing of an implantable cardioverter defibrillator in the face of normal electrolytes and no other known causes of ventricular tachydysrhythmias
- Recurrent decompensation after treatment for contributing factors that worsen heart failure and patient is *not* a candidate for research or surgical options
- Oxygen consumption of less than 14 ml/kg/min or 55% predicted for age and sex
- Relative or absolute contraindications to cardiac transplantation are:
  —Fixed pulmonary hypertension or high transpulmonary gradient
  —Morbid obesity (>140% of ideal body weight)
  —Marked cachexia (<60% ideal body weight)
  —Osteoporosis
  —Cerebral or peripheral vascular disease
  —Diabetes mellitus with organ damage
  —Psychosocial issues:
    ○ Drug or alcohol abuse
    ○ Documented nonadherence
    ○ Absence of emotional support
    ○ Depression

occurs with ACE inhibitors, angiotensin receptor blockers. Once structural heart disease is evident, even if patients are asymptomatic (stage B HF), beta-blockers are to be added to the regimen unless contraindicated. Patients are encouraged to participate in aerobic exercise. Aggravating factors are assessed and modified, medications that worsen HF are discontinued, and surgery is considered if a patient requires coronary revascularization or heart valve repair/replacement. If HF worsens

Text continued on p. 142

Table 6-2 CORE PHARMACOLOGIC THERAPIES IN CHRONIC HF MANAGEMENT

Drug Class Specific drugs indicated in HF treatment (trade name in parentheses)	Expected Actions and Rationale for Use	Precautions and Considerations
ACE-I captopril (Capoten) enalapril (Vasotec) lisinopril (Prinivil; Zestril) quinapril (Accupril) ramipril (Altace) fosinopril (Monopril)	• Blocks angiotensin II production (reduced aldosterone production and salt and water retention and improved hemodynamic actions—reduced vasoconstriction). • Enhances kinins and kinin-mediated prostaglandin synthesis (vasodilation). • Improved symptoms, such as dyspnea and reduced afterload, myocardial and vascular fibrosis. • Reduced mortality and hospitalizations.	• Use with EF <40%, regardless of symptoms. • Use caution or discontinue if hyperkalemia (>5.5 mEq/L) or high serum creatinine (>3.0 mg/dl). • Contraindicated if history of angioedema (<1% of cases), in pregnant women, and in patients in cardiogenic shock. • Titrate dose from initial to target dose; can be achieved in a short period (48 hr-2 wk, depending on agent). Target dose is the dose based on clinical trials that provided efficacy. • Full effect may take 1-2 mo; do not discontinue early because of lack of response. • If dry cough, use throat lozenges; do not discontinue unless cough prevents sleep; improves over 6-mo period. • Asymptomatic hypotension and mild renal insufficiency are *not* contraindications to use. • Symptomatic hypotension signifies marked neurohormonal activation (with depleted intravascular volume from diuresis or from advanced HF); stabilize hemodynamics after rapid diuresis. Hyponatremia (serum sodium <130 mmol/L) is associated with symptomatic hypotension. IV vasodilator such as NTP or nesiritide may be needed until serum sodium improves. • May cause worsening renal function; i.e., reduced renal perfusion and glomerular filtration. Renal function improves with reduction in diuretic dose. Reduce ACE-I dose only when diuretic dose cannot be reduced because of fluid retention. • Other side effects: rash, taste disturbances.
Beta-Blocker carvedilol (Coreg) metoprolol (Toprol XL) bisoprolol (Zebeta)	• Blunts SNS response; therefore decreases dysrhythmias, myocardial remodeling, tachycardia, ventricular volumes, myocyte apoptosis, oxidative stress, and vasoconstriction.	• Use with EF <40%, regardless of symptoms; however, initiate with caution in NYHA functional class IV patients, and initiate after euvolemic or acute volume overload has been resolved. • Start at very low dose and carefully titrate to target doses (may take 1-3 mo). • Add to ACE-I; may be used with diuretics, digoxin, and aldosterone inhibitors.

Continued

Table **6-2**   Core Pharmacologic Therapies in Chronic HF Management—cont'd

Drug Class Specific drugs indicated in HF treatment (trade name in parentheses)	Expected Actions and Rationale for Use	Precautions and Considerations
	• 3rd generation agent, carvedilol vasodilates through alpha-blockade. • Reduces mortality, hospitalizations, and symptoms. • Decreases heart rate 11-13 beats per minute, on average	• Monitor for fatigue and fluid retention when starting and titrating dose. Monitor weight daily. Do not discontinue with progressive symptoms; use diuretics to treat volume overload and adjust ACE-I if hypotensive or fatigued. Delay titration if symptomatic but attempt to reach target doses over time. • Clinical responses are delayed for 2-3 mo; even if symptoms do not improve, maintain therapy to reduce the risk of major cardiovascular events (pump failure death and SCD). • Abrupt withdrawal will lead to clinical deterioration. • Avoid with reactive airway disease, advanced heart block, and symptomatic bradycardia (without pacemaker). • Minimize risk for symptomatic hypotension by staggering schedule of ACE-I and beta-blocker administration; take 1st dose (when initiating) at bedtime. Also, reduce diuretic dose if volume-depleted.
Digitalis digoxin (Lanoxin)	• Inhibits sodium-potassium pump, thereby increases intracellular calcium to heighten myocardial contractility. • Sensitizes cardiac baroreceptors to decrease SNS out flow. • Reduces renin secretion (therefore reduces RAS activation). • Positive inotropic effect reduces symptoms and hospitalization for HF.	• Use in symptomatic HF (functional class II or greater and stage C or D HF). • Use low dose (0.125 mg/day or less) to achieve neurohormonal effects and reduce risk for toxicity. • Patient should be on ACE-I and beta-blocker before digoxin. • Do not use in sinus node or AV node block (without pacemaker). • Consider decreasing dose in patients on agents that block AV node, such as amiodarone and beta-blocker. • Side effects are usually anorexia, N/V, halo vision, yellow color perception, disorientation, and confusion. Can also cause re-entrant dysrhythmias. Maintain therapeutic serum level below 0.8 ng/μl.
Loop Diuretic furosemide (Lasix) bumetanide (Bumex) torsemide (Demadex)	• In loop of Henle, blocks co-transport of sodium, potassium, and chloride. • Reduces preload, afterload, and ventricular filling pressures. • Venous vasodilation early	• Loop diuretics induce significant diuresis and a low frequency of hypokalemia. • Use with signs and symptoms of fluid overload. • Give up to the equivalent at 480 mg/day (oral) furosemide and 1000 mg/day (IV); titrate to achieve dry weight. • Use IV in severely fluid-overloaded patients, and use continuous infusion.

after administered. • Negative effects are neurohormonal activation; patient should be on concomitant ACE-I and beta-blocker.	• Excessive diuresis can cause orthostatic hypotension, fatigue, and worsening renal function. • Begin therapy at low dose and titrate upward as needed in mildly to moderately symptomatic patients. • Never use alone. • Supplement fluid maintenance with sodium and fluid restriction and daily weight monitoring. • Side effects are potentially important; potassium and magnesium electrolyte depletion increase ventricular dysrhythmias and SCD; periodically serum electrolytes should be monitored after dosage changes.

Aldosterone Inhibitor
spironolactone (Aldactone)
eplerenone (Inspre)

• Blocks sodium reabsorption in the distal convoluted tubule and cortical collecting duct. • Acts as a competitive inhibitor to aldosterone receptor. • Retards myocardial and vascular fibrosis and vascular damage, reduces baroreceptor dysfunction, and prevents myocardial norepinephrine uptake. • Improves survival and reduces hospitalization in NYHA functional III/IV patients. (spironolactone) • Post MI patients had clinical signs of HF at time of event (eplerenone)	• Patient should be on an ACE-I, beta-blocker, digoxin, and diuretic before initiating therapy in patients with non-ischemic cardiomyopathy. • Weakly diuretic at low doses used to achieve aldosterone inhibition; however, can facilitate diuresis and decrease fluid retention. Low doses are 25 mg/day or less (spironolactone). • Do not titrate (spironolactone). • Decrease doses if hyperkalemia; carefully monitor serum potassium and decrease potassium intake (diet; salt substitutes; medications) if needed. Obtain serum potassium 7 days initiating therapy. • Most common side effects (up to 10%) and breast discomfort spironolactone gynecomastia. • Unknown response in mild or moderate HF. • Newer agent (eplerenone) decreases gynecomastia and breast pain

OTHER CARDIAC OR CARDIOVASCULAR AGENTS

ARB
losartan (Cozaar)
irbesartan (Avapro)
candesartan (Atacand)
valsartan* (Diovan)
telmisartan (Micardis)

• Angiotensin II is formed locally in tissues by the action of chymase and other enzymes. ARBs attach to the angiotensin I receptors and prevent vasoconstriction, worsening ventricular remodeling (attenuates myocyte	• Use with EF <40%, regardless of symptoms, but not as a substitute for ACE-I's. Use when cannot tolerate ACE-I and do not have significant renal dysfunction or hyperkalemia. • Use doses from clinical trials for best effect. • Symptomatic and worsening renal dysfunction: see ACE-I precautions and considerations.

Continued

Table **6-2**   Core Pharmacologic Therapies in Chronic HF Management—cont'd

Drug Class Specific drugs indicated in HF treatment (trade name in parentheses)	Expected Actions and Rationale for Use	Precautions and Considerations
	hypertrophy and fibroblast proliferation), and sodium and water retention. • Promotes vasodilation and reduces ventricular remodeling indirectly through the angiotensin II receptor. • Fewer side effects than ACE-I, especially cough and angioedema. • No mortality reduction compared with ACE-I's but reduces hospitalization.	
Direct Arterial Vasodilator hydralazine (Apresoline)	• Reduces afterload. • Improves valve regurgitation. • When used with a nitrate, combination reduces mortality but not hospitalizations and increases ejection fraction and exercise tolerance. Not as effective as ACE-I except in Africans-Americans.	• For long-term efficacy, use with isosorbide dinitrate or isosorbide mononitrate. • Use doses that provide hemodynamic benefit. • Four-times-a-day dosing may require adherence monitoring. • Combination therapy causes frequent adverse effects: headache and GI complaints. • For long-term efficacy, must be used with hydralazine.
Venous Vasodilator isosorbide dinitrate (Isordil) isosorbide mononitrate (Imdur)	• Reduces preload. • Improves valve regurgitation in patients with volume overload. • Decreases ischemia. • When used with hydralazine, combination reduces mortality but not hospitalizations and increases ejection fraction and exercise tolerance. Not as effective as ACE-I.	• Use in patients with ACE-I or ARB contraindications. • Three-times-a-day dosing might require adherence monitoring. • Do not dose around-the-clock. Allow for a 10-hour nitrate-free period to prevent nitrate tolerance. Use at nighttime to prevent paroxysmal nocturnal dyspnea (i.e., nitrate patch). • Combination therapy causes frequent adverse effects: headache and GI complaints.
Anti-Coagulation warfarin (Coumadin)	• Reduces the risk (1%-3%/yr) for thromboembolic event caused by stasis in dilated, hypokinetic ventricle; does not decrease mortality or hospitalizations.	• Use if in atrial fibrillation, prior thrombus, previous embolic event: peripheral vascular disease; or mechanical valve.
Antiplatelet agent aspirin clopidogrel (Plavix)	• Reduces the risk of major events, but no established benefits in HF. • Aspirin may attenuate the benefits of ACE-I and loop diuretics.	• Large-scale trial (WATCH) with both agents underway. • Use after MI or history of CAD. • Use low dose (81 mg/day) for secondary CV protection.

Drug class	Notes
Thiazide diuretic chlorothiazide (Diuril) hydrochlorothiazide (Microzide; Aquazide) metolazone (Zaroxolyn; Mykrox)	• Clopidogrel may not adversely interact with ACE-I. • In distal convoluted tubule, inhibits resorption of sodium and chloride. • Potentiates loop diuretics. • Use in combination with loop diuretics when patients are resistant to loop diuretics alone.
CCB amlodipine (Norvasc) felodipine (Plendil)	• Does not improve symptoms of HF or exercise tolerance; may increase mortality and worsening HF (except amlodipine and felodipine: NOTE: these two agents do not provide benefit; however, they do not cause harm). • Avoid 1st and 2nd generation CCBs in patients with HF and an ejection fraction of 50% or less. • Amlodipine or felodipine may be beneficial when ACE-I and ARB do not lower BP adequately or patient has angina from vasospasm. • Avoid all CCB post MI.
HMG-CoA Reductase Inhibitors; Statins Many	• Inhibits proinflammatory cytokines; improves cardiac remodeling. • Potential adverse effects: HF disease progression from reduced levels of ubiquinone (coenzyme Q10) and increased blood endotoxin levels. • Use for CAD and hypercholesterolemia; however, definitive, randomized, controlled clinical trials are needed. • Many non-cardiac side effects: hepatotoxicity; toxic epidermal necrolysis; skin discoloration; photosensitivity; blurred vision; photophobia; corneal micro-deposits; pulmonary fibrosis; thyroid disease (both hypothyroidism [more common] and hyperthyroidism]; involuntary movement; tremor; insomnia; nausea and vomiting.
Antidysrhythmic amiodarone (Cordarone; Pacerone)	• Class III agent with sympatholytic effect on the heart. • Does not reduce mortality, death, and hospitalization. • Reduces left ventricular ejection fraction and increases risk for worsening HF. • Not recommended to treat SCD except when used IV during CPR. • Used to suppress recurrent VT/VF.

*FDA-approved when ACE-I intolerant.

ACE-I, Angiotensin-converting enzyme inhibitor; ARB, angiotensin receptor blocker; AV, atrioventricular; CAD, coronary artery disease; CCB, calcium channel blocker; CV, cardiovascular; EF, ejection fraction; GI, gastrointestinal; HF, heart failure; HMG-CoA, 3-hydroxy-3-methylglutaryl coenzyme A; IV, intravenous; MI, myocardial infarction; NTP, nitroprusside; NYHA, New York Heart Association; N/V, nausea/vomiting; SCD, sudden cardiac death; SNS, sympathetic nervous system; RAS, renin angiotensin system; VT/VF, ventricular tachycardia/ventricular fibrillation.

Data from American College of Cardiology (ACC)/American Heart Association (AHA) Task Force. (2001). ACC/AHA guidelines for the evaluation and management of chronic heart failure in the adult. Practice Guidelines—full text available at www.acc.org/clinical/guidelines/failure/hf_index.htm; Ashton, E., Liew, D., & Krum, H. (2003). Should patients with chronic heart failure be treated with 'statins'? Heart Fail Monit, 3, 82-86; Scaffidi, R., & Gottlieb, S.S. (2001). Heart failure at the beginning of the 21st century. Cardiovascular Research & Review, 22, 467-481.

(stage C HF), administer digoxin (for persistent fatigue and exercise intolerance), diuretics (for signs and symptoms of volume overload), and restrict sodium. Patients with stage C disease who are symptomatic and in NYHA functional class III/IV have an aldosterone inhibitor (spironolactone) added to the regimen if potassium levels are normal. In addition, thiazide diuretics and nitrates are added if congestion is refractory to single diuretics. The addition of hydralizine reduces afterload and improves exercise tolerance. Stage D HF patients are considered medically refractory and should be considered for cardiac transplantation, mechanical assist devices, medical and surgical research protocols that might offer relief of symptoms and improve morbidity and mortality, or hospice care. Refer to Table 6-2 for details about pharmacologic agent classes just discussed.

Device Therapy

There are specific situations when cardiac devices are recommended in the management of HF. The two electrophysiologic devices commonly used are cardiac resynchronization therapy (CRT), using bi-ventricular pacing, and implantable cardioverter defibrillator (ICD). These devices are targeted for patients with structural heart disease and HF, but patients must meet Medicare requirements for reimbursement.

CRT. Bi-ventricular pacing restores cardiac resynchronization in patients with HF and a prolonged QRS duration and left bundle-branch block. This therapy involves placing three endocardial pacemaker leads in the heart at the right ventricular apex and right atrium, and in the left lateral cardiac vein adjacent to the left lateral or posterior ventricular wall. The device is set to sense atrial activity and paces the right and left ventricle simultaneously or sequentially to decrease septal-to-posterior left ventricular wall motion delay (intraventricular synchrony) and improve interventricular synchrony between the right and left ventricles (Albert, 2003). An emerging alternative approach is to place a pair of leads (one lead is a spare) epicardially through a thoracotomy or by a robotic surgical approach. A surgical approach requires anesthesia, chest tube placement, critical

care monitoring post-procedure, and other routine care expectations after cardiac surgery. It can be associated with early morbidity in patients with HF and requires a hospital stay averaging 4 days. Placement of an epicardial lateral-posterior wall lead is more exacting and may provide better long-term results. It is too early to determine if one method of insertion is superior to another.

Patients who meet criteria for bi-ventricular pacing are those with evidence of NYHA functional class III/IV symptoms and an ejection fraction of 35% or less, a QRS duration equal to or greater than 130 milliseconds, left ventricular end-diastolic diameter of 55 millimeters or greater, and optimized pharmacologic medical care for a minimum of 2 months before implantation. In summary, bi-ventricular therapy is considered appropriate for patients with advanced HF and prolonged QRS duration in whom traditional medical management is no longer effective.

Most studies have demonstrated at 1 year improved heart function and reduced cardiac morbidity, specifically: improvement in ejection fraction, reversal of left ventricular remodeling, reduced mitral regurgitation, improved exercise tolerance, reduced peak oxygen consumption, reduced symptoms, improved health-related quality of life, and reduced hospitalizations (Albert, 2003). The combined endpoint of mortality and hospitalization are statistically reduced in two recently reported trials (Abraham, Fisher, Smith, et al., 2002; Albert, 2003). Once the device is operational, medical therapy should not be discontinued even in the face of clinical improvement because the benefits are present only when the device is active (Yu, Chau, Sanderson, et al., 2002). In addition, it is important to educate patients about the need to maintain all medical therapies, lifestyle modification, and self-monitoring. Patients need to recognize signs and symptoms of worsening condition and continue ongoing communication with the health care team. Health care team members must assess patients to determine if HF medications can be modified. Improved ejection fraction may lead to improved renal function and better diuresis with diuretics, resulting in a need to decrease the diuretic dose. Improved ejection fraction could also decrease symptomatic hypotension with ACE inhibitors and beta-blockers, allowing practitioners to increase ACE-inhibitor and beta-blocker dosages to target levels. The electrophysiology team who inserted the device must monitor the leads at regular intervals to ensure that the electrode tips are functioning optimally and also to determine if preset pacing intervals and refractory periods should be altered to maximize ventricular synchronization. The long-term benefits of CRT (over 2 years) are unknown.

ICD. Patients with ischemic cardiomyopathy and post–myocardial infarction have a 31% reduction in mortality with prophylactic ICD implantation, compared with medical management alone (ACC/AHA, 2001; Moss, Zareba, Hall, et al., 2002). In this landmark study, the only criterion for entry was an ejection fraction of 30% or less post–myocardial infarction. This landmark study provides definitive evidence that mechanical intervention in ventricular dysrhythmias for patients with ischemic cardiomyopathy influences mortality. An ICD is larger than a standard pacemaker and is placed within the left pectoralis muscle as a pocket. The devices currently in use are single-chamber with bradycardia pacing as a backup, dual-chamber with sophisticated rate-adaptive dual-chamber pacing and atrial-based detection to reduce the number of inappropriate shocks, and dual-chamber with the ability to treat atrial fibrillation (atrial defibrillation). Dual-chamber devices offer tiered therapy: high-energy defibrillation, low-energy cardioversion, and antitachycardia pacing in addition to dual-chamber pacing or backup pacing on demand. Biphasic waveforms, which reverse polarity during energy delivery, allow for lower defibrillation thresholds, thus creating less shock intensity for patients.

The ACC, AHA, and National Association of Pacing and Electrophysiology (NASPE) recommend prophylactic ICD placement for a variety of patients with a history of structural heart disease. Ischemic cardiomyopathy patients who meet criteria are those with an ejection fraction of 30% or less, at least 1 month post–myocardial infarction and 3 months post–coronary artery revascularization surgery (ACC/AHA/NASPE, 2002). In addition, patients with non-ischemic HF also meet criteria for ICD placement if they have the following high-risk conditions (ACC/AHA/NASPE, 2002):

1. History of cardiac arrest caused by ventricular fibrillation or ventricular tachycardia not the result of transient or reversible causes or spontaneous sustained ventricular tachycardia.
2. History of nonsustained ventricular tachycardia with history of coronary artery disease and inducible or sustained ventricular tachycardia by electrophysiology study that is not suppressible by class I antidysrhythmic medications.
3. Syncope attributable to ventricular tachycardia while awaiting cardiac transplantation.
4. Syncope in which invasive and noninvasive studies have failed to find a cause.

Patients who meet criteria for both CRT and ICD therapies can have a combination device implanted. Similar to CRT pacing, patients with ICD devices must continue to receive ongoing care by both the HF and electrophysiology teams to ensure optimal cardiac care.

Core Nonpharmacologic Management

In addition to pharmacologic and device therapies, it is important for patients with HF to receive nonpharmacologic care. Specific themes of nonpharmacologic care are lifestyle modification, patient and family education, social services, communication, and ongoing monitoring for adherence to the plan of care.

Lifestyle Modification. The five key recommendations for lifestyle modification are regular exercise and activity, 2000-mg sodium diet, adherence to medications as prescribed, regular monitoring and appropriate fluid limitations, and self-monitoring for signs and symptoms of worsening HF (Grady, Dracup, Kennedy, et al., 2000; Liu, Arnold, Belenkie, et al., 2001; Uretsky, Pina, Quigg, et al., 1998). Lifestyle choices will affect risk factors (i.e., hypertension, hyperlipidemia, smoking, obesity, atherosclerosis), which will independently be detrimental to HF management and lead to relapse.

Patients should be encouraged to stay as physically active as possible, including sexual activity and regular exercise, regardless of HF stage or functional class. Clinical studies have found that mild and moderate aerobic exercise (brisk walking, bicycling, swimming) results in improved exercise tolerance and induration, less fatigue, and improved general well-being (Grady et al., 2000; Uretsky et al., 1998). The old adage that rest should be encouraged and exercise avoided is no longer good advice. It is common for HF patients to have co-morbid conditions (e.g., asthma, arthritis, diabetic neuropathy, obesity), which promote a false perception that they should not exercise. Patients may falsely believe that exercise will worsen their condition or stress the heart, causing premature death.

It is important for health care providers not only to encourage exercise and activity but also to actively *assist* in promoting exercise by conducting warm-up, cool-down, and walking exercises for patients or sending them to a cardiac rehabilitation program where they can exercise in a monitored group setting. In this way, patients will increase their confidence in exercise benefits and will receive positive feedback as they progressively improve in exercise endurance and intensity. In advanced HF, patients may be debilitated by physical deconditioning from a recent hospitalization or by worsening functional status. It is important for patients in this situation to exercise or be active every day, even if it entails moving from one chair to another chair a few feet away every hour for the first day and then slowly increasing the amount of movement and level of activity. In this way, patients will have more control over their cardiac condition and have more autonomy. In the terminal phase of HF, patients will be bedridden and will need scheduled turning and positioning and passive exercises to maintain muscle group compliance, prevent bedsores, and maintain comfort.

Although no studies have been conducted that evaluate specific diet recommendations, many researchers have reported that excessive sodium retention ranks as the primary factor that leads to hospitalization and acute exacerbation of HF (Bennett, Huster, Baker, et al., 1998; Joshi, Mohanan, Sengupta, et al., 1999; Tsuyuki, McCelvie, Arnold, et al., 2001). Volume overload because of lack of adherence to sodium restriction is the predominant precipitating factor for hospitalization in many patients. Sodium retention and volume overload are considered preventable causes for hospitalization in patients with compensated HF (Joshi, Mohanan, Sengupta, et al., 1999). The AHA and ACC recommend that patients with HF restrict sodium intake to 2000 to 3000 mg per day (ACC/AHA Task Force, 2001; Grady et al., 2000).

Patients must understand medication compliance because the ramifications of skipping doses, taking double doses, and altering the dosing schedule based on daily living plan may lead to worsening HF or drug toxicity. In a study that examined diuretic adherence, patients who had poor scheduling adherence had significantly more hospitalizations and worsened functional class (Chui, Deer, Bennett, et al., 2003). Although this phenomenon has not been studied with other medications in patients with HF, health care providers have noted the negative effects of taking all vasodilators at the same time each morning and the benefits of a staggered schedule of medications with the same pharmacologic action. Medication timing is a more complex issue than just getting patients to take the right number of drug doses each day. However, emphasis on compliance to schedule may improve quality of life and reduce morbidity, especially in patients with advanced HF and moderate to severe symptoms.

Monitoring fluid intake to maintain dry weight requires simple actions: a weight every day, attention to the daily intake of fluids, and assessment for new or worsening edema, followed by communication with the health care team when weight gain is excessive or signs or symptoms of volume overload appear or worsen. Adherence may be poor for a variety of reasons, including patient uncertainty of when and what to communicate to the health care team, the cost of a scale, poor eyesight, lack of understanding as to what "dry weight" is, and the connection between weight and fluid and sodium consumption with symptoms of HF. Patients must receive clear instructions, verbalize an understanding, and demonstrate the ability to monitor fluid status before the paradigm to managing fluid overload is introduced. Proper self-care includes alternatives to fluids when thirsty (sucking on hard candy or frozen grapes), reducing sodium intake to 1800 mg or less per day, and limiting fluid volume limited to 6 cups per day if body weight has increased by 2 pounds, and learning when it is appropriate to take extra doses of diuretic (and potassium supplement).

Patient-centered monitoring for signs and symptoms of worsening HF is an important adjunct to pharmacologic therapy. Patients must be cognizant of a symptom, such as increased fatigue, and its relationship to HF or when the symptom has another cause, such as overexertion. Because many HF symptoms and signs can have multiple causes, including aging, it is easy for patients to become too focused on their health status and develop psychologic stress caused by symptom preoccupation and over-interpretation. Patients must learn the common signs and symptoms of worsening of HF based on their particular type of HF through past experiences and based on their present functional status. Patients must understand how and when to communicate their concerns to their health care provider.

Patient and Family Education. Consistent, ongoing patient and family education promotes a stable clinical course by abrogating early relapses of HF symptoms (Cunningham & Mayet, 2002; Grady et al., 2000). Patient education involves informative materials for home use, outlined goals to reinforce key behavioral messages, frequent reminders that HF is a chronic condition, and supplementary information on the emotional impact of chronic illness on quality of life, hospital admissions, and hospital length of stay (Serxner, Muyaji, & Jeffords, 1998). Inadequate knowledge of self-care is found to be an important predictor of adherence to recommendations (Ni, Nauman, Burgess, et al., 1999). Patients should be educated to understand that HF follows a continuum of having no symptoms with activity to becoming symptomatic at rest. Details as to lifestyle modifications must be clearly understood and have a known connection to HF pathophysiology so that patients can understand the impact of self-management on HF outcomes. Educational interventions that involve a group within a classroom setting allow patients to practice new techniques, learn from mistakes, and mutually encourage one another. In addition,

patients will gain confidence in their ability to carry out the recommendations, which are more likely to continue over time.

There are many forms of patient education (e.g., one-on-one, group classes, web-based, video-centered, written handouts, audiotapes) and many settings where education can be accomplished (e.g., home, hospital, outpatient department, classroom, practice room). Each method has strengths and weaknesses, and it is often helpful to use combined approaches so that the patient's usual style of learning is enhanced; however, one-on-one education is basic to providing individualized care. No matter the education methods chosen, it is important to assess the patient's level of understanding. It is especially important for patients to understand lifestyle modifications and have an opportunity to practice new or seldom-used skills early in the course of HF so that they can realize the benefits of the recommendations. Having a favorable experience with the lifestyle modifications becomes more imperative when patients have advanced HF. Patients with advanced HF make choices that promote comfort, and these comfort options are more likely to conflict with optimal nonpharmacologic management, particularly if the patient has never realized the benefits of recommended strategies. For example, a patient's favorite comfort food is chicken noodle soup, but most commercial brands of chicken noodle soup are extremely high in sodium, which will worsen dyspnea in patients who are in a fluid overload state. Patients who understand the importance of sodium content in foods will have experienced first-hand the benefits of avoiding foods high in sodium and will choose a comfort food that is consistent with recommended HF behaviors.

Social Services. Social services as part of the management team will enhance coordination and collaboration among specialty services, which leads to a more cohesive management approach. Social services can (Uretsky et al., 1998):

1. Assess the social burden of illness on the patient and family members.
2. Clarify patient needs and facilitate communication among family members and the health care team.

3. Develop an individualized plan that takes into account the patient's physical, psychosocial, emotional, cultural, spiritual, transportation, housing, and financial issues.

4. Assist in developing or enhancing social and psychologic support for the patient and family so that individual members of the family do not experience burnout from caregiver responsibilities.

5. Aid in connecting patients and their family members to support groups that may offer respite from caregiver responsibilities or may enhance their coping ability to care for the person with HF.

There is no substitute for a thorough assessment of the patient's life situation so that pharmacologic and surgical intervention and comfort measures are implemented when they are most appropriate. In addition, a social service coordinator must have a broad perspective as to the various possibilities open to patients with HF within the community and also have great depth and expertise in handling many life issues at various stages of HF so that patients and families derive the greatest benefit of services (Uretsky et al., 1998).

Communication. Communication is often a barrier to optimal medical management of HF. Poor communication among team members affects the quality, continuity, and cost of care (Uretsky et al., 1998). Poor communication causes duplication of tests and medications and contradictory instructions to patients by various caregivers and influences decision making, especially when it omits information about allergies, co-morbid conditions, previous surgery, and lack of adherence (Uretsky et al., 1998). Specific team communication paradigms are highlighted in Figure 6-3. Systems that enhance communication and collaboration among team members will save time and energy for all parties and enhance patient outcomes, whether the focus is cure or palliation.

Ongoing Monitoring for Adherence. The therapeutic plan will be successful only if patients participate fully and adhere to recommendations. Follow-up care must include a plan for vigilant monitoring and consistent adherence to the plan of care. Nonadherence to various parts of the plan

of care is common and is often multifactorial. Patients may adhere to one recommendation but not another, so it is important to ask questions about the entire plan—medications, diet, fluid management, monitoring, and exercise and activity. Some common barriers to adherence are lack of knowledge and lack of understanding regarding lifestyle with HF, helplessness, poor motivation, denial as to severity of illness, lack of social support and social and emotional isolation, dementia, poor eyesight, finances, lack of transportation, and dependence upon others who work. Divergent expectations of outcome, frailty, and lack of insight as to life choices are additional barriers (Albert, Paul, & McCauley, 2003; Grady et al., 2000).

Health care providers and health care organizations contribute to nonadherence when recommendations differ from written materials or when written materials are unavailable to support the verbal communication. Physicians may change the plan of care without consulting the HF specialty team, or divergent goals of care may exist between physician groups. Significant others who could participate in the plan of care may be excluded from interacting with the health care team.

Patients may have challenges that influence adherence. Increasing age, co-morbid conditions, polypharmacy, and cognitive limitations can cause confusion as to priorities.

Nonadherence to office visits is common and may be caused by transportation difficulties, weather conditions, or perception that follow-up is not needed. Other barriers are long waits at the physician's office or long waits to be scheduled for an appointment, inconvenient office access such as steps or distance from the parking area, and costs.

The health care team must consider all types of nonadherence as detrimental and develop a system that addresses these important issues in the patient population they serve. Disease management programs that incorporate prevention, pharmacologic treatment, education, promotion of healthy lifestyle, vigilant monitoring, and ongoing communication have been shown to improve compliance and quality of life and to reduce hospitalization (McAlister, Lawson, Teo, et al., 2001). Disease management programs can be implemented

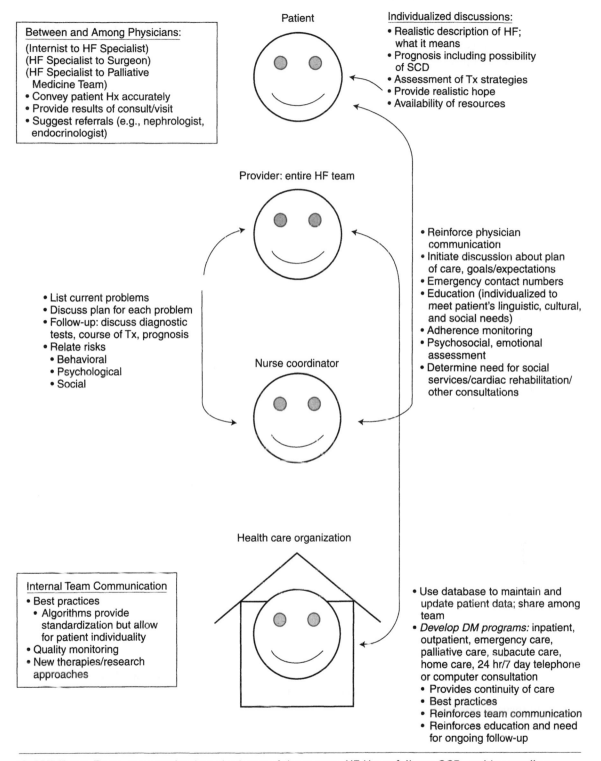

Between and Among Physicians:
(Internist to HF Specialist)
(HF Specialist to Surgeon)
(HF Specialist to Palliative
Medicine Team)
• Convey patient Hx accurately
• Provide results of consult/visit
• Suggest referrals (e.g., nephrologist,
endocrinologist)

Patient

Individualized discussions:
• Realistic description of HF;
what it means
• Prognosis including possibility
of SCD
• Assessment of Tx strategies
• Provide realistic hope
• Availability of resources

Provider: entire HF team

• List current problems
• Discuss plan for each problem
• Follow-up: discuss diagnostic
tests, course of Tx, prognosis
• Relate risks
• Behavioral
• Psychological
• Social

• Reinforce physician
communication
• Initiate discussion about plan
of care, goals/expectations
• Emergency contact numbers
• Education (individualized to
meet patient's linguistic, cultural,
and social needs)
• Adherence monitoring
• Psychosocial, emotional
assessment
• Determine need for social
services/cardiac rehabilitation/
other consultations

Nurse coordinator

Health care organization

Internal Team Communication
• Best practices
• Algorithms provide
standardization but allow
for patient individuality
• Quality monitoring
• New therapies/research
approaches

• Use database to maintain and
update patient data; share among
team
• *Develop DM programs:* inpatient,
outpatient, emergency care,
palliative care, subacute care,
home care, 24 hr/7 day telephone
or computer consultation
• Provides continuity of care
• Best practices
• Reinforces team communication
• Reinforces education and need
for ongoing follow-up

FIGURE **6-3** Team communication: the heart of the matter. *HF,* Heart failure; *SCD,* sudden cardiac death; *Tx,* treatment; *Hx,* history; *DM,* disease management.

in many environments, including within palliative and hospice care, and can offer patients the level of support they need to promote and achieve adherence to the plan of care.

END-OF-LIFE CARE
Anticipated Symptoms at End of Life

At end of life, patient symptoms are classified into one of three categories:

1. Refractory decompensated HF with symptoms of congestion, exercise intolerance, and systemic hypoperfusion
2. Symptoms of damage to liver, kidney, brain, gut, and other organs arising from systemic hypoperfusion
3. Symptoms of debility, anorexia, and cachexia (cardiac cachexia)

In a study of 66 terminally ill patients with advanced HF, the most troublesome problems were related to cardiac decompensation (58%), followed by physical debility (20%), social/functional dysfunction (14%), and psychiatric problems (8%) (Anderson, Ward, Eardley, et al., 2001). When patients were asked to identify their three most *troublesome* problems, 66 patients identified breathlessness (55%), pain/angina (32%), tiredness (27%), difficulty walking (23%), loss of independence (20%), anxiety or depression (15%), difficulty sleeping (11%), nausea or vomiting (5%), and constipation (3%). It is interesting to note that the number of symptoms identified was much higher then those just enumerated, but these did not affect the quality of life to the same degree as the troublesome problems (Anderson et al., 2001). Box 6-4 lists problems/symptoms in patients with terminal HF that occur with a frequency of 30% or more.

Managing terminal symptoms in HF is similar to managing symptoms in patients with cancer and are not discussed in this chapter. However, a few caveats are mentioned. Patients who are not on an optimal medical and nonpharmacologic regimen need to be treated to the standard of care to ensure that consensus guidelines known to improve morbidity and mortality are met before hospice referral. When patients have an acute exacerbation of HF, the goals of treatment should be aimed at reversing the congestive state. Symptom measures

Box 6-4   PROBLEMS AND SYMPTOMS SEEN IN ADVANCED HEART FAILURE

List includes symptoms with a frequency of ≥30%; (frequency in parentheses):
- Breathlessness (83%)
- Tiredness (82%)
- Difficulty walking (65%)
- Difficulty sleeping (48%)
- Dry mouth or thirst (45%)
- Cough (44%)
- Decreased sexual interest (42%)
- Pain (41%)
- Feeling depressed or anxious (41%)
- Swollen arms or legs (33%)
- Hot flushes/sweating (32%)

Data from Anderson, H., Ward, C., Eardley, A., et al. (2001). The concerns of patients under palliative care and a heart failure clinic are not being met. *Palliat Med, 15*, 279-286.

can be instituted simultaneously to improve patient comfort. The elements of good end-of-life care with HF include:

1. Providing treatments known to relieve symptoms and suffering in a timely fashion.
2. Eliminating burdensome symptoms that diminish quality of life or negatively affect a comfortable death.
3. Listening to family preferences seriously, and maintaining respect for the roles of family members, friends, and clergy. After all, the patient ultimately belongs to the family and not to the physician or health care team.
4. Eliminating gaps in communication by providing individualized care and discussing transition from cure to comfort.
5. Helping patients live their lives to their fullest potential.

Social dysfunction and barriers are an issue for patients with terminal HF. In a survey of 66 patients with advanced HF, 18% reported family concerns, 12% reported financial constraints, and 6% reported challenges to personal faith (Anderson, 2001). In a qualitative study of terminal HF patients, uncoordinated hospital care, lack of continuity, lack of social services and support, failure to address advance directives, and failed opportunity to die at home were major complaints (Murray et al., 2002). These reports highlight the need for advance care planning, coordinated services continuity, and family communication to deal with end-of-life decision making. Effective communication needs to encompass conflict resolution around withholding/withdrawing of therapy, medical futility regarding intensive interventional procedures, and expectations in the last hours of life. This will improve patients' and families' experiences and care and promote a satisfactory relationship between patients and their families and health care providers (von Gunten, Ferris, & Emanuel, 2000). The Study to Understand Prognoses and Preferences for Outcomes and Risks of Treatments (SUPPORT) provides insight into patient preferences. Among the HF population, 23% did not want to be resuscitated and 69% preferred resuscitation. Therefore it should not be assumed that patients are willing to forego resuscitation to diminish suffering (Levenson, McCarthy, Lynn, et al., 2000).

Considerations in HF: CRT and ICD Devices

Palliative care practitioners often ask how they should manage CRT and ICD devices when the end of life is imminent. Because the CRT device does not provide enough energy to create a clinically detectable shock, it should be turned off only if the refractory period and interval timing cannot be optimized to maintain or enhance electrical conduction and myocardial contractility and in situations where the device can cause potential harm. The benefits to CRT last only while the device is turned on. Within a week of discontinuation, contractility declines and by 4 weeks or less, most parameters are back to pre-therapy levels, which may lead to worsening symptoms (Yu et al., 2002). Therefore this device should be maintained without interruption if at all possible during palliation and hospice care.

An ICD device will cause pain and mental anguish if it delivers multiple shocks in bursts or with great frequency throughout the course of a day or days (appropriately or inappropriately). Some patients will request to have the device turned off, knowing that their death may be sooner, rather than worry about an impending ill-timed shock. When this situation occurs, it is important for the health care provider to assess the rationale for the patient's request. Device timing is easily altered in an electrophysiology laboratory and may relieve the patient's anxiety about multiple inappropriate shocks. When cardiac conversion by ICD is appropriate, serum electrolytes and medications should be assessed to ensure adverse effects are not leading to ventricular dysrhythmias and ICD firing. If laboratory values and medication are not contributing to dysrhythmias, then discussions must take place regarding the risk of sudden death versus pump failure death. An alternative to turning off the device is to maintain the device with the current battery, knowing it will become non-operational when the battery life ends. Another approach is to involve the patient in cognitive coping. This therapy provides patients an opportunity to voice their concerns and nurses the opportunity to help guide the patient toward appropriate steps if the ICD discharges and elicits a shock. Through cognitive therapy, the patient learns new, more effective ways of psychologically coping with a threatening situation (Dunbar & Summerville, 1997).

Left Ventricular Assist Devices. For years, left ventricular assist devices (LVAD) have been used as a bridge to cardiac transplantation. Even with the high rate of serious adverse effects, such as infection, bleeding, or mechanical failure, insertion before end-organ damage occurs will improve many clinical parameters. This led to the prospective REMATCH study, a study that used LVADs for (destination) therapy in patients who were not candidates for cardiac transplantation or other surgical options. Both the medically managed and LVAD groups experienced high mortality; however, LVAD patients clearly benefited with improved survival at all points throughout the 2-year study period as the major outcome and also demonstrated improved activity and decreased HF symptoms (Rose, Gelijns, Moskowitz, et al., 2001). The Food and Drug Administration approved these devices for destination therapy, and the Centers for Medicare and Medicaid Services (CMS) currently refining its reimbursement for LVAD. Once more centers gain experience with these devices, it will be relatively common for palliative medicine and hospice programs to encounter devices when caring for patients at the end of life with HF. These devices can be turned off if the patient chooses. Death may be quick unless the left ventricle has undergone significant recovery (reverse ventricular remodeling).

When a patient requests to have a LVAD turned off, a sequence of steps should be taken:

1. The health care provider must be sure of the patient's intent to have the device turned off and possibly removed.
2. The patient must understand the ramifications (consequences) of his or her decision to have the device discontinued.
3. The patient and family should be counseled by an ethicist, social worker, and/or clergy member who can assist in supporting the patient's decision while ensuring that everyone is fully informed of the expected outcome of such a decision.
4. The surgeon will use an echocardiogram or other diagnostic tests or will adjust the LVAD settings to determine if the ventricle has recovered enough to allow a sufficient cardiac output to sustain life.
5. If the ventricle has recovered, the patient is scheduled for surgical removal of the device.
6. If no recovery, the patient should have the device turned off within the hospital setting after being medicated to decrease symptoms that will occur after the device is turned off.

The decision to turn off an LVAD is associated with myriad responses from the patient and family, depending on the patient's individual situation. The health care team must provide support and guidance in anticipation of these varied responses throughout the discussion and action processes.

Intermittent and Continuous IV Inotropic Therapy. The ACC/AHA guideline for chronic HF management (2001) does not recommend outpatient intermittent infusions of inotropic agents for the management of HF. No placebo-controlled randomized trial has shown improvement in survival with the use of dobutamine or milrinone therapy as an intermittent infusion. In

fact, these agents have been associated with increased mortality caused by tachydysrhythmia. Therefore it is appropriate to discontinue intermittent inotropic infusions when patients enter a palliative or hospice care program.

Patients who do not tolerate weaning continuous intravenous inotropic agents during an acute exacerbation of HF may be maintained on their continuous therapy at home or other setting. CMS will reimburse for continuous inotropic therapy if patients fail to wean from inotropes, which is supported by worsening hemodynamic parameters (cardiac output). There must be documented evidence of improvement in hemodynamics when the infusion is restarted or when the rate is increased. This group of patients should be maintained on an inotropic infusion upon entering a palliative or hospice program since the infusion is used for symptom management to maintain quality of life and comfort. In general, the infusion rate is set to the level needed to maintain hemodynamics as monitored in the hospital. The palliative medicine team will not adjust up or down the infusion rate based on blood pressure. There are times when up-titration of the inotropic agent is consistent with palliation goals. Patients who are extremely symptomatic with CHF and are not responding to oral or intravenous loop diuretic therapy may derive palliative benefit with inotropic agent titration. If cardiac output increases with dose, renal perfusion will also increase and improve diuresis with diuretics. Guidelines should be established and used to determine the criteria for titration and maximum infusion dose. In addition, guidelines should also include dose reduction and discontinuation, particularly with the development of dysrhythmia.

SUMMARY

The HF literature provides evidence for guidelines as they relate to diagnosis, prognostic tests, outpatient management, acute medical management, device management, and surgical management. However, minimal data and practical information are available on care of dying patients with cardiac failure. The obvious focus over time has been to improve survival and morbidity but at the cost to patients who no longer receive benefit from aggressive interventions, even when evidence-based therapies are optimized. Once HF is diagnosed, the course is progressive and the prognosis for patients treated in the community is poor. At the end of life, unrelieved physical symptoms accentuate psychologic, social, and spiritual suffering and negatively affect quality of life and completion of life tasks for patients and families. Health care providers must understand the HF trajectory of illness and patient needs and be knowledgeable about service availability/utilization so that a foundation can be laid for optimizing of patient-centered care and future research.

Case Study

58-year-old African-American male (W.P.); body mass index equals 27 and history of sick sinus syndrome (with DDD pacemaker), gout, hyperlipidemia, and hypertension. He worked full time before recent events. Currently, hospitalized for decreasing urine output despite doubling of loop diuretics for 2 days. Weight has increased by 18 pounds in 2 weeks. Paroxysmal nocturnal dyspnea (PND), orthopnea, shortness of breath, cough, and leg edema progressively worsened. Two weeks ago, W.P. was treated in the emergency department and hospitalized for two-pillow orthopnea, cough, PND, and leg edema. Creatinine was 2.1 mg/dl at that time, and echocardiogram findings were: dilated cardiomyopathy, ejection fraction of 10%; moderate-severe mitral regurgitation (3+); moderate tricuspid regurgitation (2+-3+); severe right ventricular dysfunction, and left atrial clot.

At current admission W.P. has 3+ to 4+ lower leg edema, positive S_3 gallop, positive hepatojugular reflux, and jugular venous pressure of approximately 20 cm H_2O in addition to symptoms from prior admission. W.P.'s medications on admission were: furosemide 120 mg twice daily; carvedilol 6.25 mg twice daily; digoxin 0.25 mg daily; simvastatin 20 mg daily; potassium supplement 40 mEq twice daily; metolazone 2.5 mg daily; max oxide 400 mg daily; and allopurinol 100 mg daily. At this admission, W.P.'s serum laboratory values were: troponin 0.13 ng/ml; sodium, 136 mmol/l; potassium, 4.0 mmol/l; blood urea nitrogen (BUN), 78 mg/dl; creatinine, 4.1 mg/dl; glucose, 182 mg/dl, and BNP, 4420 pg/ml. Electrocardiogram findings were: right ventricular paced rhythm with premature ventricular contractions and atrial flutter, heart rate of 65 beats per minute; QRS interval, 182 ms; QT interval, 566 ms; and corrected QT interval, 588 ms. Initial vital signs were: blood pressure, 90/79 mm Hg; and respirations 18 breaths per minute. Hemodynamics after pulmonary artery catheter placement were: cardiac output, 3.3 L/min; cardiac index, 1.5 L/min/m²; systemic vascular resistance, 1775 dynes/sec/cm⁻⁵; pulmonary artery wedge pressure, 32 mm Hg; right atrial pressure, 26 mm Hg; and venous oxygen saturation, 52%.

Medications discontinued were: max oxide, allopurinol, carvedilol, digoxin, and metolazone. New therapies were: hydralazine 100 mg four times daily; isosorbide dinitrate 60 mg three times daily; spironolactone 25 mg daily; continuous intravenous furosemide drip at 30 ml/hour; continuous intravenous dobutamine drip at 5 mcg/kg/min; and heparin drip to maintain activated partial thromboplastin time (APTT). Simvastatin and potassium supplement were continued as previously ordered.

W.P. was admitted to the Heart Failure Specialty Care Unit and aggressively managed with intravenous and oral vasodilator therapy and intravenous dobutamine. Dobutamine drip dose decreased to 2.5 mcg/kg/min; however, attempts to wean led to worsening vital signs and symptoms of heart failure. Renal consult initiated for end-stage renal disease.

After 3 weeks of therapy, W.P. could not be evaluated for cardiac transplantation because of unresolved renal failure. What treatment options are available at this time? Should cardiac resynchronization therapy be initiated? Should evaluation for surgical repair of mitral and tricuspid regurgitation be undertaken? Should dialysis be initiated? Should hospital discharge on continuous dobutamine therapy and palliation be considered?

Currently, there is not sufficient long-term follow-up information about what to expect regarding a patient's illness trajectory, thus making it difficult for health care providers to determine the right time to begin end-of-life discussions. Prognostic indicators abound, and patients who remain highly symptomatic after optimized medical therapies, especially those with poor prognostic signs, ought to be referred to an HF specialty team for advance care options or initiated in palliative measures.

Patients with HF struggle to live with their progressively worsening condition. They experience loss of autonomy, social isolation, increased disability, and co-morbidity, which contribute to the uncertainty of relief, challenges to coping, and poor quality of life. Communication with patients during these stressful periods not only may improve patient compliance despite uncertainty in their abilities but also may offer patients a sense of hope and understanding about their life situation. In advanced HF, specialty clinics that routinely follow patients (via telephone monitoring or frequent office visits) increase adherence to treatment plans, improve short-term health-related quality of life, and decrease morbidity (McAlister et al., 2001). Depression is common, and communication facilitates a sense of community and belonging with dignity that reduces depression and improves quality of life, physical functioning, and survival.

Palliative care specialists must become experienced in the care of patients with advanced HF since the paradigms of symptom management and palliation in cancer care may not apply to cardiac patients. Internists and cardiologists must be reassured about appropriately referring patients to palliative medicine when indicated, yet there still is uncertainty about when to shift focus from a curative model to a caring/comfort promotion model. Because HF health care expenditures continue to grow, it is imperative that palliative principles be addressed. Symptom management, the role of family, health service provision, and ethical issues (e.g., use of inotropic agents, maintaining implantable defibrillator power) need to be actively addressed to improve patient outlook and outcomes despite living with a progressive terminal illness.

Objective Questions

1. Chronic systolic left ventricular dysfunction refers to:

   a. Ventricular injury with cardiogenic shock after acute myocardial infarction.
   b. Ventricular relaxation dysfunction with an ejection fraction more than 40%.
   c. Reduced ventricular contraction with low ejection fraction caused by structural heart disease.
   d. Heart failure from cardiac fibrosis and stiffness in the ventricle from hypertension.

2. Which of the following statements is *true* about ventricular remodeling:

   a. It is reversible.
   b. Cardiac muscle contracts, resulting in a diminished ventricular volume.
   c. It occurs only after myocyte necrosis from acute myocardial infarction.
   d. With progression, the sympathetic nervous system becomes less active.

3. Sympathetic nervous system and renin-angiotensin system activation leads to:

   a. Worsened cardiac output and heart function in the early stages of HF.
   b. Worsened cardiac output and heart function in the late stages of HF.
   c. No influence on cardiac output or ventricular function.
   d. Improvement early in HF but a worsening in HF with time.

4. The most frequently cited reason for rehospitalization in HF is:

   a. Unstable angina or myocardial infarction.
   b. Sodium retention and fluid overload.
   c. Hypertension.
   d. Renal dysfunction.

5. When patients are admitted to the hospital with decompensated HF, the most common profile is:

   a. Dry and warm.
   b. Wet and warm.

c. Wet and cold.
d. Cold and dry.

6. A 78-year-old female arrives in the hospital with worsening chronic heart failure. Assessment reveals an elevated jugular venous pressure of 15 cm/H$_2$0, a positive S$_3$ gallop, clear lungs, no peripheral edema, warm skin, and a blood pressure of 106/64, a pulse of 88 with a regular rhythm, and 18 respirations per minute. Initial treatment includes:

a. Oxygen and continue oral medications from home.
b. Intravenous inotropic infusion with dobutamine and discontinue beta-blocker agent.
c. Intravenous loop diuretics and continue medications from home.
d. Intravenous infusion of nitroglycerin (or other intravenous vasodilator), hold angiotensin-converting enzyme inhibitor, and maintain other home medications.

7. A 67-year-old male arrives in the hospital with worsening chronic heart failure. He has a history of coronary artery bypass surgery 3 years ago. Assessment reveals an elevated jugular venous pressure of 15 cm/H$_2$0, positive S$_3$ gallop, clear lungs but diminished breath sounds in bases, no peripheral edema, cold feet and hands, cool legs and arms, and vital signs of 126/84 blood pressure, a pulse of 88, atrial fibrillation, and respirations of 18. Initial treatment includes:

a. Oxygen and continue oral medications from home.
b. Intravenous inotropic infusion with dobutamine and discontinue beta-blocker agent.
c. Intravenous loop diuretic and continue medications from home.
d. Intravenous infusion of nitroglycerin (or other intravenous vasodilator), hold the angiotensin-converting enzyme inhibitor, change loop diuretic to parenteral and

administer the same dose immediately, and maintain other home medications.

8. Which of the following prognostic signs are most likely to predict that a patient with advanced heart failure (ejection fraction of 15%) is ready for palliative care:

a. Serum sodium level of 127 mmol/L after diuresis and stabilization.
b. BNP level of 164 pg/dl and NYHA functional class I.
c. An ejection fraction improved by 5% one month following cardiac resynchronization therapy.
d. Heart rate >100 beats per minute at rest during acute admission to hospital for decompensated HF in a patient known not to be compliant to drugs and diet.

9. You are asked to assess a patient with heart failure and fluid overload for admission to a home-based palliative medicine program. The patient is taking the following medications:

• Digoxin 0.5 mg/day
• Furosemide 60 mg/ 2 times per day by intravenous bolus
• Captopril 6.25 mg/ 3 times a day
• Intravenous dobutamine infusion (continuously) at 2.5 mcg/kg/minute
  There is no documentation of intolerance to any drug, and the patient does not have contraindications to any medications commonly used in heart failure. Your response to this request is:

a. The patient is on adequate heart failure medications and the next step in care is plan to palliation.
b. The patient cannot be in palliative care until the dobutamine infusion is discontinued and beta-blockers are started.
c. The patient should be titrated on oral furosemide before determining that palliation is the next most appropriate step in care plan.
d. The patient is not ready for palliative medicine and hospice care.

10. A patient is in a home palliative care program for end-stage heart failure, and you are the caregiver. The patient wants "comfort food." Which of the following has a low sodium content and could be offered:

a. A lean turkey sandwich made with deli meat and no condiments.

b. Pancakes from a box mix and packaged bacon.

c. Homemade chicken noodle soup using fresh chicken and vegetables and unsalted broth.

d. 1 cup of fat-free potato chips.

REFERENCES

Aaronson, K.D., Schwartz, S., Chen, T., et al. (1997). Development and prospective validation of a clinical index to predict survival in ambulatory patients referred for cardiac transplant evaluation. *Circulation, 95,* 2660-2667.

Abbate, A., Biondi-Zoccai, G.G., Bussani, R., et al. (2003). Increased myocardial apoptosis in patients with unfavorable left ventricular remodeling and early symptomatic post-infarction heart failure. *J Am Coll Cardiol, 41,* 753-760.

Abraham, W.T., Fisher, W.G., Smith, A.L., et al. (2002). Cardiac resynchronization in chronic heart failure. *N Engl J Med, 346,* 1845-1853.

ACC/AHA/NASPE. (2002). ACC/AHA/NASPE 2002 guideline update for implantation of cardiac pacemakers and antiarrhythmic devices: Summary article. *Circulation, 106,* 2145-2161.

Adams, K.F., Mathur, V.S., & Gheorghiade M. (2003). B-type natriuretic peptide: From bench to bedside. *Am Heart J, 145,* S34-S46.

Albert, N. (1999). Heart failure: The physiologic basis for current therapeutic concepts. *Crit Care Nurse,* 19(3 Suppl.), 2-13.

Albert, N.M. (2003). Cardiac resynchronization therapy through biventricular pacing in patients with heart failure and ventricular dyssynchrony. *Crit Care Nurse,* 23(3 Suppl.), 2-13.

Albert, N.M., Davis, M., & Young, J. (2002). Improving the care of patients dying of heart failure. *Cleve Clin J Med, 69,* 321-328.

Albert, N.M., Paul, S., & McCauley, K.M. (2003). Living with heart failure: Promoting adherence, managing symptoms and optimizing function. In M. Jessup & K. M. McCauley (Eds.), *Heart failure: Providing optimal care* (Chapter 10). Elmsford, NY: Blackwell Publishing.

Alla, F., Briancon, S., Juillière, Y., et al. (2000). Differential clinical prognostic classifications in dilated and ischemic advanced heart failure: The EPICAL study. *Am Heart J, 139,* 895-904.

American College of Cardiology (ACC)/American Heart Association (AHA) Task Force. (2001). *ACC/AHA guidelines for the evaluation and management of chronic heart failure in the adult.* Practice Guidelines—full text. www.acc.org/clinical/guidelines/failure/hf_index.htm.

American Heart Association (AHA). (2001). *2002 Heart and stroke statistical update.* Dallas: Author.

American Heart Association (AHA). (2002). *Heart disease and stroke statistics: 2003 Update.* Dallas: Author.

Anand, I.S. (2002). Ventricular remodeling without cellular contractile dysfunction. *J Card Fail, 8,* S401-S408.

Anderson, H., Ward, C., Eardley, A., et al. (2001). The concerns of patients under palliative care and a heart failure clinic are not being met. *Palliat Med, 15,* 279-286.

Ashton, E., Liew, D., & Krum, H. (2003). Should patients with chronic heart failure be treated with 'statins'? *Heart Fail Monit, 3,* 82-86.

Baldasseroni, S., Opasich, C., Gorini, M., et al. (2002). Left bundle branch block is associated with increased 1-year sudden and total mortality rate in 5517 outpatients with congestive heart failure: A report from the Italian Network on Congestive Heart Failure. *Am Heart J, 143,* 398-405.

Bart, B.A., Shaw, L.K., McCants, C.B., et al. (1997). Clinical determinants of mortality with angiographically diagnosed ischemic or nonischemic cardiomyopathy. *J Am Coll Cardiol, 30,* 1002-1008.

Bennett, S.J., Huster, G.A., Baker, S.L., et al. (1998). Characterization of the precipitants of hospitalization for heart failure decompensation. *Am J Crit Care, 7,* 168-174.

Berger, R., Huelsman, M., Strecker, K., et al. (2002). B-type natriuretic peptide predicts sudden death in patients with chronic heart failure. *Circulation, 105,* 2392-2397.

Chen, H.H., & Burnett, J.C. Jr. (1999). The natriuretic peptides in heart failure: Diagnostic and therapeutic potentials. *Proc Assoc Am Physicians, 111,* 406-416.

Chui, M.A., Deer, M., Bennett, S.J., et al. (2003). Association between adherence to diuretic therapy and health care utilization in patients with heart failure. *Pharmacology, 23,* 326-332.

Cleutjens, J.P., & Creemers, E.E. (2002). Integration of concepts: Cardiac extracellular matrix remodeling after myocardial infarction. *J Card Fail, 8,* S344-S348.

Cohn, J.N., Ferrari, R., & Sharpe, N. (2000). Cardiac remodeling-concepts and clinical implications: A consensus paper from an international forum on cardiac remodeling. *J Am Coll Cardiol, 35,* 569-582.

Cunningham, S.L., & Mayet, J. (2002). Modern management of heart failure: Education as well as medication. *Eur Heart J, 23,* 101-102.

Dorn, G. (2002). Adrenergic pathways and left ventricular remodeling. *J Card Fail,* S370-S373.

Dunbar, S.B., & Summerville, J.G. (1997). Cognitive therapy for ventricular dysrhythmia patients. *J Cardiovasc Nurs, 12,* 33-44.

Elkayam, U., Khan, S., Mehboob, A., et al. (2002). Impaired endothelium-mediated vasodilation in heart failure: Clinical evidence and the potential for therapy. *J Card Fail, 8,* 15-20.

Felker, G.M., Adams, K.F., Konstam, M.A., et al. (2003). The problem of decompensated heart failure: Nomenclature, classification, and risk stratification. *Am Heart J, 145,* S18-S25.

Fonarow, G.C. (2001). The treatment targets in acute decompensated heart failure. *Cardiovasc Rev, 2*(Suppl. 2), S7-S12.

Fox, E., Landrum-McNiff, K., Zhong, Z., et al. (1999). Evaluation of prognostic criteria for determining hospice eligibility in patients with advanced lung, heart, or liver disease. *JAMA, 282,* 1638-1645.

Gheorghiade, M., & Bonow, R.O. (1998). Chronic heart failure in the United States: A manifestation of coronary artery disease. *Circulation, 97,* 282-289.

Goldman, S., Johnson, G., Cohn, J.N., et al. (1993). Mechanisms of death in heart failure. The vasodilator-heart failure trials. *Circulation, 87* [Suppl. VI], VI-24–VI-31.

Goldsmith, E.C., & Borg, T.K. (2002). The dynamic interaction of the extracellular matrix in cardiac remodeling. *J Card Fail, 8,* S314-S318.

Grady, K.L., Dracup, K., Kennedy, G., et al. (2000). Team management of patients with heart failure. A statement for healthcare professionals from the cardiovascular nursing council of the American Heart Association. *Circulation, 102,* 2443-2456.

Iuliano, S., Fisher, S.G., Karasik, P E., et al. (2002). QRS duration and mortality in patients with congestive heart failure. *Am Heart J, 143,* 1085-1091.

Jain, P., Massie, B.M., Gattis, W.A., et al. (2003). Current medical treatment for the exacerbation of chronic heart failure resulting in hospitalization. *Am Heart J, 145,* S3-S17.

Jessup, M., & Brozena, S. (2003). Heart failure. *N Engl J Med, 348,* 2007-2018.

Jiang, W., Alexander, J., Christopher, E., et al. (2001). Relationship of depression to increased risk of mortality and rehospitalization in patients with congestive heart failure. *Arch Intern Med, 161,* 1849-1856.

Joshi, P.P., Mohanan, C.J., Sengupta, S.P., et al. (1999). Factors precipitating congestive heart failure: Role of non-compliance. *J Assoc Physicians India, 47,* 294-295.

Kaye, D.M., Lefkovits, J., Jennings, G.L., et al. (1995). Adverse consequences of high sympathetic nervous activity in the failing human heart. *J Am Coll Cardiol, 26,* 1257-1263.

Kearney, M.T., Fox, K.A., Lee, A., et al. (2002). Predicting death due to progressive heart failure in patients with mild-to-moderate chronic heart failure. *J Am Coll Cardiol, 40,* 1801-1808.

Khand, A., Gemmel, I., Clark, A.L., et al. (2000). Is the prognosis of heart failure improving? *J Am Coll Cardiol, 36,* 2284-2286.

Koelling, T.M., Semigran, M.J., Mijller-Ehmsen, J., et al. (1998). Left ventricular end-diastolic volume index, age, maximal heart rate at peak exercise predict survival in patients referred for heart transplantation. *J Heart Lung Transplant, 17,* 278-287.

Koglin, J., Pehlivanli S., Schwaiblmair, M., et al. (2001). Role of brain natriuretic peptide in risk stratification of patients with congestive heart failure. *J Am Coll Cardiol, 38,* 1934-1941.

Kokkonen, J.O., Lindstedt, K.A., & Kovanen, P.T. (2003). Role for chymase in heart failure: Angiotensin II dependent or independent mechanisms? *Circulation, 107,* 2522-2524.

Krüger, S., Graf, J., Kunz, D., et al. (2002). Brain natriuretic peptide levels predict functional capacity in patients with chronic heart failure. *J Am Coll Cardiol, 40,* 718-722.

Krumholz, H.M., Butler, J., Miller, J., et al. (1998). Prognostic importance of emotional support for elderly patients hospitalized with heart failure. *Circulation, 97,* 958-964.

Levenson, J.W., McCarthy, E.P., Lynn, J., et al. (2000). The last six months of life for patients with congestive heart failure. *J Am Soc Geriatr Dent, 48,* S101-S109.

Liu, P., Arnold, M., Belenkie, I., et al. from the Canadian Cardiovascular Society. (2001). The 2001 Canadian Cardiovascular Society consensus guideline update for the management and prevention of heart failure. *Can J Cardiol, 17*(Suppl. E), 5E-25E.

Loh, E. (2000). Maximizing management of patients with decompensated heart failure. *Clin Cardiol, 23*(Suppl. III), III-1–III-5.

Lucas, C., Johnson, W., Hamilton, M.A., et al. (2000). Freedom from congestion predicts good survival despite previous class IV symptoms of heart failure. *Am Heart J, 140,* 840-847.

Lüscher, T.F., & Barton, M. (2000). Endothelins and endothelin receptor antagonists: Therapeutic considerations for a novel class of cardiovascular drugs. *Circulation, 102,* 2434-2440.

MacIntyre, K., Capewell, S., Stewart, S., et al. (2000). Evidence of improving prognosis in heart failure: Trends in case fatality in 66,547 patients hospitalized between 1986 and 1995. *Circulation, 102,* 1126-1131.

Maeda K., Tsutamoto, T., Wada, A., et al. (2000). High levels of plasma brain natriuretic peptide and interleukin-6 after optimized treatment for heart failure are independent risk factors for morbidity and mortality in patients with congestive heart failure. *J Am Coll Cardiol, 36,* 1587-1593.

Mann, D. (2002). Tumor necrosis factor-induced signal transduction and left ventricular remodeling. *J Card Fail,* S379-S386.

Matsumoto, T., Wada, A., Tsutamoto, T, et al. (2003). Chymase inhibition prevents cardiac fibrosis and improves diastolic dysfunction in the progression of heart failure. *Circulation, 107,* 2555-2558.

McAlister, F.A., Lawson, F.M., Teo, K.K., et al. (2001). A systematic review of randomized trials of disease management programs in heart failure. *Am J Med, 110,* 378-384.

Moss, A.J., Zareba, W., Hall, W.J., et al. (2002). Prophylactic implantation of a defibrillator in patients with myocardial infarction and reduced ejection fraction. *N Engl J Med, 346,* 877-883.

Murray, D.R., & Freeman, G.L. (2003). Proinflammatory cytokines: Predictors of a failing heart? *Circulation, 107,* 1460-1462.

Murray, S.A., Boyd, K., Kendall, M., et al. (2002). Dying of lung cancer or cardiac failure: Prospective qualitative interview study of patients and their carers in the community. *Br Med J, 325,* 929-932.

Ni, H., Nauman, D., Burgess, D., et al. (1999). Factors influencing knowledge of and adherence to self-care among patients with heart failure. *Arch Intern Med, 159,* 1613-1619.

Nohria, A., Lewis, E., & Stevenson, L.W. (2002). Medical management of advanced heart failure. *JAMA, 287,* 628-640.

O'Connell, J.B. (2000). The economic burden of heart failure. *Clin Cardiol, 23*(Suppl. III), III-6–III-10.

Peterson, K.L. (2002). Pressure overload hypertrophy and congestive heart failure: Where is the "Achilles' heel"? *J Am Coll Cardiol, 39,* 672-675.

Poses, R.M., Smith, W.R., McClish, D.K., et al. (1997). Physicians' survival predictions for patients with acute congestive heart failure. *Arch Intern Med, 157,* 1001-1007.

Rickli, H., Kiowski, W., Brehm, M., et al. (2003). Combining low-intensity and maximal exercise test results improves prognostic prediction in chronic heart failure. *J Am Coll Cardiol, 42,* 116-122.

Rose, E.A., Gelijns, A.C., Moskowitz, A.J., et al. (2001). Long term use of left-ventricular assist device for end-stage heart failure. *N Engl J Med, 345,* 1435-1443.

Scaffidi, R., & Gottlieb, S.S. (2001). Heart failure at the beginning of the 21st century. *Cardiovascular Research & Review, 22,* 467-481.

Schrier, R.W., & Abraham, W.T. (1999). Hormones and hemodynamics in heart failure. *N Engl J Med, 341,* 577-585.

Scios, Inc. (2003). ADHERE™ Acute Decompensated Heart Failure National Registry. *4th Quarter 2002 Benchmark Report.* San Diego: Scios, Inc.

Selvais, P.L., Robert, A., Ahn, S., et al. (2000). Direct comparison between endothelin-1, N terminal proatrial natriuretic factor, and brain natriuretic peptide as prognostic markers of survival in congestive heart failure. *J Card Fail, 6,* 201-207.

Serxner, S., Muyaji, M., & Jeffords, J. (1998). Congestive heart failure disease management study: A patient education intervention. *Congest Heart Fail, 4*(3), 23-28.

Shah, M.R., Hasselblad, V., Gheorghiade, M., et al. (2001). Prognostic usefulness of the six-minute walk in patients with advanced congestive heart failure secondary to ischemic or nonischemic cardiomyopathy. *Am J Cardiol, 88,* 987-993.

Sharma, R., Al-Nasser, F., & Anker, S.D. (2001). The importance of tumor necrosis factor and lipoproteins in the pathogenesis of chronic heart failure. *Heart Fail Monit, 2,* 42-48.

Silvet, H., Amin, J., Padmanabhan, S., et al. (2001). Prognostic implications of increased QRS duration in patients with moderate and severe left ventricular systolic dysfunction. *Am J Cardiol, 88,* 182-185.

Smith, J.J., & Levine, H.J. (1999). Systolic dysfunction of the ventricle in congestive heart failure: Pathophysiology, diagnosis and therapy. *Congest Heart Fail, 5*(1), 10-26.

Spieker, L.E., Noll, G., Ruschitzka, F.T., et al. (2001). Endothelin receptor antagonists in congestive heart failure: A new therapeutic principle for the future? *J Am Coll Cardiol, 37,* 1493-1505.

Stewart, S., MacIntyre, K., Hole D.J., et al. (2001). More 'malignant' than cancer? Five-year survival following a first admission for heart failure. *Eur J Heart Fail, 3,* 315-322.

Suresh, D.P., Lamba, S., & Abraham, W.T. (2000). New developments in heart failure: Role of endothelin and the use of endothelin receptor antagonists. *J Card Fail, 6,* 359-368.

Sutton, M.G., & Sharpe, N. (2000). Left ventricular remodeling after myocardial infarction: Pathophysiology and therapy. *Circulation, 101,* 2981-2988.

Tsutamoto, T., Hisanaga, T., Wada, A., et al. (1998). Interleukin-6 spillover in the peripheral circulation increases with severity of heart failure, and the high plasma level of interleukin-6 is an important prognostic predictor in patients with congestive heart failure. *J Am Coll Cardiol, 31,* 391-398.

Tsuyuki, R.T., McCelvie, R.S., Arnold, M.O., et al. (2001). Acute precipitants of congestive heart failure exacerbations. *Arch Intern Med, 161,* 2337-2342.

Unger, T. (2000). Neurohormonal modulation in cardiovascular disease. *Am Heart J, 139,* S2-S8.

Uretsky, B.F., Pina, I., Quigg, R.J., et al. (1998). Beyond drug therapy: Nonpharmacologic care of the patient with advanced heart failure. *Am Heart J, 135,* S264-S284.

Vaccarino, V., Kasl, S.V., Abramson, J., et al. (2001). Depressive symptoms and risk of functional decline and death in patients with heart failure. *J Am Coll Cardiol, 38,* 199-205.

Von Gunten, C.F., Ferris, F.D., & Emanuel, L.L. (2000). Ensuring competency in end-of-life care. Communication and relational skills. *JAMA, 284,* 3051-3057.

Wilson, E. M., Gunasinghe, H.R., Coker, M.L., et al. (2002). Plasma matrix metalloproteinase and inhibitor profiles in patients with heart failure. *J Card Fail, 8,* 390-398.

Yamaoka-Tojo, M., Tojo, T., Inomata, T., et al. (2002). Circulating levels of interleukin 18 reflect etiologies of heart failure: Th1/Th2 cytokine imbalance exaggerates the pathophysiology of advanced heart failure. *J Card Fail, 8,* 21-27.

Yu, C.M., Chau, E., Sanderson, J.E., et al. (2002). Tissue Doppler echocardiographic evidence of reverse remodeling and improved synchrony by simultaneously delaying regional contraction after biventricular pacing therapy in heart failure. *Circulation, 105,* 438-445.

Zile, M. (2002). Structural components of cardiomyocyte remodeling: Summation. *J Card Fail,* S311-S313.

Zucker, I.H., & Pliquett, R.U. (2002). Novel mechanisms of sympatho-excitation in chronic heart failure. *Heart Fail Monit, 3,* 2-7.

CHAPTER 7

Pulmonary

James Varga
Joshua Cox

OBJECTIVES

After the completion of this chapter, the reader should be able to:

1. Recognize and understand the clinical features of COPD.
2. Understand how to diagnosis, assess, and monitor advanced pulmonary disease.
3. Recognize and understand the differential diagnosis between COPD and asthma.
4. Apply COPD management guidelines, pharmacologic treatment, and nonpharmacologic interventions.

INTRODUCTION

Chronic obstructive pulmonary disease (COPD) is currently the fourth leading cause of death in the United States and is the only disease among the top 10 whose incidence is increasing. By 2020, COPD is expected to be the third leading cause of death in the United States (Murray & Lopez, 1997). More striking is the fact that current estimates of prevalence are likely to be grossly underestimated since the insidious course of COPD goes undetected until it is moderately advanced and symptomatic. Traditionally, COPD has been thought of as a disease that affects men to a greater extent than women; however, in the year 2000, slightly more women than men died from COPD (59,936 vs. 59,118) (Mannino, Homa, Akinbami, et al., 2002). The economic and social burden of COPD is no less daunting than the prevalence. The National Heart, Lung, and Blood Institute (NHLBI) estimates that in 2001 the direct and indirect costs associated with COPD amounted to $34.4 billion (NHLBI,

2001). Economic and mortality data, however, do not reveal a complete picture of the burden of COPD on society. One way to quantify the relative social burden of disease is by using disability-adjusted life years (DALYs). DALYs is the sum of total years lost as a result of premature death and years lived with disability. In 1996, COPD was the seventh and eighth leading cause of DALYs among women and men, respectively, and is expected to be the fifth leading cause worldwide by 2020 (Lopez & Murray, 1998; Michaud, Murray, & Bloom, 2001).

Definitions

COPD has been recently defined as "...a disease state characterized by airflow limitation that is not fully reversible. The airflow limitation is usually both progressive and associated with an abnormal inflammatory response of the lungs to noxious particles or gases" (Pauwels, Buist, Calverly, et al., 2001, p. 1256). Other organizations, such as the American Thoracic Society, have defined COPD as "a disease state characterized by the presence of airflow limitation due to chronic bronchitis or emphysema; the airflow obstruction is generally progressive, may be accompanied by airway hyper-reactivity, and may be partially reversible" (American Thoracic Society, 1995, p. S78). These earlier definitions have focused largely on the terms *emphysema* and *chronic bronchitis*, whereas more recent definitions provided by the Global Initiative for Chronic Obstructive Lung Disease (GOLD), do not. These recent definitions agree that COPD is a progressive disease characterized by some degree of airflow limitation or obstruction, which is not fully reversible. In addition to airflow obstruction, patients with COPD commonly experience a complex of symptoms including chronic cough, exertional dyspnea, sputum production, and wheeze. Although some disagreement exists regarding the precise classification of patients with these symptoms, COPD typically refers to patients suffering from emphysema and chronic bronchitis, as well as a fraction of patients with concomitant asthma.

Pathogenesis

A variety of pathologic changes in the lung are believed to contribute to the eventual development of symptomatic COPD, including mucus hypersecretion, airway narrowing and remodeling, lung parenchyma destruction, and pulmonary vascular changes. These changes are a result of the inflammation, oxidative stress, proteolytic enzymes (elastases), and other processes typically initiated by the inhalation of noxious particles and gases (e.g., cigarette smoke). The following is an overview of these pathologic changes and the cells involved.

Inflammation. Inflammation has long been accepted to play a significant role in the development of airway pathology associated with COPD (Hunninghake & Crystal, 1983). However, because of differences in patient selection during clinical trials in methods used to assess inflammation, much debate still exists regarding which type of inflammatory cell plays the most important role in the damage of airways and lung parenchyma. In COPD, a majority of inflammation occurs in the peripheral airways and lung parenchyma. This inflammation, which leads to a higher concentration of macrophages, neutrophils, cytotoxic T cells, and inflammatory mediators, eventually results in the destruction of lung parenchyma.

Macrophages. Macrophages are responsible for the destruction of foreign material in the body. In the lungs, macrophages destroy and remove toxins and other matter by phagocytosis and transportation of phagocytized matter up the mucus "escalator" or through the lymphatic system before being eventually eliminated. However, bronchoalveolar lavage (BAL) findings from the lungs of smokers and patients with COPD suggest that the ability of macrophages to remove toxins is compromised when toxins increase dramatically (Tetley, 2002). Furthermore, it has been suggested that macrophages

are responsible, at least in part, for the proteinase/antiproteinase imbalance in COPD. This hypothesis is derived from the knowledge that macrophages are capable of directly releasing, or generating the release of, a variety of mediators (proteinases) such as matrix metalloproteinases (MMP). The generation of proteases in the lung leads to an imbalance such that antiproteases inadequately neutralize regional proteases, leading to the eventual destruction of collagen and elastin in lung parenchyma (Tetley, 2002). In addition to MMP, macrophages release neutrophil elastase (NE) in *in vitro* studies (Finlay, O'Driscoll, Russell, et al., 1997). Although macrophages do not synthesize NE, they are capable of internalizing the enzyme and subsequently releasing it during an inflammatory response.

However, the exact role and importance of macrophages in the development of COPD are unclear and continue to be debated. The relationship between detection in the lungs of patients with COPD and the knowledge that macrophages have the ability to destroy connective tissue together with the pathologic changes of COPD suggests that macrophages do play an important role in the pathology of COPD. Activation of macrophages may then lead to the generation of reactive oxygen species (nitric oxide) and acute inflammation (Cosio, Joaquim, & Cosio, 2002).

Neutrophils. The importance of neutrophils in the pathogenesis of COPD was first suggested in 1963 when it was observed that patients with early-onset emphysema were deficient in the serum antiproteinase, α_1-antitrypsin (α_1-AT) (Laurell & Eriksson, 1963), a protein that neutralizes neutrophil enzymes. α_1-AT protects the lungs from damage caused by neutrophil proteinases. When patients lack antiproteinase or when proteinase activity is greater than what can be neutralized by antiproteinases, the result is the destruction of lung tissue. Therefore neutrophils, recruited by macrophages (also cytokines), play a major role in proteinase/antiproteinase imbalance. Proteases released by neutrophils are capable of inducing pathologic changes consistent with emphysema (Snider, Stone, Lucey, et al., 1985; Stockley, 2002). Neutrophils, found in sputum at higher concentrations in patients with COPD than in normal individuals, directly correlates with severity of airflow obstruction (Confalonieri, Mainardi, Della, et al., 1998).

T Lymphocytes. Like the macrophage and neutrophil, the definitive role of T lymphocytes in the development of COPD has not been fully elucidated. However, bronchial biopsies demonstrate increased T lymphocytes in COPD, specifically CD8+ cells (Finkelstein, Fraser, Ghezzo, et al., 1995). T cells may contribute to lung damage by releasing cytokines, such as interleukins, which are capable of attracting and activating macrophages. T lymphocytes may cause epithelial cell apoptosis and destruction in the alveolar wall secondary to release of cytokines, such as TNF-α and perforin (Liu, Mohammed, Rice, et al., 1999).

Oxidative Stress. Oxidative stress may play a role in COPD (Repine, Bast, & Lankhorst, 1997). Markers of oxidative stress such as hydrogen peroxide, nitric oxide, and 8-isoprostane have been found in the breath, epithelial lining, and urine of patients with COPD (Dekhuijzen, Aben, Dekker, et al., 1996; Maziak, Loukides, Culpitt, et al., 1998;

Pratico, Basili, Vieri, et al., 1998). Increased concentrations of oxidants in the lungs lead to cell dysfunction by damaging a variety of cellular proteins and lipids. Oxidative stress further contributes to the destruction of tissue by contributing to the proteinase/antiproteinase imbalance through activation of MMP and inactivation of various antiproteinases and by stimulating increased production of proinflammatory cytokines such as interleukin-8 and TNF-α (Barnes & Karin, 1997). The cellular mechanism shown in Figure 7-1 has been proposed to contribute to the physiologic changes in COPD.

In addition to the aforementioned processes, a variety of other pathologic mechanisms contribute to the development of COPD or its progression. For example, the parasympathetic nervous system may play a significant role in bronchoconstriction. The vagal nerve is the major determinant of resting airway caliber, and increased vagal stimulation generates reactive airways in COPD, resulting in bronchoconstriction (Gross, 1988; Gross & Skorodin, 1984). Clearly, the pathogenesis of COPD is complex and cannot be explicitly attributed to

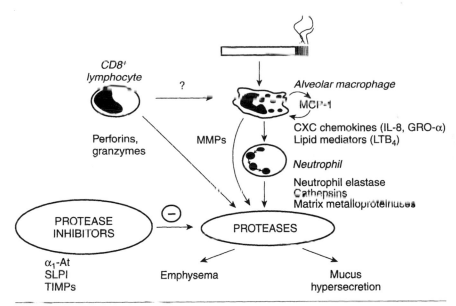

FIGURE 7-1 Mechanisms in COPD. *MCP-1,* Monocyte chemotactic protein-1; *IL-8,* interleukin-8; *MMPs,* matrix metalloproteinases; *LTB₄,* leukotriene B₄; α-*At,* α-antitrypsin; *SLPI,* secretory leukoprotease inhibitor; *TIMPs,* tissues inhibitor of metalloproteinase. (From Barnes, P.J. [2000]. Mechanisms in COPD. *Chest,* 117, 10S-14S.)

one pathologic process. It seems more likely that a variety of factors interacting over a long period brings about the symptoms and pathology of COPD.

Pathophysiology

The complex pathologic changes just described eventually result in clinically detectable physiologic abnormalities. These symptoms occur by the fifth decade of life on average. Dyspnea, initially with exertion and then eventually at rest, chronic cough, and sputum production are common complaints.

These symptoms are attributed largely to limited airflow and pulmonary hyperinflation, caused by smooth muscle hypertrophy, goblet cell hyperplasia with mucus hypersecretion, and destruction of lung parenchyma. See Figure 7-2.

Airflow Limitation and Pulmonary Hyperinflation. Expiratory airflow limitation is considered the hallmark of COPD. The airflow limitation of COPD is only partially reversible and progresses over time. The most important pathologic change responsible for airflow limitation is the narrowing and fibrosis of small airways producing

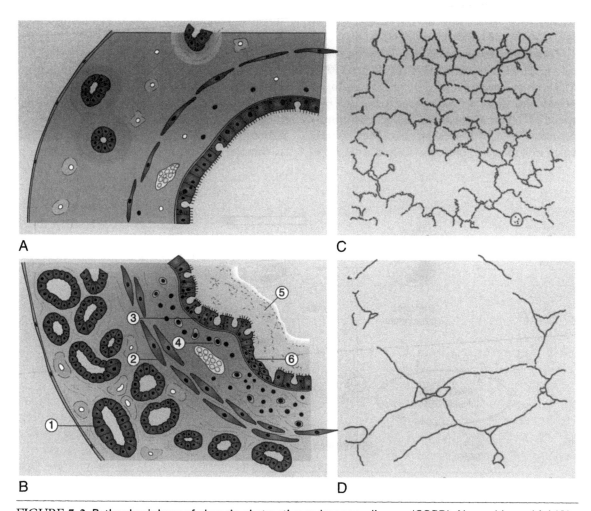

FIGURE 7-2 Pathophysiology of chronic obstructive pulmonary disease (COPD). Normal bronchial **(A)** and lung parenchyma **(C)** structures and changes seen in the airways **(B)**. **B**, *1*, Mucus gland hypertrophy; *2*, smooth muscle hypertrophy; *3*, goblet cell hyperplasia; *4*, inflammatory cell infiltrate; *5*, excessive mucus; *6*, squamous metaplasia. **D**, Parenchyma in COPD.

a fixed obstruction (Kuwano, Bosken, Pare, et al., 1993). Also contributing to increased airway resistance is the loss of the radial traction of airways, or elastic recoil, which is responsible for facilitating passive exhalation. As disease severity progresses and airflow limitation worsens, the ability to adequately exhale becomes limited during normal tidal breathing. The loss of parenchymal elastic recoil and increased airway collapsibility leads to increase residual volume and functional residual capacity (FRC) by spirometry. The expanded residual volume after "normal" expiration is known as *pulmonary hyperinflation*. As the rate and amount of lung emptying with expiration diminish, inspiration must be initiated prematurely at a higher lung volume as compensation, leading to a "dynamic" (rate-dependent) increase in FRC (dynamic hyperinflation). Dynamic hyperinflation eventually results in flattening of the diaphragm, as seen on chest radiograph. The diaphragm is forced to function on a less efficient portion of the muscle length-tension curve, resulting in an increased work of breathing and higher degree of dyspnea for level of activity and reduced maximum inspiratory pressures (Cox, Dickerson, & Petty, 2003; O'Donnell, 2000).

Impaired Gas Exchange. A ventilation-perfusion mismatch may be seen in patients with more advanced COPD. The changes in the small airways described previously result in a decrease in ventilation of distal alveoli, which are well perfused. When perfusion is maintained in the presence of regional alveolar hypoventilation, a ventilation-perfusion mismatch is established, causing hypoxemia initially and, in more advanced stages, hypercapnia. Clinically significant arterial blood gas abnormalities are rare if the forced expiratory volume is maintained above 1 liter (Lane, Howell, & Giblin, 1968). See Table 7-1.

PULMONARY FUNCTION TESTS

Pulmonary function testing (PFT) is of great importance to the diagnosis of COPD and is helpful in monitoring response to treatment and disease course. Because of the slow, insidious course of COPD and the large lung function reserve, clinical symptoms do not typically occur until the fifth or sixth decade of life, at which time a critical loss of function has occurred. Pulmonary function testing on patients with persistent or worsening dyspnea, chronic cough, chronic sputum production, or history of exposure to tobacco smoke is highly recommended for diagnosis. The measurement of lung function through the use of PFT should include a forced expiratory volume in 1 second (FEV_1), forced vital capacity (FVC), a post-bronchodilator spirometry FEV_1, diffusion capacity (DLCO), and lung volumes, as well as pulse oximetry (Evans & Scanlon, 2003). The consensus statement by the American College of Chest Physicians and the National Heart, Lung, and Blood Institute is that spirometry should be done on current smokers 45 years or older and any smoker with respiratory complaints (Evans & Scanlon, 2003).

Forced Expiratory Volume

Forced expiratory volume (FEV_1) is the volume of gas exhaled in 1 second by forced expiration from full inspiration and is the most reproducible and useful measurement in the diagnosis and follow-up in patients with obstructive lung disease. The FEV_1 is affected by changes in airway resistance caused by reversible bronchoconstriction (in asthma) or structural airway changes and lung parenchyma destruction with loss of elastic recoil in COPD. The FEV_1 can also be reduced in interstitial lung disease (Glady, Aaron, Lunau, et al., 2003).

Forced Vital Capacity

Forced vital capacity (FVC) is the volume of air that can be forcibly exhaled from the point of maximal inhalation and is not time-dependent. Diseases in which the FVC is decreased include those affecting the thoracic cage, such as ankylosing spondylitis; those affecting the respiratory muscles or respiratory muscle innervation, such as amyotrophic lateral sclerosis (ALS), muscular dystrophy, or myasthenia gravis; those affecting the pleural cavity, such as pneumothorax; and those affecting the lung itself, such as pulmonary fibrosis or diseases that cause premature closure of the airways during expiration, such as COPD (West, 1998). The ratio of FEV_1 over the FVC is a standard measure of obstruction. Airflow obstruction causes a disproportionate reduction in maximum airflow as measured by

Table 7-1 COPD Prognostic Table

Clinical Presentation	Diagnostic Evaluations	Pathophysiology
Worsening dyspnea, increased mucus secretion and cough. Repeated exacerbations and interference with quality of life. Abnormal patterns of breathing and fatigue of the respiratory muscles, cyanosis, pedal edema, increased jugular venous pressure.	Polycythemia in arterial hypoxemia—hematocrit >55%. FEV_1/FVC <70%, 30% ≤FEV_1 <50% predicted indicates severe COPD with or without chronic symptoms (cough, sputum production). Arterial blood gas tests should be performed in all patients with an FEV_1 <40% predicted. Respiratory failure or right heart failure is indicated by Pao_2 <8.0 kPa (60 mm Hg) with or without $Paco_2$ >6.7 kPa (50 mm Hg) in arterial. Very severe COPD FEV_1/FVC <70%.	Primary pathology in a severe exacerbation of COPD is a worsening of gas exchange that is produced primarily by an increased VA/Q mismatch. As the VA/Q relationship worsens in the face of an exacerbation, there is an increased work of the respiratory muscles that results in greater oxygen consumption, decreased mixed venous oxygen tension, and progressive amplication of gas exchange abnormalities. This can cause further deterioration in blood gases and contribute to respiratory acidosis. Alveolar hypoventilation contributes to hypoxemia, hypercapnia, and respiratory acidosis. Increased pulmonary artery pressures and increased volume on the right ventricle of the heart.

COPD, Chronic obstructive lung disease; FEV_1, forced expiratory volume in 1 second; *FVC,* forced vital capacity; *VA/Q*, ventilation-perfusion; Pao_2, partial pressure of oxygen in arterial blood; $Paco_2$, partial pressure of carbon dioxide in arterial blood.
Data from Global Initiative for Chronic Obstructive Lung Disease (GOLD) Guidelines. (2003).

FEV_1 relative to the volume of air the patient can eventually displace from the lungs (FVC). The ratio of FEV_1/FVC in obstructive lung disease is usually less than 70% (Evans & Scanlon, 2003).

Diffusion Capacity

Spirometry With Bronchodilators. The diffusion capacity (DLCO) is abnormal in pulmonary parenchymal disorders, pulmonary vascular abnormalities, and diseases that reduce effective alveolar ventilation as occurs in emphysema (Evans & Scanlon, 2003). The diffusion capacity of the lung will be reduced in severe COPD of the emphysematous type. This is not caused by loss of pulmonary vasculature but the ventilation in the non-perfused lung.

Patients may present late in life with asthma, which has overlapping symptoms with COPD. Performing spirometry before and after a bronchodilator will separate reversible from fixed airway obstruction. A significant bronchodilator response is considered an improvement in either FEV_1 or FVC of 0.2 liter over baseline (Evans & Scanlon, 2003).

Differential Diagnosis (Asthma vs. COPD)

As stated, COPD is a disease characterized by progressive airflow obstruction commonly associated with dyspnea, chronic cough, and a myriad of systemic manifestations including renal and hormonal dysfunction, cachexia, and peripheral muscle weakness. Only two interventions are currently recognized to decrease the rate of decline in lung function and cardiac complications—smoking cessation and long-term oxygen therapy. Therefore once a diagnosis of COPD is made, disease management is essentially palliative regardless of disease severity. It is exceedingly important for clinicians treating patients with respiratory disorders to have a thorough understanding of a differential diagnosis and disease management to optimize clinical outcomes and patients' health-related quality of life.

The diagnosis of COPD begins with the ability to recognize features that are suggestive of the disease as compared with features suggestive of asthma. Patients with COPD have a long smoking history and typically present with slowly progressive dyspnea on exertion by midlife. Asthma will start early in life although late onset is increasingly recognized. In addition, patients with COPD have largely irreversible airflow limitation as measured by spirometry before and after bronchodilation, unlike the largely reversible obstruction seen in asthma. Patients with asthma typically have a history of atopy and a positive family history. Once a patient is suspected of having COPD, the diagnosis is confirmed by measurement of airflow by spirometry. Spirometry is recommended for those individuals with risk factors for COPD, such as history of exposure to tobacco smoke or occupational dusts and chemicals.

The clinical presentation of asthma is similar to COPD, but the pathogenesis of COPD and the pathogenesis of asthma have important differences (cellular mechanisms, inflammatory mediators, inflammatory effects) and response to therapy is crucial. The appropriate assessment, management, and follow-up care for patients with either disease is different (Barnes, 2000).

Perhaps the most important dissimilarity between COPD and asthma is the type of inflammation. Although both diseases are characterized by persistent inflammation and airflow obstruction, the inflammation is mediated by different cells and mediators. The inflammation associated with asthma is mediated predominantly by eosinophils, whereas the neutrophil is the cell found in highest concentrations in the lungs of patients with COPD (Confalonieri et al., 1998). Also, bronchial biopsies in COPD demonstrate an increased concentration of mononuclear cells, especially CD8+ T lymphocytes cells, whereas CD4+ T lymphocytes are most prevalent in patients with asthma (Jeffrey, 1998). Other important differences include the location of airway damage and airway hyperresponsiveness. The inflammation associated with asthma affects all of the airways but spares lung parenchyma; in contrast, most of the airflow limitation associated with COPD is secondary to fibrosis and narrowing of the peripheral airways with permanent damage to the lung parenchyma. Patients with asthma have characteristic airway hyperresponsiveness related to eosinophilic infiltration; although patients with COPD may have some degree of hyperresponsiveness, it is certainly less significant and is believed to be caused by different mediators (Celli, 2000).

The inflammatory mediators present in the lungs of patients with COPD and asthma also are different. Cysteinyl leukotrienes are released from mast cells and eosinophils and cause bronchoconstriction in asthma; histamine, kinins, and prostaglandins are also believed to add to bronchoconstriction. In COPD, however, few of these mediators are present, which may explain the relative irreversible airflow obstruction seen with COPD compared with asthma. Moreover, increased cholinergic tone seems to be the only reversible component of COPD, which explains the observation that anticholinergic agents are more effective than β2 (beta$_2$ sympathomimetic) agonists in improving airflow obstruction in COPD, the reverse being true for asthma (Barnes, 2000). See Table 7-2.

STAGING

Current recommendations for the assessment and management of patients with COPD are based on severity of airflow obstruction. Therefore the importance of appropriate evaluation of patients with COPD cannot be overstated. A variety of staging systems exist, but the most recent guidelines published by the Global Initiative for Chronic Obstructive Lung Disease categorize patients into one of four stages of disease severity (Table 7-3).

Table 7-2 DIFFERENTIATING COPD FROM ASTHMA

Differential Diagnosis	COPD	Asthma
Age of onset	Usually >40 years	Any age
Smoking history	Yes	Minimal
Symptoms	Usually chronic, slowly progressive	Varies daily
Airway reversibility as measured by post-bronchodilator spirometry	Partially reversible	Largely reversible
Cells	Neutrophils, CD8+ lymphocytes, macrophages	Eosinophils, CD4+ lymphocytes, mast cells
Effects	Peripheral airways	All airways

Table 7-3 COPD STAGING

Stage	Description
Stage 0: At Risk	Chronic symptoms Exposure to risk factors Normal spirometry
Stage 1: Mild	FEV_1/FVC <70% FEV_1 ≥80% With or without symptoms
Stage 2: Moderate	FEV_1/FVC <70% 50% ≤FEV_1 <80% With or without symptoms
Stage 3: Severe	FEV_1/FVC <70% 30% ≤FEV_1 <50% With or without symptoms
Stage 4: Very Severe	FEV_1/FVC <70% FEV_1 <30% or presence of chronic respiratory failure or right heart failure

FEV_1, Forced expiratory volume in 1 second; FVC, forced vital capacity.

Modified from Global Initiative for Chronic Obstructive Lung Disease (GOLD) Guidelines. (2003).

Restrictive Versus Obstructive Lung Disease

Patients with restrictive lung disease present with cough, dyspnea with exertion, rest dyspnea, and tachypnea. Restrictive lung diseases include those that affect pulmonary parenchyma, cardiac disorders, pulmonary emboli, alveolar filling processes, pleural diseases, lung infections, and pulmonary granulomatous disease (Wagers, Bouder, Kaminsky, et al., 2000). Restrictive lung disease may also be associated with a reduced FEV_1 and FVC ratio; that is, the reduction of FEV_1 is the result of loss of lung volume and not airway obstruction (Balfe, Lewis, & Mohsenifar, 2002). Lung volumes will need to be measured (by helium or nitrogen washout or body plethysmography) if the FVC is less than 85% of predicted and the FEV_1/FVC ratio is more than 55% (Evans & Scanlon, 2003; Glady et al., 2003). For all values of FVC below 80% of predicted, the likelihood of a restrictive lung disease increases with the increase in FEV_1/FVC ratio (Aaron, Dales, & Cardinal, 1999).

COMMON AND FREQUENT SYMPTOMS
COPD

Among the three major airflow obstruction diseases (asthma, chronic bronchitis, emphysema), a significant overlap of signs and symptoms exists. This overlap is illustrated by the Venn diagram (Figure 7-3).

Nevertheless, the signs and symptoms of all three major diseases have been well characterized and can be identified through a thorough history and physical examination. Asthma, although acute, episodic, or even perennial, does not strictly fall under the category of COPD since its hallmark is reversible airflow obstruction. In contrast, COPD, comprising chronic bronchitis and emphysema, is not fully reversible. Despite its chronic and progressive nature, COPD may also be characterized by

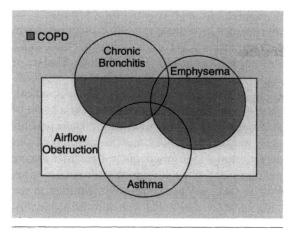

FIGURE 7-3 Venn diagram. *COPD,* Chronic obstructive pulmonary disease. (From Halpin, D.M.G. [2002]. *COPD.* Mosby International.)

exacerbations and remissions in airflow obstruction and symptoms. It is important to recognize that many of the signs and symptoms of COPD are nonspecific and can occur in other diseases such as congestive heart failure (National Lung Health Education Program [NLHEP] Executive Committee, 1998).

Restrictive Lung Disease

Patients with restrictive lung disease will present with cough, dyspnea with exertion, rest dyspnea, and tachypnea. Restrictive lung disease also can be associated with a reduced FEV_1 but without a reduction of the FEV_1/FVC ratio; that is, the reduction of FEV_1 is the result of loss of lung volume and not airway obstruction (Balfe et al., 2002). Lung volumes will need to be measured (by helium or nitrogen washout or body plethysmography) if the FVC is less than 85% of predicted. Usually the FEV_1/FVC ratio is more than 55% in restrictive lung diseases (Evans & Scanlon, 2003; Glady et al., 2003). For all values of FVC below 80% of predicted, the likelihood of a restrictive lung disease increases with the increase in FEV_1/FVC ratio (Aaron et al., 1999). The DLCO will be reduced in interstitial pulmonary diseases, which affect pulmonary parenchyma and vasculature, and usually not in asthma or chronic bronchitis (Evans & Scanlon, 2003).

Chronic Bronchitis

Chronic bronchitis is more prevalent than pure emphysema. The cardinal symptom of chronic bronchitis is a productive cough. The frequency of cough varies among individuals; some report cough only upon awakening or after smoking, whereas others cough continuously during the day and may be awakened at night by cough. The amount and type of sputum produced also vary, from small amounts of clear liquid to large volumes of thick, purulent sputum. Early in the disease, the patient may complain of a "smoker's cough," which is more prevalent in winter. The patient might also complain of frequent colds or respiratory infections. It is at this stage that patients are misdiagnosed and are frequently treated as if they were asthmatic.

The diagnosis of chronic bronchitis is based on symptoms that occur for a specified period of time and is defined as excessive sputum production with progressive cough for at least 3 months of each year for 2 consecutive years. There is technically no such thing as "asymptomatic" chronic bronchitis. However, incipient disease can be detected through spirometry before overt symptoms (Evans & Scanlon, 2003). When symptoms do occur, they correlate directly with the degree of large airway inflammation and inversely with FEV_1. In drug steady state, patients with chronic bronchitis usually have some degree of exercise limitation and dyspnea because of dynamic hyperinflation and air trapping with increased respiratory rate (O'Donnell, 2000). Over time, progression caused by changes in lung tissue interferes with gas exchange at rest. Patients with advanced chronic bronchitis will have low arterial oxygen and elevated carbon dioxide. The poor arterial oxygenation leads to tissue hypoxia and a "blue" appearance. Physicians often refer to patients with advanced chronic bronchitis as "blue bloaters" (Heath, 1993). Oxygen desaturation gives tissues a bluish tone. Chronic edema occurs from right heart failure. The normal blood flow from the heart is impeded by pulmonary hypertension. As pressure in the lung artery increases, strain occurs on the right ventricle resulting in cor pulmonale. As the right ventricle dilates, liver congestion, fluid retention, and peripheral edema follow. Fluid retention is the result of both increased intravascular pressures and reduced renal blood flow. Oxygen reduces pulmonary artery constriction and reduces right heart strain.

The signs of pulmonary hypertension are lower extremity edema, neck vein distention, hepatojugular reflux, and a loud pulmonic component of the second heart sound. Tricuspid regurgitant may also be present.

Emphysema

Chronic bronchitis is recognized based on signs and symptoms. In contrast, emphysema is defined on the basis of pathologic changes in lung tissue. Emphysema is characterized by enlarging air spaces and disappearing alveoli distal to the terminal bronchiole. The terminal bronchiole structure is destroyed. See Figure 7-4.

The diagnosis is presumptive during life and is substantiated at autopsy. The particular "symptoms of emphysema" are difficult because symptoms are not part of the definition of emphysema. However, individuals who are found to have significant emphysema can experience extreme disability. Dyspnea occurs with exertion or at rest and is gradual at onset. Emphysema is associated with cough, but this symptom usually follows the onset of dyspnea, in contrast to chronic bronchitis, in which cough is the first symptom. Cough associated with emphysema is usually nonproductive, unlike with chronic bronchitis. The pathologic changes of emphysema impair ventilation, and the normally automatic process of breathing becomes an effort. Patients lose weight and become thin as a result of the strenuous effort with each breath. These patients must use their accessory muscles to force air out of their lungs and often purse their lips during prolonged and difficult expiration. Physicians often refer to them as "pink puffers," in contrast to the "blue bloaters" associated with chronic bronchitis. In advanced disease, the patient usually has a hyperresonant chest to percussion and has limited diaphragmatic excursions. Cyanosis is not common, unlike with chronic bronchitis. The patient's respiratory rate is often rapid. During exacerbations of the disease process, tachypnea and tachycardia will be common. Patients often will position themselves upright and lean forward to catch their breath. Pursed-lip breathing causes a fall in respiratory rate and increases tidal volume, leading to a reduction in total minute ventilation, a fall in partial pressure of carbon dioxide in arterial blood ($PaCO_2$), and a rise in partial pressure of

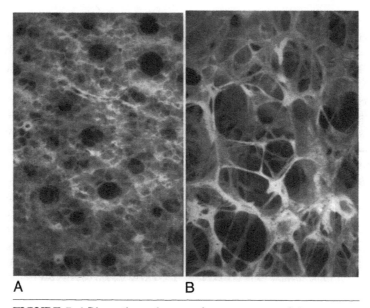

FIGURE **7-4** Dissecting microscopic appearance of the cut surface of a normal **(A)** and emphysematous **(B)** lung. (From Halpin, D.M.G. [2002]. COPD [Fig. 14, p. 25]. Mosby International.)

Table **7-4** EMPHYSEMA VERSUS COPD

Feature and Indicators of Disease	Predominantly Emphysema	Predominantly Chronic Bronchitis
Age at diagnosis	60+ years	50+ years
Dyspnea	Severe	Mild
Cough	After dyspnea appears	Before dyspnea appears
Sputum	Scanty, mucoid	Copious, purulent
Bronchial infections	Less frequent	More frequent
Episodes of respiratory insufficiency	Often terminal	Repeated
Pulmonary hypertension		
At rest	None to mild	Moderate to severe
With exercise	Moderate	Worsens
Cor pulmonale	Rare, except terminally	Common

From Braunwald, E. (Ed.). (2001). *Harrison's principles of internal medicine* (14th ed.). New York: McGraw-Hill.

oxygen in arterial blood (PaO_2). This is caused by increased airway pressures ("auto peep"), which prevent premature airway collapse. Paradoxical motion of the abdomen is frequent with advanced disease. Right ventricular failure is unusual in the emphysematous disease states until very late (NLHEP Executive Committee, 1998). Although chronic bronchitis and emphysema are distinct clinical entities, they often occur as a combined entity in the same patient. See Table 7-4.

DYSPNEA

Dyspnea is the awareness of breathlessness or shortness of breath and is among the most common symptoms associated with airflow obstruction. A variety of sensations may be experienced when breathing feels difficult. Frequently, dyspnea is experienced as "tightness" in the chest or "not able to get enough air." Patients describe the need to "really work" in order to breathe. Some patients may experience respiratory panic attacks. The subjective experience of breathing discomfort that varies in intensity is referred to as *dyspnea* (American Thoracic Society, 1995). The experience is multifactorial and encompasses physiologic, psychologic, social, and environmental factors, which may induce secondary physiologic and behavioral responses as well (American Thoracic Society, 1995).

Chronic progressive dyspnea is a hallmark of patients with COPD, whereas episodic dyspnea is more common in asthmatics. Dyspnea may also be

BOX **7-1** NON-DRUG MEASURES FOR THE TREATMENT OF DYSPNEA

- A calming presence
- Sight of other people
- Cool draught (open window, fan)
- Breathing exercises
- Relaxation therapy
- Complementary therapies (massage, visualization, acupuncture, hypnosis)

From Twycross, R. (1997). *Symptom management in advanced cancer* (2nd ed.). Oxon, U.K.: Radcliffe Medical Press.

caused by cancer, cachexia, the chemotherapy used to treat cancer, pulmonary emboli, pleural disease, or heart failure. Bronchodilators are considered to be the drug treatment of choice, although non-drug measures may be of benefit (Twycross, 1997). See Box 7-1.

EXACERBATIONS

The progressive course of COPD is complicated by acute exacerbations of increasing frequency. Exacerbations are important clinical events in COPD and are associated with mortality, frequent hospitalizations, and significant health care utilization. Exacerbations generally have three clinical manifestations: worsening dyspnea, increase in sputum purulence, and increase in sputum volume. Acute exacerbations, often called "asthmatic bronchitis," can be triggered by tracheobronchial infections or environmental exposures, although in many cases the exact cause of a severe exacerbation cannot be identified. Patients often have other co-morbid conditions, such as heart failure, extrapulmonary infections, and pulmonary embolism.

There is currently no widely accepted definition of what constitutes worsening COPD. The following working definition of COPD has been proposed (American Thoracic Society, 1995):

a sustained worsening of the patient's condition distinct from the stable state and beyond normal day-to-day variations that is acute in onset and necessitates a change in medication for relief of symptoms associated with COPD.

In severe disease, patients may not experience dyspnea because of a reduced ventilatory drive but may have symptoms related to CO_2 retention (drowsiness) and right ventricular failure (edema) and/or headache, daytime somnolence, and sleep apnea. After an episode, most patients have a decrease in quality of life, which may be transitory or permanent, and nearly half of patients discharged are readmitted to the hospital in the following 6 months. One of the main treatment goals for COPD is to reduce the number and severity of exacerbations (Rodriguez-Roisin, 2000; Snow, Lascher, Mottur-Pilson, et al., 2001).

The following have been shown to be risk factors for acute exacerbations: previous COPD hospitalization, defined as three or more COPD admissions in the previous year; underprescribing of long-term oxygen therapy; low FEV_1; and a current smoker (Garcia-Aymerich, Monso, Marrades, et al., 2001).

MONITORING

A diagnosis of COPD should be considered in any patient who has cough, sputum production, or dyspnea and/or a history of risk factors. Physical signs of airflow limitation are usually not present until significant lung impairment has occurred. Detection by physical examination has a relatively low sensitivity and specificity. Diagnosis is confirmed by spirometry. The presence of a post-bronchodilator FEV_1 less than 80% in combination with an FEV_1/FVC less than 70% confirms the presence of airflow limitation and air trapping.

In April 2001, a consensus workshop report, the Global Strategy for the Diagnosis, Management, and Prevention of COPD, was published (GOLD). The GOLD Guidelines are a collaborative effort of the National Heart, Lung, and Blood Institute and the World Health Organization (Global Initiatives for Chronic Obstructive Lung Disease [GOLD], 2003). The following components are addressed in the GOLD Guidelines published in the fall of 2003. See Box 7-2. (The 2004 Guidelines should be available at the time of this publication.)

Monitoring Disease Progression and Complications

COPD treatment goals are best ensured by ongoing monitoring and assessment of patients. The best way to detect changes in symptoms and overall health status of patients is to ask questions. The same questions should be asked of each patient, at each visit, and should cover the monitoring and assessment particulars just mentioned. See Box 7-3.

Monitoring Exposure to Risk Factors

Identification, reduction, and control of risk factors are an important step toward prevention and treatment. In the case of COPD, these factors include ongoing tobacco use, occupational exposures, and indoor and outdoor air pollution and irritants. Because cigarette smoking is the major risk factor for COPD, smoking prevention programs should be implemented and smoking cessation programs encouraged for all individuals who do smoke. See Box 7-4.

Box 7-2   COMPONENTS IN THE ASSESSMENT AND MONITORING OF COPD

- Disease progression and development of complications
- Exposure to risk factors
- Pharmacotherapy and other medical treatment
- Exacerbation history
- Co-morbidities

Data from Global Strategy for Diagnosis, Management and Prevention of COPD: GOLD Workshop Report Updated 2003. Available from www.goldcopd.org.

Box 7-3 SUGGESTED QUESTIONS TO MONITOR DISEASE PROGRESSION AND DEVELOPMENT OF COMPLICATIONS

- How much can you do before you get short of breath? (use an everyday example)
- Has your dyspnea worsened, improved, or stayed the same since our last visit?
- Have you had to reduce your activities because of dyspnea or other symptoms?
- Have any of your symptoms worsened since our last visit?
- Have you experienced any new symptoms since our last visit?
- Has your sleep been disrupted because of dyspnea or other symptoms?
- Since our last visit, have you missed any work because of your symptoms?

From Global Strategy for Diagnosis, Management and Prevention of COPD: GOLD Workshop Report Updated 2003. Available from www.goldcopd.org.

Box 7-4 SUGGESTED QUESTIONS TO MONITOR EXPOSURE TO RISK FACTORS

- Have you continued to stay off cigarettes?
- If not, how many cigarettes per day are you smoking?
- Would you like to quit smoking?
- Has there been any change in your working environment?

From Global Strategy for Diagnosis, Management and Prevention of COPD: GOLD Workshop Report Updated 2003. Available from www.goldcopd.org.

Monitoring Pharmacotherapy and Other Medical Treatment

To adjust therapy appropriately as the disease progresses, each follow-up visit should include a discussion of the current drug regimen. Dosages of various medications, compliance, inhaler technique, effectiveness of the current regimen, and side effects to treatment should be reviewed. See Box 7-5.

Box 7-5 SUGGESTED QUESTIONS TO MONITOR PHARMACOTHERAPY AND OTHER MEDICAL TREATMENTS

- What medications are you currently taking?
- How often do you take each medication?
- How much do you take each time?
- Have you missed or stopped taking any regular doses of your medications for any reason?
- Have you had trouble filling your prescriptions?
- Please show me how you use your inhaler.
- Have you tried any other medications or remedies?
- Has your medication been effective in controlling your symptoms?
- Has your medication caused you any problems?

From Global Strategy for Diagnosis, Management and Prevention of COPD: GOLD Workshop Report Updated 2003. Available from www.goldcopd.org.

Monitoring Exacerbation History

Physicians and nurses should query the patient about worsening COPD, self-medication, and/or treatment by other health care providers. Frequency, severity, and likely causes for exacerbations should be evaluated. Increased sputum volume, purulent sputum, and worsening dyspnea should be noted. Specific inquiry into unscheduled office visits, telephone calls, and the use of urgent or emergency care facilities should be included in the history. Severity of the COPD relapse can be estimated by the increased need for bronchodilators or the use of glucocorticoids and the need for antibiotics. Hospitalizations should be documented, including the facility, duration of stay, and any critical care transfers or the requirement for intubation. The clinician should request summaries of all care received to facilitate continuity of care (GOLD Guidelines, 2003). See Box 7-6. Patients are encouraged to report worsening symptoms early. Failure to report exacerbations is associated with an increased risk for hospitalization, longer recovery time, and diminished quality of life (Wilkinson, Donaldson, & Hurst, 2004).

Monitoring Co-morbidities

It is important to consider the presence of concomitant conditions such as hypertension, ischemic heart disease, congestive heart failure, lung carcinoma, tuberculosis, and sleep apnea.

Box 7-6   SUGGESTED QUESTIONS TO MONITOR EXACERBATION HISTORY

- Since our last visit, have you had any episodes/times when your symptoms were a lot worse than usual?
- If so, how long did the episode(s) last? What do you think caused the symptoms to get worse? What did you do to control the symptoms?

From Global Strategy for Diagnosis, Management and Prevention of COPD: GOLD Workshop Report Updated 2003. Available from www.goldcopd.org.

PHARMACOLOGIC TREATMENT

Therapy involves prevention and control of symptoms to reduce frequency and severity of exacerbations, improve health status, and improve exercise tolerance. It is important to realize that none of the existing pharmacotherapies have been shown to modify the long-term decline in lung function that is the hallmark of this disease. Therefore medications are used to palliate symptoms and reduce complications. The overall approach to managing stable COPD should be characterized by a stepwise increase in treatment, guided by the severity of disease. However, each treatment regimen needs to be individualized in relationship to the severity of symptoms and the air flow limitation and is influenced by other factors, such as the frequency and severity of exacerbations, the presence of complications, the presence of respiratory failure, co-morbidities, and general health status (GOLD Guidelines, 2003; Pauwels et al., 2001). The following is a step-wise approach to care. See Figure 7-5.

The following medications are listed in the order in which they would normally be introduced, based on the level of disease severity.

Old	0: At risk	I: Mild	II: Moderate		III: Severe
New	0: At risk	I: Mild	II: Moderate	III: Severe	IV: Very severe
Characteristics	• Chronic symptoms • Exposure to risk factors	• FEV_1/FVC <70 • FEV_1 ≥80% • With or without symptoms	• FEV_1/FVC <70% • 50% ≤FEV_1 <80% • With or without symptoms	• FEV_1/FVC <70% • 30% <FEV_1 <85% • With or without symptoms	• FEV_1/FVC <70% • FEV_1 <30% or presence of chronic respiratory failure or right heart failure
	Avoidance of risk factor(s); influenza vaccination				
		Add short-acting bronchodilator when needed			
			Add regular treatment with one or more long-acting bronchodilators *Add* rehabilitation		
				Add inhaled glucocorticosteroids if repeated exacerbations	
					Add long-term oxygen if chronic respiratory failure *Consider* surgical treatments

FIGURE 7-5 Therapy at each stage of COPD. *FEV₁*, Forced expiratory volume in 1 second; *FVC,* forced vital capacity. (From *Global Strategy for Diagnosis, Management and Prevention of COPD: GOLD Workshop Report Updated 2003.* Available from www.goldcopd.org.)

Bronchodilators

Bronchodilator medications are key to the symptomatic management of COPD. They may be given on an "as needed" or on a regular basis to prevent or reduce symptoms depending upon disease severity. The principal bronchodilators are anticholinergics and beta agonists. These agents reduce airway smooth muscle tone, decreasing airway resistance, which in turn decreases the work of breathing and dyspnea. Antimuscarinics may reduce mucus production, and long-acting beta-2 agonists may facilitate mucociliary transport (Tashkin & Cooper, 2004). Secondarily, theophylline, another bronchodilator, has an antiinflammatory and immunomodulatory effect at low doses (Hansel, Tennant, Tan, et al., 2004.) The outcomes of therapy should be evaluated by spirometry testing (Briggs, Kuritzky, Boland, et al., 2000).

Anticholinergics

Anticholinergic bronchodilators are considered first-line therapy for patients with COPD. Elevated cholinergic tone is responsible for bronchoconstriction and is the only reversible component of airway obstruction (Gross & Skorodin, 1984). Anticholinergic drugs work by binding to and blocking muscarinic receptors that directly cause bronchoconstriction (Littner, Ilowite, Tashkin, et al., 2000). Tiotropium, a once-daily long-acting bronchodilator, is the agent of choice for maintenance therapy. Anticholinergic bronchodilators are poorly absorbed systemically and do not cross the blood-brain barrier. Therefore side effects are minimal. The most commonly reported adverse event associated with tiotropium and ipratropium, a short-acting anticholinergic, is dry mouth. Tiotropium is a 24-hour sustained release anticholinergic inhaled once daily. Short-acting ipratropium can be used in those patients with mild to moderate COPD who require bronchodilation only as needed. The ipratropium dosing requires inhalation 4 times daily.

Beta Agonists

If response to inhaled anticholinergic therapy is not optimal, an inhaled beta agonist should be added. Short-acting and long-acting beta agonists are available. Beta agonists work by binding to beta adrenoceptors, causing increased adrenergic tone and bronchodilation. Inhaled beta agonists are readily absorbed systemically and can lead to numerous systemic side effects, including tachycardia, tremor, and dysrhythmia in susceptible patients (GOLD Guidelines, 2003; NLHEP Executive Committee, 1998). Of all currently available short-acting beta agonists, albuterol is considered the drug of choice. Albuterol has a rapid onset of action and is useful as rescue medication during acute exacerbation in patients with severe disease. In these situations, albuterol is dosed at 2 puffs every 6 hours as needed. Albuterol can also be recommended for patients with mild to moderate disease who require bronchodilation only as needed. For maintenance therapy, currently two long-acting beta agonists are available, formoterol and salmeterol (Tashkin & Cooper, 2004). Both drugs are administered by inhalation every 12 hours. Long-acting beta agonists are more effective and convenient for patients than short-acting albuterol. The choice between formoterol and salmeterol may be determined by individual patient response in terms of symptom relief and side effects. Tachyphylaxis to bronchodilator efficacy has been variably reported for long-acting beta agonists (Tashkin & Cooper, 2004).

Combination Therapy

Because of differing mechanisms of action, combination anticholinergic and beta agonist bronchodilator therapy has improved efficacy and decreased side effects compared with maximum doses of either agent alone (American Thoracic Society, 1995; Briggs, Kuritzky, Boland, et al., 2000; GOLD Guidelines, 2003; NLHEP Executive Committee, 1998). Combination therapy with or without inhaled or systemic steroids is particularly recommended for Gold levels II through IV exacerbations (Tashkin & Cooper, 2004).

Theophylline

Debate continues about the value of theophylline. Nevertheless, theophylline has been shown to benefit some COPD patients (Hansel, et al., 2004). Evening dosing of long-acting theophylline preparations has been shown to reduce overnight reductions in FEV_1 and to improve morning respiratory symptoms in patients using inhaled bronchodilators. Theophylline has also been suggested to have various other benefits, including reduced gas trapping (dynamic hyperinflation), improved respiratory muscle function, gas exchange, and enhanced mucociliary clearance, which will not be measured by FEV_1 as an outcome measure (O'Donnell, 2000). In addition, theophylline has been shown to improve the central drive to breathe. Theophylline dilates pulmonary arteries and reduces right ventricular afterload and improves exercise performance. It is important to be aware of toxicity with theophylline therapy and the various co-morbidities that may alter theophylline clearance, such as hepatic dysfunction and drug interactions. If warranted, theophylline should be given at doses that achieve serum levels in the lower therapeutic range (8 to 12 mcg/ml). Rarely, higher doses in the range of 16 mcg/ml may beneficial, although close monitoring for side effects and drug toxicity is required (NLHEP Executive Committee, 1998).

Corticosteroids

The effects of both oral and inhaled corticosteroids are much less dramatic for COPD than for asthma, and their role in the management of COPD is limited to very specific indications. Current guidelines address the use of both oral and inhaled corticosteroid therapy in the management of stable COPD, as well as in patients experiencing an acute exacerbation.

Oral Corticosteroid Therapy in Stable COPD. Little evidence supports the benefit of long-term use of oral corticosteroid therapy in stable COPD, and much evidence opposes it (Wood-Baker, 2003). Side effects of chronic oral corticosteroids are considerable and include adrenal insufficiency, cutaneous thinning, osteoporosis, peptic ulcer disease, cataracts, diabetes mellitus, hypertension, and proximal myopathy. Therefore the long-term use of oral corticosteroids therapy in the management of stable COPD cannot be recommended (Wood-Baker, 2003). Also, mounting evidence suggests that short-term oral corticosteroid therapy, as a means to identify patients who might benefit from long-term inhaled corticosteroid treatment,

should also be avoided. This recommendation is based on evidence that a short (2-week) course of oral therapy is a poor predictor of the long-term response to inhaled corticosteroid therapy (GOLD Guidelines, 2003; Lyseng-Williamson & Keating, 2002; Niewoehner, 2002; Sin, Golmohammadi, & Jacobs, 2004; Soriano, Kiri, Pride, et al., 2003).

Oral Corticosteroid Therapy in Acute Exacerbations. The use of a systemic, preferably oral, short-term corticosteroid use is recommended as a cost-effective treatment for patients experiencing an acute COPD exacerbation (Niewoehner, 2002). Treatment should not extend more than 2 weeks. The optimal dose of corticosteroids is not known (Niewoehner, 2002). Prednisone is generally considered the oral drug of choice.

Inhaled Corticosteroid Therapy in COPD. Inhaled corticosteroids have had a proven benefit in the management of asthma, but until recently, their efficacy in COPD was not evidence based (Bonay, Bancal, & Crestani, 2002). The use of inhaled corticosteroids as regular treatment is now recommended for certain patients. However, early use of an inhaled corticosteroid does not influence the course of COPD (Van Grunsven, Schermer, Akkermans, et al., 2003). The support for the use of inhaled corticosteroids is as an adjunct to bronchodilator therapy, not as a replacement (Box 7-7) (Calverley, Boonsawat, Cseke, et al., 2003; Lyseng-Williamson & Keating, 2002; Soriano, et al., 2003).

Inhaled corticosteroids do not modify the disease process with COPD but have been shown to reduce the frequency of exacerbations and

---

BOX 7-7   INDICATIONS FOR THE REGULAR USE OF INHALED CORTICOSTEROIDS IN COPD

Patients with advanced disease and repeated exacerbations
- Stage III and Stage IV severity, per GOLD guidelines
- Symptomatic patients with $FEV_1 \leq 50\%$ predicted

Data from Global Initiative for Chronic Obstructive Lung Disease (GOLD) Guidelines. (2003). www.goldcopd.org.

improve health status. Commonly prescribed inhaled corticosteroids include beclomethasone, budesonide, flunisolide, fluticasone, and triamcinolone. The pharmacology and subsequent dosing of these drugs is uniquely individual. Recent studies have focused primarily on two corticosteroids in particular—budesonide and fluticasone. Both have glucocorticoid receptor affinities that are greater than other corticosteroids. This greater affinity may lend itself to lessened systemic absorption and consequently adverse effects over time. Long-term studies to evaluate efficacy and safety of inhaled corticosteroids for advanced COPD are currently underway. The decision to use an inhaled corticosteroid long term must always be evaluated against the real risk of systemic side effects. The risk of an adverse corticosteroid event can be assumed to be greater in the COPD population (Bonay et al., 2002). See Box 7-8.

Antibiotic Therapy

In several large-scale controlled studies, prophylactic continuous antibiotics were shown to have no effect on the frequency of exacerbations in COPD. Therefore, based on present evidence, the use of antibiotics is not recommended other than for treating infections associated with exacerbations of COPD (GOLD Guidelines, 2003). In most situations, broad-spectrum antibiotics capable of

Box 7-8 PREDISPOSING RISK CHARACTERISTICS OF COPD PATIENTS

- Patients tend to be elderly.
- Patients tend to have a significant smoking history and may be currently smoking.
- Patients are relatively inactive because of dyspnea and co-morbidities.
- Patients with severe COPD have a limited life expectancy.
- Co-existing disease due to age and tobacco use as a common risk factor.

From Bonay, M., Bancal, C., & Crestani, B. (2002). Benefits and risk of inhaled corticosteroids in chronic obstructive pulmonary disease. *Drug Saf, 25*(1), 57-71.

treating *Streptococcus pneumoniae, Haemophilus influenzae,* and *Moraxella catarrhalis* are preferred (Briggs, Kuritzky, Boland, et al., 2000).

Vaccines

Patients with COPD are at risk for increased morbidity and mortality from respiratory tract infections. Influenza vaccines reduce serious illness and death by about 50%. Vaccines containing killed or live, inactivated viruses are recommended because they are more effective in elderly patients with COPD (Briggs, et al., 2000; GOLD Guidelines, 2003).

Strategic Drugs

Mucolytics. Clearance of thick, tenacious secretions can be a major problem in COPD patients. Thinning of secretions and improved sputum clearance can relieve symptoms for some COPD patients. A Cochrane systematic review that included 23 studies found that mucolytic treatment for patients with chronic bronchitis or COPD decreased yearly exacerbations by 29% (Poole & Black, 2003). In addition, patients who received mucolytics were twice as likely to remain exacerbation free.

Antitussives. Cough suppressants should be avoided or prescribed cautiously, since they may impair the clearance of secretions and could theoretically increase mucus plugging (NLHEP Executive Committee, 1998).

Antioxidant Agents. Antioxidants, in particular *N*-acetylcysteine, have been shown to reduce the frequency of exacerbations and could have a role in the treatment of patients with recurrent exacerbations. However, before their routine use can be recommended, the results of ongoing trials will have to be mature (GOLD Guidelines, 2003).

Respiratory Stimulants. Various respiratory stimulants, including medroxyprogesterone, acetazolamide, and doxapram, have been suggested as a means of improving ventilation, hypercapnia, and oxygenation in COPD patients. Unfortunately, the stimulating effects of these agents are frequently short lived. These medications can have significant side effects, and stimulation of overworked respiratory muscles leads to respiratory muscle fatigue and worsening respiratory failure (NLHEP Executive Committee, 1998).

Opioids. Opioids are beneficial in relieving dyspnea. Low doses of morphine increase exercise tolerance and reduce dyspnea in selected patients. A systematic review found a statistically positive effect of opioids on breathlessness (Jennings, Davies, Higgins, et al., 2002). A randomized double-blind placebo-controlled trial found that sustained-release morphine 20 mg twice daily provided significant improvement in dyspnea compared with placebo (Abernethy, Currow, Frith, et al., 2003). No evidence supports the use of nebulized opioids for the relief of dyspnea in COPD (Foral, Malesker, Huerta, et al., 2004).

Emerging Drug Therapy

There is an urgent need to develop new and effective treatments for COPD. As mentioned, aside from smoking cessation, existing medications do not alter the long-term outlook of COPD nor delay loss of lung function. Research is now focused on the pathologic changes and the cellular mechanisms, which are critical to disease evolution. The search for disease-modifying therapy will involve novel drug therapy. Until that time, bronchodilators are the mainstay of therapy. The following drugs are anticipated to be available in the near future.

Phosphodiesterase Inhibitors. Phosphodiesterases (PDEs) play a critical role in the regulation of cellular activity. Researchers have identified 12 distinct PDE families. The PDE 4 family is responsible for the regulation of cell types involved in pulmonary inflammation. Therefore PDE 4 inhibitors have an antiinflammatory effect in pulmonary tissue. PDE inhibitors increase intracellular cyclic adenosine monophosphate (AMP) and guanosine monophosphate (GMP), which produces bronchodilation (Vianna & Martin, 1998). The major limitation to PDE 4 inhibitors has been side effects, especially nausea and vomiting. Of all the PDE 4's currently being developed, cilomilast appears closest to FDA approval.

Montelukast. Inhibitors to leukotriene synthesis or receptor inhibitors reduce inflammation. Montelukast significantly reduces dyspnea, sputum production, wheezing, and nocturnal symptoms in patients with COPD (Rubinstein, Kumar, & Schriever, 2004).

Ciclesonide. Ciclesonide is a uniquely designed inhaled corticosteroid that has lower systemic side effects than currently available inhaled corticosteroids. Ciclesonide is a prodrug with little activity until it is enzymatically altered in the lungs to become active. Ciclesonide may prove to be a valuable treatment in those patients with severe to very severe disease that requires an inhaled corticosteroid.

NONPHARMACOLOGIC TREATMENT

Oxygen

The long-term administration of oxygen, more than 15 hours per day, has been shown to increase survival. Oxygen therapy can also have a benefit on hemodynamics, hematologic characteristics (polycythemia), exercise capacity, lung mechanics, and mental state. Long-term oxygen therapy is generally introduced in stage IV (GOLD Guidelines, 2003). See Box 7-9. Blood gases should be obtained while the patient receives oxygen to be sure that saturation is greater than 88% without an overt rise in $PaCO_2$ (Booth, Anderson, Swannick, et al., 2004).

Box 7-9   INDICATION FOR LONG-TERM OXYGEN THERAPY

Generally, introduced for patients who are in stage IV (very severe) COPD who have:
- PaO_2 at or below 7.3 kPa (55 mm Hg) or SaO_2 at or below 88%, with or without hypercapnia
- PaO_2 between 7.3 kPa (55 mm Hg) and 8.0 kPa (60 mm Hg), or SaO_2 of 89% if there is evidence of pulmonary hypertension, peripheral edema suggesting congestive cardiac failure, or polycythemia (hematocrit >55%)

Modified from Global Initiative for Chronic Obstructive Lung Disease (GOLD) Guidelines. (2003). www.goldcopd.org.

Noninvasive Positive-Pressure Ventilation (NIV)

Noninvasive ventilation (NIV) is being used in the hospital management of acute exacerbations. In a Cochrane systematic review, NIV resulted in decreased mortality, decreased need for intubation, reduced treatment failure, rapid improvement in blood gases and pH within the first hour of therapy, and improved respiratory rate (Ram, Picot, Lightower, et al., 2004). NIV is considered a first-line adjuvant therapy to standard medical management. NIV reduces breathlessness in terminally ill patients and may "buy time" while other therapies are initiated (Shee & Green, 2003).

Lung Volume Reduction Surgery

Lung volume reduction surgery (LVRS) improves respiratory mechanics of patients suffering from bullous emphysema. Algorithm for patient selection and cost efficacy have been validated in selected patients (Martinez, Flaherty, & Iannettoni, 2003). See Box 7-9.

Nutrition

Weight loss is a characteristic of advanced COPD and is associated with greater respiratory symptoms because of sarcopenia and muscle weakness. It is widely accepted that weight loss is a consequence of decreased food intake caused by breathlessness, at a time when resting energy expenditures are rising as a result of the increased work of breathing. Weight loss may also be caused by proinflammatory cytokines, which will not be reversed by nutrition (pulmonary cachexia). All tissue compartments may be affected, although loss of skeletal muscle may be particularly affected because of the wasting of respiratory muscles. COPD patients who are underweight have an increased risk of mortality, which may be reduced by appropriate nutritional support (Halpin, 2002; Eid, Ionescu, Nixon, et al., 2001).

PULMONARY REHABILITATION

All COPD patients benefit from exercise training programs. Pulmonary rehabilitation programs are designed to improve general muscle tone and respiratory efficiency in COPD patients whose exercise tolerance is poor or whose activities of daily living are hampered. The benefits derived from pulmonary rehabilitation may be both psychologic and physiologic, to increase the patient's sense of well-being. Such programs have been shown to reduce office visits, decrease telephone calls, increase exercise tolerance, increase vocational potential, and improve overall quality of life (Alberts & Rolfe, 1994). See Box 7-10.

It is important to note that, in severe disease, effective management may also include the integration of different disciplines and treatment approaches that exist within the stepped care algorithm already described. These approaches include but are not limited to patient education and specific counseling in matters relating to smoking cessation, instruction in physical exercise, nutritional advice, and continued nursing support. See Figure 7-6.

ANXIETY AND DEPRESSION

The prevalence of significant anxiety and depression in COPD patients is 50%, which is much higher than the general population (Brenes, 2003; Mikkelsen, Middelboe, Pisinger, et al., 2004). Concurrent treatment of the psychiatric disorder improves physical and psychologic well-being. Trials of nortriptyline, buspirone, and sertraline have been found to reduce anxiety (Brenes, 2003). In addition, nonpharmacologic therapy such as cognitive-behavioral programs, which focus on relationships, can reduce anxiety.

Box 7-10 COMPONENTS OF A GOOD REHABILITATION PROGRAM

- Patient and family education
- Respiratory, physical, and occupational therapy
- Exercise conditioning
- Nutritional assistance
- Psychosocial support
- Vocational rehabilitation

From Halpin, D.M.G. (2002). *COPD*. Mosby International.

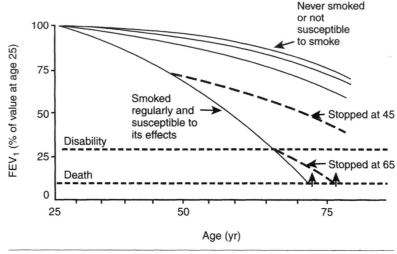

FIGURE **7-6** Smoking and function loss. *FEV₁,* Forced expiratory volume in 1 second. (From Fletcher, C., & Peto, R. [1977]. *Br Med J, 1,* 1645-1648.)

Even in individuals who have never smoked, lung function begins to decline after age 25. In patients who smoke regularly, lung function declines more rapidly. As seen in the graph, smoking cessation slows down the rate of functional loss, comparable to the rate of decline seen in nonsmokers. Therefore a survival benefit can be realized even in overt disease and at lower FEV capacities. The rate of decline in patients who persist in smoking is approximately two to four times that of nonsmokers.

SUMMARY

COPD is a significant cause of death and disability in the United States, with more than 90% of diagnosed patients having a history of smoking. The disease is characterized by a progressive airflow limitation that is not fully reversible and an abnormal inflammatory process in the lungs caused by exposure to tobacco smoke or other noxious gases. COPD includes both chronic bronchitis and emphysema. Asthma is also a disease of airflow obstruction but is a different disease from COPD. A small percent of patients have both COPD and asthma. Chronic progressive dyspnea helps distinguish the two diseases and is a hallmark in patients with COPD. In addition, COPD patients commonly experience a complex of symptoms including chronic cough, sputum production, and wheeze. The diagnosis of COPD is based on initial clinical presentation and a thorough patient history and confirmed by spirometry. As the disease progresses, acute exacerbations become more common and troublesome. Management of acute exacerbations is generally multifactorial. Management of stable disease is characterized by a stepwise increase in treatment, depending on disease severity. Evidence-based guidelines recommend both pharmacologic and nonpharmacologic interventions. Inhaled bronchodilator medications are central to symptom management in COPD. Depending on disease severity, bronchodilators are prescribed on an as-needed basis or as maintenance therapy. Treatment can improve and prevent symptoms, reduce frequency and severity of exacerbations, and improve health status and exercise tolerance. Treatment goals are best ensured by ongoing monitoring and assessment of the patient.

Objective Questions

1. Dyspnea is:

   a. A subjective sensation that appears only in patients with end stage COPD.

   b. Generally episodic in patients with COPD.

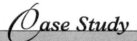
Case Study

B.L. is a 65-year-old anxious male who is being seen for complaints of dyspnea and a cough productive of white sputum. The patient's past medical history includes asthma and an 80 pack-year smoking history. The patient states he had asthma 10 to 15 years ago when he saw his physician for dyspnea on exertion and chronic cough. In addition, B.L. describes his symptoms as "off and on" but becoming more frequent and more severe over the past few years. He uses a beta-2 agonist for dyspnea, which he states seems to relieve his symptoms only temporarily.

The physical examination reveals a thin male in respiratory distress. No pallor, cyanosis, jaundice, lymphadenopathy, or clubbing is noted.

Temperature = 98°; pulse = 90; blood pressure = 130/90; respiration rate = 26/min. For most of the examination, B.L. sits on the table with his hands on his knees and breathes through pursed lips. Chest examination reveals increased chest diameter, reduced breath sounds with prolonged expiratory phase, and a few scattered expiratory wheezes.

Laboratory Data
- Chest x-ray: normal-size heart; flat diaphragms; clear, hyperinflated lungs
- Complete blood count (CBC): Hgb = 16 g/dl; white blood count = 7200/mm^3
- Arterial blood gases (ABGs): pH = 7.28; Paco$_2$ = 60 mm Hg; Pao$_2$ = 55 mm Hg

Pulmonary Function Tests

	Pre-bronchodilator	% Predicted	Post-bronchodilator
Forced expiratory volume in 1 sec (FEV$_1$)	1.2 L	39	1.3 L
Forced vital capacity (FVC)	3.0 L	68	3.0 L
FEV$_1$/FVC	40%	<70%	
TLC	8.4 L	120	

   c. The medical term for hyperinflation of the chest.

   d. A subjective sensation with causes.

2. Which of the following is most important in diagnosing COPD?

   a. EEG.

   b. Chest x-ray.

   c. Pulmonary function test (spirometry).

   d. Physical examination.

3. Pharmacologic therapy in COPD is used:

   a. To cure the underlying cause of COPD.

   b. To prevent and control the symptoms of COPD.

   c. As a last resort, because nothing modifies long-term lung function decline.

   d. As an alternative to other non-drug interventions.

4. Which of the following are believed to contribute to the pathologic changes eventually seen in patients with COPD:

   a. Various autoimmune reactions.

   b. Eosinophil-mediated inflammation caused by exposure to allergens.

   c. Oxidative stress, chronic airway inflammation, and enzyme imbalances secondary to the inhalation of noxious particles and gases.

   d. The pathogenesis of COPD has yet to be determined.

5. Current guidelines for the pharmacologic treatment of COPD recommend:

   a. The regular use of inhaled corticosteroids in all stages of disease.

   b. The use of bronchodilators as principal treatment.

   c. The prophylactic use of antibiotic therapy to prevent exacerbations.

d. The use of mucolytics, antitussives, and antioxidants as adjuvants because of their proven effectiveness in COPD patients.

6. The current epidemiology associated with COPD is consistent with the following:

    a. A decreasing prevalence, primarily the result of declining rates of cigarette smoking in our population.

    b. A prevalence of disease that is likely to be underestimated, because COPD frequently goes undetected.

    c. The global economic burden associated with COPD is fairly insignificant when compared with diseases like diabetes and hypertension.

    d. The rate of mortality caused by COPD is declining as a result of curative treatments and earlier diagnosis.

7. Diagnostic staging of COPD is defined by:

    a. The severity of airflow obstruction.

    b. The patient's age.

    c. The patient's smoking history.

    d. The patient's current medication profile.

8. Pulmonary rehabilitation in COPD is:

    a. Beneficial to only those patients with mild to moderate disease.

    b. Beneficial to only those patients with severe to very severe disease.

    c. Psychologically and physiologically helpful for all COPD patients. However, it is not considered to be cost-effective.

    d. Improves exercise tolerance and the patient's sense of well-being.

REFERENCES

Aaron, S.D., Dales, R.E., & Cardinal, P. (1999). How accurate is spirometry at predicting restrictive pulmonary impairment? *Chest, 115*(3), 869-873.

Abernethy, A.P., Currow, D.C., Frith, P., et al. (2003). Randomised, double blind, placebo controlled crossover trial of sustained release morphine for the management of refractory dyspnea. *BMJ, 327,* 1-6.

Alberts, W.M., & Rolfe, M.W. (1994). A step care approach to managing COPD. *Hosp Formul, 29*(11).

American Thoracic Society. (1995). Standards for the diagnosis and care of patients with chronic obstructive pulmonary disease. *Am J Respir Crit Care Med, 152,* S85.

Balfe, D.L., Lewis, M., & Mohsenifar, Z. (2002). Grading the severity of obstruction in the presence of a restrictive ventilatory defect. *Chest, 122*(4), 1365-1369.

Barnes, P.J. (2000). Mechanisms in COPD: Differences from asthma. *Chest, 17,* 10S-14S.

Barnes, P.J., & Karin, M. (1997). Nuclear factor-κB: A pivotal transcription factor in chronic inflammatory diseases. *N Eng J Med, 336,* 1066-1071.

Bonay, M., Bancal, C., & Crestani, B. (2002). Benefits and risk of inhaled corticosteroids in chronic obstructive pulmonary disease. *Drug Saf, 25*(1), 57-71.

Booth, S., Anderson, H., Swannick, M., et al. (2004). The use of oxygen in the palliation of breathlessness: A report of the expert working group of the Scientific Committee of the Association of Palliative Medicine. *Respir Med, 98*(1), 66-77.

Brenes, G.A. (2003). Anxiety and chronic obstructive pulmonary disease: Prevalence, impact, and treatment. *Psychosom Med, 65*(6), 963-970.

Briggs, D.D., Kuritzky, L., Boland, C., et al. (2000). Early detection and management of COPD. *J Respir Dis, 21*(9), S15-S16.

Calverley, P.M., Boonsawat, W., Cseke, Z., et al. (2003). Maintenance therapy with budesonide and formoterol in chronic pulmonary disease. *Eur Respir J, 22*(6), 912-919.

Celli, B.R. (2000). The importance of spirometry in COPD and asthma. *Chest, 117*(2), 15S-19S.

Cheer, S.M., & Scott, L.J. (2002). Formoterol: A review of its use in chronic obstructive pulmonary disease. *Am J Respir Med, 1*(4), 285-300.

Confalonieri, M., Mainardi, E., Della, P.R., et al. (1998). Inhaled corticosteroids reduce neutrophil bronchial inflammation in patients with chronic obstructive pulmonary disease. *Thorax, 53,* 583-585.

Cosio, M.G., Joaquim, M., & Cosio, M.G. (2002). Inflammation of the airways and lung parenchyma in COPD. *Chest, 121*(5), 160S-165S.

Cox, J.M., Dickerson, E.D., & Petty, T.L. (2003). Chronic obstructive pulmonary disease and depression: A Pandora's box of comorbid symptoms? *Am J Hosp Palliat Care, 20*(3), 179-181.

Dekhuijzen, P.N., Aben, K.K., Dekker, I., et al. (1996). Increased exhalation of hydrogen peroxide in patients with stable and unstable chronic obstructive pulmonary disease. *Am J Respir Crit Care Med, 154,* 813.

Eid, A.A., Ionescu, A.I., Nixon, L.S., et al. (2001). Inflammatory response and body composition in chronic obstructive pulmonary disease. *Am J Respir Crit Care Med, 164,* 1414-1418.

Evans, S.E., & Scanlon, P.D. (2003). Current practice in pulmonary function testing. *Mayo Clin Proc, 78*(6), 758-763.

Finkelstein, R., Fraser, R.S., Ghezzo, H., et al. (1995). Alveolar inflammation and its relation to emphysema in smokers. *Am J Respir Crit Care Med, 152,* 1666.

Finlay, G.A., O'Driscoll, L.R., Russell, K.G., et al. (1997). Matrix metalloproteinase expression and production by alveolar macrophages in emphysema. *Am J Respir Crit Care Med, 156,* 240-247.

Foral, P.A., Malesker, M.A., Huerta, G., et al. (2004). Nebulized opioids use in COPD. *Chest, 125*(2), 691-694.

Garcia-Aymerich, J., Monso, E., Marrades, R,M., et al. (2001). Risk factors for hospitalization for a chronic obstructive pulmonary disease exacerbation. *Am J Respir Crit Care Med*, *164*, 1003-1006.

Glady, C.A., Aaron, S.D., Lunau, M., et al. (2003). A spirometry-based algorithm to direct lung function testing in the pulmonary function laboratory. *Chest, 123*(6), 1939-1946.

Global Initiative for Chronic Obstructive Lung Disease (GOLD) Guidelines. (2003). pp. 67-77.

Gross, N.J., & Skorodin, M.S. (1984). Role of the parasympathetic system in airway obstruction due to emphysema. *N Eng J Med, 311*, 421-425.

Gross, N.J. (1988). Ipratropium bromide. *N Eng J Med, 319*, 486-494.

Halpin, D.M.G. (2002). *COPD*. Mosby International.

Hansel, T.T., Tennant, R.C., Tan, A.J., et al. (2004). Theophylline: Mechanism of action and use in asthma and chronic obstructive pulmonary disease. *Drugs Today, 40*(1):55-69.

Heath, J.M. (1993). Outpatient management of chronic bronchitis in the elderly. *Am Fam Physician, 48*(5):841-843.

Hunninghake, G.W., & Crystal, R.G. (1983). Cigarette smoking and lung destruction: Accumulation of neutrophils in the lungs of cigarette smokers. *Am Rev Respir Dis, 128*, 833-838.

Janssens, J.P., de Muralt, B., & Titelion, V. (2000). Management of dyspnea in severe COPD. *J Pain Symptom Manage, 19*(5), 381-382.

Jeffery, P.K. (1998). Structural and inflammatory changes in COPD: A comparison with asthma. *Thorax, 53*, 129-136.

Jennings, A.L., Davies, A,N., Higgins, J.P.T, et al. (2002). A systematic review of the use of opioids in the management of dyspnea. *Thorax, 57*, 939-944.

Kuwano, K., Bosken, C.H., Pare, P.D., et al. (1993). Small airways dimensions in asthma and in chronic obstructive pulmonary disease. *Am Rev Respir Dis, 148*, 1220.

Lane, D.J., Howell, J.B., & Giblin, B. (1968). Relation between airways obstruction and CO2 tension in chronic obstructive pulmonary disease. *BMJ, 3*, 707.

Laurell, C., & Eriksson, S. (1963). The electrophoretic α1-globulin pattern of serum in α1-antitrypsin deficiency. *Scand J Clin Lab Invest, 15*, 132-140.

Littner, M.R., Ilowite, J.S., Tashkin, D.P., et al. (2000). Long-acting bronchodilation with once-daily dosing of tiotropium (Spiriva) in stable COPD disease. *Am J Respir Crit Care Med, 161*(4 Pt. 1), 1136-1142.

Liu, A.N., Mohammed, A.Z., Rice, W.R., et al. (1999). Perforin-independent CD8(+) T-cell mediated cytotoxicity of alveolar epithelial cells is preferentially mediated by tumor necrosis factor-alpha: Relative insensitivity to Fas ligand. *Am J Respir Cell Mol Biol, 20*, 849.

Lopez, A.D., & Murray, C.C. (1998). The global burden of disease, 1990-2020. *Nat Med, 4*, 1241-1243.

Lyseng-Williamson, K.A., & Keating, G.M. (2002). Inhaled salmeterol/fluticasone propionate combination in chronic obstructive pulmonary disease. *Am J Respir Med, 1*(4), 273-282.

Mannino, D.M., Homa, D.M., Akinbami, L.J., et al. (2000). Chronic obstructive pulmonary disease surveillance: United States, 1971-2000. *MMWR Surveill, 51*, 1-16.

Martinez, F.J., Flaherty, K.R., & Iannettoni, M.D. (2003). Patient selection for lung volume reduction surgery. *Chest Surg Clin N Am, 13*(4), 669-685.

Maziak, W., Loukides, S., Culpitt, S., et al. (1998). Exhaled nitric oxide in chronic obstructive pulmonary disease. *Am J Respir Crit Care Med, 157*, 998.

Michaud, C.M., Murray, C.J., & Bloom, B.R. (2001). Burden of disease: Implications for future research. *JAMA, 285*, 535-539.

Mikkelsen, R.L., Middelboe, T., Pisinger, C., et al. (2004). Anxiety and depression in patients with chronic obstructive pulmonary disease (COPD): A review. *Nord J Psychiatry, 58*(1), 65-70.

Murray, C.J., & Lopez, A.D. (1997). Alternative projection of mortality by cause 1990-2020: Global burden of disease study. *Lancet, 349*,1436-1442.

National Lung Health Education Program (NLHEP) Executive Committee. (1998). Strategies in preserving lung health and preventing COPD and associated diseases. *Chest, 113* (2 Suppl.), 123S-163S.

NHLBI. (May 2001). *Data fact sheet*.

Niewoehner, D.E. (2002).The role of systemic corticosteroids in acute exacerbation of chronic obstructive pulmonary disease. *Am J Respir Med, 1*(4), 243-248.

O'Donnell, D.E. (2000). Assessment of bronchodilator efficacy in symptomatic COPD. *Chest, 117*(2), 42S-47S.

Pauwels, R., Calverley, P., Buist, A.S., et al. (2004). COPD exacerbations: The importance of a standard definition. *Respir Med, 98*(2), 99-107.

Pauwels, R.A., Buist, A.S., Calverly, P.M., et al. (2001). Global strategy for the diagnosis, management, and prevention of chronic obstructive lung disease (GOLD): Workshop summary. *Am J Respir Crit Care Med, 163*, 1256.

Pearson, M.G., Alderslade, R., Allen, S.C., et al. (1997). Diagnosis and management of stable COPD. *Thorax, 52*(Suppl. 5), S1-S28.

Petty, T.L., & Rennard, S.I. (2000). Mechanisms of COPD. *Chest, 117*(5), 219S-223S.

Poole, P.J., & Black, P.N. (2003). Preventing exacerbations of chronic bronchitis and COPD: Therapeutic potential of mucolytic agents. *Am J Respir Med, 2*(5), 367-370.

Pratico, D., Basili, S., Vieri, M., et al. (1998). Chronic obstructive pulmonary disease is associated with an increase in urinary levels of isoprostane F2a-III, an index of oxidant stress. *Am J Respir Crit Care Med, 158*, 1709-1714.

Ram, F., Picot, J., Lightower, J., et al. (2004). Non-invasive positive pressure ventilation for treatment of respiratory failure due to exacerbations of chronic obstructive pulmonary disease. *Cochrane Database Syst Rev, 1*, CD004104.

Repine, J.E., Bast, A., & Lankhorst, I. (1997). Oxidative stress in chronic obstructive pulmonary disease. *Am J Respir Crit Care Med, 156*, 341-357.

Rodriguez-Roisin, R. (2000). Toward a consensus definition for COPD exacerbations. *Chest, 117*, 398S-401S.

Rubinstein, I., Kumar, B., & Schriever, C. (2004). Long-term montelukast therapy in moderate to severe COPD: A preliminary observation. *Respir Med, 98*(2):134-138.

Shee, C.D., & Green, M. (2003). Non-invasive ventilation and palliation: Experience in a district general hospital and a review. *Palliat Med, 17*, 21-26.

Sin, D.D., Golmohammadi, K., & Jacobs, P. (2004). Cost-effectiveness of inhaled corticosteroids for chronic pulmonary disease according to disease severity. *Am J Med, 116*(5), 325-331.

Snider, G.L., Stone, P.J., Lucey, E.C., et al. (1985). Eglin C, a polypeptide derived from the medicinal leech prevents human neutrophil elastase induced emphysema and bronchial secretory cell metaplasia. *Am Rev Respir Dis, 132*, 1155-1161.

Snow, V., Lascher, S., Mottur-Pilson, C., et al. (2001). The evidence base for management of acute exacerbations of COPD: Clinical practice guideline, part 1. *Chest, 119,* 1185-1189.

Soriano, J.B., Kiri, V.A., Pride, N.B., et al. (2003). Inhaled corticosteriods with/without long-acting beta-agonists reduce the risk of rehospitalization and death in COPD patients. *Am J Respir Med, 2*(1), 67-74.

Stockley, R.A. (2002). Neutrophils and the pathogenesis of COPD. *Chest, 121*(5), 151S-155S.

Tashkin, D.P., & Cooper, C.B. (2004). The role of long-acting bronchodilators in the management of stable COPD. *Chest, 125*(1), 249-259.

Tetley, T.D. (2002). Macrophages and the pathogenesis of COPD. *Chest, 121*(5), 156S-159S.

Twycross, R. (1997). *Symptom management in advanced cancer* (2nd ed.). Oxon, U.K.: Radcliffe Medical Press.

Van Grunsven, P., Schermer, T., Akkermans, R., et al. (2003). Short- and long-term efficacy of fluticasone propionate in subjects with early signs and symptoms of chronic obstructive pulmonary disease: Results of the DIMCA study. *Respir Med, 97*(12), 1303-1312.

Vianna, E.O., & Martin. R.J. (1998). Recent innovations in asthma therapy. *Drugs Today, 34*(4), 341-351.

Wagers, S.S., Bouder, T.G., Kaminsky, D.A., et al. (2000). The invaluable pressure-volume curve. *Chest, 117*(2), 579-583.

Wedzicha, J.A., & Donaldson, G.C. (2003). Exacerbations of chronic obstructive pulmonary disease. *Respir Care, 48*(12), 1204-1213.

West, J.B. (1998). *Pulmonary pathophysiology: The essentials* (5th ed.). Baltimore, Md.: Lippincott Williams & Wilkins.

Wilkinson, T.M., Donaldson, G.C., Hurst, J.R., et al. (2004). Early therapy improves outcomes of exacerbations of chronic obstructive pulmonary disease. *Am J Respir Crit Care Med, 169*(12), 1298-1303. (Epub Feb 27 ahead of print)

Wood-Baker, R. (2003). Is there a role for systemic corticosteroids in the management of stable chronic obstructive pulmonary disease? *Am J Respir Med, 2*(6), 451-458.

Nephrology

Michael Germain

Lewis M. Cohen

OBJECTIVES

After the completion of this chapter, the reader should be able to:

1. Describe the symptom burden and limited life expectancy of many patients with chronic kidney disease (CKD).
2. Discuss common symptoms and their management by employing the unique pharmacokinetics of drug therapy in this patient population.
3. Understand the role of dialysis withdrawal at the end of life for the dialysis patient.
4. Examine advance care planning, advance directive, health care proxy, and a model do-not resuscitate policy.

INTRODUCTION

Prognosis

The National Kidney Foundation has recommended the term *chronic kidney disease* (*CKD*) to encompass all stages of renal disease. (This and other information can be found at www.kidney.org/professionals/kdoqi/guidelines_ckd/p4_class_g1.htm.) The five stages described for CKD patients are defined by the glomerular filtration rate (GFR). Stage 1 includes patients who have a normal GFR (>90 ml/min); with disease progression, stage 5 identifies patients with end-stage renal disease (ESRD) who are approaching or currently receiving dialysis or renal transplantation (GFR <15). Dialysis has traditionally been thought of as a lifesaving treatment. However, as older patients with multiple co-morbid conditions receive dialysis, it is often viewed as providing a palliative intervention. Approximately 300,000 people currently undergo

maintenance dialysis in the United States, and about 95,000 new patients initiate treatment annually. More than 65,000 patients with ESRD die annually, and the 23% annual mortality rate is at least in part due to the high number of co-morbid illnesses in patients with an average age of 65 years. As stated by Cohen and Germain (2003), "to put this in perspective, the prevalent ESRD mortality rate is comparable with that of non-Hodgkin's lymphoma, and higher than that of human immunodeficiency virus and colorectal and ovarian carcinoma. The expected prognosis of dialysis patients are one quarter to one fifth those of the same age-matched, general population" (www.usrds.org).

Perhaps because the nephrology community has focused on the "life saving" aspects of dialysis in a "culture of denial," a poor prognosis is often ignored and a palliative approach in this population is often limited (Germain & Cohen, 2001). This chapter describes the pathophysiology, symptoms, and supportive measures that can be used for the renal patient.

SYMPTOM BURDEN

Patients with CKD carry a high symptom burden, with an average of 10.5 symptoms at any given time (Merkus, Jager, Dekker, et al., 1999; Valderrqabano, Jofre, & Lopez-Gomez, 2001; Weisbord, Carmody, Bruns, et al., 2003). Before dialysis, a uremic state can affect all organ systems, thereby creating significant symptoms. Pruritus, fatigue, gastrointestinal symptoms, sexual dysfunction, neuropathy, and arthropathy are common symptoms that affect this patient population. Erythropoietin administered before dialysis can improve the fatigue and weakness often encountered in the renal-compromised patient (Robertson, Kaky, Gurthrie, et al., 1990). The initiation of dialysis can ameliorate symptoms, but unfortunately many symptoms remain problematic for the patient (Table 8-1). Ninety percent of the U.S. dialysis patients receive hemodialysis three times per week, and 40% of dialysis treatments are further complicated by intra-dialytic symptoms (Maggiore, Pizzarelli, Santoro, et al., 2002). Daily or nocturnal and peritoneal dialysis demonstrate a significant reduction in symptoms. Over 40% of ESRD patients are diabetic, and 80% are hypertensive. Cardiomyopathy, peripheral vascular disease (PVD), bone disease (e.g., Paget's), skin diseases, arthropathies, and psychiatric conditions are common co-morbidities that contribute significantly to the symptoms of these patients and ultimately interfere with their quality of life (www.usrds.org).

Table **8-1** Common Symptoms in CKD Patients

Symptom	Prevalence
Fatigue	74%-87%
Itching	53%-73%
Pain	50%-63%
Cramps	60%
Lack of appetite	25%-48%
Restless legs syndrome (RLS)	20%-40%
Nausea	30%-40%
Dry mouth	58%
Shortness of breath	50%
Dizziness	38%-45%

Data from Merkus, M.P., Jager, K.J., Dekker, F.W., et al. (1999). Physical symptoms and quality of life in patient on chronic dialysis: Results of the Netherlands cooperative study on adequacy of dialysis (NECOSAD). *Nephrol Dial Transplant, 14,* 1163-1170; Weisbord, S.D., Carmody, S.S., Bruns, F.J., et al. (2003). Symptom burden, quality-of-life, advance care planning, and the potential value of palliative care in severely ill hemodialysis patients. *Nephrol Dial Transplant, 18,* 1345-1352; Weisbord, S.D., Carmody, S.S., Bruns, F.J., et al. (2002). The prevalence, severity and physician recognition of symptoms in hemodialysis patients (abstract). *J Am Soc Nephrol, 13,* 706A.

Concomitant Diseases

CKD patients are often elderly and have concomitant (co-morbid) diseases. Diabetes, hypertension, cardiovascular disease, peripheral vascular disease, and heart failure are common disorders that can lead to significant suffering and mortality. Germain, McCarthy, Swartz, et al., 2004 discuss the treatments of these co-morbid conditions in a new publication. See Table 8-2.

Pharmaceutical Renal Metabolism

Many drugs and their metabolites are excreted by the kidney through glomerular filtration, tubular secretion, or both. Consequently, renal impairment has a significant effect on the clearance of many medications and ultimately affects the absorption, distribution, and protein binding that is associated with drug clearance (see Chapter 4). Protein binding is affected by renal impairment, which can alter drug levels and precipitate adverse effects. Serum albumin concentrations are low in patients who have a nephrotic syndrome and/or are cachexia. Therefore low serum albumin levels reduce the number of drug binding sites available for protein binding medications. As a consequence, the proportion of free drug to bound drug is systemically increased with greater fluctuations in the free drug following the administration of each dose. This can result in an increased susceptibility to adverse drug reactions and systemic toxicities.

Guidelines for specific medication dosing in CKD have been published and are available for use in this patient population. Dosages for specific medications are further articulated to support pre-dialysis and post-dialysis conditions (Aronoff, Berns, Brier, et al, 1999; Cohen & Germain, 2003; Cohen, Germain, & Tessier, 2003).

Symptom-treatment protocols could easily assist in the care of this patient population; however, their usage is underutilized and none to date have been published. One institution with eight dialysis units providing services for over 650 patients has developed specific symptom-management protocols for practice based on a current review of the literature. These protocols are available to the rounding physician and nurse practitioner within the

Table **8-2**   PROGNOSTIC TABLE

Risk factors for poor QOL, suffering, morbidity, mortality-RR, life expectancy:
- Advanced age
- Malnutrition; hypoalbuminemia. Low PCR
- Chronic inflammatory state. High CRP, homocysteine
- Severe PVD; amputations
- Calciphylaxis
- CHF
- DM

Risk Factor	1-Year Survival (%)	Relative Risk (reference <44 years old; no co-morbid disease)
Advanced age >80 yr	61% (80% in 60-yr-old)	2.68
Albumin <3.5 g/dl)	50% (86% for albumin >3.5)	7.45 for albumin <2.5 (1.0 Alb. 4.0)
Diabetes mellitus	78% vs. 83% in non-DM	1.23
Amputation AKA	27%	
Amputation BKA	49%	
Amputation toe	63%	
CHF	54%	5.5 at 6 months
Calciphylaxis	No solid data <10%	

RR, Relative risk; *QOL*, quality of life; *PCR*, protein catabolic rate; *CRP*, C-reactive protein; *PVD*, peripheral vascular disease; *CHF*, congestive heart failure; *DM*, diabetes mellitus; *AKA*, above-the-knee amputation; *BKA*, below-the-knee amputation. From Mortality of U.S. Dialysis Patients USRDS 2003. www.usrds.org/.

dialysis unit. By utilizing standardized symptom assessment tools similar to the Likert scale, these clinicians routinely evaluate the impact of symptom burden through ongoing assessment and optimal management (Poppel, Cohen, & Germain, 2003).

COMMON SYMPTOMS

In this section, suggested management approaches to some of the common symptoms in CKD patients are reviewed. The best treatment options are those that are minimally invasive and well supported by the literature. Because many drugs and toxic metabolites are cleared by the kidney, these build up in CKD patients and exacerbate systemic side effects (e.g., prolonged episodes of mental status changes, seizures). It is important when managing symptoms and choosing specific medications that the clinician does not replace one symptom with another (e.g. treating neuropathic pain with amitriptyline and precipitating restless legs syndrome [RLS]). It is advisable to always evaluate

specific precautions, warnings, and dosage adjustments for CKD based on the patient's GFR (Aronoff et al., 1999).

Intradialytic Symptoms

Intradialytic symptoms occur in approximately 40% of patients undergoing hemodialysis and occur more frequently in patients with advanced age, diabetes, and heart disease. Common symptoms include hypotension, cramps, nausea and vomiting, and pruritus. In addition, post-dialysis hypotension and a "washed out" feeling lasting up to 24 hours are prevalent. Symptoms that occur early in the dialysis treatment session are commonly related to inadequate vasoconstriction, whereas those occurring later may be caused by excessive or rapid volume removal. Many of these symptoms are easily diminished or eliminated by peritoneal dialysis or frequent, slow hemodialysis or nocturnal daily dialysis. Only a minority of patients who experience recurrent symptoms require aggressive symptom management.

Management. Recent studies have supported the value of changes in the dialysis prescription to support a decrease in the occurrence of intradialytic symptoms. Monitoring blood volume, dialysate temperature, and dialysate sodium and the ultrafiltration rates are inexpensive and effective steps to accomplish this. Symptoms that occur in the first part of the dialysis treatment may improve with a trial of low dialysate temperature (36° C) or isothermic control of the dialysis machine (Maggiore et al., 2002). If this is ineffective or not tolerated, raising the dialysate sodium with profiling, ultrafiltration profiling, or "mirroring" the sodium and ultrafiltration profiles can be helpful (Straver, De Vries, Donker, et al., 2002). Continuous blood volume monitoring has also been shown to be effective by preventing rapid or large intravascular volume changes. The addition of biofeedback control on the ultrafiltration with volume monitoring has also been used (Santoro, Mancini, Basile, et al., 2002). For sudden hypotension, a result of a loss of the autonomic nervous system control, sertraline 50 to 100 mg daily has been useful (Dheenan, Venkatesan, Grubb, et al., 1998). Midodrine, an oral alpha-adrenergic agonist, 2.5 to 10 mg pretreatment and mid-treatment, is also quite effective in preventing hypotension (Cruz, Mahnensmith, & Perazella, 1997; Flynn, Mitchell, Caruso, et al., 1996; Perazella, 2001). Intravenous carnitine (10 mg/kg) during dialysis should be considered when other therapies have failed (Eknoyan, Latos, & Linberg, 2003; Riley, Rutherford, & Rutherford, 1997).

For patients who experience symptoms later in dialysis treatment, the target dry weight may be too low. The dry weight should be raised by 0.5 kg each treatment until symptoms resolve. Continuous blood volume monitoring will be helpful when determining the appropriate dry weight.

DISCUSSION OF SPECIFIC SYMPTOMS AND THEIR MANAGEMENT
Pruritus

Uremic pruritus (Robertson & Mueller, 1996) is often difficult to manage in the renal compromised patient. Approximately 60% of dialysis patients have pruritus, which can worsen during the dialysis session. A specific etiology has not been identified, but a number of factors can contribute to this symptom. Secondary hyperparathyroidism (Massry, Popovtzer, Coburn, et al., 1968), hyperphosphatemia (Blachley, Blankenship, Menter, et al., 1985), increased calcium phosphate deposition in the skin, dry skin, inadequate dialysis (Hiroshige, Kabashima, Takasugi, et al., 1995), anemia (De Marchi, Ceddhin, Villaltgra, et al., 1992), iron deficiency, and low-grade hypersensitivity to products used in the dialysis procedure have all been identified as possible contributory factors to pruritus.

Management. The management of pruritus includes adequate dialysis, anemia management, and control of calcium, phosphorus, and parathyroid hormone levels as the first line of defense. The National Kidney Foundation's Kidney Disease Outcomes Quality Initiative (K/DOQI) guidelines provide target levels for treatment (www.kidney.org/professionals/doqi/guidelines). If a patient, for example, has xerosis, an emollient such as an oatmeal moisturizer, oil, or ammonium lactate cream should be considered. If there is only a partial response, then an emollient with an antipruritic (e.g., doxepin cream) can be trialed. Consideration should include changing the brand of heparin and/or the dialysis membrane. If pruritus continues, a sequential 2-week trial of the following interventions should be considered in the patient's plan of care:

1. Oral antihistamine therapy is safe and inexpensive, and it should be considered first line. However, most of the evidence to support the efficacy of this intervention is anecdotal.
2. Phototherapy with UVB light 3 times weekly is effective but may be inconvenient for the patient (Blachley, Blankenship, Menter, et al., 1985).
3. A trial of naltrexone has been shown to be effective in small controlled trials (Peer, Kivity, Agami, et al., 1996).
4. If the naltrexone interferes with opioids for pain or is not tolerated by the patient, then

capsaicin cream 4 times daily should be prescribed (Tarng, Cho, Liu, et al., 1996).

5. Ketotifen (mast cell stabilizer) 2 mg twice daily (available in Europe) or ondansetron (5HT3 antagonist) 4 mg twice daily has been found to be effective in limited trials (Ashmore, Jones, Newstead, et al., 2000; Balaskas, Bamihas, Karamouzis, et al., 1998; Francos, Kauh, & Grittlen, 1991).

6. Cholestyramine 5 mg twice daily (Silverberg, Ianina, & Reisin, 1997) or activated charcoal 6 g per day in 4 to 6 divided doses for 8 weeks (Giovanetti, Barsotti, & Cupisti, 1995) is effective but can interfere with the absorption of other medications.

7. Intravenous lidocaine (100 mg) use during dialysis is reserved for severe and refractory cases, because it can be associated with seizures (Tapia, Cheigh, & David, 1977).

8. Thalidomide 100 mg at bedtime has been shown to be effective in a randomized trial with refractory pruritus in dialysis patients; extraordinary care must be taken in handling pills and avoiding exposure to pregnant women (Silva, Vianna, Lagon, et al., 1994).

Anorexia

Nutrition is a major problem in dialysis patients, and anorexia is a common symptom. Anorexia is a nonspecific symptom but can be an indication of inadequate dialysis and uremia buildup. However, many other causes can contribute to anorexia, including anemia, depression, taste disorders, dry mouth, and mechanical causes. Many gastrointestinal problems can also precipitate anorexia such as nausea, constipation, diarrhea, and diabetic gastroparesis. Anorexia contributes to poor nutrition and is common in patients with co-morbidities including the geriatric subpopulation. Depression should not be ruled out as a contributory factor.

Management. Zinc deficiency can lead to taste disorders resulting in anorexia; therefore a trial of oral zinc (220 mg daily) is suggested (Vreman, Venter, Leegwater, et al., 1980). A dry mouth is also

very common in dialysis patients, and medications should be reviewed to reduce or eliminate any drugs that may be contributory. Specific medications include clonidine (antihypertensive central adrenergic blocker), prochlorperazine (phenothiazine), and amitriptyline (tricyclic antidepressant). Saliva substitutes may be used every 1 to 2 hours. Pilocarpine, saliva stimulant, 5 to 10 mg 3 times daily can be helpful (Miller, 1993). Finally, a trial of appetite stimulants such as megestrol 40 to 400 mg daily (Boccanfuso, Hutton, & McAllister, 2000; Lien & Ruffenach, 1996), dronabinol 2.5 to 5 mg 2 or 3 times a day, or prednisone 10 to 20 mg 1 or 2 times a day has been used in ESRD. Antidepressants should be considered if depression is contributing to anorexia.

Constipation

Constipation is a common complaint in the dialysis patient and is multifactorial in origin. The dietary restriction of high-potassium fruits and vegetables decreases the fiber content of food. Fluid restriction, physical inactivity, and medications, including aluminum and calcium phosphorus binders, iron supplements, and opioids, can all contribute to this symptom.

Management. Increased dietary fiber, regular exercise, and a combination of stool softener with a laxative can be effective. Osmotic laxatives such as lactulose or polyethylene glycolate are safe in CKD patients, as are stimulant laxatives like bisacodyl or casanthranol. Laxatives containing magnesium or phosphate should be avoided.

Muscle Cramping

Muscle cramps are a common complaint among patients on hemodialysis and frequently occur during the dialysis session if large amounts of fluid are removed (Canzanello & Burkart, 1992; Daugirdas, 2000).

Management. The prevention of muscle cramps is preferred (Goodling & Eisinger, 1982). Sodium "modeling" of dialysate has been shown to reduce the occurrence of abdominal cramps. This can be accomplished without post-dialysis thirst by starting with a high dialysate sodium (150-155 meq/L) and then using a programmed linear or step decrease to 135 to 140 meq/L at the end of each treatment. Quinine may prevent cramps (260-325 mg by mouth [PO] before symptoms [i.e., before dialysis or sleep]) without exceeding three doses per day (Goodling & Eisinger, 1982).

If quinine is ineffective, vitamin E 400 international units (IU) PO per day or oxazepam 5 to 10 mg 2 hours before dialysis can be tried. If cramping continues, carnitine 1000 to 2000 mg intravenous (IV) during dialysis for a 3-month trial should be considered (Ahmad, Robertson, Golpher, et al., 1990).

Excessive or too-rapid fluid removal can result in cramps secondary to intravascular volume depletion. Fluid restrictions to prevent large intradialytic fluid gains can be preventive. To abort cramps during dialysis, administer hypertonic (23.4%) saline 5 to 20 ml over 3 to 5 minutes. Hypertonic (50%) glucose (50 ml) may be preferred in nondiabetics since it will not cause post-dialysis thirst. Practical measures include stretching of the affected muscle (dorsiflexion of the foot, either manually or by standing) and the application of heat.

Insomnia

Sleep disturbances have been reported by 50% to 90% of dialysis patients (Walker, Fine, & Kryger, 1995). Research has demonstrated that these patients have a high incidence of primary sleep disorders such as sleep apnea syndrome (Kimmel, Miller, & Mendelson, 1989), periodic leg movement disorder, and restless legs syndrome. See Chapter 5 for further discussion of these symptons.

Management. If sleep apnea is suspected, the patient should be referred for diagnostic sleep studies. Caffeinated beverages, nicotine, and daytime naps should be avoided. If sleep apnea has been excluded, a hypnotic can be prescribed. Drugs with a short duration of action and reduced potential for addiction should be considered, along with behavioral techniques aimed at improving sleep hygiene. Zolpidem 5 to 10 mg at bedtime, temazepam 7.5 to 30 mg at bedtime, flurazepam 15 to 30 mg at bedtime, trazodone 50 mg at bedtime, and triazolam 0.125 to 0.25 mg at bedtime generally are safe medications for dialysis patients.

See Chapter 5 for further discussion on specific medications.

Fatigue

Fatigue is probably one of the most common complaints from dialysis patients. Persistent and unrelenting fatigue and post-dialysis fatigue have been attributed to a number of causes: the rapid osmotic changes of the extracellular fluid space during hemodialysis; depletion of specific substances (e.g., carnitine); and the effect of ultrafiltration on blood pressure, blood membrane interactions, depression, insomnia, poor nutrition, anemia, and medications (Sklar, Newman, Scott, et al., 1999; Sklar, Riesenberg, Silber, et al., 1996).

Management. To provide adequate dialysis, a near-normal hemoglobin should be the desired goal (Robertson et al., 1990). Depression and hypotension should be anticipated, and providing the patients with proactive interventions will reduce the burden of concomitant symptoms exacerbating fatigue. A decrease in physical activity can also potentiate fatigue, and therefore it is important to encourage routine activity and regular exercise throughout the day. If the patient is deconditioned, a prompt referral for an inpatient or home care physical therapy evaluation and plan of care would be beneficial. Fatigue is also influenced by poor nutrition, and encouraging adequate fluids and nutritional intake should not be ignored. A course of megestrol acetate with protein supplements may be helpful in patients who are clinically malnourished. Specific medications should be evaluated, discontinued, and/or substituted if they are considered to be contributing to fatigue. If fatigue is severe and affects the patient's quality of life, a psychostimulant such as methylphenidate should be considered. Carnitine 10 mg/kg IV may be tried after each dialysis treatment, but convincing evidence to improve fatigue is lacking (Brass, Adler, Sietsema, et al., 2001).

Peripheral Neuropathies

Uremic neuropathy is the result of both mixed motor and sensory polyneuropathy that is often distal and symmetric (Fraser & Arieff, 1988). Uremic neuropathies were previously believed to be a direct result of a deficiency of thiamine, which is often diminished during dialysis. However, with the routine replacement of water-soluble vitamins, uremic neuropathies are now believed to be a result of the inadequate removal of one or more toxins retained from uremia. Because many CKD patients are diabetic and neuropathy is a common diabetic complication, the specific etiology of the patient's neuropathy is often difficult to differentiae.

Management. The patient should be adequately dialyzed with a high-flux membrane to ensure optimal middle molecule clearance (Tattersall, Cramp, Shannon, et al., 1992). Thiamine deficiency should always be ruled out. Neuropathic pain can be treated with tricyclic antidepressants, such as amitriptyline 25 to 100 mg/day (Portenoy, 1993). Another adjuvant analgesic that can be used in this setting is gabapentin (Rose & Kam, 2002); it should be started at a low dose (100 mg every other day) with the understanding that gabapentin is excreted unchanged by the kidney and accumulates in renal failure, often creating sedation. If the patient is able to tolerate gabapentin, the dose can then be titrated to a maximum dose of 100 to 300 mg 3 times daily. Carbamazepine may also be tried, starting at a dose of 100 mg twice daily and gradually increasing in increments of 100 mg twice daily to maximum of 400 to 800 mg daily. Serum level must be monitored (Covington, 1998).

Restless Legs Syndrome

The prevalence of uremia-associated restless legs syndrome is estimated to be between 20% and 40% of dialysis patients (Callaghan, 1966). Although it is unclear as to what extent, this condition is related to uremic neuropathy. Anemia, low serum ferritin levels, low levels of parathyroid hormone, and inadequate dialysis are also associated with restless legs syndrome in dialysis patients (Collado-Seidel, Kohnen, Samtleben, et al., 1998; Roger, Harris, & Stewart, 1991; Winkelman, Cherow, & Lazarus, 1996). Medications such as tricyclic antidepressants, lithium, neuroleptics, and caffeine can aggravate this symptom (Hening, 1997). This symptom is discussed further in Chapter 5.

Management. Optimal anemia and iron management should be ensured. If symptoms

persist, then a trial of benzodiazepines (e.g., clonazepam 0.5 to 2 mg at night as needed, temazepam 7.5 to 30 mg at night as needed, or triazolam 0.125 to 0.5 mg at night as needed) is usually well tolerated and may be effective (Schenck & Mahowald, 1996). Consider a dopaminergic agent such as carbidopa-levodopa either as a regular formulation of 12.5/50 to 75/300 mg in divided doses throughout the day and at bedtime or a sustained-release preparation of 25/100 to 100/400 mg twice a day (Von Scheele & Kempe, 1990). Newer agents such as pergolide 0.1 to 1 mg at bedtime may also be effective (Silber, Shepart, & Wisbey, 1997). Other drugs that can be used include bromocriptine 2.5 to 20 mg at bedtime, gabapentin 100 to 300 mg 3 times a day, and clonidine 0.1 to 1 mg at bedtime (Thorp, Morris, & Bagby, 2001; Wagner, Walters, Coleman, et al., 1996). Should these interventions fail in resistant and severe restless legs syndrome, prescribing an opioid can be effective (Walters, Wagner, Hening, et al., 1993). Patients routinely become resistant to these medications, requiring an escalation of dose (tachyphylaxis). If this occurs, the patient can be rotated to a different agent for 3 to 4 months, and, typically, in the future they will respond to the first agent at a lower dose. Finally, restless legs syndrome is associated with anxiety and stress and can be very difficult to effectively treat (Takaki, Nishi, Nangaku, et al., 2003).

Nausea and Vomiting

The numerous causes of nausea and vomiting include uremia, fluid and electrolyte imbalances, and dialysis-associated hypotension. Other co-morbid conditions and/or side effects from specific medications may significantly contribute to nausea and vomiting.

Management. If nausea and vomiting are considered to be caused by gastroparesis, a trial of metoclopramide in a small starting dose (5 mg twice daily) that is gradually increased should be considered. Uremia along with specific medications such as opioids can stimulate the area postrema (the chemoreceptor trigger zone) and can be responsive to dopamine receptor antagonists such as haloperidol. Broad-spectrum antiemetics include prochlorperazine 5 to 10 mg orally (PO), intramuscularly (IM), or intravenously (IV) 3 times daily as needed, per rectum (PR) 25 mg 3 times daily as needed; trimethobenzamide 250 mg PO 3 to 4 times daily, PR, IM 200 mg 3 to 4 times daily; or promethazine 25 mg PO, PR 4 times daily as needed. In treatment-resistant cases, chlorpromazine 10 to 25 mg PO 3 times daily as needed, 25 mg 3 times daily PR as needed, 25 to 50 mg 3 times daily IM as needed but should be used with caution, because this can create sedation. There is evidence for the use of 5HT3 antagonists, such as ondansetron, in anesthetic-, radiation-, and chemotherapy-induced vomiting; however their use empirically in other situations, although costly, may be quite effective and is safe in this patient population.

Pain

Pain is yet another common problem for CKD patients. A recent study found that approximately 50% of hemodialysis patients report pain at any given time and 30% rate their pain as severe (Davison, 2002a). The etiology is often multifactorial and may be caused by polycystic kidney disease (Steinman, 2000), co-morbidity (e.g., diabetic nephropathy or peripheral vascular disease), or complications of renal failure as seen in calciphylaxis (Green, Green, & Minott, 2000; Mathur, Shortland, & El Nahas, 2001; Wilmer & Magro, 2002). Other causes of pain include bone pain from renal osteodystrophy, dialysis-related amyloid arthropathy, dialysis vascular access "steal syndrome," or abdominal pain from peritoneal dialysis. Peripheral neuropathies, a result of vascular disease, can become severe in patients with extensive ischemia.

Not surprisingly, dialysis patients have a high incidence of pain at the end of life (EOL). Significant data have demonstrated the incidence of pain and other distressing symptoms in the final 24 hours (Cohen, Germain, Poppel, et al., 2000a, 2000b; Cohen, Poppel, Cohen, et al, 2001; Davison & Chater, 2001). However, it is unlikely that dialysis withdrawal itself is the single reason for pain (Davison, 2002a, 2002b). Barriers to good pain control in this population include:

1. There is a lack of clinical research in the pattern and types of pain, efficacy of analgesia, toxicity, and pharmacokinetic/pharmacodynamics of

opioids and adjuvant analgesics used in this patient population.
2. The pharmacokinetics, pharmacodynamics, and metabolism of specific analgesics is altered and complicated in the CKD population. Consequently, complications and side effects are more frequent (e.g., cognitive impairment).
3. CKD patients are routinely prescribed four or more medications at any given time, which increase their risk of drug-to-drug interactions.

Management. Treatment of pain should follow the World Health Organization (WHO) analgesic ladder approach with attention to the specific issues related to renal drug clearance. The use of nonsteroidal antiinflammatory drugs (NSAIDs), for example, should be contraindicated in CKD patients who may rely on their fragile kidney function to metabolize these medications, which have the propensity to cause acute renal failure. Because there is no ceiling to opioid therapies, the clinician should assess for untoward side effects as parameters for optimal opioid dosing.

Specific Opioid Analgesics. Codeine is predominately tolerated in CKD patients. Codeine is first metabolized in the liver and its analgesic metabolites are excreted by the kidney, which can precipitate coma-like phenomena in patients who are unable to metabolize these metabolites. This is not well understood but is believed not be dose-dependent.

Dextropropoxyphene and its active metabolite *norpropoxyphene* are excreted by the kidney, and their accumulation is associated with central nervous system toxicity, respiratory depression, and cardiotoxicity. For these reasons and because of its potential for abuse (it creates more euphoria than analgesia) and its weak analgesic properties, it is not recommended in this population.

Tramadol and its metabolites are metabolized in the kidney. The suggested dose adjustments in patients with a creatinine clearance less than 30 ml/min is 50 to 100 mg twice daily.

Morphine has two associated metabolites: morphine-3-glucuronide (M3G), the major metabolite; and morphine-6-glucuronide (M6G), the minor metabolite associated with only 5% the total dose. Despite the low incidence of M6G per dose of morphine, it is the most important metabolite from morphine because of its analgesic potency (twice as potent as morphine). Because M6G is excreted by the kidney, this metabolite can accumulate in patients with renal failure (Chauvin, Sandouk, Scherrmann, et al, 1987; Sawe, & Odar-Cederlof, 1987). The accumulation of M6G most likely explains the potential for morphine-related systemic toxicities and prolonged duration of action in patients with renal impairment. The ratio of M3G and M6G to morphine may also play a significant role in toxicity. It has been found, however, that the ratio for these metabolites is lower with morphine administered parentally than with morphine administered orally. Therefore in the setting of a progressive accumulation of M3G and M6G in patients receiving oral morphine, there may be some therapeutic advantage in changing the route to parenteral morphine (Pauli-Magnus, Hofmann, Mikus, et al., 1999).

Although morphine may be well tolerated by many patients with severe renal failure or by those needing dialysis, alternative strong opioids such as hydromorphone or fentanyl may be safer because of minimal metabolite production, which is excreted by the kidneys.

Hydromorphone has a similar side effect profile to morphine; however, it is thought to produce less pruritus, sedation, and nausea. Hydromorphone is primarily metabolized in the liver to hydromorphone-3-glucuronide (H3G), and these conjugates are excreted in the kidney. Despite the buildup of H3G, this metabolite appears to be well tolerated by CKD patients (Lee, Leng, & Tiernan, 2001).

Methadone is excreted mainly in feces, with metabolism into pharmacologically inactive metabolites primarily in the liver, although about 20% is excreted unchanged in the urine. It is not removed by dialysis, but in anuric patients, methadone is excreted exclusively in feces with no accumulation in plasma. These factors would suggest that methadone may be a safe, effective analgesic for use in patients with renal impairment, if carefully monitored.

Meperidine is less potent and a shorter-acting opioid than morphine. The metabolite *normerperidine* has an analgesic activity that is significantly less than the parent compound but has twice the proconvulsive propensity. Because normerperidine is excreted in the kidney and can rapidly accumulate as a result of a prolonged half-life, meperidine is not recommended for use in chronic pain in patients with CKD. Accumulation of normerperidine contributes to severe myoclonus and seizure activity.

Oxycodone has an analgesic and side effect profile similar to that of morphine. It is metabolized in the liver to its analgesic metabolites *noroxycodone* and *oxymorphone*. It appears to be safe for use in patients with renal impairment.

Fentanyl is a potent opioid with a short onset time and short half-life ($1\frac{1}{2}$-6 hr) transdermal delivery system. Fentanyl has poor oral bioavailability; it is therefore usually administered intravenously or transdermally. There does not appear to be any clinically significant accumulation of fentanyl because of its lack of active metabolites when administered to patients with renal impairment (Bower, 1982; Mercadante, Caligara, Sapio, et al., 1997).

Buprenorphine can be given sublingually and has a long duration of action. Buprenorphine is metabolized by the liver with little unchanged drug found in the urine. The two major metabolites, *buprenorphine-3-glucuronide* (B3G) and *norbuprenorphine*, are excreted in the kidney and can accumulate in patients with renal failure, creating untoward adverse reactions (Hand, Sear, & Uppington, 1990).

Naloxone is an opioid antagonist and is metabolized mainly by conjugation in the liver with little excreted or unchanged in the urine. No dosage alteration is required in renal impairment. However, because of the accumulation of opioid metabolites in renal patients, repeat dosing may be required.

Additional Opioid Information. When patients are unable to take oral pain medication, sublingual, buccal, and rectal routes can be effective with some of the opioids if IV or subcutaneous (SQ) is not an option (Ripamonti & Bruera, 1991).

Adjuvant Analgesics for Neuropathic Pain.
Neuropathic pain unresponsive to opioid therapy often requires the addition of an adjuvant analgesic. Neuropathic adjuvant analgesics include the tricyclic antidepressants (TCA) and anticonvulsants that are well tolerated in CKD patients. Selective serotonin reuptake inhibitors (SSRIs) appear to be less effective as adjuvant analgesics in the management of neuropathic pain despite having fewer adverse reactions. Gabapentin, which has been discussed previously, is widely prescribed for neuropathic pain. Evidence suggests that it is not superior to carbamazepine. In CKD, blood levels of carbamazepine and valproate acid require frequent monitoring. Gabapentin should be started at a low dose (100 mg twice daily) and slowly titrated.

ADVANCE CARE PLANNING
Patient Attitudes

Common understanding of advance care planning (ACP) is that the patient completes an advance directive (AD), which should be a necessity for the dialysis patient. However, only 7% to 35% of this population complete their health care directives (Singer, 1999; Singer, Martin, Lavery, et al., 1998). It has been suggested that the focus might be better placed on assigning a health care proxy (HCP) and having discussion surrounding the issues of ACP with the patient, family, and his or her chosen HCP (Hines, Glover, Babrow, et al., 2001; Holley, Finucane, & Moss, 1989; Holley, Nespor, & Rault, 1992). A user-friendly ACP/AD document such as the "Five Wishes" (www.agingwithdignity.org/5wishes.html) can be used to help guide these important discussions. Completing a standardized form can help set the stage for the patient and his or her designated HCP on what specific issues should be enforced in the event the patient is unable to advocate on his or her own behalf.

A recent survey showed that many nephrologists believe that ADs facilitate decisions to withhold and withdraw dialysis (Moss, Stocking, Sachs, et al., 1993), but a major study of hospitalized nondialysis patients has failed to show a specific benefit of ACP (SUPPORT Principal Investigators, 1995). Small studies in the ESRD population suggest that ADs increase the likelihood of reconciled or

"good" deaths, and they may reduce chances of inappropriate interventions (Cohen, McCue, Germain, et al., 1997; Swartz & Perry, 1993). Patients would rather discuss their ADs with their family more frequently than with their nephrologists (Hines et al., 2001). Patients may view the role of the physician as a provider of clinical information and perhaps fear that the physician will not honor their wishes.

Professional Attitudes

Unfortunately, there is a disconnect between a dialysis patient's desire to have his or her nephrologist discuss end-of-life care (EOL) issues (Cohen et al., 1997; Cohen et al., 2000a) and the nephrologist's views about such discussions (Moss et al., 1993). Dialysis programs vary on which staff member will discuss ACP (Perry, Buck, Newsome, et al., 1995). Staff may often avoid these types of conversations for many reasons, including lack of time and training in this area of health care and the professionals' personal difficulties with the issues surrounding death and dying. Perry, Swartz, Smith-Wheelock, et al. (1996) found that professional caregivers who have experienced a positive death in their personal life are more likely to engage in EOL care discussions with their patients. In a survey of nephrologists and patients, Cohen and associates (1997) found that only 6% of patients completed an AD with their nephrologists and that 84% of patients never discussed their EOL preferences.

A Model Do-Not-Resuscitate Policy

Cardiopulmonary resuscitation (CPR) in dialysis patients is largely ineffective and futile. In one study, 8% of dialysis patients who had a cardiac/pulmonary arrest survived to hospital discharge, and only 3% of patients who were "successfully" resuscitated remained alive 6 months after discharge (Karnik, Young, Lew, et al., 2001). Despite these dire statistics, most dialysis patients want and expect to be offered CPR (Holley et al., 1989). Interesting, however, is the culture that pervades dialysis patients in supporting other patients in their personal right to have their do-not-resuscitate (DNR) request honored even if they do not believe that a DNR is in their own best interest (Moss, Hozayen, King, et al., 2001).

A model DNR policy has been developed by the ESRD Workgroup for Promoting Excellence in EOL Care (www.promotingexcellence.org/content/workgroups.html). These guidelines seek to establish the principles of autonomy in decision making by patients and their families. Practical solutions to the existing barriers that interfere with instituting this policy are offered. To date, it is uncertain if these guidelines and policies have been widely instituted but they have been disseminated and made available to the major dialysis corporations.

END-OF-LIFE AND HOSPICE CARE

Coordinated and continuous palliative care should extend into the end of life. Palliative interventions can promote the emphasis of symptom management and help implement the patient's advance directives. Palliative practices can support a referral to hospice care if needed and help identify emotional and spiritual issues that are important to the patient. Although most patients die in the hospital and the majority of deaths occur in the intensive care unit (ICU), this does not change the fact that most patients would prefer a home death (Cohen et al., 1997; Davison, 2002a). This can be facilitated by good advance care planning, advance directives, and the referral to hospice care.

There are multiple barriers to enrolling dialysis patients into hospice care. If the patient has not discontinued dialysis and the diagnosis for terminal illness is renal failure (or the diagnosis was the cause of the renal failure), the Medicare hospice benefit is required to cover all treatment options including dialysis in patients with a prognosis of 6 months or less. Most Medicare hospice programs find this cost prohibitive. However, if the admitting hospice diagnosis is other than CKD (e.g., cardiomyopathy, malignancy), hospice coverage can be instituted and dialysis is reimbursed under Medicare Part B (hospice care is reimbursed under Medicare Part A). A considerable percentage of CKD patients would benefit from hospice care and should be referred if they choose this type of care. To further add to the confusion, each Medicare fiscal intermediary throughout the country has its own interpretation of the coverage policy and different hospice organizations may make different decisions based on the enrollment of CKD patients' participation. The National Kidney Foundation has published an excellent set of guidelines and check list for end-of-life care (National Kidney Foundation, 1996).

DISCONTINUING DIALYSIS

From 1995 to 1999, 36,000 (17%) of the incident population deaths were preceded by dialysis withdrawal. Although discontinuation rates vary according to geographic region and the practice at individual clinics, dialysis discontinuation has steadily increased. Last year in New England, 32% of ESRD deaths followed treatment cessation (Santacrose, Finklestein, & Klinger, 2003).

When dialysis first became available in the 1960s, it was a scarce resource and patients were selected on the basis of age, lack of co-morbid conditions, and eligibility for transplantation. In 1972 the ESRD amendment to the Social Security Act made dialysis available to a growing population of elderly patients and those with many co-morbid conditions.

In 1986 Neu and Kjellstrand's article on dialysis withdrawal began a debate in the dialysis community concerning the ethics associated with this practice (Neu & Kjellstrand, 1986).

The principles of autonomy and self-determination led to the right to refuse therapy, and this led professionals in the renal community to examine their practices and standards more critically. In 1991 the Institute of Medicine suggested that clinical practice guidelines be developed to evaluate patients for whom the burdens of renal replacement therapy substantially outweighed the benefits. Data are now collected routinely from the ESRD death forms about the use of dialysis withdrawal and the rationale to support dialysis withdrawal. These data are reported by the United States Renal Data System (USRDS) and can be found at www.USRDS.org. Cessation of dialysis has become recognized as being an appropriate decision when the burdens of therapy outweigh the benefits (Cohen & Germain, 2003; Cohen, Germain, & Brennan, 2003; Cohen, McCue, Germain, et al., 1995; Klinger & Finklestein, 2003).

Guidelines for Withholding and Withdrawing Dialysis

The Renal Physicians Association (RPA) and American Society of Nephrology recently published practice guidelines for the withholding and withdrawing of dialysis (Moss, 2001; Renal Physicians Association [RPA] & American Society of Nephrology, 2000). These guidelines identify the challenges that arise when initiating dialysis in severely ill patients with a poor prognosis. The guidelines were developed with a formal evidence-based approach that included an extensive review of the literature. These guidelines can be found on-line at www.renalmd.org and have nine tenets that begin with a patient-physician relationship promoting shared decision making. The decision-making process entails preparatory psychologic consideration and planning, followed by the decision to terminate dialysis, and then further efforts directed at achieving a "good" death.

Bereavement Care

A bereavement program is an important component for palliative practice in the renal patient. An opportunity to grieve as a community is important to the deceased patient's family, the health care team, and surviving patients. Dialysis clinics can institute rituals to acknowledge death. They may include displaying a flower, a copy of the obituary, or a picture of the patient. It is important for surviving patients to come to terms with their own mortality and for staff to take this opportunity to answer questions that are stimulated by the death. An annual memorial service for family, staff, and patients is considered a valuable service for many families of renal patients (Poppel et al., 2003).

Communication Skills

The ability to communicate sensitive issues to patients and family requires a special set of skills by health care professionals (Buckman, 1992). Empathetic listening (Coulehan, Platt, Egener, et al., 2001), understanding cultural differences, and knowing when the individual is ready to contemplate difficult decisions are critical components (Levinson, Cohen, Brady, et al., 2001).

FUTURE RESEARCH

We have only begun to rigorously study palliative care issues in CKD. Greater understanding of the incidence, cause, and treatment of common symptoms in these patients is greatly needed. More studies into the pharmokinetics, pharmacodynamics, and metabolism of specific medications used for symptom relief in CKD are required. The effectiveness of different interventions, such as bereavement services, advance care planning, and dialysis withdrawal needs to be studied. Only through such endeavors will the promise of a better life and death experience for these patients be realized.

Objective Questions

1. The life expectancy of an 80-year-old dialysis patient with CHF is:

    a. 1 month.
    b. 6 months.
    c. 2 years.
    d. 5 years.

2. Patients who choose to stop dialysis survive on the average of:

    a. 8 days.
    b. 2 weeks.
    c. 3 weeks.
    d. 4 weeks.

3. Dialysis withdrawal:

    a. Is associated with significant fluid gains and therefore fluid intake should be restricted.
    b. Requires that opioid pain medicine not be given because of decreased renal clearance.
    c. Is considered euthanasia and is not ethical practice.
    d. Takes place in 20% of all deaths in dialysis patients.

4. The following medication should not be given because of toxic metabolites that can accumulate in renal patients:

    a. Meperidine.
    b. Metoclopramide.

Case Study

P.A., a 92-year-old retired Italian-American businessman, presented 5 years ago with a glomerular filtration rate (GFR) of 14 ml/min. He has had a positive history of ischemic cardiomyopathy with a left ventricular ejection fraction of 25%. His chief complaint bringing him to the clinic is distressing pruritus. Despite his previous trial of antihistamines and moisturizing creams, he cannot sleep because of excessive itching. UVB light treatments were initiated and ultimately provided P.A. with some relief. Also at the time of presentation in the clinic, erythropoietin was prescribed for his new complaint of fatigue; his hemoglobin was 9 gm/dl. He began hemodialysis 4 years prior because his GFR dropped below 10 ml/min.

Throughout the past 4 years of hemodialysis, P.A. has experienced restless legs syndrome, post-dialysis hypotension, and fatigue, particularly 24 hours post-dialysis. Recently, severe back pain secondary to osteoarthritis has been particularly bothersome for him and interfering with his daily walks around the neighborhood. His symptoms have been optimally controlled with palliative interventions, and he has remained at home with his wife without hospital admissions. Shortly after his clinic visit, he fell at home, which required a brief hospitalization followed by transfer to a rehabilitation facility.

Since the beginning of hemodialysis, P.A., his wife, and his two daughters have all participated in conversations regarding dialysis withdrawal. This conversation was again initiated during his recent hospitalization. P.A. and his family have decided to remain on dialysis, despite his congestive heart failure and a left ventricular ejection fraction (LVEF) of less than 20%.

One week after the discussion on dialysis withdrawal, P.A. announced he had enough and decided to stop dialysis. He was discharged home with hospice care and died 4 days later. His wife, daughters, and a visiting nephrologist were present during his death. His symptoms were well managed and just minutes before his death, he was reminiscing about his life and looking at old photographs. At the moment of his death he was holding the nephrologist's hand and he appeared to drift off to sleep. There was no perceptible transition between life and death as he quietly slipped away.

   c. Hydromorphone.

   d. Chlorpromazine.

5. The following statement is true:

   a. Because dialysis is a life-sustaining treatment, do-not-resuscitate (DNR) orders are not in effect during a dialysis session.

   b. The most common symptom for dialysis patients is fatigue.

   c. Pruritus is the most common symptom in dialysis patients.

   d. In general, a dialysis patient will require half of the usual dose of opioids because of poor renal clearance of these drugs.

6. When queried, most dialysis patients would prefer to die:

   a. At home.

   b. In an ICU.

   c. On a hospital ward.

   d. In a nursing home.

7. The majority of dialysis patients die:

   a. At home.

   b. In an ICU.

   c. On a hospital ward.

   d. In a nursing home.

8. All the following statements are true EXCEPT:

   a. The Medicare hospice benefit provides services to dialysis patients who discontinue therapy.

   b. The Medicare hospice benefit provides reimbursement for services for patients with a diagnosis of severe cardiomyopathy (ejection fraction of 10%) who do not stop dialysis.

c. The Medicare hospice benefit provides reimbursement for patients who do not discontinue dialysis and have a prognosis of 6 months or less.

d. The Medicare hospice benefit provides reimbursement for a pancreatic cancer patient who continues with peritoneal dialysis.

9. The strongest prognostic factor for survival in dialysis patients is:

a. Age.

b. Race.

c. Congestive heart failure (CHF).

d. Malnutrition.

10. Most dialysis patients want to discuss advance directives with their:

a. Nephrologist.

b. Social worker.

c. Dialysis nurse.

d. Family.

REFERENCES

Ahmad, S., Robertson, H.T., Golpher, T.A., et al. (1990). Multicenter trial of L-carnitine in maintenance hemodialysis patients: Clinical and biochemical effects. *Kidney Int, 38*(5), 912.

Aronoff, G.R., Berns, J.S., Brier, M.E., et al. (1999). *Drug prescribing in renal failure* (4th ed.). Philadelphia: American College of Physicians.

Ashmore, S.D., Jones, C.H., Newstead, C.G., et al. (2000). Ondansetron therapy for uremic pruritus in hemodialysis patients. *Am J Kidney Dis, 35*, 827-831.

Balaskas, E.V., Bamihas, G.I., Karamouzis, M., et al. (1998). Histamine and serotonin in uremic pruritus: Effect of ondansetron in CAPD-pruritus patients. *Nephron, 78*, 395-402.

Blachley, J.D., Blankenship, M., Menter, A., et al. (1985). Uremic pruritus: Skin divalent ion content and response to ultraviolet therapy. *Am J Kidney Dis, 5*(5), 237.

Boccanfuso, J.A., Hutton, M., & McAllister, B. (2000). The effects of megestrol acetate on nutritional parameters in a dialysis population, *J Ren Nutr, 10*, 36.

Bower, S. (1982). Plasma protein binding of fentanyl: The effect of hyperlipoproteinemia and chronic renal failure. *J Pharm Pharmacol, 34*, 102-106.

Brass, E., Adler, M., Sietsema, M., et al. (2001). Intravenous L-Carnitine increases plasma carnitine, reduces fatigue, and may preserve exercise capacity in hemodialysis patients, *Am J Kidney Dis, 37*, 1018.

Buckman, R. (1992). *How to break bad news: A guide for health care professionals.* Baltimore: Johns Hopkins University.

Callaghan, N. (1966). Restless legs syndrome in uremic neuropathy. *Neurology, 16*, 359.

Canzanello, B.J., & Burkart, J.M. (1992). Hemodialysis associated muscle cramps. *Semin Dial, 5*, 299.

Chauvin, M., Sandouk, P., Scherrmann, J.M., et al. (1987). Morphine pharmacokinetics in renal failure. *Anesthesiology, 66*, 327-331.

Cohen, L.M., & Germain, M.J. (2003). Palliative and supportive care. In H. Brady & C. Wilcox (Eds.), *Therapy of nephrology and hypertension: A companion to Brenner's The Kidney* (2nd ed., pp. 753-756). Orlando, Fla.: Harcourt.

Cohen, L.M., Germain, M., & Brennan, M. (2003). End-stage renal disease and discontinuation of dialysis. In R.S. Morrison, D.E. Meier, & C.F. Capello (Eds.), *Geriatric palliative care* (pp. 192-202). London: Oxford University Press.

Cohen, L.M., Germain, M., Poppel, D.M., et al. (2000a). Dialysis discontinuation and palliative care. *Am J Kidney Dis, 36*, 140-144.

Cohen, L.M., Germain, M., Poppel, D.M., et al. (2000b). Dying well after discontinuing the life-support treatment of dialysis. *Arch Intern Med, 160*, 2513-2518.

Cohen, L.M., Germain, M.J., & Tessier, E.G. (2003). Neuropsychiatric complications and psychopharmacology of end-stage renal disease. In H. Brady & C. Wilcox (Eds.), *Therapy of nephrology and hypertension: A companion to Brenner's The Kidney* (2nd ed., pp. 731-746). Orlando, Fla.: Harcourt.

Cohen, L.M., McCue, J., Germain, M., et al. (1995). Dialysis discontinuation: A "good" death? *Arch Intern Med, 155*, 42-47.

Cohen, L.M., McCue, J.D., Germain, M., et al. (1997). Denying the dying: Advance directives and dialysis discontinuation. *Psychosomatics, 38*, 27-34.

Cohen, L.M., Poppel, D.M., Cohen, G.M., et al. (2001). A very good death: Measuring quality of dying in end-stage renal disease. *J Palliat Med, 4*, 167-172.

Collado-Seidel, V., Kohnen, R., Samtleben, W., et al. (1998). Clinical and biochemical findings in uremic patients with and without restless legs syndrome. *Am J Kidney Dis, 31*, 132.

Coulehan, J.L., Platt, F.W., & Egener, B., et al. (2001)."Let me see if I have that right...": Words that help build empathy. *Ann Intern Med, 135*, 221-227.

Covington, E.C. (1998). Anticonvulsants for neuropathic pain and detoxification. *Cleve Clin J Med, 65*, 121.

Cruz, D.N., Mahnensmith, R.L., & Perazella, M.A. (1997). Intradialytic hypotension: Is midodrine beneficial in symptomatic hemodialysis patients? *Am J Kidney Dis, 30*, 772.

Daugirdas, J.T. (2000). Acute hemodialysis prescription. In J.T. Daugirdas & T.S. Ing (Eds.), *Handbook of dialysis* (3rd ed., pp. 192-220). Boston: Little, Brown.

Davison, S.N. (2002a). Pain in hemodialysis patients: Prevalence, etiology, severity, and analgesic use. *J Am Soc Nephrol, 13*, 587A.

Davison, S.N. (2002b). Quality end-of-life care in dialysis units. *Semin Dial, 15*, 41-44.

Davison, S.N., & Chater, S. (2001). Severe pain in hemodialysis patients requiring palliative care. *J Am Soc Nephrol, 322A.

De Marchi, S., Ceddhin, E., Villaltgra, D., et al. (1992). Relief of pruritus and decreases in plasma histamine concentrations during erythropoietin therapy in patients with uremia. *N Engl J Med, 326*, 969.

Dheenan, S., Venkatesan, J., Grubb, B.P., et al. (1998). Effect of sertraline hydrochloride on dialysis hypotension. *Am J Kidney Dis, 31*(4), 624-630.

Eknoyan, G., Latos, D., & Linberg, J. (2003). Practice recommendations for the use of L-carnitine in dialysis-related carnitine disorder. National Kidney Foundation Carnitine Consensus Conference. *Am J Kidney Dis, 41*(4), 868-876.

Flynn, J.J., Mitchell, M.C., Caruso, F.S., et al. (1996). Midodrine treatment for patients with hemodialysis hypotension. *Clin Nephrol, 45,* 261.

Francos, G., Kauh, V., & Grittlen, S. (1991). Elevated plasma histamine in chronic uremia: Effects of ketotifen on pruritus. *Int J Dermatol, 30,* 884.

Fraser, C.L., & Arieff, A.I. (1988). Nervous system complications in uremia. *Ann Intern Med, 109*(2), 143.

Germain, M.J., & Cohen, L. (2001). Supportive care for patients with renal disease: A time for action. *Am J Kidney Dis, 38,* 884-886.

Germain, M.J., McCarthy, S., Swartz, R., et al. (in press). Symptom assessment and treatment. In J. Chambers, E. Brown, & M. Germain (Eds.), *Supportive care for the renal patient.* New York: Oxford University Press.

Giovanetti, S., Barsotti, G., & Cupisti, A. (1995). Oral activated charcoal in patients with uremic pruritus. *Nephron, 70,* 193.

Goodling, K.A., & Eisinger, R.P. (1982). Acute therapy of hemodialysis-related muscle cramps. *Am J Kidney Dis, 2*(2), 287-288.

Green, J.A., Green, C.R., & Minott, S.D. (2000). Calciphylaxis treated with neurolytic lumbar sympathetic block: Case report and review of the literature. *Reg Anesth Pain Med, 25,* 310-312.

Hand, C.W., Sear, J.R., & Uppington, J. (1990). Buprenorphine disposition in patients with renal impairment: Single and continuous dosing, with special reference to metabolites. *Br J Anaesth, 64,* 276-282.

Hening, W.A. (1997). Therapeutic approaches to restless legs syndrome and periodic limb movement disorder. *Hospital Medicine, 33,* 135.

Hines, S.C., Glover, J.J., Babrow, A.S., et al. (2001). Improving advance care planning by accommodating family preferences. *J Palliat Med, 4,* 481-489.

Hiroshige, K., Kabashima, N., Takasugi, M., et al. (1995). Optimal dialysis improves uremic pruritus. *Am J Kidney Dis, 25,* 413-419.

Holley, J.L., Finucane, T.E., & Moss, A.H. (1989). Dialysis patients' attitudes about cardiopulmonary resuscitation and stopping dialysis. *Am J Nephrol, 9,* 245-251.

Holley, J.L., Nespor, S., & Rault, R.A. (1992). Comparison of reported sleep disorders in patients on chronic hemodialysis and continuous peritoneal dialysis. *Am J Kidney Dis, 19*(2), 156.

Karnik, J.A., Young, B.S., Lew, N.L., et al. (2001). Cardiac arrest and sudden death in dialysis units. *Kidney Int, 60,* 350-357.

Kimmel, P.L., Miller, G., & Mendelson, W.B. (1989). Sleep apnea in chronic renal disease. *Am J Med, 86,* 308.

Klinger, A., & Finklestein, F. (2003). Which patient to choose to stop dialysis? *Nephrol Dial Transplant, 18,* 869-871.

Lee, M.A., Leng, M.E., & Tiernan, E.J. (2001). Retrospective study of the use of hydromorphone in palliative care patients with normal and abnormal urea and creatinine. *Palliat Med, 15,* 26-34.

Levinson, W., Cohen, M.S., Brady, D., et al. (2001). To change or not to change: "Sounds like you have a dilemma." *Ann Int Med, 135,* 386-391.

Lien, Y.H., & Ruffenach, S.J. (1996). Low dose megestrol increases serum albumin in malnourished dialysis patients. *Int J Artif Organs, 19,* 147.

Maggiore, Q., Pizzarelli, F., Santoro, A., et al. (2002). The effects of control of thermal balance on vascular stability in hemodialysis patients: Results of the European randomized clinical trial. *Am J Kidney Dis, 40*(2), 280-290.

Massry, S.G., Popovtzer, M.M., Coburn, J.W., et al. (1968). Intractable pruritus as a manifestation of secondary hyperparathyroidism in uremia. *N Engl J Med, 279,* 697.

Mathur, R.V., Shortland, J.R., & El Nahas, A.M. (2001). Calciphylaxis. *Postgrad Med J, 77,* 557-561.

Mercadante, S., Caligara, M,, Sapio, M., et al. (1997). Subcutaneous fentanyl infusion in a patient with bowel obstruction and renal failure. *J Pain Symptom Manage, 13,* 241-244.

Merkus, M.P., Jager, K.J., Dekker, F.W., et al. (1999). Physical symptoms and quality of life in patient on chronic dialysis: Results of the Netherlands cooperative study on adequacy of dialysis (NECOSAD). *Nephrol Dial Transplant, 14,* 1163-1170.

Miller, L.J. (1993). Oral pilocarpine for radiation-induced xerostomia. *Cancer Bull, 45,* 549.

Moss, A.H. (2001). Shared decision-making in dialysis: The new RPA/ASN guideline on appropriate initiation and withdrawal of treatment. (Clinical conference; journal article). *Am J Kidney Dis, 37*(5), 1081-1091.

Moss, A.H., Hozayen, O., King, K., et al. (2001). Attitudes of patients toward cardiopulmonary resuscitation in the dialysis unit. *Am J Kidney Dis, 38,* 847-852.

Moss, A.H., Stocking, C.B., Sachs, G.A., et al. (1993). Variation in the attitudes of dialysis unit medical directors toward decisions to withhold and withdraw dialysis. *J Am Soc Nephrol, 4,* 229-234.

National Kidney Foundation. (1996). *Initiation or withdrawal of dialysis in end stage renal disease: Guidelines for the health care team.* New York: Author.

Neu, S., & Kjellstrand, C.M. (1986). Stopping long-term dialysis: An empirical study of withdrawal of life-supporting treatment. *N Engl J Med, 314,* 14-20.

Pauli-Magnus, C., Hofmann, U., Mikus, G., et al. (1999). Pharmacokinetics of morphine and its glucuronides following intravenous administration of morphine in patients undergoing continuous ambulatory peritoneal dialysis. *Nephrol Dial Transplant, 14,* 903-909.

Peer, G., Kivity, S., Agami, O., et al. (1996). Randomized crossover trial of naltrexone in uremic pruritus. *Lancet, 348,* 1552.

Perazella, M.A. (2001). Pharmacologic options available to treat symptomatic intradialytic hypotension. *Am J Kidney Dis, 38*(4 Suppl. 4), S26-36. Review.

Perry, E., Buck, C., Newsome, J., et al. (1995). Dialysis staff influence patients in formulating their advance directives. *Am J Kidney Dis, 25,* 262-268.

Perry, E, Swartz, R, Smith-Wheelock, L., et al. (1996). Why is it difficult for staff to discuss advance directives with chronic dialysis patients? *J Am Soc Nephrol, 7*(10), 2160-2168.

Poppel, D.M., Cohen, L.M., & Germain, M.J. (2003). The renal palliative care initiative. *J Palliat Med, 6,* 321-326.

Portenoy, R.K. (1993). Adjuvant analgesics in pain management. In D. Doyle, G.W. Hanks, & N. MacDonald (Eds.), *Oxford textbook of palliative medicine* (pp. 187-203). New York: Oxford University Press.

Renal Physicians Association (RPA), & American Society of Nephrology. (2000). *Shared decision-making in the appropriate initiation of and withdrawal from dialysis* (pp. 41-43). Washington, D.C.: RPA.

Riley, S., Rutherford, S., & Rutherford, P.A. (1997). Low carnitine levels in hemodialysis patients: Relationship with functional activity status and intra-dialytic hypotension. *Clin Nephrol, 48,* 3.

Ripamonti, C., & Bruera, E. (1991). Rectal, buccal, and sublingual narcotics for the management of cancer pain. *J Palliat Care, 7*(1), 30-35.

Robertson, H., Kaky, N., Gurthrie, M., et al. (1990). Recombinant erythropoietin improves exercise capacity in anemic hemodialysis patients, *Am J Kidney Dis, 4,* 325.

Robertson, K., & Mueller, B. (1996). Uremic pruritus. *Am J Health Syst Pharm, 53,* 2159.

Roger, S.D., Harris, D.C.H., & Stewart, J.H. (1991). Possible relation between restless legs and anemia in renal dialysis patients. *Lancet, 337,* 1551.

Rose, M.A., & Kam, P.C. (2002). Gabapentin pharmacology and its use in pain management. *Anaesthesia, 158,* 451.

Santacrose, S., Finklestein, F., & Klinger, A. (2003). *Dialysis withdrawal in a large peritoneal dialysis population.* Poster presentation at the ESRD Network of New England. 10/2/2003.

Santoro, A., Mancini, E., & Basile, C. (2002). Blood volume controlled hemodialysis in hypotension-prone patients: A randomized, multicenter controlled trial. *Kidney Int, 62*(3), 1034-1045.

Sawe, J., & Odar-Cederlof, I. (1987). Kinetics of morphine in patients with renal failure. *Eur J Clin Pharmacol, 32,* 377-382.

Schenck, C.H., & Mahowald, M.W. (1996). Long-term, nightly benzodiazepine treatment of injurious parasomnias and other disorders of disrupted nocturnal sleep in 170 adults. *Am J Med, 100,* 333.

Silber, M.H., Shepart, J.W. Jr., & Wisbey, J.A. (1997). Pergolide in the management of restless legs syndrome: An extended study. *Sleep, 20*(1), 878.

Silva, S.R.B., Vianna, P.C.F, Lagon, N.V., et al. (1994). Thalidomide for the treatment of uremic pruritus: A crossover randomized double-blind trial. *Nephron, 67,* 270-274.

Silverberg, D., Ianina, A., & Reisin, E., (1997). Cholestyramine in uremic pruritus. *Br Med J, 1,* 752.

Singer, P.A. (1999). Advance care planning in dialysis. *Am J Kidney Dis, 33,* 980-991.

Singer, P.A., Martin, D.K., Lavery, J.V., et al. (1998). Reconceptualizing advance care planning from the patient's perspective. *Arch Int Med, 158,* 879-884.

Sklar, A., Newman, N., Scott, R., et al. (1999). Identification of factors responsible for postdialysis fatigue. *Am J Kidney Dis, 34,* 464.

Sklar, A, Riesenberg, L.A., Silber, A.K., et al. (1996). Postdialysis fatigue. *Am J Kidney Dis, 28,* 732.

Steinman, T.I. (2000). Pain management in polycystic kidney disease. *Am J Kidney Dis, 35,* 770-772.

Straver, B., De Vries, P.M., Donker, A.J., et al. (2002). The effect of profiled hemodialysis on intradialytic hemodynamics when a proper sodium balance is applied. *Blood Purif, 20*(4), 364-369.

Swartz, R.D., & Perry, E. (1993). Advance directives are associated with "good deaths" in chronic dialysis patients. *J Am Soc Nephrol, 3,* 1623-1630.

SUPPORT Principal Investigators. (1995). A controlled trial to improve care for seriously ill hospitalized patients (SUPPORT). *J Am Med Assoc, 274,* 1591-1598.

Takaki, J., Nishi, R., Nangaku, M., et al. (2003). Clinical and psychological aspects of restless legs syndrome in uremic patients on hemodialysis. *Am J Kidney Dis, 41*(4), 833-839.

Tapia, L. Cheigh, H., & David, D. (1977). Pruritus in dialysis patients treated with parenteral lidocaine. *N Eng J Med, 296*(5), 261.

Tarng, D.C., Cho, Y.L., Liu, H.N., et al. (1996). Hemodialysis-related pruritus: A double-blind, placebo-controlled, crossover study of capsaicin 0.025% cream. *Nephron, 72*(2), 617.

Tattersall, J.E., Cramp, M., Shannon, M., et al. (1992). Rapid high flux dialysis can cure uremic peripheral neuropathy. *Nephrol Dial Transplant, 7,* 539.

Thorp, M.L., Morris, C.D., & Bagby, S.P. (2001). A crossover study of gabapentin in treatment of restless legs syndrome among hemodialysis patients. *Am J Kidney Dis, 38,* 104.

Valderrqabano, F., Jofre, R., & Lopez-Gomez, J.M. (2001). Quality of life in end-stage renal disease patients. *Am J Kidney Dis, 38,* 443-464.

Von Scheele, C., & Kempe, V. (1990). Long-term effect of dopaminergic drugs in restless legs: A 2-year follow-up. *Arch Neurol, 47,* 1223.

Vreman, H.F., Venter, C., Leegwater, J., et al. (1980). Taste, smell and zinc metabolism in patients with chronic renal failure. *Nephron, 26,* 163.

Wagner, M.L., Walters, A.S., Coleman, R.G., et al. (1996). Randomized, double-blind, placebo-controlled study of clonidine in restless legs syndrome. *Sleep, 19*(1), 52.

Walker, S., Fine, A., & Kryger, M.H. (1995). Sleep complaints are common in a dialysis unit. *Am J Kidney Dis, 28,* 372.

Walters, A.S., Wagner, M.L., Hening, W.A., et al. (1993). Successful treatment of the idiopathic restless legs syndrome in a randomized double-blind trial of oxycodone versus placebo. *Sleep, 16*(32), 82.

Weisbord, S.D., Carmody, S.S., Bruns, F.J., et al. (2003). Symptom burden, quality-of-life, advance care planning, and the potential value of palliative care in severely ill hemodialysis patients. *Nephrol Dial Transplant, 18,* 1345-1352.

Wilmer, W.A., & Magro, C.M. (2002). Calciphylaxis: Emerging concepts in prevention, diagnosis, and treatment. *Semin Dial, 15,* 172-186.

Winkelman, J.W., Cherow, G.M., & Lazarus, J.M. (1996). Restless legs syndrome in end-stage renal disease. *Am J Kidney Dis, 28,* 372.

CHAPTER 9

Oncology

Mary Magee Gullatte
Roberta Kaplow
Debra E. Heidrich

OBJECTIVES

After the completion of this chapter, the reader should be able to:

1. Describe the pathophysiology of advanced malignancies and their associated symptomatology.
2. Utilize prognostic indicators in identifying patients with advanced malignancy who can benefit from palliative intervention.
3. Review oncologic emergencies and their management.
4. Describe common symptoms that accompany advanced malignancies and their management.

INTRODUCTION

Cancer is the second leading cause of mortality in the United States (American Cancer Society [ACS], 2004). Illustrated in Tables 9-1 and 9-2 are the top five cancer diagnoses for adult men and women and mortality rates in the United States for the year 2004. The estimated number of patients who will have cancer in the year 2004 in the United States identified by the American Cancer Society (ACS) is 1,368,030, with an expected mortality of 563,700. The National Cancer Institute (NCI) estimated that 8.9 million Americans were living with a diagnosis of cancer in January 1999 (ACS, 2003a). The 5-year relative survival rate for all cancers is 62%. This percentage represents individuals living with disease. Cancer survivors are defined to include any person with a diagnosis or history of cancer regardless of stage, treatment, recovery, or cure. The ACS's goal is to reduce the cancer mortality by the year

The authors would like to acknowledge the work done by Valarie Pompey, MS, APRN, BC-PCM, OCN, on this chapter.

2015. There continues to be an unacceptably high mortality associated with almost all malignancies.

Palliative medicine includes a broad multidiscipline subspecialty, which encompasses the physical, social, psychologic, and spiritual care of supporting patients and their families throughout the trajectory of disease (Hightower & Vaughn, 2003). This chapter covers advanced cancers and prognostic indicators, oncologic emergencies, common symptoms, and their management.

Cancer is not a disease just of the elderly; however, the elderly do have a higher incidence of cancer. Cancer has been considered a disease of aging. Yet the burden of cancer frequency in the elderly varies by type and incidence. LaVecchia, Lucchini, Negri, et al. (2001) reported that pancreatic cancer mortality rates increased in the elderly of both sexes in Western Europe and Japan, whereas it has decreased in the United States. However, female breast cancer mortality in the elderly has declined over the past decade by 8% in the United States and 3% in Western Europe but has increased in Eastern Europe and Japan (LaVecchia et al., 2001).

THE COST OF CANCER

The costs associated with cancer are staggering. Cancer can strike those in the prime of life during their productive years, which has an impact on the national workforce. In 2002 the NCI estimated that the economic impact of cancer prevention, screening, and detection was in excess of $171 billion independent of treatment (ACS, 2003a).

Table 9-3 shows the national cancer treatment expenditures for 1963 through 1995. Cancer treatment accounted for about $41 billion in 1995. This is just under 5% of the total U.S. spending for

Table **9-1**　ESTIMATED NEW CANCER CASES BY SITE AND BY SEX, 2004

Cancer Site	Estimated Cases	Cancer Site	Estimated Cases
Male		Female	
Prostate	230,110 (33%)	Breast	215,990 (32%)
Lung/Bronchus	93,110 (13%)	Lung/Bronchus	80,660 (12%)
Colon/Rectum	73,620 (11%)	Colon/Rectum	73,320 (11%)
Urinary Bladder	44,620 (6%)	Uterine Corpus	40,320 (6%)
Melanoma of Skin	29,900 (4%)	Ovary	25,580 (4%)

Data from Jemal A., Tiwari, R.C., Murray, T., et al. (2004). Cancer statistics. *CA Cancer J Clin, 54*(1), 9-11.

Table **9-2**　ESTIMATED CANCER DEATHS BY SITE AND BY SEX, 2004

Cancer Site	Estimated Cases	Cancer Site	Estimated Cases
Male		Female	
Lung/Bronchus	91,930 (33%)	Lung/Bronchus	68,510 (25%)
Prostate	29,900 (10%)	Breast	40,110 (15%)
Colon/Rectum	28,320 (10%)	Colon/Rectum	28,410 (10%)
Pancreas	15,440 (5%)	Pancreas	15,830 (6%)
Non-Hodgkin's lymphoma	10,390 (4%)	Ovary	16,090 (6%)

Data from Jemal A., Tiwari, R.C., Murray, T., et al. (2004). Cancer statistics. *CA Cancer J Clin, 54*(1), 9-11.

Table **9-3**　NATIONAL CANCER TREATMENT EXPENDITURES IN BILLIONS OF DOLLARS, 1963-1995

Year	Cancer Treatment Spending (billions)	Total Health Care Spending (billions)	% of Cancer Treatment Spending to Total
1963	$ 1.3	$ 29.4	4.4%
1972	$ 3.9	$ 78.0	5.0%
1980	$13.1	$217.0	6.0%
1985	$18.1	$376.4	4.8%
1990	$27.5	$614.7	4.5%
1995	$41.2	$879.3	4.7%

Data from Brown, M.L., Lipscomb, J., & Snyder, C. (2001). The burden of illness of cancer: Economic cost and quality of life. *Annu Rev Public Health, 22,* 91-113; *Cancer Progress Report 2001*(Table 1, p. 59). www.progressreport.cancer.gov/; National Cancer Institute, National Institutes of Health, U.S. Dept. of Health and Human Services.

medical treatment (National Cancer Institute [NCI], 2001).

The cost associated with palliative treatment continues to escalate for both Medicare and non-Medicare expenditures. While inpatient expenditures constitute a large portion of end-of-life costs, the use of palliative services and hospice by terminally ill patients has declined over the past 2 decades (Garber, MaCurdy, & McClellan, 1999; Lubitz & Riley, 1993; Scitovsky, 1994; Temkin-Greener, Meiners, Petty, et al., 1992). Of the inpatient care expenditure, 51% has been found to occur in the final month of life (Hoover, Crystal, Kumar, et al., 2002).

Improved utilization of palliative services for advanced malignancies that are integrated throughout the course of disease could be expected to have a significant impact on reducing the overall cost of care. Are early assessment of symptoms and prompt intervention by clinicians could also have a positive impact on quality of life and reduce health care expenditures for patients with advanced malignancies.

CULTURALLY COMPETENT PALLIATIVE PRACTICES

Cultural competence refers to being sensitive and responsive to issues related to culture, race, ethnicity, gender, age, socioeconomic status, and sexual orientation (Oncology Nursing Society [ONS], 1994). Cultural competence requires the translation of cultural awareness into appropriate behaviors.

A patient's worldview combines culture; race; religious, spiritual orientation; and social and ethnic beliefs and practices. These factors coupled with the family structure are important considerations when planning and delivering palliative interventions. Living with cancer takes on different meanings for patients based on their sociocultural and spiritual beliefs and practices. The astute, compassionate health care professional can include the patient and family in the decision making and advance care planning.

The heightened awareness around culturally appropriate care prompts greater exploration into ways of tailoring the needs of individualized care (Kavanagh & Kennedy, 1992). The Oncology Nursing Society (ONS) has published guidelines

for cultural competence. A goal when providing competent care is to establish rapport and build trust with the patient and family (ONS, 1999). Although it is important that the practitioner consider cultural relevance, treatment decisions should be based on multifactorial issues—not just age and culture.

Age-appropriate considerations of care should also be followed since most patients with cancer, as mentioned, are older. With guidance from the Administration on Aging, the Department of Health and Human Services developed several focused areas for the care of the elderly population. Reducing the prevalence of diseases such as arthritis, osteoporosis, cancer, diabetes, and kidney disease is the focus of diagnostic concern for the elderly (*Healthy People 2010*). Often the elderly will experience greater toxicity from chemotherapy and other treatment modalities because of co-morbid conditions, which are consequences of aging (*Healthy People 2010*). Individual practitioners should evaluate each patient as an individual by applying a multidimensional approach and making appropriate treatment decisions in collaboration with the patient and the family. Often elderly patients are under-treated as a result of age and other co-morbidities. This has been found in the management of lung, colorectal, and breast carcinomas and lymphomas (Dale, 2003). Chemotherapy doses should be adjusted based on organ function and measured by pharmacokinetics and liver and kidney function rather than age. Myelosuppression is the most severe complication of age and a risk factor for developing neutropenia, which may lead physicians to under-dose chemotherapy in treating older cancer patients (Balducci, 2003).

HEALTH DISPARITIES

Despite some overall declines in mortality and morbidity for some cancers, the incidence of cancer among minority groups and the poor is increasing (Freeman, 2004). In addition, the Institute of Medicine (IOM) published a study, *The Unequal Burden of Cancer*, which found that minorities and the poor are underrepresented in NCI-funded clinical trials (Stinson, 2000). There disparities are explained by an advanced stage of disease at the time of diagnosis. Additional risk factors include lifestyle choices, such as diet; racial and ethnic disparities; and access to health care (Ward, Jemal, Cokkinides, et al., 2004). Breast cancer in African-American women is not as prevalent as in Caucasian women, yet they are more likely to die from the disease once it is detected (Ross, 2000). This may reflect unique tumor biology in African-Americans as well as a delay in diagnosis. This finding has implications for the use of palliative medicine as minority groups may be overrepresented in the advanced cancer population. Drawing inferences from the IOM report and general medical services and practice, it is possible that the quality of care for minorities and poor patients with advanced malignancies is inadequate.

CELLULAR PATHOPHYSIOLOGY OF ADVANCED CANCER

Cancer is an abnormal and uncontrolled growth of cells triggered by genetic mutations. These cells lose their ability to modulate growth differentiation and cellular cohesion and down-regulate cell growth. Abnormal clones of cells proliferate in the absence of cell cycle control. Loss of adhesion to cells permits these cells to spread outside their site of origin through lymphatics and blood vessels. In addition, cancer cells develop the ability to form new blood vessels (angiogenesis), which permits the growth of large metastasis. Metastatic spread and local invasion are the hallmarks of this life-threatening disease. Table 9-4 depicts the tumor-host interactions

Table **9-4** TUMOR HOST INTERACTION DURING THE METASTATIC CASCADE

Tumor	Interaction
1. Tumor initiation	Carcinogenic insult, oncogene activation or depression, chromosome rearrangement
2. Promotion and progression	Karyotypic, genetic, and epigenetic instability, gene amplification, promotion-associated genes and growth factors, mutation or loss of suppressor gene products
3. Uncontrolled proliferation	Autocrine growth factors or their receptors, receptors or most hormones, such as estrogens
4. Angiogenesis	Multiple angiogenesis factors, including known growth factors
5. Invasion of local tissues, blood, and lymphatic vessels	Serum chemoattractants, autocrine motility factors, attachments receptors; degradative enzymes, loss of expression of proteinase inhibitors
6. Vulcrating tumor cell arrest and extravasation:	Tumor cell homotypic or stereotypic aggression
a. adherence to endothelium	Tumor cell interaction with fibrin, platelets, and clotting factors, adhesion to RGN-type receptors
b. retraction of endothelium	Platelet factors, tumor cell factors
c. adhesion to basement membrane	Receptors for laminin, thrombospondin, and types of IV collagen
d. dissolution of basement membrane	Metalloproteinases, serine proteinases, herapinase, cathepsin
e. locomotion	Autocrine motility factors, chemotaxis factors
7. Colony formation at secondary site	Receptors for local tissue growth factor, angiogenesis factors, mutation, or loss of metastasis suppressor genes
8. Evasion of host defenses and resistance to therapy	Resistance to killing by host macrophage, natural killer cells, and activated T cells, failure to express or block tumor-specific antigens; amplification of drug-resistant genes

Data from Liotta, L.A., & Kohn, E.C. (2000). Invasion and metastases. In R.C. Bast, D.W. Kufe, R.E. Pollock, et al., *Cancer medicine* (5th ed., p. 122). Hamilton, Ontario Canada: B.C. Decker.

during the metastatic cascade. During unregulated growth, the cancer cells can generate their own blood supply. Angiogenesis utilizes vascular endothelial growth factor (VEGF) to cause young endothelial cells to migrate into new, small metastatic deposits (Tortorice, 2003).

The role of angiogenesis in malignant cell growth is of particular interest to cancer researchers because it is believed to hold the key to limiting cancer cell growth. Experimental and clinical evidence suggests that targeting angiogenesis will interrupt the blood flow to the tumor, thereby reducing tumor burden; this is referred to as *antiangiogenic therapy* (Folkman, 2000). Vascular endothelial growth factor and basic fibroblast growth factor (bFGF) are two potent angiogenic factors targeted in new drug development studies (Weidner & Folkman, 1997). Blocking angiogenesis can induce apoptosis of normal cells and promote tumor regression (Manley, Bold, Bruggen, et al., 2004; Mukhopadhyay & Datta, 2004; Verheul & Pimedo, 2003).

Another neoplastic process that prompts metastatic spread of cancer is stromal proteolysis (extracellular matrix and degradation). This process is accomplished by several matrix metalloproteinase (MMP) enzymes that are catalytic in the presence of zinc and calcium (Brooks, Stromblad, & Sanders, 1996). Degradation of extracellular matrix by MMPs promotes tumor invasion and metastasis (Ramnath & Creaven, 2004). The direct role of these enzymes in the treatment of malignant spread is currently under investigation.

Malignant tumors can arise from nearly every body tissue. A malignant transformation is the end result of an irreversible genetic mutation (or mutations) that occurs in promoter genes or structural genetic transformation into a cancer (Mathlouthi, Aberl, Schug, et al., 2003). Regulator genes that govern cellular division and processes may be influenced in cancer by hypermethylation, which prevents gene DNA expression (Herman & Baylin, 2003). Malignant transformation leads to direct extension and implantation into adjacent tissues and organs and vascular and/or lymphatic invasion. Other means of spreading are via peritoneal seeding. Peritoneal seeding is the implantation of

malignant cells on serosal surfaces as a result of a contiguous spread from the primary site; this usually arises within the abdominal or peritoneal cavity. Seeding may occur during an operative procedure for debulking the primary tumor or as a result of the intrinsic biology of the cancer. Once within the peritoneum, the cancer spreads throughout the peritoneal cavity, resulting in malignant ascites and other local complications such as bowel obstruction, constipation, nausea, and vomiting.

When malignant cells invade the blood-brain barrier and develop growth, patients will exhibit signs and symptoms of central nervous system disruption such as headache, confusion, and focal motor or sensory deficits. The signs and symptoms associated with invasive cancer are discussed later in this chapter.

CANCER STAGING

Cancer staging is based on the anatomic extent of the malignancy and metastasis by incorporating the primary site of origin, regional lymphatic spread, and distant metastasis. The two types of staging are *clinical* and *pathologic*. Clinical staging is determined without pathologic (histologic) confirmation of stage. Pathologic staging is preferred and is more accurate because it is based on tissue that is obtained during surgery or biopsy. Cancer staging determines the treatment plan (e.g., surgery, specific cytotoxic agents, radiation) and prognosis. The American Joint Committee on Cancer (AJCC) has identified a staging classification for cancers as the Tumor, Node, Metastasis (TNM) classification. These three components constitute the depth of penetration of the tumor, (or in some cases the tumor sizes), the presence or absence of lymphatic involvement, and the presence or absence of distant metastases. TNM staging is the most appropriate for solid malignant neoplasms and lymphomas and is not used in staging hematologic malignancies. When other staging or grading methods are used relative to a specific malignancy in this chapter, the method is discussed in more detail. Table 9-5 outlines the nomenclature for AJCC-TNM staging.

For purposes of palliative discussion, this chapter focuses on advanced-stage malignancies: primarily stages III and IV. The grade of cancer reflects the

Table **9-5**   American Joint Committee on Cancer Staging

(T) Tumor	(N) Regional Lymph Node	(M) Distant Metastases
T_X: Cancer cannot be assessed	NX: Cannot be assessed	MX: Cannot be assessed
T0: Cannot be found	N0: No nodal involvement	M0: No distant metastasis
Tis: Carcinoma in situ		M1: Metastasis present
T1, T2, T3, T4: Increasing size or depth of tumor invasion	N1, N2, N3: Increasing involvement of regional lymph nodes	

Data from American Joint Committee on Cancer (AJCC). (2002). *AJCC staging manual* (6th ed.).

degree of malignant differentiation and is important in determining prognosis. High-grade cancers (grades 3 and 4) usually have greater malignant behavior (ability to spread, invade, and establish tumor deposits at distant sites from the primary site). Patients may have low-stage cancer with a high histologic grade and thus have a poorer prognosis. Grades 3 and 4 (in the case of Gleason's grade used in prostate staging) have a greater risk of recurrence with a poor prognosis. There is a direct correlation between the higher stage of disease and grade in advanced disease.

METASTATIC SITES AND ASSOCIATED SYMPTOMS

Disease metastasis is a leading cause of all cancer-related deaths. A minority of patients will have symptoms from treatment, but most will experience symptoms from their advanced disease. Five prevalent symptoms reported by Potter (2004) include pain (64%), anorexia (34%), constipation (32%), weakness (32%), and dyspnea (31%).

The prognosis for cancer patients changes over time as a result of disease-related events modified by exacerbations and therapeutic interventions (Mackillop, 2001). The patient outlook will change during palliation, and patients' involvement in decisions regarding their treatment options and expected outcomes in advanced cancer is critical to patient autonomy and satisfaction. A more detailed discussion related to disease and prognosis of common malignancies in the adult population follows.

Lung Cancer

Head, neck, lung, and esophageal malignancies are among the most medically challenging of all cancers.

These malignancies share a common etiology—tobacco. Lung cancer most often spreads beyond the primary site at the time of diagnosis. Stages III and IV malignancies account for 60% to 70% of lung cancer presentations. Surgical intervention in this patient population can be performed in those patients who present with stage I or II. However, patients usually present with stage III or IV disease when surgical intervention is not a consideration. Surgical intervention is usually extensive and involves either a lobectomy or pneumonectomy.

Although the 1-year survival for lung cancer has increased from 34% in 1975 to 42% in 1998, the 5-year survival for all stages is 15%. Lung cancer remains the leading cause of cancer mortality in both men and women in the United States (ACS, 2004). Only one in seven patients with non–small cell lung cancer (NSCLC) can be cured, most of whom have early staging and resectable lesions (Karp & Thurer 2003). Lung cancers include two primary types: small cell (SC) and non–small cell (NSC). NSCLCs (adenocarcinoma and squamous cell carcinoma) constitute the highest percentage of all lung cancers. Sixty percent of small cell carcinomas and 30% to 40% of non–small cell carcinomas present with stage IV metastatic disease (Smith & Khuri, 2004). More than 80% of small cell lung cancers present with extension beyond or into the main stem or lobar bronchi at diagnosis (Merchant & Schiller, 2003).

Without treatment, the median survival for small cell lung cancer (SCLC) from diagnosis is only 2 to 4 months (Merchant & Schiller, 2003). Clinical presentation of both SCLC and NSCLC includes:
• Local symptoms (cough, shortness of breath on mild exertion, chest pain,

pleural effusion, hemoptysis, dyspnea, pneumonitis)
- Distant symptoms (anorexia, cachexia, fatigue)
- Paraneoplastic (syndrome of inappropriate antidiuretic hormone secretion [SIADH], Cushing's syndrome)
- Bone metastases (pain, fractures, hypercalcemia)

The prognosis for SCLC and NSCLC depends on several factors. These factors include TNM stage, gender, functional performance score, and the histologic type of lung cancer. See Table 9-6.

Breast Cancer

Breast cancer has the second highest frequency of occurrence of cancer among women in Western countries (ACS, 2004). Breast cancer accounts for 32% of cancers found in women and is second only to lung cancer as the leading cause of cancer deaths in women (ACS, 2004). There is an unequal ethnic burden of breast cancer; African-American women have a higher mortality compared with Caucasian women. The disparities might be attributed to poverty, high-fat diet, limited access to health care, inadequate treatment, and delayed diagnosis, although, as mentioned earlier, ethnic differences in breast cancer biology may also be a factor (Bach, Schrag, Brawley, et al., 2002; Bradley, Givens, & Roberts, 2001; Shavers & Brown, 2002; Smedley, Stith, & Nelson, 2002).

Risk factors for the development of breast cancer include advanced age and female gender, personal and family history, early menarche, late menopause, and a high-fat diet. The controversy continues related to exogenous hormone use and the development of breast cancer in light of the cardiovascular and skeletal benefits (Chen & Schnitt, 1998; Davidson, 1995). Other environmental factors might include cigarette smoking and alcohol consumption.

The course or natural history of invasive breast cancer varies among patients. Mutated suppressor genes have been related to an increased risk for

Table 9-6   Prognostic Table for Lung Cancer

Advanced Malignancy	Signs and Symptoms of Advanced Malignancy	Metastatic Site(s)	Prognostic Indicators
SMALL CELL LUNG CANCER			
• **Limited**—disease is restricted to one hemithorax with regional lymph node metastasis, including the hilar, ipsilateral and contralateral mediastinal, or supraclavicular nodes, and including ipsilateral pleural effusion regardless of cytology. • **Extensive**—disease is beyond the above definitions and may involve metastasis to liver, bone, bone marrow, brain, adrenals, and lymph nodes.	Shortness of breath Dyspnea Bone pain Pathologic fractures Swelling of neck and face Asthenia Fatigue Anemia Increased respiratory secretions	Chest wall Lung Bone Brain Liver	Histologic type Poor performance status Malignant pleural effusion Bone metastasis Brain metastasis Liver metastasis
NON–SMALL CELL LUNG CANCER			
• Stage III • Stage IV			

Data from American Joint Committee on Cancer (AJCC). (2002). *AJCC staging manual* (6th ed.); Daniel, B.T. (2001). Malignant lymphoma. In S. Otto, (Ed.), *Oncology nursing* (4th ed.), St. Louis: Mosby; Gullatte, M. (2001). Cancer prevention, screening and early detection, In S.E. Otto (Ed.), *Oncology nursing* (4th ed.). St. Louis: Mosby; Mellott, A., & Gordon, L.I. (2003). Intermediate and high grade lymphoma. In B. Furie, P.A. Cassileth, M.B. Atkins, et al. (Eds.), *Clinical hematology and oncology*. Philadelphia: Churchill Livingston.

developing breast cancer. The two major genes associated with familial breast cancer are BRCA1 and BRCA2 (Marcus, Watson, Page, et al., 1996). Another mutated gene, p53, associated with regulating cell cycling, has also been identified as a risk factor for breast cancer. Most p53 mutations are spontaneous somatic mutations except in patients with germline p53 mutations (Li Fraumeni syndrome) (Fitzgibbons, 2001). Loss of normal cell cycle regulation can lead to additional mutations, which can result in breast cancer (Elledge & Allred, 1994). The overexpression of *epidermal growth factor* (EGF) type II (HER-2/neu), a glycoprotein found on breast epithelial membranes, in some breast cancer patients can influence both prognosis and response to hormones (Burnnell, Winer, & Garber, 2003) .

Breast cancer often presents as a palpable lesion, found by the patient on self-examination, by physician-initiated clinical breast examination, or through radiographies (mammography). Other unusual presentations are breast pain, nipple discharge, rash or erythematous skin changes, nipple retraction, ulceration, breast dimpling, (peau d'orange), dermal changes, and/or arm lymphedema.

Several prognostic factors are used to determine treatment response and patient outcome. The prognosis for long-term survival from breast cancer is determined by presence and extent of axillary lymph node involvement, tumor size, inflammatory dermal changes (Table 9-7), hormone receptor status (estrogen [ER] and progesterone [PR] status), HER-2/neu overexpression, age, race, and treatment response (Burnnell et al., 2003; Elledge, Green, Ciocca, et al., 1998).

Colorectal Cancer

Among African-Americans and Caucasians, cancers of the colon and rectum are the third leading cause of cancer mortality. Among Hispanics, it is the second leading cause of cancer mortality. There is a difference in mortality between men and women. Colon cancer is the second leading cause of death from cancer in males and the third leading cause of cancer death in females (ACS, 2004).

The etiology of colorectal cancer has been associated largely with excessive dietary habits. Colorectal cancer is associated with consumption of foods high in animal fat and low in fiber. Slow transit time through the gastrointestinal (GI) tract is assumed to be a promoting factor. Potential

Table **9-7** PROGNOSTIC TABLE FOR BREAST CANCER

Advanced Malignancy	Signs and Symptoms of Advanced Malignancy	Metastatic Site(s)	Prognostic Indicators
Stages IIIB, IV, and recurrent	Weight loss Asthenia Bone pain Fatigue Dyspnea Shortness of breath Unsteady gait Lymphedema Lymphadenopathy Immobility Ascites Pleural effusion	Chest wall Lung Liver Bone Brain	Age Poor performance status Disease progression Bone metastasis Liver metastasis Hypercalcemia Spinal cord compression Superior vena cava syndrome

Data from Bociek, G., & Armitage, J.O. (2003). Low-grade non-Hodgkin's lymphoma. In B. Furie, P.A. Cassileth, M.B. Atkins, et al. (Eds.), *Clinical hematology and oncology: Presentation, diagnosis, and treatment* (p. 638). Philadelphia: Churchill Livingston; Gullatte, M. (2001). Cancer prevention, screening and early detection. In S.E. Otto (Ed.), *Oncology nursing* (4th ed.). St. Louis: Mosby.

carcinogens have longer contact time with the gut mucosa. Age is also a risk factor for developing colorectal cancer; more that 90% of all individuals with colon cancer are older than 50 years (ACS, 2004). A history of colorectal polyps in the patient and familial history are also risk factors for the potential development of colorectal cancer. Twenty percent of patients with colorectal cancer have a strong family history of the same cancer (Mayer, 2003). Patients with prolonged or chronic inflammatory bowel disease and patients with high alcohol consumption are at greater risk. More than 50% of colon cancers occur in the rectum, rectosigmoid, or sigmoid colon although there is a recent trend of cancers occurring with increasing frequency in the right colon (Bruckner, Pitrelli, & Merrick, 2000). Most colorectal cancers are histologically adeno-carcinomas.

Clinical presentation is often related to the location of the malignancy. The colon is identified by quadrants: right or ascending colon, transverse colon, left or descending colon, and the rectum (Table 9-8). Prognosis depends on the initial stage of disease determined by the extent of bowel wall invasion and the number of involved lymph nodes, grade, vascular or lymphatic invasion, serum chorio-embryonic antigen level, and tumor genetics (Burnnell et al., 2003; Mayer, 2003).

The staging classification is either the AJCC/TNM or Dukes' classification (formally the most widely used to stage colon cancers). The Dukes' staging system has been modified over the years, and in recent times is used with reduced frequency by cooperative groups (Table 9-9). Staging is a key determinant to specific treatment. Cure with surgery is possible in 70% of patients with early-stage disease. The 5-year survival rate for cancer limited to the mucosa approaches 90%; with extension into the muscularis propria, 80%; and with regional lymph node spread it decreases to 30% to 50%, depending on the number of nodes involved (Beers & Berkow, 1999).

Prognostic indicators for advanced cancer of the colon are listed in Table 9-10. Palliative oncology approaches to treat local or regional metastasis and/or recurrent colon cancer that has metastasized to the liver can include hepatic artery infusions of

Table 9-8 CLINICAL PRESENTATION OF COLON AND RECTAL CANCERS

Anatomic Location	Signs and Symptoms
Right/ascending colon	Anemia Gastrointestinal bleeding Persistent lower abdominal pain Right lower quadrant mass Fatigue and weakness
Transverse colon	Obstructive constipation Rectal bleeding Anemia
Left/descending colon	Cramps, abdominal pain Gross blood in the stool Excessive bloating and flatulence Decrease in stool caliber Changes in bowel habits (constipation, diarrhea)
Rectum	Constipation Hematochezia Tenesmus Feeling of incomplete evacuation Rectal pain Prolapse of rectal mass

Data from Beers, M.H., & Berkow, R.(Eds.). (1999). Gastrointestinal disorders. *The Merck manual: Centennial edition* (pp. 327-328). New Jersey: Merck Research Laboratories; Bruckner, H.W., Pitrelli, J.P., & Merrick, M. (2000). Adenocarcinoma of the colon and rectum. In R.C. Bast, D.W. Kufe, R.E. Pollock, et al. (Eds.), *Cancer medicine* (p. 1472). Hamilton, Ontario Canada: B.C. Decker; Gullatte, M. (2001). Cancer prevention, screening and early detection. In S.E. Otto (Ed.), *Oncology nursing* (4th ed.). St. Louis: Mosby; Mayer, R.J. (2003). Colorectal cancer. In B. Furie, P.A. Cassileth, M.B. Atkins, et al. (Eds.), *Clinical hematology and oncology: Presentation, diagnosis, and treatment.* Philadelphia: Churchill Livingston.

chemotherapy and/or hepatic resection or resections of isolated non-hepatic metastasis. Approaches to improve local disease control with initial therapy include preoperative, intraoperative, or postoperative radiation therapy for rectal cancers located below the peritoneal reflection or cancers adherent to adjacent structures (T4 lesions) (Willett, Fung,

Table **9-9**   CLASSIFICATION AND STAGING OF COLORECTAL CANCERS

AJCC-TNM Staging	Dukes' Classification
Stage 0: Carcinoma in situ. (T_{is}, N_0, M_0) *Stage I:* *IA* confined to the mucosa or submucosa. (T_1, N_0, M_0) *IB* involves the muscularis propria. (T_2, N_0, M_0)	*A:* Tumor confined to the mucosa or submucosa *B:* Involving multiple layers of the bowel wall *C:* Lymphangitic spread *D:* Distant metastases
Stage II: Involves all layers of the bowel wall with or without invasion of the immediate structures. (T_3, N_0, M_0) *Stage III:* Any degree of bowel wall involvement with regional node metastasis. (any T, N_{1-3}, M_0) Extends beyond the contiguous tissue or immediately adjacent organs with no regional lymph node metastasis. (T_4, N_0, M_0) *Stage IV:* Any invasion of the bowel wall with or without regional lymph node metastasis but with evidence of distant metastasis. (any T, any N, M_1)	

AJCC, American Joint Committee on Cancer; *TNM,* tumor, node, metastases.
Data from American Joint Committee on Cancer (AJCC). (2002). *AJCC staging manual* (6th ed.); Mayer, R.J. (2003).
Colorectal cancer. In B. Furie, P.A. Cassileth, M.B. Atkins, et al. (Eds.), *Clinical hematology and oncology: Presentation, diagnosis, and treatment.* Philadelphia: Churchill Livingston.

Table **9-10**   PROGNOSTIC TABLE FOR COLORECTAL CANCER

Advanced Malignancy	Signs and Symptoms of Advanced Malignancy	Metastatic Site(s)	Prognostic Indictors
Stages III and IV and recurrent	Weight loss Anorexia Abdominal pain Bone pain Constipation Diarrhea Erectile dysfunction Lower extremity edema Elevated carcinoembryonic antigen level Asthenia Neuropathy Ascites Bowel obstruction	Liver Omental seeding Bone Lymph nodes Brain Adrenal glands Genitourinary organs Lungs	Disease progression Poor performance status Bowel obstruction Ascites Hypercalcemia Spinal cord compression Bone metastasis Liver metastasis

Data from Gullatte, M. (2001). Cancer prevention, screening and early detection. In S.E. Otto (Ed.), *Oncology Nursing* (4th ed.). St. Louis: Mosby; Mayer, R.J. (2003). Colorectal cancer. In B. Furie, P.A. Cassileth, M.B. Atkins, et al. (Eds.), *Clinical hematology and oncology: Presentation, diagnosis, and treatment.* Philadelphia: Churchill Livingston.

Kaufman, et al., 1993). Radiation therapy is ineffective for cancers above the peritoneal reflection.

Prostate Cancer

Cancer of the prostate is the most prevalent cancer in males. Prostate cancer is second only to lung cancer as the leading cause of cancer mortality in men in the United States. The ACS estimates that 230,110 new cases of prostate cancer will occur in 2004, with an expected 29,900 prostate cancer deaths (ACS, 2004). Prostate cancer is known as a disease primarily of older men. There is a disproportionate increased incidence of prostate cancer among African-American men, which may reflect an ethnic predisposition. Between 1995 and 1999, prostate cancer increased by 60% in African-American men compared with Caucasian men (ACS, 2003b).

The prostate is an integral part of the male reproductive system. It is a walnut-shaped gland located at the base of the bladder encompassing the urethra. The three zones of the prostate are the peripheral, the central, and the transitional zones; most cancers are found in the peripheral zone (Scher, Issacs, Zelefsky, et al., 2000). The prostate consists of epithelial, stromal, basal, and neuroendocrine cells. The epithelial cells are the source of cancer and the site of prostate-specific antigen (PSA) and prostate-specific acid phosphatase (PAP) production and secretion (Scher et al., 2000).

Factors associated with the development of prostate cancer include age, race, familial history, and a high-fat diet. Several studies have demonstrated a positive correlation between a high-fat diet and levels of circulating testosterone. One study indicated that a 30% decrease in circulating testosterone was found in men who stopped eating a high-fat diet in favor of a vegetarian, low-fat diet (Dennis & Resnick, 2000; Kolonel, 1996). However, it is not known if altering diet can affect the incidence of cancer. The highest risk of prostate cancer is in men with a familial history of this disease (i.e., father, brother), particularly if it occurred before age 65 (Ko & Bubley, 2003).

The clinical presentation of prostate cancer is dominated by local or regional invasion. Signs and symptoms may include hematuria, pain, an elevated PSA and PAP, and an abnormally hard, asymmetric, enlarged prostate on digital rectal examination (DRE). The DRE and PSA have been used to screen and detect early prostate cancer. The PSA has three measures: total PSA, which measures the serum PSA bound to protease inhibitors; free PSA, a measure of serum PSA unbound to protease inhibitor; and complexed PSA, a measure of PSA with various protease inhibitors (Brawer, Cheli, Neaman, et al., 2000). The influence on survival of the practice of PSA screening has not been determined.

Prognostic indicators for prostate cancer include race, age, stage of disease, tumor grade by Gleason score, and treatment response to hormonal ablation. TNM clinical staging is often used in conjunction with the Gleason histologic grading system for prognosis and treatment decisions. The "histologic Gleason scoring system assigns a grade based on histologic differentiation—one each to the predominant pattern contained within the specimen: 1 (well differentiated) to 5 (poorly differentiated)" (Ko & Bubley, 2003, p. 861). The Gleason biopsy score is 1 through 10 (Table 9-11).

Non-Hodgkin's Lymphoma

Non-Hodgkin's lymphoma (NHL) ranks as sixth in cancer incidence among American men and women but is the fourth leading cause of cancer deaths in men and fifth in women (ACS, 2004). Among African-Americans, it is fourth in incidence among males and eighth in incidence among females and Hispanic men and women.

NHL is the eighth leading cause of cancer deaths in African-American men and seventh in Hispanic men and women; it is tenth among African-American women (ACS, 2003b, 2003c). Overall, the incidence of NHL is increasing. NHL is a malignant monoclonal proliferation of lymphoid cells, usually within lymph nodes, bone marrow, and spleen but also in extranodal sites such as the liver and gastrointestinal system (Beers & Berkow, 1999). The histologic classification of NHL is based on the overall pattern of lymph node architecture and cytologic classification of individual neoplastic cells (Freedman & Nadler, 2000). The classification and staging of lymphomas has undergone several modifications over the past several decades. The World Health Organization (WHO) has proposed

Table **9-11** PROGNOSTIC TABLE FOR PROSTATE CANCER

Advanced Malignancy	Signs and Symptoms of Advanced Malignancy	Metastatic Site(s)	Prognostic Indictors
Stages III, IV, and recurrent Gleason score >8 *The Gleason score is the total sum of the primary and secondary pattern of heterogeneity of prostate cancer (the range of each is 1-5):* • *GX grade: cannot be assessed* • *GI: well differentiated (Gleason 2-4)* • *G2: moderately differentiated (Gleason 5-6)* • *G3-4: poorly differentiated (Gleason 7-10)*	Bone pain (pelvic and lower back) Weakness Paralysis Urinary incontinence Anemia Erectile dysfunction Pathologic fractures	Bone Bladder	Age at diagnosis Disease progression TNM clinical stage Poor performance status Bone metastasis Hypercalcemia PSA score Gleason score Molecular markers (p53 and bcl-2)

TNM, Tumor, node, metastases; *PSA,* prostate-specific antigen.
Data from American Joint Committee on Cancer (AJCC). (2002). *AJCC staging manual* (6th ed.); Gullatte, M. (2001). Cancer prevention, screening and early detection. In S.E. Otto (Ed.), *Oncology nursing* (4th ed.). St. Louis: Mosby; Ko, Y.J., & Bubley, G.J. (2003). Prostate cancer. In B. Furie, P.A. Cassileth, M.B. Atkins, et al. (Eds.), *Clinical hematology and oncology: Presentation, diagnosis, and treatment* (p. 860). Philadelphia: Churchill Livingston.

a new classification system that does not follow the usual TNM staging system used for solid tumors. The major classification of NHLs is B cell, T cell, and NK (natural killer) cell neoplasms. NHL is then divided by histologic grades based on nodal architecture and cellular appearance. The NHLs are grouped in three categories: low-grade (indolent), intermediate-grade, and high-grade. Extranodal lymphomas (lymphomas arising in non-nodal tissue) may be classified as T, B or NK cell lymphomas, mantle cell (B cell lymphoma), and marginal zone (B cell lymphomas).

Although there are no definitive causes of NHL, numerous associations have been cited: immunodeficiency disorders (human immunodeficiency virus [HIV] infections), autoimmune disorders, infectious agents (Epstein-Barr virus and *Helicobacter pylori),* and environmental/occupational factors such as lead, paint thinners, hair dyes, benzene, herbicides, and styrene. Staging is generally based on the Ann Arbor Staging System: I, II, III, and IV (Table 9-12).

Clinical features of NHL include painless lymphadenopathy, vague abdominal discomfort, back pain, recurrent fevers, night sweats, decreased appetite with resultant weight loss, and gastrointestinal complaints (Daniel, 2001; Gullatte, 2001). Clinical features, along with histology, help guide treatment decisions. Prognostic factors are histology, age, stage of disease, lactate dehydrogenase (LDH) levels, and immunologic subtype (Table 9-13).

Understanding prognosis and risk of recurrence is essential when making treatment decisions. In the future, prognostication in oncology is likely to increase as micro-array technology allows us to better understand tumor behavior in relationship to genetic mutations and can provide clinicians and patients with better tools to address prognosis and therapeutic options.

ONCOLOGIC EMERGENCIES

Patients with advanced malignancies often develop complications related to the disease process or

Table **9-12** ANN ARBOR STAGING SYSTEM FOR ADVANCED NHL

Stage	Anatomic Description
Stage III	Involvement of lymph node regions on both sides of the diaphragm without (III) or with (IIIE) localized involvement of an extralymphatic organ or site
Stage IV	Diffuse involvement of one or more extralymphatic organ or site, with or without lymphatic involvement

NOTE: Systemic involvement is denoted by an "A" or a "B" after the stage to convey presence or absence of symptoms: fever, night sweats and weight loss. A = Absent; B = Present. Stage notation with "B" denotes further advanced disease.

Data from Bociek, G., & Armitage, J.O. (2003). Low-grade non-Hodgkin's lymphoma. In B. Furie, P.A. Cassileth, M.B. Atkins, et al. (Eds.), *Clinical hematology and oncology: Presentation, diagnosis, and treatment* (p. 638). Philadelphia: Churchill Livingston.
NHL, Non-Hodgkin's lymphoma.

Table **9-13** PROGNOSTIC TABLE FOR NON-HODGKIN'S LYMPHOMA

Advanced Malignancy	Signs and Symptoms of Advanced Malignancy	Metastatic Site(s)	Prognostic Indictors
Ann Arbor stages III & IV	Superior vena cava syndrome Spinal cord invasion Elevated LDH levels	Bone marrow involvement GI tract Bone CNS involvement	Histologic type Extent of disease Age Poor performance status Response to treatment Number of extranodal sites

LDH, Lactic dehydrogenase; *GI*, gastrointestinal; *CNS*, central nervous system.
Data from Bociek, G., & Armitage, J.O. (2003). Low-grade non-Hodgkin's lymphoma. In B. Furie, P.A. Cassileth, M.B. Atkins, et al. (Eds.), *Clinical hematology and oncology: Presentation, diagnosis, and treatment* (p. 638). Philadelphia: Churchill Livingston; Freedman, A.S., & Nadler, L.M. (2000). Non-Hodgkin's lymphomas. In R.C. Bast, D.W. Kufe, R.E. Pollock, et al. (Eds.), *Cancer medicine* (p. 2034). Hamilton, Ontario Canada: B.C Decker.

related to treatment interventions. These complications can be life threatening; therefore, prompt assessment and management of these complications will affect both survival and patient-perceived quality of life.

Oncologic complications are classified into one of three categories—metabolic, structural, or hormonal. Hormonal complications and some metabolic complications are most often related to tumor products, whereas structural complications are related to tumor location. Clinical manifestations of these oncologic emergencies may be insidious or rapid in onset. Clinicians should be knowledgeable and clinically aware of the potential development of specific emergencies. The goals of treatment are to avert morbidity and mortality and reduce the symptom burden often associated with these complications.

HYPERCALCEMIA OF MALIGNANCY
Introduction and Definition

Hypercalcemia is the most common paraneoplastic syndrome associated with cancer. It occurs in approximately 10% of patients with cancer and poorly relates to tumor bulk or stage. Up to 30% of all cancer patients develop hypercalcemia during their disease. Approximately 10% to 20% of all patients with cancer experience hypercalcemia each year.

Hypercalcemia is defined as a serum calcium level greater than 10.5 mg/dl though this is relative to serum albumin levels. Calcium is released from bone at a rate that surpasses bone formation and renal excretion (Barnett, 1999).

Etiology

Many risk factors predispose the patient to the development of hypercalcemia. Bone destruction and immobility can potentiate hypercalcemia. Humoral-induced increased osteoclast activity with consequent release of calcium into the bloodstream is a common cause. The hypercalcemia of malignancy is often associated with elevated parathyroid hormone (PTH)–related protein produced by the cancer and reduced serum levels of PTH. Hypercalcemia is most often associated with primary tumors of the breast, lung, head and neck, kidney, cervix, lymphomas, and melanoma (Gucalp & Dutcher, 2001; Reid-Finlay & Kaplow, 2001).

Other factors that contribute to the occurrence of hypercalcemia include (1) inordinate consumption of calcium and vitamin D in alternative diets and (2) dehydration, which reduces the renal excretion of sodium and calcium.

Antineoplastic therapies such as estrogen, antiestrogen agents, and all-trans retinoic acid may transiently cause hypercalcemia from the tumor before treatment response (Reid-Finlay & Kaplow, 2001).

Associated Symptoms

Hypercalcemia affects the neurologic, gastrointestinal, renal, and cardiovascular systems. The clinical manifestations of hypercalcemia are nonspecific but usually related to the effects of calcium on smooth, skeletal, and cardiac muscle and the loss of cell membrane polarization. The severity of signs and symptoms is related to the serum level of calcium, rate of rise, the patient's general stamina, stage of disease, kidney function, and extent of skeletal metastasis (Barnett, 1999) (Box 9-1). Most patients with hypercalcemia have advanced cancer, although some will have early-stage disease. Signs and symptoms of hypercalcemia cluster, with

Box 9-1   SYMPTOMS OF HYPERCALCEMIA

NEUROLOGIC
Lethargy, personality and behavioral changes, confusion, stupor,[1] convulsions, disorientation, restlessness, headache, CNS depression → coma[1,2]

CARDIAC
Shortened QT segment, depressed T waves, bradycardia,[2] tachycardia,[3] heart blocks, ventricular dysrhythmias (if severe), increased contractility, bundle branch block, dehydration

GASTROINTESTINAL
Nausea, vomiting, constipation, anorexia, abdominal pain

RENAL
Renal insufficiency, kidney stones, polyuria, polydipsia, decreased ability to concentrate urine

MUSCULOSKELETAL
Fatigue, generalized muscle weakness, bone pain, decreased deep tendon reflexes, ataxia

MISCELLANEOUS
Hypophosphatemia

[1]If rapidly advancing hypercalcemia.
[2]Late sign.
[3]Early sign.
CNS, Central nervous system.

symptoms that resemble terminal illness and include cognitive changes, nausea, constipation, and weakness (Barnett, 1999).

Diagnosis

Hypercalcemia is screened with serum calcium levels and compared with serum albumin. Patients may have "normal" serum calcium levels but low albumin levels and be hypercalcemic.

Interventions

The management of hypercalcemia is related to the severity of symptoms and the trajectory and treatment of the underlying disease. Tumor reduction is the only long-term effective measure for reversing the hypercalcemia of malignancy. Chemotherapy, radiation therapy, and surgery may be used depending on tumor type and location (Barnett, 1999). Chemotherapy can effectively reverse the hypercalcemia of breast cancer, lymphoma, and multiple myeloma. However, not all patients with moderate (≤2 mg/dl) hypercalcemia require treatment. Treatment will depend on the patient's quality of life, symptoms, and options for further treatment (Gucalp & Dutcher, 2001). Some patients with hyperparathyroidism as an incidental finding to their cancer can develop hypercalcemia on the basis of a benign parathyroid adenoma. In these individuals the serum PTH is usually elevated, unlike cancer-associated hypercalcemia.

Emergency medical intervention should begin for patients who are symptomatic or who have a serum calcium of 13 mg/dl or more or with elevated creatine. Severe hypercalcemia with cognitive failure or renal failure is a medical emergency requiring vigorous hydration with isotonic saline (0.9%) for volume repletion to enhance calcium excretion by the kidneys. At least 3 L/day, and possibly as much as 8 L/day, may be required to restore the normal volume of fluid in the extracellular space. Diuretics should not be given initially.

Patients with elevated calcium levels are usually dehydrated as a result of nausea, vomiting, polyuria, and the calcium-induced inability to concentrate urine. Hydration reduces calcium and promotes saluresis and urinary calcium excretion (Reid-Finlay & Kaplow, 2001).

Administration of furosemide promotes sodium diuresis and, in turn, promotes calcium diuresis while preventing circulatory overload and hypernatremia. The use of diuretics should be restricted to the patient who has been rehydrated. Diuretic administration can worsen hypercalcemia in dehydrated patients by promoting additional depletion of extracellular fluid, resulting in increased calcium reabsorption.

Corticosteroids and bisphosphonates are the mainstay of treatment. Phosphorus supplementation may be necessary in some, but phosphates in hypercalcemia patients may result in soft tissue calcification (malignant soft tissue calcification). Bisphosphonates are necessary to decrease the rate of bone resorption and to prevent worsening or recurrence of hypercalcemia in patients with metastatic bone disease. Numerous agents are available or are undergoing clinical trials. Some of these agents are listed in Table 9-14. Antiresorptive

Table **9-14** ANTIRESORPTIVE AGENTS

Drug	Mechanism of Action	Dosage
Calcitonin	Suppresses bone reabsorption by inhibiting activity of osteoclasts	2-8 International Units/kg IM or subcutaneous q 6-12 hr
Plicamycin (Mithramycin, Mithracin)	Blocks parathyroid hormone action on osteoclasts	25 mcg/kg/day over 4-6 hr. Repeat q 24-48 hr × 3-4 days
Gallium nitrate (Ganite)	Stops the release of calcium from bone by blocking bone breakdown	Severe hypercalcemia: 200 mg/m²/day IV × 5 days Mild hypercalcemia: 100 mg/m²/day IV × 5 days
Etidronate (Didronel)	Strengthens bone and inhibits bone removal by osteoclasts	7.5 mg/kg IV infusion over 4 hr × 3-7 days
Pamidronate (Aredia)	Binds to bone and may block resorption; inhibits osteoclast activity	90 mg IV infusion over 2-4 hr given on a monthly basis
Zoledronic acid (Zometa)	Inhibits osteoclast bone resorption	4-8 mg IV infusion over ≥15 min q 3-4 wk

IM, Intramuscular; *IV,* intravenous; *q,* every.

therapy should commence once the patient has been rehydrated (Barnett, 1999; Ross, Saunders, Edmonds, et al., 2004).

Corticosteroids are most often used in hypercalcemia related to lymphoma, multiple myeloma, and breast cancer and as an adjunct to salmon calcitonin. They inhibit bone resorption, increase urinary calcium excretion, and decrease GI absorption of calcium. Concomitant use of calcitonin with glucocorticoids works quickly and can be safely used in patients with renal failure (Barnett, 1999).

The course of hypercalcemia associated with malignancy can be quick. Death can occur within 12 hours. Fortunately, fewer than 5% of patients have life-threatening levels of calcium.

Identifying patients at risk for elevated serum calcium levels is of paramount importance. Patients require observation for signs and symptoms of hypercalcemia, and changes in the patient's clinical status consistent with hypercalcemia should be followed by measuring serum calcium levels. Cardiac, renal, and GI function should be monitored during fluid resuscitation through assessment of shortness of breath, monitoring breath sounds, and assessing intake and output and hemodynamic status. This is especially important for patients who have heart failure or who have received cardiotoxic therapies (e.g., anthracyclines). Bisphosphonates may be renally toxic and therefore require ongoing serum creatinine evaluation. Ancillary serum chemistry values (e.g., potassium, phosphorus, magnesium) should also be evaluated. If clinically appropriate, efforts to eliminate contributory causes to hypercalcemia (e.g., prolonged immobilization, thiazide diuretics) should be made (Reid-Finlay & Kaplow, 2001). Patients failing to respond to bisphosphonates and salmon calcitonin will respond to gallium nitrate (Leyland-Jones, 2003).

Care of the patient with hypercalcemia entails symptom management. Patients should be mobilized and have constipation evaluated and treated. Bone pain should be managed, but nonsteroidal antiinflammatory agents (NSAIDS) should be avoided in patients using bisphosphonates due to extensive renal excretion.

Patients and families should recieve psychosocial support and education on the recurrence of hypercalcemia, what symptoms to observe, and the importance of reporting these symptoms early. Preventive measures can include preventing dehydration, weight-bearing activities, managing pain, and avoiding calcium-containing antacids and thiazide diuretics (Barnett, 1999).

SYNDROME OF INAPPROPRIATE ANTIDIURETIC HORMONE SECRETION (SIADH)

Introduction and Definition

Antidiuretic hormone (ADH) is normally produced in the hypothalamus, stored in the neurohypophysis, and released to govern serum osmolality (Keenan, 1999). When ADH is secreted, water reabsorption is stimulated in the distal convoluted tubules and collecting ducts of the kidney. This results in decreased free water excretion and the production of concentrated urine (Verbalis, 2003). Plasma, therefore, becomes more dilute, resulting in a decrease in plasma osmolality and hyponatremia (Reid-Finlay & Kaplow, 2001). Urinary sodium levels are increased as a response to volume expansion.

Inappropriate secretion of ADH results in hyponatremia and clinical water intoxication. The syndrome of inappropriate antidiuretic hormone secretion (SIADH) usually does not produce edema or symptomatic hypovolemia.

Etiology

The causes for SIADH are (1) cancer, (2) neurologic diseases, (3) benign lung disease, and (4) a wide variety of drugs (Baylis, 2003). SIADH is another paraneoplastic syndrome. It is caused by production of arginine vasopressin (AVP, ADH) by tumor cells (Flounders & Ott, 2003). The most common malignancies associated with the development of SIADH are neuroendocrine cancers, which include small cell lung cancer (two thirds of patients with SCLC have impaired water excretion), pancreatic, prostate, esophageal, colon, duodenal, uterine, or bladder cancers, thymoma, lymphomas (Hodgkin's and non-Hodgkin's), leukemias, carcinoid, breast, and squamous cell carcinoma of the head and neck (Gucalp & Dutcher, 2001; Reid-Finlay & Kaplow, 2001). Brain tumors will cause release of AVP from the pituitary gland as a result of increased intracranial pressure. Other tumors such as neuroblastoma, bladder, and mesothelioma have been reported to contribute to SIADH (Keenan, 1999). Administration of antineoplastic therapies such as vincristine, vinblastine, cyclophosphamide, ifosfamide, cisplatin, and melphalan can cause hyponatremia and elevated AVP levels (Gucalp & Dutcher, 2001).

Associated Symptoms

Most patients with SIADH are symptomatic (Gucalp & Dutcher, 2001). The types of symptoms depend on the degree and rapidity of hyponatremia (Baylis, 2003). The hallmark signs of SIADH are hyponatremia, serum hypoosmolality, and inappropriately concentrated urine for serum osmolality. Patients may have mild fluid retention, weight gain, nausea, vomiting, and central nervous system (CNS) manifestations (e.g., confusion, agitation, hallucinations, lethargy, pseudofocal deficits, seizures, coma) (Baylis, 2003). These findings are related to water excess from resultant hyponatremia and the movement of free water intracellularly. Advanced cancer can mimic water intoxication and hyponatremia. Therefore prompt attention to early signs such as anorexia, depression, irritability, lethargy, confusion, muscle weakness, and personality changes is important.

If a serum sodium level is less than 120 mmol/L and develops acutely, cerebral edema can be a risk.

These patients will present with headache, nausea, restlessness, irritability, muscle cramps, hyporeflexia, confusion, coma, seizures, and brain damage and eventual death (Langfeldt & Cooley, 2003). Common signs of chronic hyponatremia, when serum sodium levels reach 115 to 125 mEq/L, include anorexia, nausea, vomiting, headache, and abdominal cramps. Additional findings are listed in Table 9-15.

Diagnosis

Diagnosis of SIADH is based on laboratory data and through the exclusion of other contributing factors of hyponatremia. The clinician should have a high index of suspicion based on the presence of risk factors in a patient who is hyponatremic, such as euvolemic with an absence of edema, orthostatic hypotension, or signs of dehydration, normal renal function, or elevated urinary sodium concentration (>40 mEq/L) and urine osmolality greater than plasma osmolality (Janicic & Verbalis, 2003; Verbalis, 2003).

Interventions

If possible, treatment of the underlying malignancy is essential for the long-term management and resolution of SIADH. Treatment may entail combination of chemotherapy, radiation therapy, or corticosteroids (Keenan, 1999). The mainstay of treatment is fluid restriction with strict monitoring of intake and output (Baylis, 2003). Fluid is limited to an intake of less than 800 to 1000 ml/day until hyponatremia improves. The degree of fluid restriction is less than urinary output and insensible loss combined.

Table **9-15** Signs of SIADH in Relation to Serum Sodium Levels

Mild Hyponatremia: (125-135)*	Headache, lethargy, behavioral changes, ataxia, peripheral edema, muscle cramps, anorexia
Moderate Hyponatremia: (118-124)*	Irritability, disorientation, weakness, somnolence, hallucinations, tremors, nausea, vomiting, diarrhea, weight gain, oliguria
Severe Hyponatremia: (112-117)*	Obtundation, coma, seizures, inability to maintain a patent airway and mobilize secretions, death
Serum Sodium <110*	Areflexia, coma, convulsion, death

*Measurement should be mEq/L.
SIADH, Syndrome of inappropriate antidiuretic hormone secretion.

Fluid restriction alone, however, may not be successful. Administration of demeclocycline 600 to 1200 mg/day in divided doses is recommended. Demeclocycline induces nephrogenic diabetes insipidus by decreasing renal tubular response to ADH and should be used cautiously in patients with diabetes mellitus.

Patients with acute hyponatremia who manifest severe confusion, seizures, or coma should also receive hypertonic (3%) saline at a rate of 300 to 500 ml intravenously (IV) over 4 to 6 hours. This rate should be adequate to increase serum sodium levels by 2 mEq/L/hour and should continue until the patient's serum sodium reaches 125-130 mEq/L (Crook, 2002). If the patient has been hyponatremic for more than 48 hours, the rate of correction should be slow (0.5-1 mEq/L/hour) to avoid cerebral complications and rapid fluid shifts, pulmonary edema, hypernatremia, and seizures (Gucalp & Dutcher, 2001; Kozniewska, Podlecka, & Rafalowska, 2003; Reid-Finlay & Kaplow, 2001).

Administration of loop diuretics to decrease urine concentration and augment clearance of free water is recommended. This will enable the clinician to liberalize fluid intake. Thiazide diuretics should not be used because they can precipitate SIADH (Gucalp & Dutcher, 2001). Vasopressin V_2 receptor antagonists represent a promising new treatment for SIADH (Verbalis, 2002).

The key to managing SIADH is early detection to prevent complications (Keenan, 1999). Monitoring fluid status may require urine specific gravity, daily weights, serum and urine electrolytes, and strict intake and output (I/O). Patients receiving hypertonic saline require ongoing assessment for overcorrection and/or fluid overload (Keenan, 1999). Patients with hyponatremia will complain of thirst and xerostomia; oral hygiene and small amounts of ice chips may alleviate their discomfort. Monitoring neurologic status is essential because sudden changes in mentation may indicate worsening hyponatremia coupled with rapid changes in sodium. If the patient's mental status is already impaired because of hyponatremia, the clinician should consider the propensity for the development of delirium.

INCREASED INTRACRANIAL PRESSURE
Introduction and Definition

Increased intracranial pressure (ICP) is defined as an increased pressure above 15 mm Hg, which impinges on brain tissue and is transmitted through cerebrospinal fluid (CSF) (Hickman, 1998). ICP is proportionate to the volume within the cranium. If ICP increases, this places additional pressure on the brain, which results in a shift and can affect structures such as the cerebellum (seen in tonsillar herniation) or the cerebrum (seen in falx herniation) (www.nlm.nih.gov). Patients with midline shifts within the brain structures may exhibit brain herniation with a pronounced reduction in cerebral blood flow and brain ischemia compared with those with local compression (Nakayama, Tanaka, Kumate, et al., 1996).

Three factors determine intracranial volume: the brain, blood, and CSF. The brain has a fixed volume of 1400 ml and floats on the CSF. Blood volume and CSF are normally 150 ml each but can increase or decrease, resulting in pressure changes. Blood volume usually remains stable. CSF is produced by the chorioid plexus at an approximate rate of 20 ml/hour and flows downward over the spinal cord and up over the cerebral hemispheres, ultimately being absorbed by arachnoid granulations (Hickman, 1998).

Pressures increase when an underlying disorder increases intracranial volume and the boney skull cannot accommodate changes in volume (Hickman, 1998). Therefore, if volume increases (through brain metastases, destructed CSF flow, or cerebral bleed), the brain is shifted to accommodate these changes. Compensation for the increased volume can involve displacement of blood and CSF. When compensatory mechanisms can no longer accommodate pressures, the small volume change will dramatically increase pressures, leading to a shift in brain structure and sudden neurologic deficits (Hickman, 1998).

An ICP greater than 15 mm Hg leads to decreased cerebral blood flow, which can result in ischemia. Herniation in the anterior compartment or through the foramen magnum as in a tonsillar herniation will result in focal neurologic changes, altered consciousness, and eventual death (Groenwald, Frogge, Goodman, et al., 1998; Madden, 2001).

Etiology

Increased ICP is caused by several mechanisms. For the patient with advanced cancer, brain tumor or metastases from other extra-cranial sites are often the cause. Patients with brain tumors are at particular risk for the development of increased ICP when the tumor causes cerebral edema or obstructs CSF flow (Groenwald et al., 1998). Increased ICP is most often caused by an increasing tumor burden or by a bleed from the brain metastasis. Brain tumors that cause obstruction to CSF flow through the third and fourth ventricle can contribute to increases in ICP (Hickman, 1998). Leptomeningeal metastases can produce focal deficit but can also obstruct CSF flow out of the third and fourth ventricle or prevent CSF absorption through arachnoid granulation (Abrey, 2002). Cancer-associated coagulopathies, disseminated intravascular coagulopathies, or cerebral venous occlusion can cause increased intracranial pressure (Rogers, 2003). Either intracerebral bleeding, subarachnoid bleeds, or subdural bleeds ultimately lead to cerebral herniation caused by shifting pressures.

Brain tumors associated with increased ICP are located in cerebellar, pineal, midbrain, and ventricular areas. Histologies include medulloblastoma, ependymoma, hemangioblastoma, pinealoma, gliomas, and craniopharyngioma (Hickman, 1998). Primary tumors that often are associated with cerebral metastasis include breast, lung, colon, kidney, thyroid, prostate, and melanoma (Hickman, 1998).

Associated Symptoms

Signs and symptoms of increased intracranial pressure are listed in Box 9-2. Patients with tumors that gradually cause an increase in pressures may remain asymptomatic until the tumor or tissue becomes large enough to produce a shift in the brain with associated functional significance (Hickman, 1998). Signs and symptoms are related to the nerve tracts compressed within the cranial vault or foramen as a result of pressure shifts. The clinical triad of

Box 9-2 SIGNS AND SYMPTOMS OF INCREASED INTRACRANIAL PRESSURE

Headache* (increases in intensity later)
Vomiting
Mental status changes:
  Drowsiness*
  Altered level of consciousness
  Lethargy*
  Restlessness*
  Disorientation*
  Obtundation
  Confusion
  Somnolence[†]
  Stupor[†]
  Coma[†]
  Short-term memory loss*
  Personality changes (usually gradual in onset)
  Disorderly conduct
  Impaired mental faculties
  Decreased attention span*
  Poor judgment
  Mood changes
  Decreased intellectual functioning
Papilledema[†]
Changes in vital signs[†] (increased SBP, decreased DBP, widening pulse pressure)
Seizures
Blurred vision*
Decreased visual acuity*
Diplopia*

*In early stages.
[†]In late stages.
[‡]Unusual except just before death.
SBP, Systolic blood pressure; *DBP,* diastolic blood pressure.

hypertension, bradycardia, and irregular respirations (Cushing's reflex) reflect the influence of pressures on brainstem function (www. neurologyindia.com).

Cognitive changes are initially identified. Seizures can occur and may become focal (Jacksonian) or generalized. They are more common in meningiomas, slow-growing astrocytomas, and oligodendrogliomas (gliomas involving oligodendrocytes).

Papilledema is a later sign of increased ICP and is caused by an increase in CSF pressure on the optic nerve. This contributes to impaired outflow of blood from the retina causing edema and swelling and can be evaluated in the retina through a funduscopic examination (Hickman, 1998).

Headaches associated with increased ICP can be bilateral and located in the frontal or occipital regions. Cerebellar metastases produce headaches more frequently and are usually more intense in the morning and diminish upon rising. Bending, coughing, or Valsalva maneuver may produce a worsening in headaches, which are often described by patients as being dull, sharp, or throbbing (Hickman, 1998).

Diagnosis

The diagnosis of increased ICP is suspected based on the patient's history and physical findings. Accurate diagnosis can be made by measuring the ICP. Transcranial Doppler ultrasound is a safe, noninvasive means of measuring critical changes in intracranial pressures. Computed tomography (CT) of the head or magnetic resonance imaging (MRI) will demonstrate an intracranial mass or cerebral edema (www.neurologyindia.com). Lumbar puncture should be done with extreme caution and only after imaging studies are completed. The presence of multiple masses or bleed is a contraindication (Reinhard, Petrick, Steinfurth, et al., 2003).

Interventions

Increased intracranial pressure can be fatal and requires prompt intervention. The acute monitoring and treatment of intracranial pressure should be conducted in an intensive care unit (http://cpmcnet.columbia.edu).

Treatment of the underlying malignancy is essential. Tumor debulking should control pressures (Hickman, 1998). The modality of treatment depends on the underlying cause and the severity of pressure. The use of chemotherapy or radiation therapy may be indicated, depending on tumor histology, but the response time to these procedures is slow. Radiation therapy is indicated with several metastatic lesions and also indicated when

surgery is contraindicated as a result of the patient's condition/functional status or location of tumor (Hickman, 1998). Temporizing procedures such as removal of CSF via ventriculostomy or mannitol infusion can reduce intracranial pressure. If a ventricular catheter is placed, 5 to 10 ml of CSF is removed at a single setting (www.neurologyindia.com). In addition to whole-brain radiation, stereotactic radiosurgery, gamma knife radiation, or intensity modulated radiation may be used for single offending lesions in patients who are not surgical candidates (Kanner, Suh, Siomin, et al., 2003; Lutterbach, Cyron, Henne, et al., 2003; Noel, Simon, Valery, et al., 2003).

There is controversy in the literature regarding the optimal position; there is, however, a general consensus that the head of bed should be elevated 15 to 30 degrees to decrease cerebral venous pressure and decrease ICP. This is considered safe practice as long as cerebral perfusion pressure is maintained at 70 mm Hg (www.neurologyindia.com). One study suggests that the head should be kept flat and was preferred to elevating the head of bed (Rosner, Rosner, & Johnson, 1995).

Parenteral fluids should not include free water (e.g., ½ NS, D_5W); this may increase brain edema and precipitate neurologic complications. Isotonic solutions (e.g., 0.9% NS) is preferred. There is currently no data to support colloid administration over crystalloids to maintain cerebral perfusion pressure. Serum osmolality should be maintained within the normal range.

Fever should be evaluated and controlled because elevated temperatures can potentiate intracranial hypertension, decrease cerebral metabolism, and increase cerebral blood flow. Use of acetaminophen or ice water gastric lavage is recommended if the patient has a temperature higher than 101° F. Indomethacin may also be considered as an antipyretic. Hypothermia intervention should be initiated if all other measures to control ICP have failed.

Seizures can also increase cerebral blood flow and therefore increase ICP. Prophylactic phenytoin can be considered; however, there is little data to support the preventive use of anticonvulsants. A loading dose of phenytoin 15 to 20 mg/kg with maintenance dosing at 100 to 300 mg/day can be considered for those who have had seizures or who are seizure-prone (Forsyth, Weaver, Fulton, et al., 2003).

Other symptoms such as anxiety, fear, tachycardia, and hypertension can contribute to an increase in cerebral blood flow and ICP. Administration of anxiolytics is suggested in this situation and should be titrated until the patient is calm and non-agitated. Labetalol and nicardipine are considered the antihypertensive agents of choice as they do not cause cerebral vasodilation (Olsen, Svendsen, Larsen, et al., 1995; Vaughan & Delanty, 2000). Administration of high-dose pentobarbital has been suggested to decrease cerebral blood flow and volume by causing vasoconstriction and lowering ICP (Hickman, 1998). Data suggest, however, that pentobarbital can produce cerebral hypoxia, and it has been suggested that patients receiving this therapy should concomitantly receive vasopressors to maintain cerebral perfusion pressure above 70 mm Hg (Cruz, 1996). Barbiturate therapy is indicated for severe elevations in ICP that have not responded to other interventions (Hickman, 1998).

Intravenous mannitol (1 gm/kg of 20% solution, followed by 0.25-0.5 gm/kg, PRN) is administered with corticosteroids (dexamethasone or prednisone) as a temporizing measure (Sarin & Murthy, 2003). Steroids may be used if the increased ICP is caused by a brain tumor. Corticosteroids decrease the area of edema, thereby reducing symptoms. They may also improve the blood-brain barrier by reducing the permeability of vessel leakage into the brain (Pollmiller, 2001). Mannitol can accumulate in the brain with repeated doses and can cause rebound increases in ICP (Kaufmann & Carduso, 1993). Mannitol administration should be withheld once ICP is normal because further treatments lose their effectiveness with prolonged use (Sarin & Murthy, 2003).

If the patient is comatose and has signs of increased ICP, management includes intubation with mechanical ventilation to hyperventilate the patient to a partial pressure of carbon dioxide in arterial blood ($PaCO_2$) of 26 to 30 mm Hg. Hyperventilation causes cerebral vasoconstriction and reduces ICP. Bicarbonate levels of 30 mm Hg

are associated with a reduced ICP, which occurs within minutes. One to three minutes after intubation and mechanical ventilation, there is evidence of tachyphylaxis to hyperventilation, a result of compensatory mechanisms (Muizelaar, Marmaroli, Ward, et al., 1991). Once ICP has been stabilized, hyperventilation can be slowly decreased over 6 to 12 hours.

Some patients with brain tumors will experience neurologic symptoms, which exacerbate with standing. These transient symptoms are related to acute elevations of ICP that occur despite dexamethasone. Acetazolamide, which reduces CSF production, can reduce or prevent further episodes (Watling & Cairncross, 2002). Additional activities that can elevate the ICP include Valsalva maneuver, isometric muscle contractions, emotional outbursts, head rotation, neck flexion and extension, sneezing, coughing, hip flexion, and prone position (Groenwald et al., 1998).

Accurate neurologic assessments will play a significant role in the selection of treatments. A baseline and ongoing neurologic assessment include changes in consciousness, degree of orientation, motor strength, vital signs, and pupillary response and size (Hickman, 1998).

A patent airway is maintained and adequacy of ventilation is assessed. The head of the bed should be kept at the prescribed level (either flat or elevated 15-30 degrees) Cheyne-Stokes respirations are a sign of increased ICP (Hickman, 1998). Monitoring vital signs, intake and output, specific gravity, and serum electrolytes and osmolality are an indirect way of evaluating intravascular volume (Hickman, 1998).

Patients require mobilization and compression stockings to prevent complications associated with immobility-related thrombosis. Turning and positioning, passive range-of-motion exercises, and implementation of a bowel regimen will prevent pressure ulcers, muscle weakness, and constipation (Hickman, 1998).

SPINAL CORD COMPRESSION
Introduction and Definition

Spinal cord compression (SCC) is an oncologic emergency that occurs with variable frequency depending on the primary origin of cancer.

The cumulative probability of experiencing an SCC in the 5 years preceding death is 2.5% and varies from 0.2% for pancreatic cancer patients to 7.9% for myeloma patients (Loblaw, Laperriere, & Mackillop, 2003). Tumors usually arise from the anterior vertebral body and extend into the epidural space, compressing the spinal cord and vasculature leading to ischemic damage to motor and sensory pathways and associated gray matter. Immediate, assessment, and intervention prevent permanent disability (Flounders & Ott, 2003).

Etiology

Epidural metastasis is the most common site of SCC; however, tumor growth on the dural surface or directly implanted within the spinal cord can produce the same constellation of symptoms (Schiff, 2003; Yalamanchili & Lesser, 2003). A fortyfold variation exists in the cumulative incidence of SCC among different cancers (Loblaw et al., 2003). Lung, breast, and prostate cancers and multiple myeloma are cancers most often associated with SCC (Gucalp & Dutcher, 2001). Other malignancies include melanoma and GI and renal cancers. The thoracic spine is the most common site, followed by lumbosacral, and cervical spine (70%, 20%, and 10%, respectively) because of the narrowness of the spinal cord canal within the thoracic spine (Guncalp & Dutcher, 2001). Multiple sites of metastasis spread can often occur in patients with breast or prostate cancer (Gucalp & Dutcher, 2001).

Paravertebral tumor extension through the intervertebral foramen usually occurs with lymphoma, myeloma, or a pediatric tumor. It is important to note that standard radiographs of the spine will be normal in these malignancies, yet patients often present with neurologic deficits from SCC.

Associated Symptoms

Clinical presentation of SCC is related to location and invasion of the spinal cord or spinal roots (Flounders & Ott, 2003). Sudden neurologic deficits may occur from decreased blood flow in the spinal cord with infarct or vertebral collapse (Gucalp & Dutcher, 2001). Signs and symptoms of SCC progress quickly within 24 hours. The clinical

features are listed in Box 9-3. Pain is the most common early complaint and is described as being localized, radicular, or medullary in nature (Bucholtz, 1999; Flounders & Ott, 2003; Levack, Graham, Collie, et al., 2002). Pain reported with SCC may be experienced for days or months before other signs and symptoms appear and may persist for 3 months before sensory deficits. Other characteristic features include pain with movement, coughing, or sneezing or when the patient is in a supine position (Gucalp & Dutcher, 2001). Discomfort can be induced by straight leg raising or by neck flexion. Localized pain and tenderness are a result of the involvement of the vertebrae by tumor, perosseous and osseous nerve stimulation, and an increased pressure in the epidural space (Gucalp & Dutcher, 2001; Reid-Finlay & Kaplow, 2001). It is important for the clinician to appreciate the patient's complaint of pain and not directly correlate pain with the site of compression (Levack et al., 2002).

Patients may lose sensation to pinprick, vibration, or position. Motor and sensory loss usually occur before loss of sphincter function. Sensory deficits can include numbness and paresthesia,

> **Box 9-3** SIGNS AND SYMPTOMS OF SPINAL CORD COMPRESSION
>
> Back pain
> Pain radiating from the back
> Loss of sensation in lower part of body
> Autonomic dysfunction:
>   Urinary retention or incontinence, hesitancy, overflow
>   Constipation or diarrhea
>   Impotence
> Weakness or paralysis of body below level of cord that is being compressed:
>   Sensory loss—loss of sensation of touch, pain, and temperature over area of body below level of compression
> Numbness and paresthesias in extremities or trunk
> Brisk deep tendon reflexes
> Ataxia
> Tingling
> Feelings of coldness

which radiate to the site of SCC (Levack et al., 2002). Autonomic dysfunction is manifested by decreased anal tone, bladder distention, and urinary retention, creating overflow and incontinence (residual volume >150 ml) (Gucalp & Dutcher, 2001). The presence of autonomic dysfunction, however, is a poor prognostic indicator. Weakness and sensory abnormalities are late findings and frequently irreversible.

Diagnosis

The diagnosis of SCC is initially based on the presence of clinical signs and symptoms that are elicited from a neurologic examination. Confirmation is made with either a CT scan or MRI of the spine. Spinal radiographs are rarely diagnostic but may reveal erosion and lesions of the vertebral body and pedicle or vertebral body collapse into the epidural spaces (Levack et al., 2002). X-rays will not reveal SCC in its early phase because 50% of bone must be destroyed before lesions are detectable (Flounders & Ott, 2003). Plain films and bone scans accurately predict spinal cord level 20% of the time (Levack et al., 2002). MRI of the entire spine is the diagnostic procedure of choice to define the extent of spinal involvement (Husband, Grant, & Romaniuk, 2001; Loughrey, Collins, Todd, et al., 2000). Initially, the MRI in an emergency setting does not require administration of contrast media (Flounders & Ott, 2003). However, contrast-enhanced images are necessary if an MRI is not available or if the unenhanced appearances do not correspond to clinical findings or suggest intradural or intramedullary metastases (Loughrey et al., 2000). CT scan is used to confirm spinal cord compression and fully define the level and extent of the lesion. Bone scan may detect abnormalities of the vertebral column not detected by x-ray (Flounders & Ott, 2003).

Interventions

Treatment is aimed at pain relief, recovery of neurologic function, regression of the underlying malignancy, and prevention of permanent damage (Flounders & Ott, 2003). Management of SCC is often palliative and is frequently associated with metastatic disease (Flounders & Ott, 2003). In fact,

the median survival after the first episode of SCC is 2.9 months (Loblaw et al., 2003).

Therapeutic modalities for SCC involve treatment of the underlying disease and depend on tumor type, location, aggressiveness, and radiosensitivity (Flounders & Ott, 2003). This may include surgery, radiation therapy, glucocorticoids, chemotherapy, or a combination. The efficacy of treatment will depend on the extent of damage to the spinal cord and prompt interventions. The best outcomes occur in patients who are diagnosed early and treated expeditiously and aggressively.

Corticosteroids. High-dose corticosteroids (oral or IV dexamethasone) should be given promptly to provide an antiinflammatory response on the offending tumor. Corticosteroids are often used in conjunction with other treatments. The goal of corticosteroids therapy is to reduce pedal edema and relieve pain (Reid-Finlay & Kaplow, 2001).

Radiation Therapy. If the patient is functional and the tumor is radiosensitive, immediate radiation therapy may be the treatment of choice to prevent further neurologic deficits. Doses of radiation are 3000 to 4000 cGy over 2 to 4 weeks in fractionated doses. Pain may be relieved shortly after radiation treatment is initiated. Approximately 85% of patients report adequate pain relief (Loblaw et al., 2003). Radiotherapy is the treatment of choice in most circumstances.

Surgery. Surgery is indicated for (1) rapid, deteriorating neurologic deficits, (2) unstable bony spine caused by vertebral metastases destruction, (3) vertebral bone fragments that impinge upon the spinal cord, (4) cord compression occurring in a previously radiated field, (5) progressive neurologic deficits during radiation, and (6) doubt about diagnosis and the need to obtain tissue (Bartanusz & Porchet, 2003; Maranzano, Trippa, Chirico, et al., 2003). Spinal radiation before surgical decompression is associated with a threefold increased risk for a major wound complication (Ghogawala, Mansfield, & Gorges, 2001). In the past, laminectomy was the customary surgical procedure. Unfortunately, many patients who did benefit short-term from surgery had destabilized spines. Current surgical recommendations include resection of the tumor and anterior vertebral body with subsequent spinal stabilization (Maranzano et al., 2003; Seol, Chung, & Kim, 2002). Favorable results, including decreased mortality rates, have been reported although this depends on the histology and extent of cancer metastasis (Gucalp & Dutcher, 2001).

Chemotherapy. Chemotherapy is indicated in patients with chemosensitive tumors, such as lymphoma, small cell lung cancer, or germ cell tumors, or in patients who are not surgical or radiation therapy candidates (Gucalp & Dutcher, 2001). Certain tumors such as breast cancer and prostate cancer are responsive to hormonal therapy (Bucholtz, 1999).

SUPERIOR VENA CAVA SYNDROME
Introduction and Definition

Superior vena cava syndrome (SVCS) was once thought to be a life-threatening oncologic emergency. The SVCS is caused by obstruction of the superior vena cava (SVC) above or below the azygous vein, which impedes blood flow from the superior vena cava to the right atrium (Hemann, 2001; Markman, 1999; Wudel & Nesbitt, 2001). Because of the anatomic location of the superior vena cava, the fact that it is thin-walled, surrounded by non-compressible structures, and that the blood flow in the superior vena cava is under low pressure, when the regional nodes or aorta enlarge, the superior vena cava can be easily compressed, blood flow becomes sluggish, and occlusion frequently follows (www.meb.uni-bonn.d/cancer.gov).

Etiology

Obstruction of the SVC can occur as a result of an intravascular clot, aortic aneurysm, benign lymphadenopathy, or tumor (Thirlwell & Brock, 2003). In the United States, more than 90% of the cases of SVCS are caused by malignancy and 80% of SVCSs are secondary to lung cancer (adenocarcinoma and squamous cancer and non-Hodgkin's lymphoma) (Thirlwell & Brock, 2003). Lymphoma causes 15% of SVCS cases. A minority of SVCSs are caused by metastasis from testicular or breast primaries. A certain subtype of leukemia, T cell leukemia, causes mediastinal adenopathy and thymic enlargement, which can compress the SVC.

Nonmalignant causes of SVCS are infections such as tuberculosis, indwelling central catheters, or pacemaker wires (Yellin, Rosen, Reichert, et al., 1990). A rare cause of SVCS is fibrosing mediastinitis (idiopathic or related to mediastinal histoplasmosis) (Goodwin, Nickell, & DesPrez, 1972). Rare causes reported in the literature are Kaposi's sarcoma, esophageal cancer, mesothelioma, thymoma, and Hodgkin's disease (Yahalom, 1993).

Associated Symptoms

Signs and symptoms of SVCS are listed in Box 9-4. Symptoms may vary, depending on the extent and location of the obstruction. Few, if any, signs and symptoms are present early in the course of SVCS

Box 9-4 SIGNS AND SYMPTOMS OF SUPERIOR VENA CAVA SYNDROME

NEUROLOGIC
Headache, dizziness/lightheadedness, syncope, lethargy, obtundation,[‡] confusion, mental status changes, stupor, blurred vision, coma

CARDIOVASCULAR
Jugular venous distention (variable degree), chest pain,[†] hypotension, thoracic vein distention, feelings of fullness in head

RESPIRATORY
Dyspnea,[*] cough, orthopnea, swelling of tongue, cyanosis,[†] nasal congestion/stuffiness, epistaxis, tachypnea, right-sided pleural effusion, hoarseness,[†] dysphagia,[†] hemoptysis,[†] paralyzed vocal cord,[†] glossal or laryngeal edema, stridor[‡]

MISCELLANEOUS
Swelling and erythema of neck and face (especially around the eyes), reddish face or cheeks (plethora), reddish palms and mucous membranes, pain, periorbital edema, swelling in trunk or extremity, tightness of the neck (Stokes' sign), Horner's syndrome[†]

*Most common complaint.
[†]Rare complaints.
[‡]In more severe cases.

and may progress slowly and allow for collateral circulation to develop, which compensates for the obstruction (Gucalp & Dutcher, 2001). The severity of SVCS further depends on the rapidity of obstruction and location (above or below the azygous vein). The quicker the onset, the more severe the symptoms since collateral circulation does not have enough time to accommodate the obstructed blood flow (Netter, 1980). Symptoms include dyspnea and headache, as well as face, arm, and upper chest edema (Gucalp & Dutcher, 2001).

Diagnosis

The diagnosis of SVCS is based on clinical findings coupled with the presence of an abnormal chest radiograph and a mediastinal mass or lymphadenopathies. Pleural effusions occur in 25% of patients, often located in the right hemothorax. Chest CT scan can provide a diagnosis and can help define the location of mediastinal nodes (Gucalp & Dutcher, 2001). Doppler ultrasonography can also detect superior vena cava occlusion in patients who cannot tolerate CT (Benenstein, Nayar, Rosen, et al., 2003).

A CT scan with contrast is used to assess venous patency and the presence of thrombi. Venography and MRI may be beneficial in assessing the site of the obstruction (Gucalp & Dutcher, 2001). Venography, although not usually required, can facilitate the treatment of SVCS. If there is clot, thrombolysis may be done through the same catheter.

Interventions

The treatment of SVCS depends on the etiology of the obstruction, severity of symptoms, prognosis of the patient, patient preference, and the goals of therapy (Markman, 1999; Wudel, 2001). A diagnosis of SVCS should be substantiated before initiating therapy (Hemann, 2001; Wudel & Nesbitt, 2001). Radiation therapy and chemotherapy should be withheld until the etiology of the obstruction is understood (Hemann, 2001; Ostler, Clarke, Watkinson, et al., 1997; Wudel & Nesbitt, 2001). If the patient has adequate collateral circulation and symptoms are minimal, treatment may not be necessary.

Ongoing assessment and maintenance of a patent airway are of utmost importance in patients with SVCS. Airway compromise or tracheal obstruction caused by extrinsic compression of the trachea associated with SVC is possible, although not common. Some relief from dyspnea may occur with upright posture. Oxygen may provide some temporary relief of symptoms (Gucalp & Dutcher, 2001; Thirlwell & Brock, 2003).

Corticosteroids. Glucocorticoid administration will decrease edema surrounding the tumor (Thirlwell & Brock, 2003). Either methylprednisolone 125 to 250 mg IV (loading dose) followed by 0.5 to 1 mg/kg/dose every 6 hours for up to 5 days (maintenance dose) or prednisone 5 to 60 mg/day PO or in divided doses (BID-QID) can be administered and tapered over 2 weeks as symptoms resolve.

Chemotherapy. Chemotherapy is the treatment of choice for small cell lung cancer or lymphoma (Gucalp & Dutcher, 2001; Thirlwell & Brock, 2003). Partial response rates of greater than 80% to chemotherapy in patients with SVCS and small cell lung cancer have been reported (Thirlwell & Brock, 2003). Symptomatic relief has been reported in 7 to 10 days, with complete elucidation of symptoms in 2 weeks in most cases (Haapoja & Blendowski, 1999).

Radiation Therapy. Radiation therapy is often considered in chemosensitive malignancies (i.e., prostate cancer). Up to 46% of patients with non–small cell lung cancer treated with radiation have relief from concomitant symptoms (Urban, Lebeau, Chastang, et al., 1993). The dose of radiation depends on the histology of the tumor and the goals of treatment (palliative or curative). Positioning patients for radiation may be problematic because many will have worsening dyspnea in the supine position (necessary for radiation).

Diuretics. Diuretics may be administered to decrease venous return to the heart and thereby reduce right-sided preload, reduce pressure on the superior vena cava, and provide symptomatic relief of edema. However, diuretics may cause dehydration and should therefore be used with caution (Abner, 1993). In addition, if the patient has associated pericardial effusion with tamponade, diuretics

Box 9-5 SIGNS AND SYMPTOMS OF
         PERICARDIAL TAMPONADE

NEUROLOGIC
Weakness, anxiety, lightheadedness, drowsiness, malaise, restlessness, confusion, obtundation, fatigue, altered mental status (varying degrees of consciousness)

CARDIOVASCULAR
Jugular venous distention, edema, decreased cardiac output, circulatory collapse, decreased stroke volume, pulsus paradoxus, electrical alternans (pulse waves alternating between those of greater and lesser amplitude with successive beats), chest pain, tachycardia, muffled heart sounds, poorly palpable apical pulse, friction rub, cold extremities, hypotension, palpitations, narrowed pulse pressure, elevated central venous pressure, circulatory collapse, cardiac arrest

RESPIRATORY
Dyspnea on exertion, cyanosis or pallor, tachypnea, dyspnea, hiccups, hoarseness, orthopnea, cough, hypoxia

GASTROINTESTINAL
Hepatomegaly, dysphagia, abdominal pain

RENAL
Oliguria or anuria

MISCELLANEOUS
Diaphoresis, low-grade fever

should not be given (Box 9-5). Furosemide (Lasix) 20 to 80 mg PO may be administered and repeated in 6 to 8 hours, as needed. Steroids and diuretics are used if the patient's airway is compromised. Intubation and internal stenting may be necessary (Reid-Finlay & Kaplow, 2001).

Thrombolytic Therapy. Thrombus that partially occludes the SVC lumen may be treated with thrombectomy. This procedure may be done with or without thrombolytic therapy (e.g., tissue plasminogen activator, streptokinase, urokinase) (Netter, 1980). SVC related to this central catheter should warrant removal of the catheter, and anticoagulant therapy should be initiated (Thirlwell & Brock, 2003). Thrombolytic therapy should be initiated within a few days of onset of symptoms to be effective. The greatest success occurs when treatment is initiated within 2 days (Haapoja & Blendowski, 1999).

Stent Placement. Insertion of an intravascular stent to reopen the superior vena cava has been reported as a treatment method for SVCS with positive response rates of 90% and greater (Chatziioannou, Alexopoulos, Mourikis, et al., 2003; Dinkel, Mettke, Schmid, et al., 2003; Gucalp & Dutcher, 2001; Marcy, Magne, Bentolila, et. al., 2001; Nicholson, Ettles, Arnold, et al., 1997). Stent placement results in immediate relief of symptoms (Haapoja & Blendowski, 1999; Thirlwell & Brock, 2003).

Surgery. Surgery has been used to bypass and relieve the pressure associated with an obstructed SVC. Tumor resection and vein grafting have been successful in patients with neoplastic SVCS (Lequaglie, Conti, Brega-Masson, et al., 2003). However, surgery is indicated for benign causes of SVCS (Thirlwell & Brock, 2003).

The 30-month mortality rate of SVCS is 90%. Prognosis for relief of symptoms is satisfactory with radiation therapy. Symptoms will usually resolve within 1 month of radiation therapy. Survival depends on the status of the patient's disease and tumor type (Gucalp & Dutcher, 2001).

Patients with SVCS should be maintained with the head of bed elevated. Oxygen therapy may be indicated for dyspnea (Haapoja & Blendowski, 1999; Thirlwell & Brock, 2003). The patient should be protected from fluid overload, which can exacerbate symptoms of SVCS. Upper extremity venous catheters should be avoided as a result of venous stasis, particularly when giving chemotherapy.

Both the patient and family should be educated regarding the signs and symptoms of SVCS. Prompt symptom management can prevent needless suffering, airway compromise, and cerebral hypoxia (Reid-Finlay & Kaplow, 2001).

TREATMENT-RELATED ONCOLOGIC EMERGENCIES
Tumor Lysis Syndrome
Patients with a large tumor burden and/or rapidly proliferate cancer that is extremely sensitive to

chemotherapy or radiation are at a significant risk for tumor lysis syndrome (TLS). The acute release of intracellular cations into systematic circulation as a result of cancer cell death produces life-threatening hyperkalemia within 6 to 72 hours of chemotherapy initiation (Altman, 2001). The ensuing complication can lead to cardiac conduction abnormalities, dysrhythmias, and sudden death (Altman, 2001). Common electrocardiogram abnormalities include peaked T waves and a wider QRS complex.

Tumor lysis also releases large quantities of phosphate from intracellular stores. Phosphate binds to calcium, thereby causing hypocalcemia and deposition of calcium phosphate in soft tissues (Altman 2001). Nucleic acids, another normal intracellular component, are released into the bloodstream when malignant cells are destroyed. Nucleic acids are further converted into uric acid by the liver. This results in hyperuricemia, which usually occurs within 48 to 72 hours after cytotoxic therapies (Altman, 2001).

Patients at risk are those with B cell and T cell non-Hodgkin's lymphoma and acute myeloid leukemia (Nicolin, 2002). A number of clinical features are associated with a high risk for TLS and include bulky abdominal disease; an elevated pre-treatment uric acid and LDH; and decreased urinary output (Nicolin, 2002). Patients with tumor lysis syndrome may exhibit paresthesia, weakness, lethargy, nausea and vomiting, latent tetany, oliguria, edema, and hypertension (Nicolin, 2002).

The three tenets to treatment are hydration, urinary alkalinization, and uric acid reduction (Nicolin, 2002). Hydration should be started at 3 L/day and adjusted according to potassium, phosphate, and uric acid levels. Loop diuretics are given to maintain urine output of 3 mL/kg/hr (Nicolin, 2002). Thiazide diuretics or potassium-sparing diuretics should be avoided. Exuberant use of bicarbonate leads to precipitation of calcium phosphate in tissues and can precipitate the symptoms of hypocalcemia.

Allopurinol is a xanthine oxidase inhibitor, and the recommended dosing is 100 mg every 8 hours or 150 mg every 12 hours. The use of allopurinol is for prevention as well as treatment of hyperuricemia. The dose should be reduced in the presence of renal failure. Allopurinol is also available in intravenous form if the patient is unable to tolerate oral medications. The dose of IV allopurinol is 200 to 400 mg/m^2/day, up to 600 mg/day. If allopurinol is ineffective in reducing uric acid levels, a recombinant urate oxidase such as rasburicase may be given. Rasburicase converts uric acid into the highly soluble allantoin. Doses of rasburicase are 50 to 100 units/kg IV over 30 minutes daily.

Ancillary measures are aluminum hydroxide 50 mg/kg every 8 hours to bind phosphate; polystyrene sulfonate resin 0.25 gm/kg every 6 hours for hyperkalemia; and parenteral calcium gluconate 10% 0.3 to 0.5 ml/kg slow IV bolus for symptomatic hypocalcemia (Nicolin, 2002). The combination of glucose 1 gm/kg plus regular insulin 0.25 units/kg will rapidly reduce life-threatening serum potassium levels by driving potassium intracellularly (Nicolin, 2002).

Nursing care for patients with TLS is critical. Patients should be monitored for mental status changes, urinary output, paresthesia, and nausea and vomiting. Strict intake and output records must be kept, and patients should be weighed daily. Patients require dose monitoring for fluid overload. Laboratory monitoring includes electrolytes, calcium, creatinine, and phosphate every 6 hours for patients in overt TLS until stability or resolution. Patient compliance to the medications is extremely important to avoid catastrophic complications.

Neutropenic Sepsis

Febrile neutropenia is a common complication of cancer chemotherapy, and if it is left untreated, has a high morbidity and mortality (Thirlwell & Brock, 2003). Neutropenic fever is defined as a fever of 38° C or higher for at least 2 hours and a neutrophil count below 1000/mm³. The degree of neutropenia directly correlates with the risk of sepsis (i.e., myelosuppression) and its duration (Thirlwell & Brock, 2003).

Initial treatment includes hydration and resuscitation if shock is present. Blood cultures, urine culture, and physical examination are important (Thirlwell & Brock, 2003). A chest radiograph may be initially normal despite having pneumonia because most of the infiltrate with pneumonia seen on chest radiography is caused by migrating leukocytes. Biochemical tests for liver and kidney function should be obtained with blood cultures (Thirlwell & Brock, 2003).

Initial treatment may include empiric antibiotics with an aminoglycoside, and either a third-generation cephalosporin or semisynthetic broad-spectrum penicillin monotherapy with a cephalosporin. Vancomycin may be added if gram-positive organisms are cultured. If no response after 48 to 72 hours and the patient remains neutropenic, an antifungal (usually amphotericin B) is empirically started (Thirlwell & Brock, 2003).

The key to management of neutropenic fever is prompt institution of antibiotics. Patients require close monitoring for signs of shock such as hypotension, dyspnea, and reduced urinary output. Changing mental status probably reflects uncontrolled infection and the possibility of evolving multiple organ failure. A complete blood count should be obtained daily. Colony-stimulating factors usually do not significantly alter the course of neutropenia once occurred, although for desperately ill patients, the marginal benefits may outweigh the risk.

Patients with cancer may develop a plethora of symptoms during the disease trajectory. Many of these symptoms are related to one or more oncologic complications associated with advanced neoplastic disease. These complications are life-threatening and add to their symptom burden.

Goals of Care

Although patients with advanced cancer may benefit from the diagnosis and treatment of oncologic emergencies, many of the interventions may be considered too aggressive in the face of advanced disease and impaired function. Some patients believe they may benefit from interventions that treat oncologic emergencies and extend their lives, but others will defer for personal reasons (i.e., advance directives).

It is essential that a multidisciplinary approach of care be developed for patients with advanced cancer who have developed an oncologic emergency. The team should formulate appropriate therapeutic goals, considering the patient's functional status, prognosis related to the underlying malignancy, patient preferences for therapy, and probable outcome of treatment. Informed choices require compassionate communication about the realistic outcomes to treatments (see Chapter 2: "Advance Care Planning"). It is imperative that patients understand the consequences of their choices and alternative care options.

SYMPTOM MANAGEMENT IN ADVANCED MALIGNANCY

Patients with advanced cancer are at risk for a plethora of uncomfortable symptoms that profoundly impair quality of life. These symptoms are more likely to be present with advanced cancer rather than with earlier stages of disease. Interventions are instituted to prevent and manage symptoms, and others are initiated to minimize suffering. This section addresses six common symptoms seen in advanced cancer. Pain and dyspnea are common symptoms in this population and are further discussed in Chapter 7: "Pulmonary" and Chapter 10: "Cancer Pain."

Cachexia

Incidence and Etiology. The cancer cachexia syndrome is characterized by a loss of appetite and involuntary weight loss that is centered on wasting of muscle and fat and potentiates a poor performance status (Inui, 2002; MacDonald, Easson, Mazurak, et al., 2003; Strasser, 2003). This syndrome is common in advanced cancer, affecting more than 80% of persons with cancer at the end of life (Bruera, 1997; Davis & Dickerson, 2000; Waller & Caroline, 2000). Cachexia is associated with poor clinical outcomes, decreased survival, compromised quality of life, and poor response to chemotherapy (Inui, 2002). Many factors contribute to weight loss including anorexia, increased resting energy expenditures, altered fat and protein metabolism (cancer cachexia), mechanical interference with nutritional intake or absorption, treatment-related side effects, altered taste, and psychosocial factors

(MacDonald et al., 2003). Cancer cachexia is recognized to be different from starvation principally because, during starvation, energy expenditures are reduced and proteins are conserved (Davis, 2002; MacDonald et al., 2003; Strasser, 2003).

The anorexia associated with cancer cachexia is likely caused by the activity of cytokines that are produced either by the tumor or by the host in response to the tumor, which interfere with appetite signals within the anterior hypothalamus (Davis, 2002). Tumor necrosis factor-α, interleukin-1, interleukin-6, and ciliary neurotrophic factors are all proinflammatory cytokines involved in various processes that decrease appetite despite weight loss (Davis, 2004; Inui, 2002; Strasser, 2003). Some of these cytokines may also increase the metabolic rate by inducing thermogenesis and muscle wasting to the point that food intake is not adequate to offset energy expenditures. This is done by increasing uncoupling proteins within the muscle and liver, which leads to heat generation rather than adenosine triphosphate (ATP). Energy expenditures are also increased when the large amounts of lactate produced by solid tumors are converted to glucose, because gluconeogenesis from lactate is extremely energy inefficient (Strasser, 2003; Tisdale, 2000a).

Other metabolic changes in persons with cachexia include alterations in fat and protein metabolism. Some cytokines likely interfere with the ability of adipocytes to extract fat for storage, whereas others cause a loss of lipids from adipose tissues (Davis, 2002; Inui, 2002). Together these alterations lead to severely depleted fat storage that cannot be corrected by supplying additional dietary fats (McCarthy, 2003; Winter, 2002). Persons with cachexia show reduced rates of muscle protein synthesis coupled with increased rates of protein degradation, leading to a decrease in lean body mass. This may be caused by a chronic, systemic inflammatory response seen with certain cancer diagnoses, resulting in high hepatic synthesis of acute-phase proteins. The demand for amino acids to manufacture these acute-phase proteins may be met by the breakdown of skeletal muscle tissue, causing muscle wasting (Barber, Ross, & Fearon, 1999; Inui, 2002; Martignoni, Kunze, & Friess, 2003; Strasser, 2003). This information leads some experts

to propose that cancer cachexia is a chronic inflammatory condition rather than a nutritional aberration (McCarthy, 2003). Tumor-specific factors that contribute to muscle wasting include production of proteolysis-inducing factor and lipid-mobilizing factor by tumors, which interfere with muscle and fat anabolism (Tisdale, 2000b).

Some persons with cancer have an added tumor burden that can interfere with the ability to chew, swallow, or digest food, such as dysphasia with head/neck, esophageal, pancreatic, bowel, and genitourinary cancers. Side effects of cancer treatments, such as mucositis, xerostomia, taste changes, nausea and vomiting, and diarrhea also interfere with adequate intake of nutrients (MacDonald et al., 2003).

The somatic signs and symptoms of cancer cachexia include weight loss and fatigue and can often resemble depression. It may be difficult to determine if the person with cachexia is experiencing depression. The profound weakness associated with cachexia certainly interferes with activities of daily living, which may contribute to feelings of worthlessness. The loss of self-worth may further contribute to loss of appetite. Thus depression may be both a result of and a contributing factor to cachexia. In fact, depression from advanced cancer may have its origins from the same cytokines that are responsible for cancer cachexia (Lanquillon, Krieg, Bening-Abu-Shach, et al., 2000).

Management. The summary that was just presented provides an understanding of the complex mechanisms involved in cachexia and helps explain why simply providing high-calorie, high-fat feedings does not overcome the muscle and fat wasting of cancer cachexia (McCarthy, 2003). Indeed, many studies evaluating aggressive nutritional support for patients with malignancy show no benefit on mortality and some increased risks (Klein, Kinney, Jeejeebhoy, et al., 1997; Winter, 2000). The outcome of aggressive nutritional support is likely related to whether weight loss is from caloric deprivation or cancer cachexia. For example, those whose weight loss is from interference with the ability to ingest food but who still feel hungry (e.g., head and neck or esophageal cancers) will more likely benefit from enteral nutrition than those individuals with no appetite and rapidly progressing cancer.

As more is learned about the pathophysiology of cachexia, it may be possible to improve the efficacy of nutritional support by using medications that alter the mechanisms leading to cachexia (Davis, 2002). Box 9-16 summarizes some of the medications in clinical trials that may be used to palliate cachexia in the future.

Despite the social pressure to increase food intake, this does not reverse cachexia nor does it extend or improve the patient's quality of life (Winter, 2000). For some patients and their families, the act of eating is an important sign of hope, whereas for others, eating is no longer important. Assessing the individual's desires and goals is essential to determine the best intervention in each situation, such as the choice of appetite stimulants in cancer cachexia.

Reversible factors contributing to decreased nutritional intake should be sought. Nausea and vomiting, constipation, diarrhea, and depression should be treated, which if successful may increase caloric intake.

- Early satiety and poor appetite should initially be treated with metoclopramide before using an appetite stimulant (Davis & Dickerson, 2000):
  - Encourage small, frequent foods throughout the day instead of three larger meals, and keep snacks within reach.
  - Separate medication times from meals (except for medications that must be taken with food).
  - Make mealtime enjoyable by encouraging socialization; evaluate the pros and cons of sitting at a table with family for dinner (i.e., increased energy expenditure vs. improved socialization and nutritional intake).
  - Make the environment as pleasant as possible, paying attention to lighting, view, noise level, and odors (Davis & Dickerson, 2000; Waller & Caroline, 2000).
  - Consider the use of an appetite stimulant.
  - Corticosteroids improve appetite and sense of well-being but show no significant effect on body weight. Corticosteroids in fact will increase muscle metabolism. Use for more than 2 months for appetite stimulation is not recommended because there is concern about

the side effects of long-term use of steroids (Barber, Ross, and Fearon, 1999; Davis & Dickerson, 2000; Tyler & Lipman, 2000a; Waller & Caroline, 2000).
  - Progestational drugs (e.g., megestrol acetate) lead to weight gain and improve appetite and well-being. There is no difference in survival for patients treated with megestrol (Tyler & Lipman, 2000a; Waller & Caroline, 2000). Many untoward side effects are possible; those occurring in up to 10% of patients include peripheral edema, nausea, impotence, and diarrhea (Davis & Dickerson, 2000; Tomiska, Tomiskova, Salajka, et al., 2003; Tyler & Lipman, 2000a).
- Cannabinoids improve appetite and lead to weight gain, but many patients find the CNS effects intolerable (Grotenhermen & Muller-Vahl, 2003; Tyler & Lipman, 2000a).
- Taste changes:
  - Teach and encourage good mouth care before meals.
  - Persons who have received chemotherapy often report red meats have a metallic taste. Try marinating meats before cooking.
  - Sweet foods may taste "sickeningly" sweet. Try foods with tart flavors.
  - Serve foods at room temperature.
  - Encourage patient to try a variety of foods, even some that were not favorites in the past.
- Mucositis/xerostomia:
  - Teach and encourage good mouth care, including use of artificial saliva for xerostomia.
  - Treat any infections (e.g., oral candidiasis).
  - Encourage soft, moist, bland foods and milk.
  - Avoid acidic or spicy foods and beverages.
  - Use chewing gum (sugarless), pilocarpine, or saliva substitutes for xerostomia.

Anorexia and weight loss are often distressing to patients and family members. The continued weight loss is a visible reminder of progressive disease. Often family members believe that if they can just get their loved ones to eat, the patients will feel better and live longer. In the advanced stages of cancer, many patients do not feel like eating and actually feel worse when they do eat. When family members persist in their demand to eat, everyone becomes frustrated. Educating both patients and family members that the weight loss of advanced cancer is very different from starvation and that eating more does not reverse this process is fundamental. An honest, supportive discussion may avert the feelings of guilt for both patients and family members (Fainsinger & Pereira, 2003).

Fatigue/Asthenia

Incidence and Etiology. Fatigue is the most common symptom of advanced cancer, seen in 60% to 90% of persons in palliative care (Conill, Verger, Henriquez, et al., 1997; Klinkenberg, Willems, Wal, et al., 2004; Sweeney, Neuenschwander, & Bruera, 2003). There is no universally accepted definition of fatigue. Although some authors differentiate between fatigue and asthenia, the terms are often considered synonymous in practice. The experience of fatigue is subjective and multidimensional. The sensory, affective, behavioral, and cognitive components of fatigue include generalized weakness and feeling tired, negative or unpleasant emotions, decreased activity, and mental exhaustion demonstrated by impaired concentration or loss of memory (Sweeney et al., 2003; Visovsky & Schneider, 2003).

Fatigue used to be considered part of other symptom complexes, such as cachexia or depression, but is now recognized as a syndrome with its own complex pathology that may occur alone or in combination with other symptoms (Tyler & Lipman, 2000b). Many factors contribute to fatigue (Escalante, 2003; McKinnon, 2002; Potter, 2004; Sweeney et al., 2003; Tyler & Lipman, 2000b):

- Persons with preexisting conditions such as stroke or congestive heart failure have fewer reserves and will fatigue more easily (Visovsky & Schneider, 2003).
- Cytokine (interleukin-6) production by tumors may directly cause fatigue. Indirectly, cytokines may contribute to fatigue by causing cachexia and muscle wasting (Ahlberg, Ekman, & Gaston-Johansson, 2004).
- Physiologic states that stress the body contribute to fatigue, including pain, infection, dehydration, hypoxia, anemia, and malnutrition.

- The most common paraneoplastic syndromes—hypercalcemia and the syndrome of inappropriate antidiuretic hormone secretion (SIADH)—cause fatigue.
- Muscle abnormalities that occur with deconditioning as a result of immobility or cachexia cause persons to tire easily (Barsevick, Dudley, Beck, et al., 2004).
- Chemotherapy, radiation therapy, surgery, and biotherapy may cause fatigue directly (e.g., interferon) or indirectly (e.g., anemia, increased energy for healing). Persons on combination therapy likely experience more fatigue than those on monotherapy (Gelinas & Fillion, 2004; Mock & Olsen, 2003).
- Some medications have fatigue or sedation as a side effect, including opioids, hypnotics, anxiolytics, antihistamines, antiemetics, and antihypertensives.
- Emotional and psychologic issues, such as anxiety, depression, and stress, also contribute to fatigue.

Management. Fatigue has a profound negative impact on quality of living (Visovsky & Schneider, 2003). Persons experiencing fatigue do not have the energy to participate in activities of importance to them, such as joining the family for dinner at a table, attending religious services, and performing activities of daily living. The mental fatigue makes it difficult for the individual to participate in conversations and make decisions. The combination of physical and mental fatigue puts the individual at risk for isolation and loneliness.

A thorough assessment to determine the causative factors involved in the fatigue is critical to appropriate intervention. Whenever possible, interventions are aimed at eliminating the underlying cause(s). Preexisting conditions cannot be eliminated, but management of these conditions may lessen fatigue. The person with congestive heart failure may benefit from changes in medications to better manage the activity intolerance associated with that disease.

As noted earlier in the discussion of treating cachexia, corticosteroids and megestrol can improve the sense of well-being. The mechanism of action leading to improved functional levels and well-being is not clear but may be due to effects on cytokine release (Sweeney et al., 2003). Because the mechanisms of action for the medications listed in Table 9-16 involve inhibition of cytokines, these medications may also be indirectly helpful for the treatment of fatigue. Preliminary studies using thalidomide and omega-3 fatty acids are promising but additional study is needed (Barber, Ross, Voss, et al., 1999; Bruera, Neumann, Pituskin, et al., 1999; Moses, Slater, Preston, et al., 2004). Symptoms that cause physiologic or emotional distress, such as pain, infection, dehydration, hypoxia, and anemia, must be assessed and managed appropriately. Likewise, identification and proper treatment of hypercalcemia and SIADH can improve fatigue (as well as other symptoms).

Abundant literature supports the use of exercise to combat fatigue for patients undergoing active cancer therapies (Visovsky & Schneider, 2003). Most of these study participants had early-stage disease, and most of the studies have been in women with breast cancer. The role of exercise to treat fatigue in advanced stages of cancers has not been studied. However, the author's clinical experience is that mild exercise (e.g., going for a walk) improves mood and sleep patterns in the subset of palliative care patients who are physically able to perform the exercise. Ongoing assessment is required to evaluate when the exercise may be more of a burden than a benefit.

Consultation with a clinical pharmacist can be very helpful to identify medications contributing to fatigue. It may be possible to eliminate some medications; others may be effective at lower doses. If opioids are contributing to fatigue and sedation, methylphenidate may be helpful (Tyler & Lipman, 2002b; Rozans, Dreisbach, Lertora, et al., 2002).

Malaise and decreased activity level are common with depression as well as with advanced cancer. Because of this overlap, depression is often underdiagnosed in patients with advanced cancer (Breitbart, Chochinov, & Passik, 2003). Again, careful assessment is required. If depression is the cause of the fatigue, appropriate treatment of the depression is required. Methylphenidate is effective in reducing both cancer-related fatigue and depression (Homsi, Nelson, Sarhill, et al., 2001; Sarhill, Walsh, Nelson, et al., 2001). Methylphenidate is started at 2.5 mg to 5 mg and administered at 8 AM and noon. Doses are titrated to response.

Anxiety and stress are tiring and they interfere with sleep, making the situation worse. These symptoms must be skillfully assessed and addressed. Interventions may range from active listening to pharmacologic management. As noted, anxiolytics and hypnotics cause fatigue, so their use must be evaluated carefully.

Energy conservation is used for all causes of fatigue. Pacing activities and setting priorities are helpful in decreasing energy-requiring activities (Barsevick, Whitmer, Sweeney, et al., 2002). An analogy many patients find helpful is the concept of an "energy checkbook," requiring energy "deposits" (rest times) in order to "make withdrawals" (participate in activities). Recognizing that some activities require bigger withdrawals from the energy account helps individuals choose those activities of most importance. Keeping needed items within reach and using assistive devices, such as walkers or bedside commodes, are helpful in decreasing the energy requirements of everyday activities.

Keeping the mind active (even if the body cannot be) increases the ability to concentrate. Breast cancer

Table **9-16** PROMISING MEDICATIONS FOR THE MANAGEMENT OF CACHEXIA

Medication	Proposed Mechanism of Action
Omega-3 fatty acids	Inhibition of TNF, interleukins-1, -2, -4, -6, & interferon-γ,
Nonsteroidal antiinflammatory drugs	Decreases production of C-reactive protein
Melatonin	Inhibition of TNF
Thalidomide	Inhibition of TNF

TNF, Tumor necrosing factor.
Data from Bruera, E., & Sweeney, C., (2003). Pharmacological interventions in cachexia and anorexia. In D. Doyle, G. Hanks, N. Cherny, et al. (Eds.), *Oxford textbook of palliative medicine* (3rd ed.). New York: Oxford University Press.

patients who participated in an activity such as walking, gardening, or bird-watching after surgery (Chimprich, 1993) and those who participated in virtual reality distraction while receiving chemotherapy (Schneider, Ellis, Coombs, et al., 2003) experienced less fatigue than their matched control groups. Although not studied in palliative care settings, it makes sense that activities aimed at restoring attention are helpful. Playing card, board, or electronic games, conversing with colleagues, and working on favorite crafts are examples of attention-restorative activities that do not require the expenditure of a great deal of physical energy. Keep in mind that the plan of care will change as the disease progresses and energy levels are further decreased.

Nausea and Vomiting

Incidence and Etiology. Nausea and vomiting unrelated to chemotherapy occur in 40% to 70% of persons with advanced cancer (Davis & Walsh, 2000; Griffie & McKinnon, 2002; Komurcu, Nelson, & Walsh, 2001; Waller & Caroline, 2000). Nausea alone interferes with intake and causes emotional distress, taking a toll on quality of life. When accompanied by vomiting, the impact can be severe.

Figure 9-1 shows the mechanisms involved in nausea and vomiting. The vomiting center is located in the brainstem within the blood-brain barrier and receives stimulation from at least five

areas: the central pattern generator (CPG), nucleus tractus solitarius (NTS), motor complex and postrema, pharyngeal afferents, and the vestibular apparatus (Mannix, 2003; Waller & Caroline, 2000). The postrema lies outside the blood-brain barrier as a circumventricular organ and is exposed to substances from the circulation. Emetogenic substances likely stimulate dopamine receptors within NTS and CPG (Hornby, 2001; Twycross & Back, 1998); the CPG then stimulates the associated voluntary and involuntary motor nuclei to coordinate the retching and vomiting reflex. The NTS stimulates the CPG in the presence of anxiety and stress and with increased intracranial pressure. Vagal afferents ending in the vagal motor complex are stimulated by irritation in the gastrointestinal tract. Likewise, irritation of the glossopharyngeal nerves activates the vagal afferents. Nausea and vomiting often are preceded by dizziness if the vestibular apparatus is stimulated, which, in turn, stimulates the CPG. Multiple receptors are involved in vomiting and nausea: serotonin ($5HT_2$ and $5HT_3$), dopamine, cholinergic, histaminergic, and neurokinin (Davis & Walsh 2000; Hornby, 2001). The common causes of nausea and vomiting in palliative care are identified in Box 9-6.

Management. The management of nausea and vomiting requires careful assessment to determine the underlying cause and mechanism of stimulation to the vomiting center. Interventions to eliminate the cause are the first step to management. When the underlying cause is not treatable or while the evaluation to determine cause is ongoing, appropriate interventions to control the symptom should be initiated.

Discontinue or decrease the dose of offending medications. A review of the medication list by a clinical pharmacist can help identify offending medications as well the combinations of medications. Medications that were previously well-tolerated (e.g., digoxin) may become toxic and cause nausea and vomiting because of reduced renal and hepatic function. High levels of serum calcium or low sodium also trigger the chemoreceptor trigger zone (CTZ); assess for and treat hypercalcemia and SIADH appropriately. For example, use of bisphosphonates is appropriate when correcting the

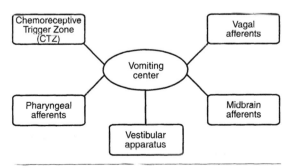

FIGURE **9-1** Mechanisms leading to nausea and vomiting. (From Griffie, J., & McKinnon, S. [2002]. Nausea and vomiting. In K. Kuebler, P. Berry, & D. Heidrich [Eds.], *End of life care clinical practice guidelines* [p. 343]. St. Louis: Saunders.)

Box 9-6   Common Causes of Nausea and Vomiting in Palliative Care

CHEMORECEPTOR TRIGGER ZONE MEDIATED
- Medications:
  —Opioids
  —Antibiotics
  —Chemotherapy
  —Corticosteroids
  —Digoxin
  —Nonsteroidal antiinflammatory drugs
  —Iron
- Metabolic:
  —Hypercalcemia
  —Hyponatremia
  —Uremia

MIDBRAIN AFFERENTS
- Emotional factors:
  —Anxiety
  —Fear
  —Pain
- Increased intracranial pressure
- Primary or metastatic brain tumors
- Meningitis

VAGAL AFFERENTS
- Gastrointestinal distention, stasis, or obstruction
- Constipation
- Gastritis
- External pressure ("squashed stomach syndrome")

PHARYNGEAL AFFERENTS
- Thick sputum
- Oral infection (e.g., candidiasis)
- Chronic cough
- Unpleasant tastes

VESTIBULAR APPARATUS
- Motion sickness
- Brain tumors
- Opioids

Data from Griffie, J., & McKinnon, S. (2002). Nausea and vomiting. In K. Kuebler, P. Berry, & D. Heidrich (Eds.), *End of life care clinical practice guidelines* (pp. 333-343). St. Louis: Saunders; Mannix, K. (2003). Palliation of nausea and vomiting. In D. Doyle, G. Hanks, N. Cherny, et al. (Eds.), *Oxford textbook of palliative medicine* (3rd ed., pp. 459-468). New York: Oxford University Press.

calcium level and improves quality of living; Patients whose quality of life is unlikely to improve even with a normal calcium level may achieve better symptom management with antiemetics instead of the bisphosphonate.

Identifying situations during which nausea and vomiting occur can help determine if emotional factors are contributing to these symptoms. Listen to concerns, address fears, and treat pain. Anxiolytics are used only when psychosocial and emotional support are not effective. Opioids are sometimes blamed for nausea when the real problem is under-treated pain, resulting in continued nausea and vomiting and worsening of pain.

When increased intracranial pressure is the cause of nausea, corticosteroids are the first line of treatment. Patients with brain tumors may achieve some relief with radiation therapy (Mannix, 2003), depending on the tumor type and previous treatments. Keep in mind that increased intracranial pressure may actually worsen with initiation of radiation therapy due to inflammation and edema (Hoskin, 2003). It is important to adjust the dexamethasone dosage as needed throughout treatment and recovery from radiation side effects.

Prokinetic agents are helpful for gastric stasis and early satiety. Metoclopramide promotes gastric peristalsis and shortens the gastric and upper intestinal transit time. Patients with partial bowel obstruction may develop gastric colic from metoclopramide (Mannix, 2003), so patient response requires careful, ongoing evaluation. External pressure on the gastric outlet with ascites or hepatomegaly can cause a "squashed stomach syndrome." Patients report feeling full and nauseous after eating and may do better with small, frequent meals, with or without the addition of metoclopramide. Management of constipation is important since a full rectum reduces gastric motility through the rectogastric reflex. Bowel obstruction produces crescendo nausea, which peaks with vomiting followed by a period of relief.

Thick sputum may cause nausea by stimulating the pharyngeal afferents. Inhalation therapy with saline or a commercial mucolytic (e.g., acetylcysteine) may be helpful. When appropriate, encourage the patient to drink more fluids to help thin secretions. Prolonged coughing also stimulates pharyngeal afferents and responds to antitussive medications. Encourage good oral hygiene to eliminate unpleasant tastes, and treat any oral infections.

When the cause of nausea and vomiting cannot be eliminated, empiric antiemetics are instituted. Selection of the appropriate medication is based on the mechanism involved in the vomiting reflex. Table 9-17 lists antiemetics based on their mechanism of action. The serotonin antagonists are very effective to treat the nausea and vomiting associated with highly emetogenic chemotherapy but have little benefit in palliative practices. Little information is available on the use of the medications for other causes of nausea and vomiting. Initial choices are either metoclopramide or haloperidol with dose titration to response. In patients who have nausea that fails to respond, consider the addition of a corticosteroid alternatively or a broad-spectrum atypical antipsychotic like olanzapine. Other options are tetrahydrocannabinoids or the combination of a 5HT$_3$ receptor antagonist and a phenothiazine (Davis & Walsh, 2000).

Another criterion to consider when selecting antiemetics is the route of administration. Patients with persistent vomiting need a route other than oral. Rectal or parenteral routes may be required, at least until the vomiting is under control. The dose must be titrated to effectiveness while assessing for side effects (Mannix, 2003). If nausea persists, look for other potential causes. Consider switching medications if a different etiology is identified, or consider adding an antiemetic from a different class if no new cause is found (Davis & Walsh, 2000).

Constipation

Incidence and Etiology. Constipation is a common problem in persons with advanced cancer. In a prospective study of 197 palliative care patients with cancer, the incidence of constipation increased from 49% at first interview (2 to 10 weeks before death) to 55% in the last 48 hours of life (Conill et al., 1997). Other studies suggest the incidence of constipation in advanced cancer ranges between 40% and 45% (Bennett & Cresswell, 2003). This is significantly higher than the general population but is still likely an underestimate of the incidence

Table **9-17** ANTIEMETIC SELECTION BY NAUSEA AND VOMITING MECHANISM

Mechanism	Receptor Site	Examples
CTZ stimulation	Dopamine antagonists	Haloperidol Metoclopramide Prochlorperazine
	Serotonin antagonists	Ondansetron Granisetron Dolasetron mesylate
Midbrain afferents:		
—Anxiety	Anxiolytics	Lorazepam
—Increased intracranial pressure	Corticosteroids	Dexamethasone
Vagal afferents	Prokinetic drugs	Metoclopramide
	Antisecretory agents	Octreotide
Vomiting center	Antihistamines	Diphenhydramine Hydroxyzine
	Anticholinergics	Scopolamine

CTZ, Chemoreceptor trigger zone.
Data from Griffie, J., & McKinnon, S. (2002). Nausea and vomiting. In K. Kuebler, P. Berry, & D. Heidrich (Eds.), *End of life care clinical practice guidelines* (pp. 333-343). St. Louis: Saunders; Mannix, K. (2003). Palliation of nausea and vomiting. In D. Doyle, G. Hanks, N. Cherny, et al. (Eds.), *Oxford textbook of palliative medicine* (3rd ed., pp. 459-468). New York: Oxford University Press; Tyler, L. (2000). Nausea and vomiting in palliative care. In A. Lipman, K. Jackson, & L. Tyler, (Eds.), *Evidence based symptom control in palliative care* (pp. 163-181). New York: Pharmaceutical Products Press.

in advanced cancer (Sykes, 2003). The term *constipation* implies that (1) the frequency of bowel movements is unsatisfactory, (2) there is a sensation of incomplete evacuation, (3) consistency of the stools is hard, and (4) stool is passed with discomfort (Klaschik, Nauck, & Ostgathe, 2003). Constipation is uncomfortable; unmanaged constipation leads to impaction and symptoms of bowel obstruction (referred to as *opioid bowel syndrome*) (Pappagallo, 2001).

Factors contributing to constipation with advanced cancer include immobility; dietary changes; medications, including opioids and anticholinergics; chemical imbalances, such as hypercalcemia; pressure on the bowel from tumors, ascites, or adhesions; changes to GI tract innervation from spinal cord compression, surgical damage, or chemotherapy-induced neuropathies; or psychosocial concerns, including stress, anxiety, and embarrassment (Bennett & Cresswell, 2003; Heidrich, 2002; Klaschik et al., 2003; Sykes, 1998).

Management. Whenever possible, treat the underlying cause of constipation. The first step in assessing constipation is to be sure that the patient does not have a bowel obstruction (Klaschik et al., 2003). Encouraging activity (when fatigue or pain does not interfere) will stimulate the bowels. Isometric and range-of-motion exercises may be helpful for patients who are bed-bound (Basta & Anderson, 1998; Klaschik et al., 2003).

Dietary and fluid intake are assessed and evaluated based on the individual's goals and prognosis. Instruct the patient with a normal appetite to drink at least 8 glasses of fluids daily and encourage a diet high in fiber (Beckwith, 2000; Klaschik et al., 2003). Note, however, that the amount of fiber required to treat constipation is rarely tolerated by persons with advanced cancer (Sykes, 2003). Diet intake that promotes motility includes salad, dates, and fruits. Constipating foods include flour products, chocolate, bananas, and tea (Klaschik et al., 2003).

Sitting in an upright position for bowel movements maximizes the muscle strength required for defecation (Basta & Anderson, 1998). Avoid bedpans and use bedside commodes for patients unable to ambulate to the bathroom. Allow for privacy during toileting. This can be especially challenging in acute

care settings or when the bed and bedside commode are in the living room in the home setting. Whenever possible, medications contributing to constipation are discontinued. However, commonly used analgesic medications such as opioids, tricyclic antidepressants, and anticholinergics may be required to control pain (Klaschik et al., 2003).

It is rare for the just-mentioned prophylactic interventions alone to manage the constipation associated with advanced cancer. Routine administration of stool softeners and laxatives is often necessary. The choice of laxative depends on the characteristics of the patient's stool and the individual's response to therapy. Hard, dry stool requires more softener; overly soft stool, causing fecal incontinence or leakage, requires less softener. Stool that is difficult to pass requires more stimulant; persons experiencing abdominal cramping may require less stimulant (Beckwith, 2000; Sykes, 2003). Many types of softeners and laxatives are available (Tables 9-18).

Osmotic laxatives are heterogenous, but the common denominator is that they are not reabsorbed during bowel transit. They transfer extracellular fluid into the bowel, and this shift in fluid may further dehydrate the patient. Therefore fluid intake is imperative if osmotic laxatives are used (Klaschik et al., 2003).

Saccharine laxatives (lactulose) pass to the colon unabsorbed and are fermented by bacteria into short-chained fatty acids. The intraluminal pH decreases, which stimulates peristalsis. Water is retained within stool and is drawn into the lumen, causing colonic distention and reflex emptying. Common side effects with saccharine laxatives are flatulence, cramps, and bloating (Klaschik et al., 2003).

Polyethylene glycol, commonly used for preparing a bowel for colonoscopy, hydrates hardened stool, increases stool volume, decreases transit time, and increases peristalsis. It is not metabolized, it does not lower lumen pH, and it does not cause migration of extracellular fluid into the bowel lumen. There is a linear dose-response relationship with polyethylene glycol, and it does not produce tachyphylaxis (Klaschik et al., 2003).

Stimulating laxatives usually consist of anthracenes (sennosides) and diphenols (bisacodyl).

Table 9-18 STOOL SOFTENERS AND LAXATIVES

Type	Action	Comments
Lubricant softeners: —Mineral oil	Penetrates stool and prevents water absorption	Less palatable than some others
Bulk-forming laxatives: —Methylcellulose —Psyllium —Polycarbophil	Resists bacterial breakdown, increasing bulk and shortening transit time	Must maintain fluid intake of 1½-2 liters of fluid per day
Emollient/surfactant softeners: —Docusate sodium	Increases water penetration	Increased transit time caused by opioids negates action of these laxatives
Osmotic laxatives: —Lactulose —Sorbitol —Glycerin	Creates osmotic gradient in the intestine	High oral doses for effectiveness may cause bloating, cramping, and diarrhea
Saline laxatives: —Magnesium citrate —Magnesium hydroxide —Sodium bisphosphate/sodium phosphate	Creates an immediate osmotic gradient in the intestine	Oral forms are effective in ½-3 hr; enemas often effective within 15 min
Stimulant laxatives: —Senna —Cascara sagrada —Bisacodyl	Stimulates submucosal nerve plexus to increase motility	May cause cramping; often used in combination with a softener

Data from Basta, S., & Anderson, D. (1998). Mechanisms and management of constipation in the cancer patient. *J Pharmaceutical Care Pain Symptom Control, 6*(3), 21-40; Beckwith, M. (2000). Constipation in palliative care patients. In A. Lipman, K. Jackson, & L. Tyler, (Eds.), *Evidence based symptom control in palliative care* (pp. 47-57). New York: Pharmaceutical Products Press; Sykes, N. (2003). Constipation and diarrhoea. In D. Doyle, G. Hanks, N. Cherny, et al. (Eds.), *Oxford textbook of palliative medicine* (3rd ed., pp. 483-496). New York: Oxford University Press.

Stimulating laxatives inhibit water reabsorption and induce an inflow of sodium, chloride, calcium, and water into the bowel lumen (similar to saccharine laxatives). Sennosides directly stimulate the myenteric plexus (Klaschik et al., 2003).

Persons with advanced cancer, especially those on opioids, require combinations of softener and stimulant laxatives. Regular assessment of the amount and consistency of stools, as well as ease and frequency of defecation, will help identify problems early (Box 9-7). If the rectum is full of soft stool, a stimulating suppository is given with a laxative. If stool is hard, a softening suppository or enema (olive oil, cotton seed oil) is used.

Patients are often embarrassed to describe bowel movements to the health care team. Teach the importance of prevention and early management of constipation. Allow for privacy during these conversations.

Diarrhea

Incidence and Etiology. Diarrhea occurs much less frequently than constipation. Approximately 5% to 10% of persons with advanced cancer report diarrhea. Most often it is an acute diarrhea lasting for only a few days (Sykes, 2003; Waller & Caroline, 2000). Overuse of laxatives is a common cause of diarrhea in advanced cancer. This tends to occur when laxative doses are progressively increased to treat a long-standing constipation. When the distal stool finally passes, it is followed by a large amount of very soft stool in a bowel stimulated by laxatives (Sykes, 2003).

Listening to bowel sounds; performing a rectal examination; identifying associated symptoms such as pain, colic, and nausea; and determining the time since the patient's last bowel movement will assist in determining the cause of diarrhea.

Box 9-7   Guidelines for Managing Constipation

1. Rule out obstruction.
2. Manually disimpact bowel, if necessary.
3. Initiate bowel regimen using emollient softener $\pm$ stimulant laxative (e.g., senna [Senokot-S]), depending on the assessment of the stool and ease of defecation.
4. If no bowel movement over 2 to 3 days, add a stimulant (e.g., bisacodyl [Dulcolax]). If the extra stimulant works, evaluate the stool and increase the daily stimulant, softener, or both.
5. If no bowel movement after additional stimulant, use a saline enema (e.g., sodium biphosphate/sodium phosphate [Fleets Enema]). If enema is effective, evaluate the stool and increase the daily stimulant, softener, or both.
6. If enema is not effective, use an oral saline (e.g., magnesium citrate) or osmotic laxative (lactulose). If this step is effective, evaluate the stool and increase the daily stimulant, softener, or both. If this step is not effective, repeat unless the patient experienced cramping or bloating.

Data from Heidrich, D. (2002). Constipation. In K. Kuebler, P. Berry, & D. Heidrich (Eds.), *End of life care clinical practice guidelines* (pp. 221-233). St. Louis: Saunders.

Keep in mind that the rectum can be empty if the impaction is higher in the colon (Klaschik et al., 2003; Waller & Caroline, 2000).

Inflammation of the mucosa from radiation therapy, chemotherapy, or infection causes a release of prostaglandins. These prostaglandins stimulate bowel secretions and inhibit absorption of liquid from the bowel. The resulting diarrhea tends to be high-volume and watery (Mercadante, 2002). This is sometimes referred to as *secretory diarrhea*. This type of diarrhea with carcinoid syndrome could also be seen as a result of neuroendocrine hormone stimulation, which can often respond to somatostatin (Waller & Caroline, 2000).

Biliary and pancreatic obstruction cause fat malabsorption as does gastrectomy and ileal resection. The resulting steatorrhea is characterized by large-volume, pale, foul-smelling feces that float in the toilet (Waller & Caroline, 2000). Short bowel syndrome occurs with total or almost total colectomy and loss of the ileocecal valve, resulting in watery stools.

Management. Interventions for diarrhea are based on the cause. Diarrhea caused by overuse of laxatives requires a medication adjustment. This most frequently occurs after severe constipation (Sykes, 2003). It may take some trial and error, with a pendulum swing between constipation and diarrhea, before finding the right combination and laxative dose for the individual.

(It may also take some time to regain the patient's trust.) The liquid oozing around an impaction requires removal of the impaction followed by careful titration of laxatives to prevent future impactions. Premedicate the patient for pain before disimpaction.

Antibiotics for infections may cause diarrhea as a result of altered bowel flora. The patient requires monitoring for signs of dehydration and syncope. Metronidazole may be necessary for the treatment of *Clostridium difficile* colitis.

When increased transit time through the GI tract is contributing to diarrhea as occurs with short bowel syndrome or from chemotherapy or radiation therapy, antidiarrheal medications such as loperamide, diphenoxylate, codeine, or tincture of opium are often helpful. Nonsteroidal antiinflammatory drugs and bismuth subsalicylate interfere with prostaglandin synthesis and can be helpful in treating diarrhea mediated by this mechanism. *Clostridium difficile* colitis is worsened by antimotility agents; hence the patient should be screened for colitis.

Octreotide is an effective but expensive intervention for secretory diarrhea. The somatostatin analogue inhibits mucosal secretion and peristalsis (Sykes, 2003; Waller & Caroline, 2000). Because of its high cost, octreotide is not a first-line treatment for diarrhea but should be considered when other interventions fail.

Steatorrhea is treated with pancreatic enzymes, and the diarrhea caused by malabsorption of bile salts can be treated with cholestyramine (Waller & Caroline, 2000).

Dietary changes can lessen diarrhea. These include eating smaller, more frequent meals; avoiding spicy foods, milk products, fatty foods, whole grains, fresh fruits, fresh vegetables, and caffeine; avoiding temperature extremes in foods; and broadening the diet slowly. Acceptable foods can be remembered using the mnemonic "BRAT"—bananas, rice or rice cereals, applesauce, and toast (Heidrich, 2002).

Bowel Obstruction

Incidence and Etiology. Bowel obstruction occurs in 3% of cancer patients, 16% of colon cancer patients, and 42% of women with ovarian cancer (Hirst & Regnard, 2003). Obstruction can be caused by intraluminal, intramural, or extramural tumor that compresses the bowel lumen, or it can be the result of a motility disorder secondary to interruption of the gastrointestinal nervous system (Davis & Nouneh, 2000; Hirst & Regnard, 2003).

Signs and symptoms of obstruction depend on the site of obstruction. The higher the obstruction in the gastrointestinal tract, the more symptoms the patient will have but the fewer the signs. Ninety percent of patients will have abdominal pain caused by mesenteric or peritoneal or retroperitoneal tumor infiltration, and 75% will have intermittent colic. Most will have nausea and vomiting (Davis & Nouneh, 2000; Hirst & Regnard, 2003). Abdominal bloating and distention are seen with small bowel and colic obstruction but not with gastric outlet obstruction. Vomiting occurs later in the course of illness when obstruction is occurring in the distal ileum or colon (Hirst & Regnard, 2003).

Management. The differential diagnosis should be made between a malignant bowel obstruction, opioid bowel obstruction, and opioid bowel syndrome (Davis & Nouneh, 2000). Additional considerations may include an ileus from anticholinergic medications, infections, and/or uremia (Hirst & Regnard, 2003).

A radiographic evaluation includes a supine and upright plain abdominal x-ray. The absence of air in the rectum and air fluid levels within the bowel lumen are helpful findings. Plain radiographs are also helpful and offer some sensitivity and reliability when attempting to differentiate a bowel obstruction from opioid bowel syndrome or an ileus. However, radiographs poorly predict the site of obstruction (Davis & Nouneh, 2000).

Multi-slice spiral CT, CT colonography, and MRI are more accurate than plain radiographs and can determine the extent of intraabdominal cancer (an important factor in determining if a patient is a surgical candidate) (Low, Chen, & Barone 2003; Taourel, Kessler, Lesnik, et al., 2003).

Patients who are candidates for surgical correction of bowel obstruction should be nutritionally sound, with minimal detectable abdominal disease and treatment options after operation (Davis & Nouneh, 2000; Pothuri, Vaidya, Aghajanian, et al., 2003; Smothers, Hynan, Fleming, et al., 2003). Stenting of obstruction lesions can be done for patients who are either being prepared for surgery or in lieu of surgery (Law, Choi, & Chu, 2003; Law, Choi, & Lee, 2004; Saida, Sumiyama, Nagao, et al., 2003). Combined stenting of biliary and duodenal obstruction can be done for relief of jaundice and nausea and vomiting in the case of pancreatic cancer (Profili, Feo, Meloni, et al., 2003; Tang, Allison, Dunkley, et al., 2003). Stenting will fail to relieve symptoms if there are multiple points of obstruction or if dysmotility is the primary cause for nausea and vomiting (Davis & Nouneh, 2000). Stenting has a reduced complication rate compared with surgical bypass and equal efficacy, at least in palliating malignant pyloroduodenal obstruction (Mittal, Windsor, Woodfield, et al., 2003).

The four major symptoms of malignant bowel obstruction can be managed by three medications. Opioids are used for continuous pain, either glycopyrrolate or hyoscine butylbromide for colic, and haloperidol for nausea and vomiting (Davis & Nouneh, 2000; Hirst & Regnard, 2003). Metoclopramide may be used for partial small obstruction in patients who do not have colic or complete obstipation (Davis & Nouneh, 2000; Hirst & Regnard, 2003). Medications to be added in case of incomplete response are dexamethasone and octreotide. Successful management is pain control, absence of nausea, and vomiting limited to once daily.

Patients who have symptoms that fail to respond to medical management should have either percutaneous gastrostomy placed by endoscopy (PEG) or fluoroscopy (PFG) or percutaneous transesophageal gastrostomy (PTEG) done for drainage. The PTEG can be done in patients who have had a previous gastric resection or ascites (Brooksbank, Game, & Ashby, 2002; Jolicoeur & Faught, 2003; Oishi, Shindo, Shirotani, et al., 2003).

Nursing concerns include wound care, catheter drainage, and pain management. Patients need to be mobilized soon after operation to reduce the risk of lower extremity thrombosis and pneumonia. Patients who undergo gastrostomy will need instructions on caring for the catheter and entrance site. Some patients may be able to be fed through their gastrostomy or will require it to be opened only intermittently to reduce nausea and vomiting.

Medications will need to be reviewed with the patient and family. Some patients will require home parenteral medications and perhaps hydration. The purpose of each medication and dose should be given to the patient in written form. Most of the drugs used to palliate the symptoms of bowel obstruction (morphine, glycopyrrolate, and haloperidol) can be combined in a single infusion, which will simplify home care.

Depression

Incidence and Etiology. The conditions for which the term *depression* is used can be viewed as being on a continuum, with reactive depression at one end, adjustment disorder with depressed mood in the middle, and major depressive disorder at the other end. Box 9-8 identifies the criteria for the diagnosis of a major depressive disorder. Reports on the incidence of depression in advanced cancer are difficult to interpret because the definition of depression that is being used is not always clear.

It is probably safe to say that patients with advanced cancer have experienced reactive depression. It seems evident that whether talking about a mood state or a depressive disorder, persons with cancer experience more depression than the general population and that the incidence of depression increases as the disease progresses (Massie & Popkin, 1998). Cited rates for depression are found to be between 10% to 47% (Breitbart et al., 2003; Massie & Popkin, 1998).

One of the problems in identifying depression in patients with advanced cancer is that so many of the symptoms of depression often overlap with expected symptoms of cancer. Weight loss (cachexia), fatigue, and diminished ability to concentrate (attentional fatigue) are common to depression and advanced malignancy. In addition to these criteria, further assessment should include

---

Box 9-8 CRITERIA FOR MAJOR DEPRESSIVE EPISODE

At least five of the following symptoms have been present most of the day, or almost every day, for at least 2 weeks. At least one of the symptoms must be item 1 or 2.
1. Depressed mood (feeling sad or empty; appears tearful).
2. Markedly decreased interest or pleasure in all, or almost all, activities.
3. Significant weight loss.
4. Insomnia or hypersomnia.
5. Psychomotor agitation or retardation.
6. Fatigue or loss of energy.
7. Feelings of worthlessness or excessive or inappropriate guilt.
8. Diminished ability to think or concentrate, or indecisiveness.
9. Recurrent thoughts of death (not just fear of dying), recurrent suicidal ideation, or suicide attempt.

Data from American Psychiatric Association (2000). *Major depressive disorder: A patient and family guide.* Washington D.C.: Author; American Psychiatric Association (2000). *Practice guidelines for the treatment of patients with major depression* (2nd ed.). Washington D.C.: Author.

(1) depressed mood or (2) decreased interest or pleasure in activities.

Abnormal levels of the neurotransmitters responsible for depression include serotonin, norepinephrine, and gamma-aminobutyric acid (GABA), as well as elevated cytokines. It is not clear if these abnormalities are the cause or the result of depression (Much & Barsevick, 1999; Sterling, 1999).

Management. An interdisciplinary approach is essential for the optimal management of depression. Patients with reactive depression need the emotional support offered by nurses, social workers, physicians, and spiritual counselors. A clinical psychiatrist should be consulted when caring for persons with major depression (American Psychiatric Association [APA], 2000) for the pharmaceutical management. Treatment for depression includes supportive psychotherapy, cognitive-behavioral supportive therapies, and antidepressant medications. Selective serotonin reuptake inhibitors (SSRIs) are frequently prescribed because they have fewer side effects than the older tricyclic antidepressants (APA, 2000). However, drug interactions are a significant problem and weeks are required before benefits occur.

Because standard antidepressants may take several days to weeks to reach peak effectiveness, psychostimulants (e.g., methylphenidate) are sometimes used for a rapid response. These medications not only have a rapid onset of action but also are energizing with few drug interactions (Breitbart et al., 2003). Potential side effects include tremor, tachycardia, insomnia, nightmares, and psychosis (Massie & Popkin, 1998; Waller & Caroline, 2000). Psychostimulants can be combined with SSRIs and then tapered once SSRIs begin to have their effect.

Persons with advanced cancer have a suicide risk twice that of the general population (Massie & Popkin, 1998). Risk factors include uncontrolled symptoms; feelings of hopelessness; delirium; history of substance abuse, psychiatric disorder, or suicide attempt; family history of suicide; social isolation; or recent death of a loved one. Assessing the seriousness of suicide intent includes asking the following question and proceeding to the rest if the patient responds affirmatively:

- "Have you ever thought about ending your own life?"
- "Are you thinking about it now?"
- "Have you ever thought about how you might do this?"
- "Do you have the means (pills, weapon, etc.) to kill yourself?"

Patients with the intent and the means to commit suicide should be immediately referred for a psychiatric evaluation. Some persons make a rational decision to end their lives—and it is legally acceptable to do so in Oregon. The psychiatric evaluation is not meant to interfere with the rational person's choice but to ensure that the treatable illness like depression is not influencing that choice.

SUMMARY

This chapter reviews the pathophysiology of advanced malignancies as well as discusses clinical symptoms and recommended management. Palliative practices are critical to cancer patient management throughout the trajectory of the disease. As palliative medicine in cancer care continues to evolve and be implemented, an increase in the overall quality patient care and satisfaction should become evident. Managing the physical, emotional, and spiritual needs of the patient throughout disease and treatment will likely mean less acute care interventions requiring symptomatic hospitalization. Early assessment and ensuring that the patients and their families are part of the care team are integral to achieving overall quality of life for the patient with advanced malignancy.

Clinicians should consider hospice referral as appropriate for this patient population. Initiate discussions early on with the patient and family regarding prognosis and end-of-life care. Engage the oncology patient care team, including the clinical social workers and case managers, in discussing the patient's prognosis and the overall individualized plan of care. The team can identify resource and support needs of the patient and family before the patient care conference to discuss the plan of care with the patient and family. Preliminary planning and thoughtful discussions will send a clear message to the patient and family that they are cared for by a compassionate team of professionals committed to partnering with them throughout their disease until death.

Case Study

T.S. is a 20-year-old college student who presented to the ED with complaints of profound weakness, fatigue, and dizziness. A CBC and a comprehensive metabolic profile were obtained and revealed that T.S. was severely anemic with a low hemoglobin, leucopenia, and a differential remarkable for circulating blasts. An oncologist was consulted, and a bone marrow biopsy was performed that revealed a B cell acute lymphocytic leukemia.

T.S. was immediately transferred to a large academic hospital and chemotherapy was initiated. His first cycle of chemotherapy was completed without significant side effects. After a brief break, T.S. was readmitted to begin his second round of treatments. A central line was placed, and chemotherapy of methotrexate 1000 mg/m^2 on day 1 and cytarabine (Ara-C) 1500 mg/m^2 every 12 hours, starting on day 2. During this hospitalization, T.S. also received methotrexate 15 mg IT for one dose. T.S.'s hospital course was basically uneventful with the exception of the development of a pilonidal cyst. He began a course of antibiotics; the cyst was incised and drained. T.S. was discharged home. Before discharge, it was determined that T.S. would be closely monitored by his oncologist with twice-weekly clinic visits that would include a CBC evaluation. He was discharged home on the following medications: ciprofloxacin 500 mg PO BID for 3 weeks; acyclovir 400 mg PO BID for 3 weeks; chlorhexidine gluconate (Peridex) solution 15 ml QID; and filgrastim (Neupogen) 480 mcg subcutaneously before discharge.

On T.S.'s first follow-up visit in the oncology clinic he was feeling well and his KPS score was 100. His vital signs and physical examination were unremarkable. T.S., now day 8 of his second cycle of chemotherapy, had the following laboratory results: WBC 0.57; RBC 2.90; Hgb 8.5; Hct 25.7; MCV 88.6; PLT 110; RDW 15.1. Differential: neutrophils 42.2; lymphocytes 54.2; monocytes 1.8; eosinophils 1.8; basophils 0.0; ANC 240.

Because of T.S.'s low WBC count and neutrophils, he was instructed to closely follow neutropenic precautions due to his propensity to develop an infection.

T.S. contacted the clinic 5 days after his last visit and informed the office nurse that he had been experiencing fever of 101.8° F. He was instructed to immediately report to the ED for an emergent evaluation. His physical examination and review of systems were unremarkable. His CBC was also unremarkable with the exception of his WBC count at 260, Hgb 6.2, PLT count less than 10,000 with an ANC of 0. Because of this ANC and fever, he was immediately admitted into the acute care setting with a diagnosis of pancytopenia and neutropenic fever and to rule out sepsis.

Blood and urine cultures were obtained, a chest radiograph was ordered, and IV fluids and empiric antibiotics were started, which included imipenem/cilastatin (Primaxin) 500 mg every 8 hours and vancomycin 1gm every 12 hours. T.S. also was restarted on filgrastim (Neupogen) 480 mcg subcutaneous injection daily. An infectious disease specialist was consulted, and a full work-up began to rule out the source of infection.

During his hospital stay, his blood counts began to recover and his condition began to stabilize. Preliminary blood cultures were positive for staphylococcus, with final cultures positive for MRSA. T.S.'s central venous catheter was identified as the source of infection after the line was discontinued for use and the tip culture returned positive. Imipenem/cilastatin (Primaxin) was discontinued, and he continued a full course of antibiotic therapy with vancomycin 1 gm every 12 hours. As a precaution, a cardiologist was consulted and a transesophageal echocardiogram was obtained to rule out a diagnosis of endocarditis. The cardiac evaluation was negative, and T.S. was discharged home with IV vancomycin to be given by a community home care agency.

ED, Emergency department; *CBC,* complete blood count; *IT,* intrathecally; *PO,* by mouth; *BID,* twice a day; *QID,* four times a day; *KPS,* Karnofsky Performance Scale; *WBC,* white blood cell count; *RBC,* red blood cell count; *Hgb,* hemoglobin; *Hct,* hematocrit; *MCV,* mean corpuscular volume; *PLT,* platelet; *RDW,* red blood cell distribution; *ANC,* absolute neutrophil count; *IV,* intravenous; *MRSA,* methicillin-resistant *Staphylococcus aureus.*

Objective Questions

1. The most life-threatening aspect of the neoplastic cascade is:

    a. Frequency of palliative symptoms.
    b. Disease progression and metastatic spread.
    c. Response to clinical trials.
    d. Karnofsky Performance Status.

2. Prognostic indicators in advanced cancer are important to:

    a. Determine cancer treatment modality.
    b. Determine placement in palliative care bed or hospice center.
    c. Guide palliative interventions in advanced malignancies.
    d. Notify the patient's family when it is time to refer to hospice.

3. Fifty one percent of inpatient care expenses occur during:

    a. The final month of life.
    b. The last 6 months of life.
    c. The diagnosis and treatment phases of care.
    d. Inpatient hospice care.

4. The Institute of Medicine report on health disparities in cancer mortality among the poor and underserved found that:

    a. Minorities and the poor are underrepresented in cancer clinical trials.
    b. Palliative care is not available to the poor and underserved.
    c. Minorities and the poor are less compliant and are lost to follow-up.
    d. Minorities and the poor have advanced disease.

5. The over-expression of this glycoprotein found in some breast cancers has given them a role in predicting treatment response to chemotherapy:

    a. p53 and EGFR.
    b. NK cells.
    c. BCRA1 and BCRA2.
    d. EGFR and HER-2/neu.

6. While still under investigation, omega-3 fatty acid supplementation may interfere with the cancer cachexia syndrome by:

    a. Decreasing the production of C-reactive protein.
    b. Inhibiting lipid mobilizing factor.
    c. Inhibiting tumor necrosis factor.
    d. Preventing protein degradation and muscle wasting.

7. The initial choice of a medication to treat early satiety and poor appetite should be:

    a. Dexamethasone.
    b. Dronabinol.
    c. Megestrol acetate.
    d. Metoclopramide.

8. The following is true regarding the symptom of fatigue:

    a. Fatigue occurs only in the presence of other pathology such as cachexia and depression.
    b. Fatigue in advanced cancer is most often caused by anemia.
    c. Persons with fatigue should not exercise because this depletes the individual's already limited energy reserves.
    d. Cytokine production by tumors may directly cause fatigue.

9. When the cause of nausea and vomiting cannot be eliminated, the initial choice of an antiemetic in the palliative care setting is:

    a. Metoclopramide.
    b. Prochlorperazine.
    c. Ondansetron.
    d. Scopolamine.

10. The first step in assessing constipation is to:

    a. Assess the patient's activity level.
    b. Evaluate fluid and food intake.
    c. Review current laxative use.
    d. Rule out a bowel obstruction.

11. The following medication is sometimes used to get a rapid response in a patient

with depression:

   a. Amitriptyline.
   b. Fluoxetine.
   c. Methylphenidate.
   d. Venlafaxine

12. Which of the following is a primary intervention that can decrease neurologic damage related to spinal cord compression?

   a. Encouraging the patient to ambulate as tolerated.
   b. Administering narcotics for relief of back pain.
   c. Logrolling the patient during repositioning.
   d. Identifying the underlying cause of the compression.

13. Symptom management of patients with SIADH can be promoted by:

   a. Encouraging patients to increase their fluid intake during episodes of thirst.
   b. Administering narcotics for pain management.
   c. Encouraging/providing frequent oral hygiene.
   d. Administering thiazide diuretics.

14. The initial treatment for palliation of symptoms of superior vena cava syndrome should be:

   a. Glucocorticoids.
   b. Chemotherapy.
   c. Streptokinase.
   d. Radiation therapy.

15. Management of the patient with increased intracranial pressure should include which of the following?

   a. Isometric exercises to minimize risks of complications related to immobility.
   b. Clustering of nursing activities to increase periods of uninterrupted rest.
   c. Encouraging neck flexion and head rotation to minimize stiffness.

   d. Protecting the patient from exposure to others with a "common cold."

REFERENCES

Abner, A. (1993). Approach to the patient who presents with superior vena cava syndrome. *Chest, 103*(4), 3945-3975.

Abrey, L.E. (2002). Leptomeningeal neoplasms. *Curr Treat Options Oncol, 4*(2), 147-156.

Ahlberg, K., Ekman, T., & Gaston-Johansson, F. (2004). Levels of fatigue compared to levels of cytokines and hemoglobin during pelvic radiotherapy: A pilot study. *Biol Res Nurs, 5*(3), 203-210.

Altman, A. (2001). Acute tumor lysis syndrome. *Semin Oncol, 28*(2 Suppl. 5), 3-8.

American Cancer Society (ACS). (2003a). *Cancer facts & figures 2003.* Atlanta: American Cancer Society.

American Cancer Society (ACS). (2003b). *Cancer facts & figures for African Americans 2003-2004* (p. 4). Atlanta: American Cancer Society.

American Cancer Society (ACS). (2003c). *Cancer facts & figures for Hispanics/Latinos 2003-2005* (p. 4). Atlanta: American Cancer Society.

American Cancer Society (ACS). (2004). *Cancer facts & figures 2003.* Atlanta: American Cancer Society.

American Psychiatric Association (APA). (2000). *Practice guidelines for the treatment of patients with major depression* (2nd ed.). Washington D.C.: Author.

Bach, P.B., Schrag, D., Brawley, O.W., et al. (2002). Survival of blacks and whites after a cancer diagnosis. *JAMA, 287*(16), 2106-2113.

Balducci, L. (2003). Geriatric oncology. *Crit Rev Oncol Hematol, 46*(3), 211-220.

Barber, M., Ross, J., & Fearon, K. (1999). Cancer cachexia. *Surg Oncol, 8,* 133-141.

Barber, M., Ross, J., Voss, A., et al. (1999). The effect of an oral nutritional supplement enriched with fish oil on weight loss in patients with pancreatic cancer. *Br J Cancer, 81,* 80-86.

Barnett, M.L. (1999). Hypercalcemia. *Semin Oncol Nurs, 15*(3), 190-201.

Barsevick, A.M., Dudley, W., Beck, S., et al. (2004). A randomized clinical trial of energy conservation for patients with cancer-related fatigue. *Cancer, 100*(6), 1302-1310.

Barsevick, A.M., Whitmer, K., Sweeney, C., et al. (2002). A pilot study examining energy conservation for cancer treatment-related fatigue. *Cancer Nurs, 25,* 333-341.

Bartanusz, V., & Porchet, F. (2003). Current strategies in the management of spinal metastatic disease. *Swiss Surg, 9*(2), 55-62.

Basta, S., & Anderson, D. (1998). Mechanisms and management of constipation in the cancer patient. *J Pharmaceutical Care Pain Symptom Control, 6*(3), 21-40.

Baylis, P.H. (2003). The syndrome of inappropriate antiidiuretic hormone secretion. *Int J Biochem Cell Biol, 35*(11), 1495-1499.

Beckwith, M. (2000). Constipation in palliative care patients. In A. Lipman, K. Jackson, & L. Tyler, (Eds.), *Evidence based symptom control in palliative care* (pp. 47-57). New York: Pharmaceutical Products Press.

Beers, M.H., & Berkow, R. (Eds.). (1999). Gastrointestinal disorders. *The Merck manual: Centennial edition* (pp. 327-328). New Jersey: Merck Research Laboratories.

Benenstein, R., Nayar, A.C., Rosen, R., et al. (2003). Doppler diagnosis of acute occlusion of the superior vena cava. *Echocardiography, 20*(1), 97-98.

Bennett, M., & Cresswell, H. (2003). Factors influencing constipation in advanced cancer patients: A prospective study of opioid dose, dantron dose and physical functioning. *Palliat Med, 17*(5), 418-422.

Bradley, C.J., Givens, C.W., & Roberts, C. (2001). Disparities in cancer diagnosis and survival. *Cancer, 91*(1), 178-188.

Brawer, M.K., Cheli, C.D., Neaman, I.E., et al. (2000). Complexed prostate-specific antigen provides significant enhancement of specificity with total prostate-specific antigen for detecting prostate cancer. *J Urol, 163,* 1476-1480.

Breitbart, W., Chochinov, H., & Passik, S. (2003). Psychiatric symptoms in palliative medicine. In D. Doyle, G. Hanks, N. Cherny, et al. (Eds.), *Oxford textbook of palliative medicine* (3rd ed., pp. 746-771). New York: Oxford University Press.

Brooks, P.C., Stromblad, S., Sanders, L.C., et al. (1996). Localization of matrix metalloproteinase MMP-2 to the surface of invasive cells by interactions with integrin alpha-v-beta 3. *Cell, 85,* 683-693.

Brooksbank, M.A., Game, P.A., & Ashby, M.A. (2002). Palliative venting gastrostomy in malignant intestinal obstruction. *Palliat Med, 16*(6), 520-526.

Bruckner, H.W., Pitrelli, J.P., & Merrick, M. (2000). Adenocarcinoma of the colon and rectum. In R.C. Bast, D.W. Kufe, R.E. Pollock, et al. (Eds.), *Cancer medicine* (p. 1472). Hamilton, Ontario Canada: B.C. Decker.

Bruera, E. (1997). Anorexia, cachexia and nutrition. *Br Med J, 315,* 1219-1222.

Bruera, E., Neumann, C., Pituskin, E., et al. (1999). Thalidomide in patients with cachexia due to terminal cancer: Preliminary report. *Ann Oncol, 10,* 857-859.

Bucholtz, J.D. (1999). Metastatic epidural spinal cord compression. *Semin Oncol Nurs, 15*(3), 150-159.

Burnnell, C.A., Winer, E.P., & Garber, J.E. (2003). Breast cancer: Staging and prognosis. In B. Furie, P.A. Cassileth, M.B. Atkins, et al. (Eds.), *Clinical hematology and oncology: Presentation, diagnosis, and treatment* (pp.719-722). Philadelphia: Churchill Livingston.

Chatziioannou, A., Alexopoulos, T., Mourikis, D., et al. (2003). Stent therapy for malignant superior vena cava syndrome: Should be first line therapy or simple adjunct to radiotherapy. *Eur J Radiol, 47*(3), 247-250.

Chen, Y.Y., & Schnitt, S.J. (1998). Prognostic factors for patients with breast cancer 1cm and smaller (review). *Breast Cancer Res Treat, 51,* 209-225.

Chimprich, B. (1993). Development of an intervention to restore attention in cancer patients. *Cancer Nurs, 16,* 83-92.

Conill, C., Verger, E., Henriquez, I., et al. (1997). Symptom prevalence in the last week of life. *J Pain Symptom Manage, 46,* 328-331.

Crook, M. (2002). Vasopressin V_2 receptor antagonists. *J Clin Pathol, 55,* 883.

Cruz, J. (1996). Adverse effects of pentobarbital on cerebral venous oxygenation of comatose patients with acute traumatic brain injury. *J Neurosurg, 85,* 758-761.

Dale, D.C. (2003). Poor prognosis in elderly patients with cancer: The role of bias and under-treatment. *Supportive Oncology, 1*(2), 11.

Daniel, B.T. (2001). Malignant lymphoma. In S.E. Otto (Ed.), *Oncology nursing* (4th ed., p. 420). St. Louis: Mosby.

Davidson, N.E. (1995). Hormone-replacement therapy: Breast versus heart versus bone (Editorial comment). *N Engl J Med, 332,* 1638-1639.

Davis, M.P. (2002). New drugs for the anorexia-cachexia syndrome. *Curr Oncol Rep, 4*(3), 264-274.

Davis, M.P., & Dickerson, D. (2000). Cachexia and anorexia: Cancer's covert killer. *Support Care Cancer, 8*(3), 180-187.

Davis, M.P., & Nouneh, C. (2000). Modern management of cancer-related intestinal obstruction. *Curr Oncol Rep, 2*(4), 343-350.

Davis, M.P., & Walsh, D. (2000). Treatment of nausea and vomiting in advanced cancer. *Support Care Cancer, 8,* 444-452.

Dennis, L.K., & Resnick, M.I. (2000). Analysis of recent trends in prostate cancer incidence and mortality. *Prostate, 42,* 247-252.

Dinkel, H.P., Mettke, B., Schmid, F., et al. (2003). Endovascular treatment of malignant superior vena cava syndrome: Is bilateral wall stent placement superior to unilateral placement? *J Endovasc Ther, 10*(4), 788-797.

Elledge, R.M., & Allred, D.C. (1994). The p53 tumor suppressor gene in breast cancer. *Breast Cancer Res Treat, 32,* 39-47.

Elledge, R.M., Green, S., Ciocca, D., et al. (1998). HER-2 expression and response to tamoxifen in estrogen receptor-positive breast cancer. A Southwest Oncology Group Study. *Clin Cancer Res, 4,* 7-12.

Escalante, C.P. (2003). Treatment of cancer-related fatigue: An update. *Support Care Cancer, 11,* 79-83.

Fainsinger, R., & Pereira, J. (2003). Clinical assessment and decision-making in cachexia and anorexia. In D. Doyle, G. Hanks, N. Cherny, et al. (Eds.), *Oxford textbook of palliative medicine* (3rd ed., pp. 533-546). New York: Oxford University Press.

Fitzgibbons, P.L. (2001). Breast cancer. In M.K. Gospodarowicz (Ed.), *Prognostic factors in cancer.* London: Wiley-Liss.

Flounders, J.A., & Ott, B.B. (2003). Oncology emergency modules: Spinal cord compression. *Oncol Nurs Forum, 30*(1), on-line exclusive, E17-23.

Folkman, J. (2000). Tumor angiogenesis. In Bast, R.C., Kufe, D.W., Pollock, R.E., et al. (Eds.), *Cancer medicine* (5th ed., pp. 133-134). Hamilton, Ontario: B.C. Decker.

Forsyth, P.A., Weaver, S., Fulton, D., et al. (2003). Prophylactic anticonvulsants in patients with brain tumour. *Can J Neurol Sci, 30*(2), 106-112.

Freedman, A.S., & Nadler, L.M. (2000). Non-Hodgkin's lymphomas. In Bast, R.C., Kufe, D.W., Pollock, R.E., et al. (Eds.), *Cancer medicine* (p. 2034). Hamilton, Ontario: B.C. Decker.

Freeman, H.P. (2004). Poverty, culture, and social injustice determinates of cancer disparities. *CA Cancer J Clin, 54*(2), 72-77.

Garber, A.M., MaCurdy, T., & McClellan, M. (1999). Medical care at the end of life: Diseases, treatment patterns and costs. In A. Garber (Ed.), *Frontiers in health policy research* (vol 2). Cambridge, Mass. MIT Press.

Gelinas, C., & Fillion, L. (2004). Factors related to persistent fatigue following completion of breast cancer treatment. *Oncol Nurs Forum, 31*(2), 269-278.

Ghogawala, Z., Mansfield, F.L., & Borges, L.F. (2001). Spinal radiation before surgical decompression adversely affects outcomes of surgery for symptomatic metastatic spinal cord compression. *Spine, 26*(7), 818-824.

Goodwin, R.A., Nickell, J.A., & DesPrez, R.M. (1972). Mediastinal fibrosis complicating healed primary histoplasmosis and tuberculosis. *Medicine, 51*(3), 227-246.

Griffie, J., & McKinnon, S. (2002). Nausea and vomiting. In K. Kuebler, P. Berry, & D. Heidrich (Eds.), *End of life care clinical practice guidelines* (pp. 333-343). St. Louis: Saunders.

Groenwald, S.L., Frogge, M.H., Goodman, M., et al. (1998). *Clinical guide to cancer nursing* (4th ed.). Boston: Jones & Bartlett.

Grotenhermen, F., & Muller-Vahl, K. (2003). IACM 2nd conference on cannabinoids in medicine. *Expert Opin Pharmacother,* 4(12), 2367-2371.

Gucalp, R., & Dutcher, J. (2001). Oncologic emergencies. In E. Braunwald, A.S. Fauci, D.L. Kasper, et al. (Eds.), *Harrison's principles of internal medicine* (15th ed., pp. 642-650). New York: McGraw Hill.

Gullatte, M. (2001). Cancer prevention, screening and early detection, In S.E. Otto (Ed.), *Oncology nursing* (4th ed.). St. Louis: Mosby.

Haapoja, I.S., & Blendowski, C. (1999). Superior vena cava syndrome. *Semin Oncol Nurs,* 15(3), 183-189.

Healthy People 2010 goals and objectives. www.health.gov/healthypeople

Heidrich, D. (2002). Constipation. In K. Kuebler, P. Berry, & D. Heidrich (Eds.), *End of life care clinical practice guidelines.* St. Louis: Saunders.

Hemann R, (2001). Superior vena cava syndrome. *Clin Excell Nurse Pract,* 5(2), 85-87.

Herman, J.G., & Baylin, S.B. (2003). Gene silencing in cancer in association with promoter hypermethylation. *N Engl J Med,* 349(21), 2042-2054.

Hickman, J.L. (1998). Increased intracranial pressure. In C.C. Chernecky & B.J. Berger (Eds.), *Advanced and critical care nursing: Managing primary complications.* Philadelphia: Saunders.

Hightower, D., & Vaughn, P. (2003, July 25). *Survivorship and the changing role of palliative care.* Retrieved August 29, 2003, from http://cancer.gov/BenchMarks/archives/2003_06/feature-print.html

Hirst, B., & Regnard, C. (2003). Management of intestinal obstruction in malignant disease. *Clin Med,* 3(4), 311-314.

Homsi, J., Nelson, K.A., Sarhill, N., et al. (2001). A phase II study of methylphenidate for depression in advanced cancer. *Am J Hosp Palliat Care,* 18(6), 403-407.

Hoover, D.R., Crystal, S., Kumar, R., et al. (2002). Medical expenditures during the last year of life: Findings from the 1992-1996 Medicare current beneficiary survey (Cost of care). *Health Serv Res,* 37(6), 1625-1642.

Hornby, P.J. (2001). Central neurocircuitry associated with emesis. *Am J Med,* 111(Suppl. 8A), 106S-112S.

Hoskin, P. (2003). Radiotherapy in symptom management. In D. Doyle, G. Hanks, N. Cherny, et al. (Eds.), *Oxford textbook of palliative medicine* (3rd ed., pp. 239-255). New York: Oxford University Press.

Husband, D.J., Grant, K.A., & Romaniuk, C.S. (2001). MRI in the diagnosis and treatment of suspected malignant spinal cord compression. *Br J Radiol,* 74, 15-23.

Inui, A. (2002). Cancer anorexia-cachexia syndrome: current issues in research and management. *CA Cancer J Clin,* 52, 72-91.

Janicic, N., & Verbalis, J.G. (2003). Evaluation and management of hypo-osmolality in hospitalized patients. *Endocrinol Metab Clin North Am,* 32(2), 459-481.

Jolicoeur, L., & Faught, E. (2003). Managing bowel obstruction in ovarian cancer using a percutaneous endoscopic gastrostomy (PEG) tube. *Can Oncol Nurs J,* 13(4), 212-219.

Kanner, A.A., Suh, J.H., Siomin, V.E., et al. (2003). Posterior fossa metastases: Aggressive treatment improves survival. *Stereotact Funct Neurosurg,* 80(1-4 Pt. 2), 18-23.

Karp, D.D., & Thurer, R.L. (2003). Non-small cell lung cancer. In B.Furie, R. Mayer, P. Cassileth, et al. (Eds.), *Clinical hematology and oncology: Presentation, diagnosis and treatment* (pp. 958-962). Philadelphia: Churchill Livingston.

Kaufmann, A.M., & Carduso, E.R. (1993). Aggravation of vasogenic cerebral edema by multiple dose mannitol. *J Neurosurg,* 44, 584-589.

Kavanagh, K.H., & Kennedy, P.H. (1992). *Promotion cultural diversity: Strategies for health care professionals.* London: Sage Publications.

Keenan, A.M. (1999). Syndrome of inappropriate secretion of antidiuretic hormone in malignancy. *Semin Oncol Nurs,* 15(3), 160-167.

Klaschik, E., Nauck, F., & Ostgathe, C. (2003). Constipation: Modern laxative therapy. *Support Care Cancer,* 11, 679-685.

Klein, S., Kinney, J., Jeejeebhoy, K., et al. (1997). Nutrition support in clinical practice: A review of published data and recommendations for future research directions. Summary of a conference sponsored by the National Institutes of Health, American Society for Parenteral and Enteral Nutrition, and American Society for Clinical Nutrition. *Am J Clin Nutr,* 66(3), 683-706.

Klinkenberg, M., Willems, D., Wal, G., et al. (2004). Symptom burden in the last week of life. *J Pain Symptom Manage,* 27, 5-13.

Ko, Y.J., & Bubley, G.J. (2003). Prostate cancer. In B. Furie, P.A. Cassileth, M.B. Atkins, et al. (Eds.), *Clinical hematology and oncology: Presentation, diagnosis, and treatment* (p. 860). Philadelphia: Churchill Livingston.

Kolonel, L.N. (1996). Nutrition and prostate cancer. *Cancer Causes Control,* 7, 83-94.

Komurcu, S., Nelson, K., & Walsh, D. (2001). The gastrointestinal symptoms of advanced cancer, *Support Care Cancer,* 9, 32-39.

Kozniewska, E., Podlecka, A., & Rafalowska, J. (2003). Hyponatremic encephalopathy: Some experimental and clinical findings. *Folia Neuropathol,* 41(1), 41-45.

Kuebler, K. (2002). Depression. In K. Kuebler, P. Berry, & D. Heidrich (Eds.), *End of life care clinical practice guidelines.* St. Louis: Saunders.

Langfeldt, L.A., & Cooley, M.E. (2003). Syndrome of inappropriate antidiuretic hormone secretion in malignancy: Review and implications for nursing management. *Clin J Oncol Nurs,* 7(4), 425-430.

Lanquillon, S., Krieg, J.C., Bening-Abu-Shach, U., et al., (2000). Cytokine production and treatment response in major depressive disorder. *Neuropsychopharmacology,* 22(4), 370-379.

LaVecchia, C., Lucchini, F., Negri, E., et al. (2001). Cancer mortality in the elderly, 1960-1998: A worldwide approach. *Oncology Spectrum,* 2(6), 386-394.

Law, W.L., Choi, H.K., & Chu, K.W. (2003). Comparison of stenting with emergency surgery as palliative treatment for obstructing primary left-sided colorectal cancer. *Br J Surg,* 90(11), 1429-1433.

Law, W.L., Choi, H.K., & Lee, Y.M. (2004). Palliation for advanced malignant colorectal obstruction by self-expanding metallic stents: Prospective evaluation of outcomes. *Dis Colon Rectum,* 47(1), 39-43.

Lequaglie, C., Conti, B., Brega-Massone, P.P., et al. (2003). The difficult approach to neoplastic superior vena cava syndrome: Surgical option. *J Card Surg,* 44(5), 667-671.

Levack, P., Graham, J., Collie, D., et al. (2002). Don't wait for a sensory level—listen to the symptoms: A prospective audit of the delays in diagnosis of malignant cord compression. *Clin Onc, 14*(6), 472-480.

Leyland-Jones, B. (2003). Treatment of cancer-related hypercalcemia: The role of gallium nitrate. *Semin Oncol, 30*(2 Suppl. 5), 13-19.

Loblaw, D.A., Laperriere, N.J., & Mackillop, W.J. (2003). A population-based study of malignant spinal cord compression in Ontario. *Clin Onc, 15*(4), 211-217.

Loughrey, G.J., Collins, C.D., Todd, S.M., et al. (2000). Magnetic resonance imaging in the management of suspected spinal canal disease in patients with known malignancy. *Clin Radiol, 55*(11), 849-855.

Low, R.N., Chen, S.C., & Barone, R. (2003). Distinguishing benign from malignant bowel obstruction in patients with malignancy: Findings at MR imaging. *Radiology, 228*(1), 157-165.

Lubitz, J.D., & Riley, G.F. (1993). Trends in Medicare payments in the last year of life. *N Engl J Med, 328*(15), 1092-1096.

Lutterbach, J., Cyron, D., Henne, K., et al. (2003). Radiosurgery followed by planned observation in patients with one to three brain metastases. *Neurosurgery, 52*(5), 1066-1073.

MacDonald, N., Easson, A.M., Mazurak, V.C., et al. (2003). Understanding and managing cancer cachexia. *J Am Coll Surg, 197*(1), 143-161.

Mackillop, W.J. (2001). The importance of prognosis in cancer medicine. Accessed July, 26, 2003, from www.mrw.interscience.wiley.com.

Madden, L.K. (2001). Invasive neurologic monitoring. In H.M. Schell & K. Puntillo (Eds.), *Critical care nursing secrets* (pp. 240-247). Philadelphia: Hanley & Belfus.

Manley, P.W., Bold, G., Bruggen, J., et al. (2004). Advances in the structural biology, design and clinical development of VEGF-R kinase inhibitors for the treatment of angiogenesis. *Biochim Biophys Acta, 1697*(1-2), 17-27.

Mannix, K. (2003). Palliation of nausea and vomiting. In D. Doyle, G. Hanks, N. Cherny, et al. (Eds.), *Oxford textbook of palliative medicine* (3rd ed., pp. 459-468). New York: Oxford University Press.

Maranzano, E., Trippa, F., Chirico, L., et al. (2003). Management of metastatic spinal cord compression. *Tumori, 89*(5), 469-475.

Marcus, J.N., Watson, P., Page, D.L., et al. (1996). Hereditary breast cancer: Pathobiology, prognosis, and BRCA 1 and BRCA 2 gene linkage. *Cancer, 77*, 697-709.

Marcy, P.Y., Magne, N., Bentolila, F., et al. (2001). Superior vena cava obstruction: Is stenting necessary? *Support Care Cancer, 9*(2), 103-107.

Markman, M. (1999). Diagnosis and management of superior vena cava syndrome. *Cleve Clin J Med, 66*(1), 59-61.

Martignoni, M., Kunze, P., & Friess, H. (2003). Cancer cachexia. *Mol Cancer, 2*, 36.

Massie, J., & Popkin, M. (1998). Depressive disorders. In J. Holland (Ed.), *Psycho-oncology.* New York: Oxford University Press.

Mathlouthi, R., Aberl, S., Schug, N., et al. (2003). Assessing optimal promoter activity for constructs in gastrointestinal gene therapy. *Anticancer Res, 23*(5A), 4015.

Mayer, R.J. (2003). Colorectal cancer. In B. Furie, P.A. Cassileth, M.B. Atkins, et al. (Eds.), *Clinical hematology and oncology: Presentation, diagnosis, and treatment.* Philadelphia: Churchill Livingston.

McCarthy, D.O. (2003). Rethinking nutritional support for persons with cancer cachexia. *Biol Res Nurs, 5*(1), 3-17.

McKinnon, S. (2002). Fatigue. In K. Kuebler, P. Berry, & D. Heidrich (Eds.), *End of life care clinical practice guidelines* (pp. 317-326). St. Louis: Saunders.

Mercadante, S. (2002). Diarrhea, malabsorption, and constipation. In A. Berger, R. Portenoy, & D. Weissman (Eds.), *Principles and practice of palliative and supportive oncology* (2nd ed., pp. 233-249). Philadelphia: Lippincott Williams & Wilkins.

Merchant, J.J., & Schiller, J.H. (2003). Small cell lung cancer. In B. Furie, P.A. Cassileth, M.B. Atkins, et al. (Eds.), *Clinical hematology and oncology: Presentation, diagnosis and treatment.* London: Churchill Livingston.

Mittal, A., Windsor, J., Woodfield, J., et al. (2003). Matched study of three methods for palliation of malignant pyloroduodenal obstruction. *Br J Surg, 91*, 205-209.

Mock, V., & Olsen, M. (2003). Current management of fatigue and anemia in patients with cancer. *Semin Oncol Nurs, 19*(4 Suppl. 2), 36-41.

Moses, A.W., Slater, C., Preston, T., et al. (2004). Reduced total energy expenditure and physical activity in cachectic patients with pancreatic cancer can be modulated by an energy and protein dense oral supplement enriched with n-3 fatty acids. *Br J Cancer, 90*(5), 996-1002.

Much, J., & Barsevick, A. (1999). Depression. In C. Yarbro, M. Frogge, & M. Goodman (Eds.), *Cancer symptom management* (2nd ed., pp. 594-607). Sudbury, Mass.: Jones & Bartlett.

Muizelaar, J.P., Marmaroli, A., Ward, J.D., et al. (1991). Adverse effects of prolonged hyperventilation inpatients with severe head injury: A randomized clinical trial. *J Neurosurg, 75*, 731-739.

Mukhopadhyay, D., & Datta, K. (2004). Multiple regulatory pathways of vascular permeability factor/vascular endothelial growth factor (VPF/VEGF) expression in tumors. *Semin Cancer Biol, 14*(2), 123-130.

Nakayama, Y., Tanaka, A., Kumate, S., et al. (1996). Cerebral blood flow in normal brain tissue of patients with intracranial tumors. *Neurol Med Chir (Tokyo), 36*(10), 709-714.

National Cancer Institute (NCI). (2001). 2001 cancer progress report: Life after cancer—costs of cancer care. Retrieved December 14, 2003, from http://progressreport.cancer.gov/doc.asp?pid=1&did=21&chid=13&coid=33&mid=vpco

Netter, F.H. (1980). Superior vena cava syndrome. In F.H. Netter. *The CIBA collection of medical illustrations: Respiratory system.* Newark, N.J.: CIBA Pharmaceutical.

Nicholson, A.A., Ettles, D.F, Arnold, A., et al. (1997). Treatment of malignant superior vena cava syndrome: Metal stents or radiation therapy. *J Vasc Interv Radiol, 8*(5), 781-788.

Nicolin, G. (2002). Paediatric update: Emergencies and their management. *Eur J Cancer, 38*, 1365-1377.

Noel, G., Simon, J.M., Valery, C.A., et al. (2003). Surgical management of cerebral metastases from non-small cell lung cancer. *Tumori, 89*(3), 292-297.

Oishi, H., Shindo, H., Shirotani, N., et al. (2003). A nonsurgical technique to create an esophagostomy for difficult cases of percutaneous endoscopic gastrostomy. *Surg Endosc, 17*, 1224-1247.

Olsen, K.S., Svendsen, L.B., Larsen, F.S., et al. (1995). Effect of labetalol on cerebral blood flow, oxygen metabolism and autoregulation in healthy humans. *Br J Anaesth, 75*(1), 51-54.

Oncology Nursing Society (ONS). (1994) *Multicultural advisory council: Strategies for inclusion.* Pittsburgh: Author.

Oncology Nursing Society (ONS). (1999). *Multicultural outcomes: Guidelines for cultural competence.* Pittsburgh: Oncology Nursing Press.

Ostler, P.J., Clarke, D.P., Watkinson, A.F., et al. (1997). Superior vena cava obstruction: A modern management strategy. *Clin Oncol (R Coll Radiol), 9*(2), 83-89.

Pappagallo, M. (2001). Incidence, prevalence, and management of opioid bowel dysfunction. *Am J Surg, 182*(5A Suppl.), 11S-18S.

Pollmiller, K. (2001). Brain tumors. In R.A. Gates & R.M. Finks (Eds.). *Oncology nursing secrets* (2nd ed., p. 203). Philadelphia: Hanley & Belfus.

Pothuri, B., Vaidya, A., Aghajanian, C., et al. (2003). Palliative surgery for bowel obstruction in recurrent ovarian cancer: An updated series. *Gynecol Oncol, 89*(2), 306-313.

Potter, J. (2004). Fatigue experience in advanced cancer: A phenomenological approach. *Int J Palliat Nurs, 10*(1), 15-23.

Profili, S., Feo, C.F., Meloni, G.B., et al. (2003). Combined biliary and duodenal stenting for palliation of pancreatic cancer. *Scand J Gastroenterol, 38*(10), 1099-1102.

Ramnath, N., & Creaven, P.J. (2004). Matrix metalloproteinase inhibitors. *Curr Oncol Rep 6*(2), 96-102.

Reid-Finlay, M., & Kaplow, R. (2001). Oncologic emergencies. In H.M. Schell & K. Puntillo (Eds.), *Critical care nursing secrets* (pp. 216-225). Philadelphia: Hanley & Belfus.

Reinhard, M., Petrick, M., Steinfurth, G., et al. (2003). Acute increase in intracranial pressure revealed by transcranial Doppler sonography. *J Clin Ultrasound, 31*(6), 324-327.

Rogers, L.R. (2003). Cerebrovascular complications in cancer patients. *Neurol Clin, 21*(1), 167-192.

Rosner, M.J., Rosner, S.D., & Johnson, A.H. (1995). Cerebral perfusion pressure: Management protocol and clinical results. *J Neurosurg, 83*, 949-962.

Ross, H. (2000). *Lifting the unequal burden of cancer on minorities and the undeserved: Closing the gap* (p. 1). Washington, D.C.: Office of Minority Health.

Ross, J.R., Saunders, Y., Edmonds, P.M., et al. (2004). A systematic review of the role of bisphosphonates in metastatic cancer. *Health Technol Assess (Rockv), 8*(4), 1-176.

Rozans, M., Dreisbach, A., Lertora, J.J., et al. (2002). Palliative uses of methylphenidate in patients with cancer: A review. *J Clin Oncol, 20*(1), 335-339.

Saida, Y., Sumiyama, Y., Nagao, J., et al. (2003). Long-term prognosis of preoperative "bridge to surgery" expandable metallic stent insertion for obstructive colorectal cancer: Comparison with emergency operation. *Dis Colon Rectum, 46*(10 Suppl.), S44-S49.

Sarhill, N., Walsh, D., Nelson, K.A., et al. (2001). Methylphenidate for fatigue in advanced cancer: A prospective open-label pilot study. *Am J Hosp Palliat Care, 18*(3), 187-192.

Sarin, R., & Murthy, V. (2003). Medical decompressive therapy for primary and metastatic intracranial tumours. *Lancet, 2*(6), 357-365.

Scher, H.I., Issacs, J.T., Zelefsky, M.J., et al. (2000). Prostate cancer. In M.D. Abeloff, J.O. Armitage, A.S. Licher, et al. (Eds.), *Clinical oncology* (pp. 1823-1884). New York: Churchill Livingstone.

Schiff, D. (2003). Spinal cord compression. *Neurol Clin, 21*(1), 67-86.

Schneider, S.M., Ellis, M., Coombs, W.T., et al. (2003). Virtual reality intervention for older women with breast cancer. *Cyberpsychol Behav, 6*(3), 301-307.

Scitovsky, A.A. (1984). The high cost of dying: What do the data show? *Milbank Q, 62*(4), 591-608.

Seol, H.J., Chung, C.K., & Kim, H.J. (2002). Surgical approach to anterior compression in the upper thoracic spine. *J Neurosurg, 97*(3 Suppl.), 337-342.

Shavers, V.L., & Brown, M.L. (2002). Racial and ethnic disparities in the receipt of cancer treatment. *J Natl Cancer Inst, 94*(5), 334-357.

Smedley, B.D., Stith, A.Y., & Nelson, A.R. (Eds.). (2002). *Unequal treatment: Confronting racial and ethnic disparities in health care.* Committee on Understanding and Eliminating Racial and Ethnic Disparities in Health Care. Institute of Medicine. Washington, D.C.: National Academy Press.

Smith, W., & Khuri, F.R. (2004). The care of the lung cancer patient in the 21st century: A new age. *Semin Onc, 31* (2 Suppl. 4), 11-15.

Smothers, L., Hynan, L., Fleming, J., et al. (2003). Emergency surgery for colon carcinoma. *Dis Colon Rectum, 46*(1), 24-30.

Sterling, L. (1999). Pharmacological review of SSRIs in panic disorder. In *Therapeutic spotlight: Psychiatric illness in primary care* (A supplement to clinician review, p. 10-13).

Stinson, N. (2000). *Working together to better understand cancer-related health disparities: Closing the gap* (Editorial, p. 3). Washington, D.C.: Office of Minority Health.

Strasser, F. (2003). Pathophysiology of the anorexia/cachexia syndrome. In D. Doyle, G. Hanks, N. Cherny, et al. (Eds.), *Oxford textbook of palliative medicine* (3rd ed., pp. 520-533). New York: Oxford University Press.

Sweeney, C., Neuenschwander, H., & Bruera, E. (2003). Fatigue and asthenia. In D. Doyle, G. Hanks, N. Cherny, et al. (Eds.), *Oxford textbook of palliative medicine* (3rd ed., pp. 560-568). New York: Oxford University Press.

Sykes, N.P. (1998). The relationship between opioid use and laxative use in terminally ill cancer patients. *Palliat Med, 12*, 375-382.

Sykes, N.P. (2003). Constipation and diarrhoea. In D. Doyle, G. Hanks, N. Cherny, et al. (Eds.), *Oxford textbook of palliative medicine* (3rd ed., pp. 483-496). New York: Oxford University Press.

Tang, T., Allison, M., Dunkley, I., et al. (2003). Enteral stenting in 21 patients with malignant gastroduodenal obstruction. *J R Soc Med, 96*(10), 494-496.

Taourel, P., Kessler, N., Lesnik, A., et al. (2003). Helical CT of large bowel obstruction. *Abdom Imaging, 28*(2), 267-275.

Temkin-Greener, H., Meiners, E.A., Petty, E.A., et al. (1992). The use and cost of health services prior to death: A comparison of the Medicare-only and the Medicare-Medicaid elderly populations. *Milbank Q, 70*(4), 111-120.

Thirlwell, C., & Brock, C.S. (2003). Emergencies in oncology. *Clin Med, 3*(4), 306-310.

Tisdale, M. (2000a). Metabolic abnormalities in cachexia and anorexia. *Nutrition, 16*, 1013-1014.

Tisdale, M. (2000b). Protein loss in cancer cachexia. *Science, 289*, 2293-2366.

Tomiska, M., Tomiskova, M., Salajka, F., et al. (2003). Palliative treatment of cancer cachexia with oral suspension of megestrol acetate, *Neoplasma, 50*(3), 227-233.

Tortorice, P.V. (2003). Chemotherapy: Principles and practice. In C.H. Yarboro, M.H. Frogge, M. Goodman, et al. (Eds.), *Cancer nursing principles and practice* (5th ed., p. 366). Boston: Jones & Bartlett.

Twycross, R., & Back, O. (1998). Nausea and vomiting in advanced cancer. *Eur J Palliat Care, 5*, 39-45.

Tyler, L., & Lipman, A. (2000a). Anorexia and cachexia in palliative care patients. In A. Lipman, K. Jackson, & L. Tyler, (Eds.), *Evidence based symptom control in palliative care* (pp. 11-22). New York: Pharmaceutical Products Press.

Tyler, L., & Lipman, A. (2000b). Fatigue in palliative care patients. In A. Lipman, K. Jackson, & L. Tyler (Eds.), *Evidence based symptom control in palliative care* (pp. 129-141). New York: Pharmaceutical Products Press.

Urban, T., Lebeau, B., Chastang, C., et al. (1993). Superior vena cava syndrome in small cell lung cancer. *Arch Intern Med, 153*(3), 384-387.

Vaughn, C.J., & Delanty, N. (2000). Hypertensive emergencies. *Lancet, 356*(9227), 411-417.

Verbalis, J.G. (2002). Vasopressin V$_2$ receptor antagonists. *J Mol Endocrinol, 29*(1), 1-9.

Verbalis, J.G. (2003). Disorders of body water homeostasis. *Best Pract Res Clin Endocrinol Metab, 17*(4), 471-503.

Verheul, H.M., & Pimedo, H.M. (2003). Vascular endothelial growth factor and its inhibitors. *Drugs Today, 39*(Suppl. C), 81-93.

Visovsky, C., & Schneider, S. (2003). Cancer-related fatigue. *Online J Issues Nurs, 8*(3), 8. www.nursingworld.org/ojin/hirsh/topic3/tpc3_1.htm.

Waller, A., & Caroline, N. (2000). *Handbook of palliative care in cancer* (2nd ed.). Boston: Butterworth-Heinemann.

Ward, E., Jemal, A., Cokkinides, V., et al. (2004) Cancer disparities by race/ethnicity and socioeconomic status. *CA Cancer J Clin, 54*(2), 78-93.

Watling, C.J., & Cairncross, J.G. (2002). Acetazolamide therapy for symptomatic plateau waves in patients with brain tumors: Report of three cases. *J Neurosurg, 97*(1), 224-226.

Weidner, N., & Folkman, J. (1997). Tumor vascularity as a prognostic factor in cancer. *Principles and Practice Oncology Update, 11*, 1-5.

Willett, C.G., Fung, C.Y., Kaufman, D.S., et al. (1993). Postoperative radiation therapy for high-risk colon carcinoma. *J Clin Oncol, 11*(6), 1112-1117.

Winter, S.M. (2002). Terminal nutrition: Framing the debate for withdraw of nutritional support in terminally ill patients. *Am J Med, 109*(9), 723-726.

Wudel, L.J. Jr., & Nesbitt, J.C. (2001). Superior vena cava syndrome. *Curr Treat Options Oncol, 2*(1), 77-91.

Yahalom, J. (1993). Oncologic emergencies: Superior vena cava syndrome. In V.T. Devita, S. Hellman, & S.A. Rosenberg (Eds.), *Cancer: Principles and practice in oncology* (4th ed., pp. 2111-2118). Philadelphia: Lippincott.

Yalamanchili, M., & Lesser, G.J. (2003). Malignant spinal cord compression. *Curr Treat Options Oncol, 4*(6), 509-516.

Yellin, A., Rosen, A., Reicher, N., et al. (1990). Superior vena cava syndrome: The myth—the facts. *Am Rev Respir Dis, 4*(5), 1114-1118.

10 Cancer Pain

Mellar P. Davis
Jan L. Frandsen

OBJECTIVES

After the completion of this chapter, the reader should be able to:
1. Differentiate cancer pain syndromes.
2. Describe how to use pain assessment tools when assessing the cancer patient in pain.
3. Examine how to use opioids and adjuvant analgesics when optimally managing the patient experiencing cancer-related pain.

INTRODUCTION

Pain is one of the most common symptoms that accompany the experience of cancer and one of the main reasons that the Institutes of Medicine recently identified advanced cancer pain management as a priority for practice improvement in the United States (Levenson, 2001). The International Association for the Study of Pain (IASP) defines pain as an unpleasant sensation or emotional experience that is associated with actual or potential tissue damage or described in terms of such damage (Merskey, 1979). Even though pain is often associated with tissue destruction, the pain intensity experienced by the patient is not always proportional to the severity of tissue destruction (Portenoy, 1989, 1992). Pain is classified by several systems that include:

- Temporally acute intermittent pain
- Chronic continuous pain
- Pathophysiologic nociceptive sensations, which are seen in visceral or somatic pain
- Neuropathic pain

The authors would like to acknowledge the work done by Maribeth B. Kowalski, PharmD, RPh, on this chapter.

Pain Intensity

Pain severity or intensity can be modulated at several different locations within the central nervous system: (1) the dorsal horn; (2) through descending neural tracts from the bulbar periaqueductal grey and rostral ventral medulla; (3) at the level of the thalamus; and (4) within the prefrontal cortex cingulate gyrus and within limbic cortex (Basbaum, Clanton, & Fields, 1976; Basbaum & Fields, 1978, 1984; Fields & Basbaum, 1978; Julius & Basbaum, 2001; Melzack & Wall, 1965). Pain intensity is also influenced by the patient's past experiences, present expectations, cognition, and/or mood (Turk, 2002). Psychologic factors rarely initiate the pain experience but can certainly contribute to the intensity of the patient's pain. Pain therefore is intensified in the setting of fear, anxiety, and depression.

Prevalence of Cancer-Related Pain

The recent evidence report "Management of Cancer Symptoms: Pain, Depression, and Fatigue" published by the Agency for Healthcare Research and Quality (AHRQ) (2002) (Lipman, 2003) identified that despite the advances in cancer biology and an overwhelming array of treatment options, cancer continues to create suffering for the many patients and their families who are affected. Despite the World Health Organization's (WHO's) methods for the treatment of cancer pain, pain is generally not eliminated despite access to multiple analgesic therapies (AHRQ, 2002). The likelihood of intensified cancer pain occurs in the advancement of the disease process. Minorities, women, and the elderly are most at risk for poor pain control (AHRQ, 2002). The impact of an aging population will also affect the increased incidence and prevalence of cancer, and this will create a challenge for clinicians to understand how to promote an optimal quality of life and improved function for many patients over the next few decades.

Pain correlates directly with the stage of cancer. For instance, 6% to 17% of patients will experience pain in the early stages of a cancer diagnosis. Pain occurs in 20% to 50% of patients undergoing anti-tumor therapy and up to 75% to 80% of patients living and dying from advanced cancer (Bonica, 1980; Twycross, 2002; Twycross, Harcourt, & Bergl, 1996). Overall, 85% of pain is directly attributable to the cancer. Of patients with cancer, 17% will have pain related to cancer treatment and/or side effects (e.g., mucositis, radiation), 9% will have pain caused by general debility (e.g., decubitus ulcers, inactivity), and 9% will have pain as a result of a co-morbid illness (e.g., diabetes, osteoarthritis) (Grond, Zech, Diefenbach, et al., 1996).

Of 154 consecutive patient referrals to the Cleveland Clinic palliative medicine service, 100 were reported to have significant pain. There were 150 separate painful sites recorded, and 88% of patients with pain had a maximum of two separate pain syndromes (e.g., somatic, neuropathic). Somatic pain syndromes from solid tumor were reported in 68% of these patients. Somatic pain was experienced by 52%, 22% experienced visceral pain syndrome, 10% experienced neuropathic pain syndrome, and 16% had mixed pain (more than one pain syndrome) (Gutgsell, Walsh, Zhukovsky, et al., 2003). Intermittent breakthrough pain occurred, and 48% described having continuous pain. Intermittent pain was related to activity in 30% (incident pain), non-incident pain occurred in 26%, and 16% experienced end-of-dose anal-gesic failure. A group of patients experienced mixed incident and non-incident flares of breakthrough pain (Gutgsell et al., 2003).

In a larger study of 2000 cancer patients, more than 75% reported pain of severe intensity. Somatic pain was most frequently reported in patients with a diagnosis of breast, genitourinary, lymphoreticu-lar, and bone primary cancers, whereas head and neck cancers were often associated with mixed nociceptive and neuropathic pain. Patients with gastrointestinal cancers had a high frequency of visceral pain complaints. A third of these patients had a single site of pain, a third reported two sites of pain, and a third had three or more sites of pain (Grond et al., 1996). Fifty percent of the patients who reported pain in this study revealed a somatic pain syndrome in origin, whereas 20% to 35% reported neuropathic pain, and a small subset of patients had visceral pain. Pain from cancer treatment occurred in 10% to 20% of the patients, and fewer than 10% had pain associ-ated with co-morbid diseases (Grond et al., 1996).

PAIN SYNDROMES

Pain assessment is much more complex than rating pain intensity on a scale of 0 to 10 and should also include the location, quality, radiation, and ampli-fying factors (Davis & Walsh, 2000). The pattern of pain requires a comprehensive assessment and if done properly will provide the clinician with the probable cause and associated pain pathophysiology (Twycross, 2002). Delays in identifying a specific pain syndrome either from inaccurate assessment or lack of skill can prolong patients' suffering, decrease their functional capabilities, and increase the risk for further complications. The following discussion summarizes common cancer-associated pain syndromes.

Somatic Bone Pain

Patients with bone metastases experience pain with the greatest frequency. Bone pain is common with advanced breast, kidney, lung, and prostate cancer and multiple myeloma (Mercandate, 1997). Patients often describe bone pain as being well-localized, dull, aching, progressive, and often nocturnal. The intensity of bone pain worsens with weight-bearing activity, particularly when metastases are located within the lower extremities or in the axial skeleton.

Bone metastases are usually found in well-vascularized bone such as the proximal extremi-ties, skull, and spinal column. Metastases to bone are blastic, lytic, or mixed as determined by radio-graphic appearance. Blastic or lytic bone lesions are determined by the balanced activity of the osteoclasts and osteoblasts. For example, if the osteoclast activity overrides osteoblastic activity, the bone lesion will be lytic in character. Prostate cancer patients may not complain of pain despite widespread bony metastases, and for most patients only a minority of bone metastases will be painful (Nielsen, Munro, & Tannock, 1991).

Vertebral metastases can cause midline pain on initial presentation. Vertebral metastases require careful and ongoing assessment to prevent paraplegia from epidural tumor extension, which is a devastating experience for the patient and his or her family (Davis & Nouneh, 2000; Portenoy, 1992; Twycross, 2002). Most patients will have involvement of multiple vertebral bodies. The most common site is the thoracic spine, followed by the lumbar spine, and rarely the cervical neck. This is because of the anatomy of the thoracic spine, which has a narrower spinal canal and a higher blood flow than other areas of the spine. Metastasis to the vertebral column usually begins within the posterior vertebral body and extends anterior to the pedicle and epidural space. This is seen on magnetic resonance imaging (MRI) as posterior vertebral body destruction, whereas on plain radiographs pedicle destruction is often observed first.

Epidural extension of vertebral metastasis creates radicular pain, a result of nerve root compression (Twycross, 2002). Radicular pain is mostly unilateral in the cervical and lumbar spine and bilateral from the thoracic spine. Specific metastatic vertebral syndromes include (Davis & Walsh, 2000; Portenoy, 1989):

- Atlantoaxial metastases produce occipital headaches and radiating pain to the vertex of the skull. Pain worsens with neck flexion.
- C7-T1 vertebrae metastases cause pain to radiate to the intrascapular area where radiographs appear to be normal and often mislead clinicians.
- T12-L1 vertebral metastases are associated with pain that radiates to the sacral iliac crest.
- Sacral metastases produce posterior thigh, buttock, and perineal pain, which worsens with sitting or lying and improves with standing.

Pain from vertebral metastases increases with cough, sneeze, or Valsalva maneuvers (bowel movement). Unlike degenerative disk disease, metastatic vertebral pain worsens in the supine position (Caraceni & Portenoy, 1999; Nielsen & Skovgaard

Poulsen, 1989; Portenoy, 1992). Sudden sensory deficits, motor weakness, funicular extremity pain, incontinence of bowel or bladder, and Lhermitte syndrome (lightning-like pain with head flexion) herald a spinal cord compression and warrant rapid assessment and aggressive interventions (see Chapter 11) to prevent paraplegia or quadriplegia.

Nonmalignant Bone Disease

Diseases common to the elderly such as degenerative disk disease, osteomyelitis, osteoporosis, and Paget's disease will mimic metastatic bone disease. Positive radiographs should be followed with an MRI for patients who have a radicular pain or neurologic deficits despite what appears to be degenerative spine disease. Bone scans are not helpful in the evaluation of spinal cord compression; however, they provide valuable information about the extent of metastases (Portenoy, 1989).

Cranial Syndromes

Cranial syndromes generally consist of a combination of headaches, neuropathic pain, and cranial nerve deficits, which can be difficult to differentiate from leptomeningeal metastases (Jaeckle, 1993). Tumors most commonly associated with cranial syndromes are nasopharyngeal carcinomas and metastases from breast, lung, and prostate cancers (Twycross, 2002). Orbital lesions produce blurred vision, chemosis, external ophthalmoplegia, proptosis, and a loss of sensation in the distribution of the trigeminal nerve. Perisellar and cavernous sinus metastases produce signs similar to those of orbital lesions but also produce visual field cuts from compression of the optic chiasm. Metastatic disease that compresses the jugular foramen refers pain to the mastoid, which can also radiate down the neck to the shoulder. Metastases within the jugular foramen are associated with cranial nerve deficits involving cranial nerves IX, X, and XI. The "numb chin" syndrome is caused by metastases within the lingual canal of the mandible, which interrupts the submentel nerve. This is frequently seen in systemic spread of breast, prostate, and lung cancer. Tumors of the skull may directly invade the lateral or sagittal sinus causing thrombosis, resulting in increased intracranial pressure and neurologic deficits, which resemble brain metastasis (Davis & Walsh, 2000; Portenoy, 1992).

Plexopathies

Advanced breast and lung malignancies will cause brachial plexopathies, as will sequelae from radiotherapy. With cancer-associated plexopathy, pain radiates to the shoulder, scapula, and anterior chest wall and down the arm to the elbow and fifth finger. This type of pain often worsens with abduction of the arm and external rotation of the shoulder. Patients will often carry their arm in front of them (Davis & Nouneh, 2000; Jaeckle, 1991; Mukherkji, Castillo, & Wagle, 1996). Radiation-induced brachial plexopathy is usually less painful and follows the distribution of the C6 nerve.

Apical lung cancers (pancoast tumors) are the most common malignancy to produce a brachial plexopathy. The ulnar nerve root from the C7-T1 foramen is compressed or infiltrated by cancer, which causes radiating pain to the little finger. An ulnar nerve entrapment neuropathy will mimic a brachial plexopathy. Supraclavicular metastases from breast cancer and lymphomas will produce a similar pain syndrome. The differential diagnosis to brachial plexopathy includes radiation-associated brachial plexus injury. Radiation usually damages the C5-6 nerve roots, resulting in weakness and sensory deficit over the shoulder in a cape-like distribution, but it is not nearly as painful as a plexopathy caused by tumor (Olsen, Pfieffer, Johannsen, et al., 1993). As tumor grows into the cervical neck, a brachial pan-plexopathy and a Horner's syndrome will be seen clinically.

Lumbar plexopathies occur with equal frequency between genders. The usual cause is an extension of colorectal cancer, genitourinary cancer, lymphoma, or sarcoma into the retroperitoneal space. Most lumbar plexopathies develop within 3 years of the diagnosis (Davis & Walsh, 2000; Jaeckle, 1991). The initial presentation of a lumbar plexopathy is lower back pain that radiates to the thigh and with accompanied sensory and motor deficits may resemble a lumbar epidural cord compression.

Upper lumbar plexopathies involve L1 and L2 nerve roots with pain referred to the lower abdomen, groin, or thigh. Lumbar plexopathies are often accompanied by lower extremity lymphedema,

which provides a clue toward the diagnosis. Cancer that invades the sacral plexus involves the nerves from S2 to S4. These patients will often present with urinary retention, a flaccid bladder, bowel or bladder incontinence, and/or impotence (Davis & Walsh, 2000).

Neuropathies

Neuropathies are the result of an imbalance of afferent input to modulatory influences (interneurons and descending tracts) into the dorsal horn, which accentuate the pain experience through a wide range of dynamic neurons leading to hypersensitivity, hyperpathia, and allodynia. Abnormal neural growth and irregular synaptic growth may result in cross-connections between motor neurons and nociceptors, creating a painful reaction to touch or pressure (allodynia). Another theory gives rise to an abnormal neuroinflammatory response or a loss of opioid receptors or function from injury to the nerve (Galer & Dworkin, 2000). Certain receptors (*N*-methyl-D-aspartate [NMDA]) are up-regulated. Patients with neuropathic pain may describe the quality of their pain as burning, aching, shooting, sharp, lancinating, and elicited easily by touch or pressure. Paradoxically, there may be numbness in the distribution of pain.

Neuropathies from cancer will arise from central nervous system metastases or central neuroplasticity, which are caused by chronic peripheral sensory stimulation (barrage) resulting in central processing adoptions over time (Davis & Walsh, 2000; Twycross, 2002). Patients with neuropathic pain frequently require higher doses of opioids for pain relief because of reduced opioid receptors and increased counter–opioid receptor activity.

Leptomeningeal Metastases

Leptomeningeal metastases produce a pattern of multiple noncontiguous neurologic deficits and pain, which is often associated with headache and/or cognitive changes (Olson, Chernik, & Posner, 1971, 1974). Brain metastases will produce morning headache, particularly if located within the posterior fossa (Jaeckle, 1993). Cognitive changes for both leptomeningeal and brain metastases may be subtle and mistaken for a medication side effect. Unilateral motor or sensory deficits with apraxia, aphasia, agraphia, and/or agnosia will be seen on physical examination with brain metastases, depending on location of tumor within the brain (dominant or nondominant hemisphere). Physical examination will demonstrate simultaneous visual or tactile deficits on the side of the body opposite the side of metastatic disease.

Visceral Pain

Visceral pain is not well localized and is difficult for patients to characterize as to location or painful origin. Pain is not usually prominent with hepatic metastases until tumor extends to the hepatic capsule, because the hepatic parenchyma does not contain sensory fibers. Sensory nerves are located only within the liver capsule. When pain does occur, it is usually in the right upper quadrant and in the hypochondrium and worsens with standing or walking as a result of pressure on the hepatic ligament (Twycross, 2002).

Pancreatic pain occurs from obstruction to the pancreatic duct, infiltration of pancreatic capillaries, or involvement of regional nerves in the celiac plexus. Visceral pain is more common with cancers that arise from the head of the pancreas versus the tail or body (Krech & Walsh, 1991).

Pain associated from a bowel obstruction occurs as a result of external or internal occlusion of the bowel's lumen or extension into surrounding tissue, which influences nerve conduction generated from the myenteric plexus. Abdominal distention, hyperactive bowel sounds, nausea, vomiting, and obstipation are symptoms of a bowel obstruction (Davis & Nouneh, 2000). An important differential diagnosis to mechanical bowel obstruction is opioid-induced obstipation and paraneoplastic pseudo-obstruction, which is a result of destruction to the gut nervous system or smooth muscle (Davis & Nouneh, 2000).

Treatment-Related Pain

Post-thoracotomy pain is neuropathic in nature and associated with sensory loss in the area of the surgical incision. Dysesthesia, allodynia, or lancinating pain in the area of numbness is common. Pain usually diminishes over time. If pain intensity recurs after resolution, recurrent cancer should be suspected (Davis & Walsh, 2000; Twycross, 2002).

Post-mastectomy pain occurs in 20% of breast cancer patients and is directly related to the axillary dissection rather than the mastectomy. Axillary dissection interrupts the intercostobrachial nerve, which induces numbness in the medial arm and axilla (Stevens, Dibble, & Miaskowski, 1995). Pain is usually superficial or burning in character and is located in both the chest wall and medial arm. Chest wall pain may also arise from nerve entrapment within the postoperative scar. Phantom breast pain from central neuroplasticity has also been described (Jamison, Wellisch, Katz, et al., 1979; Kwekkeboom, 1996).

Post-radical neck dissection causes a mixed neuropathic and nociceptive pain, which radiates into the jaw, ear, neck, and shoulder (Davis & Walsh, 2000; Jaeckle, 1993). Shoulder pain is caused by interruption of the 11th cranial nerve. The patient may describe his or her pain as burning, hot, or stabbing in character.

Phantom limb pain is disabling, centrally derived neuroplastic pain, which is difficult to manage. It occurs in a small subset of cancer amputees, many of whom experienced severe limb pain preoperatively (Weinstein, 1994).

PAIN ASSESSMENT

Pain assessment is an integral and key component to good pain management. Failure to properly assess pain is one of the most common causes for poorly controlled pain (Von Roenn, Cleeland, Gonin, et al., 1993). On average, the recording of symptoms by physicians and nurses is poorly done and the use of standardized (simple) pain scales is consistently performed only by a few (AHRQ, 2002; Stromgren, Groenvold, Pedersen, et al., 2001; Weber & Huber, 1999). The American Society of Clinical Oncology recommends the use of at least one simple quantitative assessment scale to be recorded in the chart on a regular basis throughout the patient's treatment (Joint Commission on Accreditation of Healthcare Organizations [JCAHO], 2003). The Agency for Healthcare Research and Quality (AHRQ) recommends pain scales that are simple to use and that are both reliable and valid (instruments that measure accurately what they intended to measure) (AHRQ, 2002).

The Joint Commission on Accreditation of Healthcare Organizations (JCAHO) places pain assessment and its management on the top of its agenda for hospital accreditation and as a target for quality outcome (Simmons, 2001). Quality improvement guidelines that include assessment of pain relief have been developed by the American Pain Society (APS) and serve as models for JCAHO in their accreditation process (American Pain Society [APS], 1995).

Pain Intensity

Total pain includes sensory, affective (emotional), and cognitive components. Pain intensity directly interferes with patients' activities of daily living and their perception of their quality of life. A pain intensity of less than 4 on a numerical rating scale (NRS) of 0 to 10 (0 no pain, and 10 the worst pain imaginable) does not generally interfere with daily activity. A pain rating of 5 or greater, however, dramatically interferes with the functional abilities and quality of life of patients (Cleeland, Nakamura, Mendoza, et al., 1996; Serlin, Mendoza, Nakamura, et al., 1995). A patient's mood and the meaning that they give to their pain experience will directly interface with self-reported pain intensity. Numerical pain intensities are further clustered into categories:

- *Mild pain* is rated 0 through 4.
- *Moderate pain* is rated 5 through 7.
- *Severe pain* is rated 8 through 10.

Pain intensities expressed by patients poorly correspond to perceived pain intensities recorded by formal and informal caregivers. The greater the pain intensity is for the patient, the worse the correlation between the patient and his or her caregiver (Grossman, Scheidler, Swedeen, et al., 1991). The patient-perceived pain severity is under-appreciated by physicians and nurses. Pain intensity must be what the patient says it is, and self-assessment is the most reliable marker of pain intensity (Grossman et al., 1991).

Barriers Associated With Pain Assessment

Patients are to be encouraged to give a realistic appraisal of their pain experience. Patients do not like to be considered "complainers." They may fear that complaints of pain will draw attention away from treating their underlying cancer, or they fear that the pain means that their cancer is growing and death will soon follow (Sandkuhler, 2002). Many patients fear psychologic dependence and opioid side effects and will often be stoic and/or minimize their pain. Family members also play a big part in the barriers associated with optimal pain management; they may become disturbed by the patient's progressive pain or may fear the treatment with opioids will hasten their loved one's death. Often the patient will not report his or her pain to spare the family of anxiety. The financial burden of pain management may be a concern, particularly if families have limited income and no insurance to pay for expensive opioids that are prescribed (Grossman 1994; Institute of Medicine [IOM], 2004; Turk, 2002).

Pain Assessment Tools

The routine use of pain assessment tools promotes a heightened sense of awareness about the patient's pain and facilitates communication between the patient and his or her health care team (Faries, Mills, Goldsmith, et al., 1991; Lanser & Gesell, 2001; Merboth & Basnason, 2000). Systematic pain assessment leads to optimal prescribing, resulting in reduced pain compared with those whose pain is not routinely recorded (Jamison & Brown, 1991; Lynch, 2001). Vital signs are not to be considered the basis for which to dose opioids (Chuk, 1999). A well-recorded pain pattern of the patient's corresponding pain intensity should be considered the basis for appropriate opioid dosing. The following discussion highlights some of the common pain assessment tools used in clinical practice.

Unidimensional Pain Assessment Tools

The three unidimensional pain assessment tools most commonly used are the numerical rating scale (NRS), the verbal rating scale (VRS), and the visual analog scale (VAS). The VRS pain rating by the patient should be used most frequently by elderly or cognitively challenged patients. These categories of pain include:

- None
- Mild

- Moderate
- Severe

The VAS utilizes a horizontal line measuring 100 millimeter. The patient is asked to draw a vertical line perpendicular to the horizontal line at the point that best matches his or her pain intensity. The clinician using a centimeter ruler can measure the patient's mark along the horizontal axis from 0 (no pain) to 100 millimeters (the worst severity).

The NRS uses a 0 to 10 scale (0 = no pain, and 10 = worst pain imaginable). All three tools are valid and reliable measures that are used in conjunction with the WHO analgesic ladder guidelines to assess pain response (Chapman, Casey, Dubner, et al., 1985).

Multidimensional Pain Assessment Tools

Multidimensional pain assessment tools measure both the pain intensity and its impact on the patient's function, mood, and quality of life. These assessment tools are more time-consuming than unidimensional scales yet provide extensive and more complete information about the experience of pain (Cleeland, Nakamura, Mendoza, et al., 1996; Cleeland & Ryan, 1994). These scales include the Wisconsin Brief Pain Questionnaire, the McGill Pain Questionnaire, and the Memorial Pain Questionnaire Card (Daut, Cleeland, & Flanery, 1983; Fishman, Pasternak, Wallenstein, et al., 1987; Graham, Bond, Gerkovich, et al., 1980). The use of a multidimensional pain assessment tool is usually reserved for research purposes or as initial evaluation with unidimensional scales and pain-relief scales used for measuring pain response during analgesic treatment.

Quality-of-Life Assessment

Several global quality-of-life assessment tools specific to cancer include an assessment of pain. Examples of these assessment tools include (Aaronson, Ahmedzai, Bergman, et al., 1993; Bruera, MacMillian, Hanson, et al., 1989; Cella, Tulsky, Gray, et al., 1993; De Haes, van Knippenberg, & Neijt, 1990; Schipper, Clinch, McMurray, et al., 1984; Sloan, Loprinizi, Kuross, et al., 1999):

- Functional Living Index Cancer (FLIC) scale
- Edmonton Symptom Assessment Scale (ESAS)

- Spitzer Uniscale
- Rotterdam Symptom Checklist
- European Organization for Research and Treatment of Cancer Quality-of-Life Scale (QLQ-C30)
- Functional Assessment of Cancer Therapy (FACT) scale

Assessment of Pain History and Physical Examination

A pain history consists of the date of onset, rate of pain progression, quality, location, radiation, severity, temporal pain sequence, and associated symptoms, along with specific interventions that help relieve pain.

Pain intensity is the most important factor to determine therapeutic decision making. Severe or crescendo pain warrants an urgent investigation of the underlying etiology while aggressively managing the pain. A patient with bone metastasis from prostate cancer may suddenly develop pain radiating from his lower back into the thigh, indicating a spinal cord compression, which requires both prompt evaluation and treatment.

A detailed pain history will facilitate the determination of probable cause of pain (Bruera & Watanabe, 1994). Pain intensity will modulate during the day and should be cataloged as to its average intensity, at its worst, at its best, and its progression or regression over several days to weeks (Portenoy, 1989). Additional assessment should query pain interference with daily activities. A comprehensive pain history also includes trials of medications prescribed in attempt to reduce pain; these include any over-the-counter medications and nonpharmacologic approaches. A complete list of the patient's medications is necessary to avoid drug-to-drug incompatibilities and to facilitate proper analgesic selection. The patient's past medical and social history are important in the evaluation of pain. Alcohol abuse is screened through the CAGE questionnaire. This identifies patients with a positive alcohol abuse history and the need for supportive services by experienced medical social workers and the use of benzodiazepines to avoid the withdrawal syndrome (Bruera & Watanabe, 1994).

A comprehensive physical examination should also consider the patient's psychologic status. Evaluation of the patient's ability to maintain eye contact may help identify depression (if eye contact is culturally acceptable, because avoiding eye contact is not unnatural for Native Americans and some African-Americans). The tone and inflection of voice and posture can be indicators of withdrawal or apprehension. It is important to routinely evaluate the patient for signs and symptoms of depression by directly asking if he or she is depressed.

Physical assessment includes the identification of abnormal skin lesions, lymphadenopathy, pericardial rubs, pulmonary rales, hepatosplenomegaly, periumbilical or pelvic masses, and/or peripheral edema, all of which are useful findings when the patient's source of pain is uncertain. If the patient describes neuropathic pain or cognitive changes (or if relatives volunteer that they have observed changes in the patient's mentation), a neurologic examination should follow.

The site of pain identified by the patient should be manually palpated. Maneuvers to elicit or relieve pain help determine the cause of pain and streamline the ordering of radiographic tests. Because bone metastases are the most common cause of cancer pain, physical evaluation should include:

• Joint motion
• Percussion
• Bone tenderness
• Muscle symmetry
• Joint appearance (e.g., red and swollen may indicate gout)

Radiographic imaging should be based on history and physical examination guided by the trajectory of illness and the goals of care. For instance, if the plan of care is to manage symptoms in a patient with known metastatic bone disease, a plain radiograph will confirm the origin of pain. On the other hand, if the patient's pain is acutely worsening and a pathologic fracture is suspected, plain radiographs and MRI would be warranted. However, dying patients should not be subjected to uncomfortable testing and should have their pain aggressively managed as the goal of therapy.

Standard radiographs should not be bypassed for computer tomography (CT) or MRI. Information gleaned from plain radiographs may be enough to direct therapy. Bone scans and positron tomography are good for staging many malignancies (e.g., lung, colon, prostate, breast) but rarely add to other imaging studies and are not as accurate in determining the origin of pain. Electrophysiologic studies can separate radiculopathies, peripheral neuropathies, and entrapment neuropathies. However, electrophysiologic studies may be normal in the face of non-myelinated neuronal disease.

Pain Diaries

Included in pain assessment is the patient's pain diary. If the patient is instructed properly on its use, the pain diary can provide the physician with important information about the severity and fluctuation of the patient's pain, breakthrough episodes, and treatment effectiveness. A one-time pain assessment during an outpatient appointment does not accurately account for the patient's total pain experience. Patients who are able to document their daily pain intensity and percentage of relief with opioid analgesics or non-opioid analgesics on an average of four times a day will provide the clinician with important information that will objectively improve pain management. Diaries should contain the frequency of breakthrough pain and the effective analgesic dose with the timing of these episodes and/or any adverse analgesic side effects (Smith & Safer, 1993). To effectively utilize a pain diary, patients should be instructed on unidimensional pain assessment tools. They should understand the importance of documenting their pain intensity and breakthrough medication and then again enter pain intensity with the specific intervention. Patients should be given a choice of an assessment tool to use that is convenient and easy to use at home. Additional benefits to pain diaries are a sense of control by patients, which leads to improved coping skills and self-management (de Wit, van Dam, Abu-Saad, et al., 1999).

Successful pain management is usually incremental as analgesic doses are initially adjusted to the pattern of pain. Effective analgesia will lead to increased activities with relief of pain and will improve sleep and appetite. Paradoxically, levels of alertness increase despite opioid dose escalation as pain resolves. It is important to maintain ongoing assessment by telephone conversation between patient and provider. Telephone contact within 1 to 3 days of initiating analgesics is usually sufficient, followed with a clinic evaluation within 1 to 2 weeks.

Patients who continue to experience uncontrolled pain despite following an analgesic regimen should return to the clinic for further evaluation. Patients should be seen expeditiously because this will reduce unnecessary suffering and anxiety. Simultaneous expedited pain assessment and pain management are required in cases of crescendo pain.

Patients require education on the purpose and use of opioids, the dose schedule, and fundamentals to the management of opioid side effects. The patient should have telephone numbers to call if pain worsens or adverse effects become problematic. A list of all medications and the pain diary should be available with each clinic visit.

Clinicians must do their part to help coordinate the patient's care by accurately documenting on the medical record the analgesic changes and dosages used by the patient. A comprehensive and systematic record improves communication for all involved in the patient's care.

TREATMENT

Cancer pain can be relieved in 80% of cancer patients by using the WHO analgesic ladder as a guide (Benedetti, Brock, Cleeland, et al., 2000; Bruera, & Lawlor, 1997; Cleeland et al., 2000; Stjernsward, Colleau, & Ventafridda, 1996; Twycross, 2002; Ventafridda & Stjernsward, 1995; Walker, Hoskin, Hanks, et al., 1988; Walsh, 2000; Zech, Grond, Lynch, et al., 1995). The recommendations of the WHO for patients are:

- **Step I:** Mild pain (pain subjectively rated at a 0-4 on a NRS) should be treated with a nonsteroidal antiinflammatory drug (NSAID) or acetaminophen with or without other adjuvant analgesics.
- **Step II:** Moderate pain (pain rated at a 5-7) should be treated with a "weak" opioid (e.g., tramadol, codeine), a combination analgesic with a NSAID, or low doses of a potent opioid.

- **Step III:** Severe pain (rated at a 7-10) should be treated with potent opioids (e.g., fentanyl, morphine, methadone, hydromorphone), and weak opioids are discontinued. The NSAID or acetaminophen with or without other adjuvant analgesics is continued.

Patients presenting with severe pain initially should be started on the stronger opioids rather than started at step I or step II. The drawback to the WHO analgesic ladder is that it does not provide a guide to adjuvant analgesic choices or analgesic scheduling according to pain pattern. Multiple drug changes should not be made simultaneously unless there are extenuating circumstances. Either route, dose or drug and their response should be noted before making changes in the patients drug regimen (Walsh, 2000). Changing drug, route, and dose simultaneously will make it difficult for the prescriber to discern which change lead to the relief of pain or, particularly, the adverse side effects. Changing one element of pain management (dose, route, or drug) at a time builds patient confidence and ensures patient compliance and successful dosing strategies (Walsh, 2000). Analgesic doses and schedule will need to be reviewed closely, perhaps as often as every 30 minutes for severe pain or daily for those starting on analgesics. Case management by a skilled nurse clinician who can monitor pain response, opioid adverse effects, and compliance, as well as provide education for family and patients, is essential to good cancer pain management (Walsh, 2000). For monitoring purposes, the following questions are important: (1) What analgesic was given? (2) At what dose did response occur? (3) How much was pain relieved by the dose? and (4) What was the duration of response? (Walsh, 2000). Because patients usually have multiple pains (i.e., visceral, somatic, neuropathic), it is important to assess each pain syndrome individually and to assess response to specific medications.

Common clinical errors that lead to ineffective pain management include (Kochhar, LeGrand, Walsh, et al., 2003):
- Failure to carefully assess the pain pathophysiology leading to inappropriate adjuvant choices

- Failure to quantify pain response with a pain assessment tool
- Under-dosing pain (usually by prescribers)
- Delaying the analgesic dose (usually by nursing staff)
- Fear of opioid toxicity or addiction
- Inappropriate dosing schedules such as "as needed" analgesics for chronic pain versus around-the-clock dosing with an "as needed" dose for breakthrough pain
- Failure to consider opioid equianalgesia when rotating or converting opioids or changing routes
- Failure to use adjuvants appropriately and early
- Failure to provide laxatives as part of an opioid dosing regimen
- Failure to monitor opioid adverse effects
- Polypharmacy or the simultaneous use of several analgesics from the same class (two opioids, two NSAIDs, an NSAID and a corticosteroid)
- Failure to properly educate the family and patient

An effective pain management schema that limits the possibility of errors is having just one prescriber and assigning a single nurse who is familiar with the patient and the plan of care.

Opioids

Morphine remains the opioid of choice, and preemptive around-the-clock dosing is the cardinal strategy for chronic cancer pain management (Levy, 1996). Prescribing as-needed dosing for chronic pain is an "after the fact" strategy that only increases the patient's suffering and will most likely lead to larger opioid dose requirements with an increased risk of systemic opioid side effects to regain pain control (Levy, 1996; Walsh, 2000). Such dosing strategies lead to short periods of opioid withdrawal symptoms, which increase patient suffering. Sustained-release opioids improve patient compliance with continuous 12-hour dosing. Breakthrough doses with the same opioid should be with 5% to 10% of the 24-hour dose (Mercandante, Radbruch, Caraceni, et al., 2002; Walsh, 2000).

Diurnal (circadian) variations in pain require asymmetric opioid dosing patterns for effective pain control (i.e., higher doses at night or in the afternoon). For example, the patient may be frequently awakened at night by pain but does well with pain throughout the day. A sustained-release dose, which is higher in the evening and lower in the morning, would be appropriate in this circumstance.

There is little need for weak opioids in countries where potent analgesics are readily available. Certain potent opioids such as meperidine and the opioid agonist-antagonist should be avoided. Combination analgesics (e.g., hydrocodone/acetaminophen, hydrocodone/ibuprofen) usually have ceiling doses because of the acetaminophen or NSAID in the combination, and although they are commonly used as step II analgesics, these analgesics lack the versatility of low-dose potent opioids. If a patient cannot tolerate morphine, other strong opioids are considered: methadone, oxycodone, hydromorphone, and fentanyl.

The response to opioids is determined by two variables—the patient and opioid pharmacology (Wilder-Smith, 2001). Patient factors include individual pharmacogenetics involving opioid receptors and metabolizing enzymes (cytochrome P-450 and conjugates) (see Chapter 4), age, body mass, co-morbid illnesses, psychologic make-up, and hepatic or renal function (Wilder-Smith, 2001). Co-medications can significantly interact with either opioid pharmacodynamics or kinetics. Several reviews on opioids have recently been published and are available as references in the literature (Bruera, 2002; Davis, 2003; Davis & Walsh, 2001; Donnelly, Davis, Walsh, et al., 2002; Peng & Sandler, 1999; Sarhill, Walsh, & Nelson, 2001; Wantanabe, Periera, Hanson, et al., 1998). Opioid choices will have to be modified in the face of organ failure and co-medications (Table 10-1).

Initial dosing for an opioid-naïve patient is morphine 10 mg, oxycodone 5 to 10 mg, or hydromorphone 2 mg every 4 hours by mouth. For frail elderly patients, 5 mg of morphine or oxycodone is a safe starting dose. Sustained-release morphine or oxycodone can be started at 15 to 30 mg or 10 to 20 mg every 12 hours, respectively. Methadone doses for opioid-naïve patients are 3 to 5 mg every 8 hours.

Table **10-1** Drug Metabolism and Interaction

Opioid	Metabolism	Potency (Relative to Morphine)	Drug Interactions	Dose Modification for Renal/Hepatic Failure
Tramadol	CYP2D6	100:1	SSRI (paroxetine, fluoxetine)	+++ renal +++ hepatic
Codeine	CYP2D6	130:1	SSRI (paroxetine, fluoxetine)	+++ renal +++ hepatic
Morphine	UGT2B7 UGT1A3	1:1	Kaolin, rifampin, tricyclic Ciprofloxacin Levofloxacin	++ renal + hepatic
Oxycodone	CYP2D6	1:1 to 1:1.5	Cyclosporin Rifampin Sertraline	+++ renal ++ hepatic
Hydromorphone	UGT2B7	1:5	(Same as morphine)	++ renal + hepatic
Methadone	CYP3A4 CYP2D6 CYP1A2 CYP2C9 CYP2C19	1:4 (<90 mg/day) 1:8 (90-300 mg/day) 1:12 (>300 mg/day)	Classic antiseizure Azoles Tricyclic antidepressant, fluvoxamine	− renal + hepatic
Fentanyl	CYP3A4	1:70	Erythromycin Grapefruit juice Rifampin (Same as methadone)	+ renal + hepatic

SSRI, Selective serotonin reuptake inhibitor.

+++, Severe metabolism; ++, moderate metabolism; +, mild metabolism; −, none.

Initial parenteral opioid doses include morphine 0.5 to 1.0 mg/hour, fentanyl 25 mcg/hour, or hydromorphone 0.1 to 0.2 mg/hour. Methadone doses are initiated at 0.1 mg/hour but must be monitored closely because of the risk of accumulation and wide individual differences in methadone metabolism.

Opioid-Conversion, Opioid-Rotation, and Opioid-Sparing Strategies.

Opioid Conversion. In certain clinical situations, the patient may not be able to take oral medications and an alternative route becomes necessary to maintain optimal pain relief. Patients with intractable nausea and vomiting, a bowel obstruction, dysphagia, or changes in cognition may require parenteral conversion from an oral dose. Several opioids can be administered rectal, subcutaneous, parenteral injection or infusions (Davis, Walsh, LeGrand, et al., 2002; Ripamonti, Zecca, & De Conno, 1998). Converting parenteral opioids is also a means of extending the opioid therapeutic index, as is opioid rotation. Parenteral conversion is often recommended when patients experience an acute exacerbation of pain or in the setting of severe pain in an attempt to rapidly titrate opioids. The versatility of an opioid (e.g., morphine, methadone, hydromorphone) is influenced by its ability to be administered through multiple routes.

The conversion ratio from oral to a parenteral route (either subcutaneous or intravenous) is 1:3 for morphine, 1:2 for methadone and oxycodone, and 1:5 for hydromorphone. The conversion ratio from an oral opioid to rectal is a 1:1 ratio.

Opioid Rotation. Opioid rotation should be considered when patients are experiencing unacceptable side effects from a specific opioid and have poor pain control. For those patients with poor pain control, increasing doses before opioid rotation is usual practice. Opioid rotation takes advantage of the non–cross tolerance (pharmacodynamic differences) between opioids. This requires a skillful knowledge of opioid dose equivalence (equianalgesia). Rotating opioids should be considered for uncontrolled pain rather than side effects management and should be dosed at equianalgesic recommendations. Rotations for side effects management rather than for poor pain control should be dosed at 50% to 70% of an equianalgesic dose.

Opioid equivalences are subject to individual differences in receptor genetics and metabolizing enzyme genetics, disease process, co-medications, and residual organ function, which ultimately influence opioid dynamics and clearance (Davis, 2003; De Stoutz, Bruera, & Suarez-Almazor, 1995; Mercandante, 1999; Pereira, Lawlor, Vigano, et al., 2001).

Opioid Sparing. Opioid-sparing strategies include the addition of an adjuvant analgesic to facilitate analgesia and opioid dose reduction (simultaneously). It is important that only one adjuvant analgesic is added and titrated to effect while reducing opioid doses (Walsh, 2000). Adjuvants such as an NSAID or corticosteroids added to an opioid for patients who experience nociceptive and nerve compression pain are "opioid sparing" since it may be possible to reduce or stabilize the opioid dose while improving analgesia.

Adjuvants are added for difficult-to-manage pains such as neuropathic or incident pain. Neuroleptics such as haloperidol and olanzapine may curtail a rapid escalation of opioid dose caused by poorly controlled pain in a delirious or anxious patient (Khojainova, Santiago-Palma, Kornick, et al., 2002). Further discussion on the use of specific adjuvant analgesics follows.

Side Effects of Opioid Use.

Constipation. Opioid-induced constipation occurs as a result of the contraction of the circular muscle and inhibition of longitudinal smooth muscle, which leads to segmental contractions without peristalsis. The prolonged transit time in the large bowel leads to more fluid extracted from stool, resulting in a dry, hard stool and an uncomfortable, colicky patient. Inactivity, dehydration, and certain co-medications (e.g., anticholinergics) with opioids increase the risk for constipation. Bowel regimens should include a wetting agent such as Docusate and a stimulant (bisacodyl or senna) and should be prescribed at the time that opioids are initiated. Polyethylene glycol has an advantage in that it does not draw fluid into the bowel from extracellular spaces and prevents dehydration unlike bisacodyl and senna. Patients with colostomies require a bowel regimen, but patients with ileostomy do not (McNicol, Horowicz-Mehler, Fisk, et al., 2003; Walsh, 2000). Persistent constipation correlates with reduced performance status but not the opioid dose (Fallon & Hanks 1999; McNicol et al., 2003) (Table 10-2).

Nausea and Vomiting. The incidence of nausea and vomiting occurs in 10% to 40% of patients who are prescribed opioids (McNicol et al., 2003). Opioids exert their emetogenic effects through several mechanisms and anatomic sites: (1) gastrostasis; (2) medullary central pattern generator; and (3) vestibular stimulation. Nausea is usually transient and occurs in a minority of patients; therefore, antiemetics should not be given prophylatically but rather if nausea occurs (see Table 10-2).

Cognitive Changes. Opioid neurotoxicity ranges from mild, transient, mental cloudiness to

Table 10-2 OPIOID SIDE EFFECTS AND MANAGEMENT

Side Effect	Management
Constipation	Prophylactic use of docusate 100 mg TID plus magnesium hydroxide 30 ml or bisacodyl 5-10 mg if no stool and titrate.
	Reduce or eliminate tricyclic antidepressants and anticholinergics.
	Hydrate.
	Rescue enemas, osmotic laxatives, oral naloxone, senna.
Dry mouth, urinary retention, blurred vision	Sodium bicarbonate, citrus candies, artificial saliva, pilocarpine.
	Catheterization.
Nausea and vomiting	Check for reversible co-morbidities (hypercalcemia, increased intracranial pressure, obstipation, emetogenic drugs).
	Metoclopramide 10 mg IV AC and HS or 40-60 mg CI over 24 hours.
	Haloperidol, prochlorperazine, diphenhydramine, transdermal scopolamine patch, ondansetron.
	Opioid rotation or conversion.
Delirium and hallucinations	Check for central nervous system metastasis, hypercalcemia, hyponatremia.
	Reduce or eliminate central acting medications (tricyclic antidepressants, benzodiazepines).
	Reduce opioid dose if no pain.
	Opioid convert, rotate, or spare.
	Haloperidol, chlorpromazine, olanzapine.
Sedation	Reduce antihistaminics, antidepressants, anxiolytics.
	Check for central nervous system metastasis and metabolic disturbances.
	Methylphenidate 5 mg 9 AM and noon and titrate.
	Opioid convert, rotate, or spare.
Myoclonus	Check for metabolic disturbances, renal and hepatic failure.
	Eliminate antidepressants and antipsychotics.
	Clonazepam, dantrolene, midazolam, gabapentin.
	Opioid convert, rotate, or spare.
Pruritus	Cool compresses, moisturizers.
	Diphenhydramine, hydroxyzine, cyproheptadine.
	Ondansetron, propofol.
	Opioid rotate.
Respiratory depression	Check for co-morbidities if on stable doses (central nervous system metastasis, renal or hepatic failure).
	Discontinue around-the-clock doses; provide as-needed opioid.
	Naloxone 0.4 mg every 3 minutes until responds to verbal stimuli and respiratory rate ≥10 per minute.

TID, Three times/day; *AC,* before meals; *HS,* at bedtime; *CI,* continuous infusion.

full-blown delirium with visual and tactile hallucinations. Patients may have mild hallucinations and myoclonus but not volunteer these symptoms. If patients are on stable chronic doses of opioids at the time of cognitive failure, cancer-related complications such as brain metastases, renal or hepatic failure, or dehydration should be suspected as a cause rather than the opioid. Psychotomimetic drugs such as benzodiazepines or anticholinergics may precipitate delirium while the patient is on opioids. Previous strokes, dementia, and advanced age are also contributing factors to the development of delirium (see Table 10-2).

Myoclonus. Myoclonus is a relatively common side effect and is usually mild and clinically unappreciated. It can occur at the onset of sleep (twilight jerks). Many patients do not complain of this symptom or associate it with their opioid. Myoclonus is a spinal cord reflex and is not associated with seizures with the exception of patients using meperidine (McNicol et al., 2003). The differential to myoclonus includes partial seizures, which are usually localized clonic jerks to one extremity, whereas myoclonus is more generalized. Symptomatic myoclonus usually requires opioid rotation or requires clonazepam, valproic acid, or gabapentin for patients for whom opioid rotation is not feasible (see Table 10-2).

Pruritus. Intrathecal and subdural opioids are associated with the greatest risk for pruritus. Peripherally, morphine stimulates mast cells to degranulate and release histamine, which initiates pruritus. Central opioid administration initiates pruritus either through opioid or through serotonin receptors. Dry skin is common with advanced cancer and is the important differential. Co-morbidities such as renal dysfunction or biliary obstruction will also cause severe pruritus in advanced organ failure (McNicol et al., 2003).

Respiratory Depression. Respiratory depression is the most feared complication of opioids and is one of the side effects for which tolerance develops most rapidly. However, rapid parenteral opioid titration or large bolus dosing without monitoring and without regard to half-life will cause hypoventilation. Administering small, frequent opioid doses for uncontrolled severe pain using opioids with a short half-life is a safe dosing strategy and rarely leads to respiratory depression. Opioid-induced hypoventilation leads to CO_2 retention, which will in fact increase the respiratory rate as a compensation despite shallow breathing. The respiratory rate may be maintained although there is ineffective minute ventilation; hence monitoring respiratory rate alone during opioid titration may inadequately detect hypoventilation until late. Sedation with opioids usually precedes overt respiratory depression. If a patient has fewer than 10 breaths per minute but is alert and oriented, opioid toxicity is unlikely and dose reduction is unnecessary. The oral route of administration and gradual dose titration minimize the risk of opioid-induced respiratory depression (McNicol et al., 2003). Pain is an antidote to respiratory depression as a result of stimulation of the brainstem respiratory center by way of spinoreticular tracts that arise from dorsal horn neurons. If respiratory depression does occur while the patient is on stable doses of opioids, there may be secondary causes such as pneumonia, pulmonary embolism, cardiomyopathy, heart failure, or sedative co-medications (McNicol et al., 2003).

Systematic reviews and recommendations for managing opioid side effects have been previously published and are well worth reviewing (McNicol et al., 2003; Walsh, 2000); they are outlined in Table 10-2.

Adjuvant Analgesics

The skilled and prudent use of adjuvant analgesics reduces the need for opioid conversion or titration (Walsh, 2000). Adjuvant analgesics such as acetaminophen and NSAIDs combined with opioids are termed *co-analgesics*. Other agents such as antidepressants and antiseizure drugs not formally classified as analgesics can be used to reduce several pain states as potentiators of opioid analgesia. Unlike opioids, adjuvants have (1) a "ceiling dose," (2) a therapeutic drug level, (3) a potential for end-organ damage, (4) a limited spectrum of activity (nociceptive or neuropathic), and (5) limited routes of administration (lack of versatility) (Guay, 2001; Walsh, 2000). Adjuvants are

used when (Walsh, 2000):
- Pain is poorly responsive to opioids.
- Opioid doses need to be reduced to curtail side effects and treat unmanaged pain.
- There are complex pain syndromes that warrant a diagnostic and therapeutic maneuver to investigate the pain pathophysiology.

Adjuvants may produce responses at lower-than-therapeutic doses, and titration to therapeutic levels may not be necessary for all patients. Adjuvant dose titration and rescue dosing are part of an analgesic strategy but are less important than with opioids (Walsh, 2000).

Nonsteroidal Antiinflammatory Drugs. NSAIDs have both a peripheral and a central action centered on inhibition of prostaglandin metabolism. Several classes of NSAIDs are available that are non–cross tolerant. The recent development of selective cyclooxygenase-2 specific inhibitors (Cox-2 inhibitors) and nitric oxide (NO)–donating NSAIDs expands the therapeutic index of NSAIDs by limiting gastrointestinal toxicity (Emery, 1999; Rigas, Kalofonos, Lebovics, et al., 2003). Both the NSAIDs and Cox-2 inhibitors are being explored clinically as chemopreventive agents and in combination with chemotherapy as antitumor adjuvants, which may facilitate tumor response (Dicker, 2003; Tarnawski & Jones, 2003). These medications should be carefully prescribed in the setting of renal insufficiency and with a positive history of gastrointestinal ulcers.

Acetaminophen and non-acetylated aspirin have reduced renal and gastrointestinal toxicity but also lower efficacy. Acetaminophen should be limited to 4 grams daily as a general rule to avoid hepatic toxicity. Cox-2 selective agents inhibitors have reduced gastrointestinal side effects compared with the NSAIDs, but their benefits as an adjuvant are selective (Lashbrook, Ossipov, Hunter, et al., 1999; McCormack & Twycross, 2001).

Naproxen and parenteral ketorolac are the first choices of NSAIDs for those with no contraindicators to their use—these include patients with a history of gastrointestinal bleeding within the past 2 years, renal failure, corticosteroid therapy, or peptic ulcer disease (Walsh, 2000). Although it is reported that NSAIDS do not relieve neuropathic pain, both

in animal models and clinically, NSAIDS have been identified as effective analgesics in managing neuropathic pain (Hefferan, O'Reilly, & Loomis, 2003; McCleane, 2003; Ripamonti, Ticozzi, Zecca, et al., 1996).

Tricyclic Antidepressants. Tricyclic antidepressants effectively relieve pain associated with diabetic neuropathy and postherpetic neuralgia as well as post–cerebrovascular accident (CVA) and central mediated pain (Gonzales, 1995; Guay, 2001; Magni, 1991). However, the benefits from tricyclics in the management of cancer neuropathic pain are not well documented.

Additional benefits from tricyclic antidepressants include improved mood and decreased insomnia. Secondary amine tricyclic antidepressants such as despiramine and nortriptyline have less anticholingeric side effects and are preferred for use in the older population (Watson, Vernich, Chipman, et al., 1998). Tricyclics should be used cautiously or not at all in patients with angle-closure glaucoma, urinary retention, severe constipation, limited liver function, or advanced cardiovascular disease. Tricyclics, however, can prolong the QTc interval noted on electrocardiogram, which can be problematic for patients with a positive history of cardiac dysrhythmia (Guay, 2001).

Dexamethasone. Dexamethasone is a Cox-2 inhibitor, a leukotriene inhibitor, and inhibits the expression of nitric oxide synthase necessary for NMDA receptor activity. There is no ceiling dose to dexamethasone, unlike the NSAIDs. Dexamethasone reduces pain in "compressive" neuropathies (cord compression and plexopathies), visceral pain, and pain arising from widespread bony metastases (Wantanabe & Bruera, 1994). Additional benefits include the relief of nausea, improved appetite, euphoria, and improved sense of well-being. Dexamethasone has an "opioid-sparing" benefit, which may dramatically relieve pain when added to an opioid regimen. This can lead to opioid toxicities and necessitate a reduction in opioid doses (Walsh, 2000). Peptic ulcers are less frequent with dexamethasone as well as other corticosteroids (prednisolone) compared with non-selective or Cox-2 agents; however, combining corticosteroids with NSAIDs significantly increases the risk of gastrointestinal ulcer and bleeding compared with NSAIDs alone. Long-term side effects with corticosteroids are problematic and include (1) cataracts, (2) psychosis, (3) Cushingoid syndrome, (4) diabetes, (5) osteoporosis, and (6) proximal myopathy.

A single 20-mg test dose of dexamethasone may produce a rapid response and can be used before instituting long-term therapy. Doses should be tapered to the lowest effective dose to maintain benefit or should be discontinued if there is no response within 1 week (i.e., 8 mg twice/day and taper)(Walsh, 2000).

Antiseizure Medications. Antiseizure medications are sodium channel blockers, which prevent spontaneous depolarization from injured nerves. Certain antiseizure medications also potentiate the gamma aminobutyric acid (GABA) antinociceptive activity within the dorsal horn. Others are calcium channel blockers, which block a central or peripheral neuropathic pain (Bowsher, 1996). Carbamazepine, a sodium channel blocker, has traditionally been used for trigeminal neuralgia but also reduces cancer-associated neuropathic pain (Guay, 2001). Carbamazepine is inexpensive but has a large number of drug interactions due to hepatic CYP3A4 leading to accelerated clearance of multiple drugs.

Gabapentin has fewer side effects than those of carbamazepine and few drug interactions, but it has limited versatility. Fortunately gabapentin neither stimulates nor inhibits hepatic cytochrome enzymes. However, gabapentin must be given multiple times during the day, is highly dependent upon renal function, and is expensive. Gabapentin is a calcium channel blocker and prevents the release of the neuroactive amino acid *glutamate,* which binds to NMDA receptors.

Valproic acid is an inexpensive antiseizure medication with fewer side effects and drug interactions than those of carbamazepine but more than those of gabapentin. Valproic acid can be dosed once or twice daily (Hardy, Rees, Gwilliam, et al., 2002) (Table 10-3). Common side effects to all antiseizure medications include somnolence, dizziness, and nystagmas. Valproic acid rarely causes hepatic toxicity. Carbamazepine suppresses bone marrow production and induces hyponatremia.

The newer antiseizure medication, lamotrigine, blocks sodium channels and inhibits the release of glutamate (Canavero & Conicalzi, 1997; Devulder, 2000; Eisenberg, Alon, Ishay, et al., 1998; Harbison, Dennehy, & Keating, 1997; McCleane, 2000). Lamotrigine has demonstrated effectiveness in

Table **10-3**   CEILING DOSES OF SPECIFIC MEDICATIONS

Drug	Initial Dose	Maximum Dose	Type of Pain
Naproxen	250 mg BID	500 mg TID	Somatic, visceral
Ketorolac	15 mg q12hr	30 mg q6hr	Somatic, visceral
Acetaminophen	650 mg QID	1 g QID	Somatic, visceral
Amitriptyline	10-25 mg qHS	150 mg daily	Neuropathic
Desipramine	10-25 mg qHS	150 mg daily	Neuropathic
Dexamethasone	2-4 mg daily	100 mg daily	Neuropathic, somatic, visceral
Carbamazepine	100 mg BID	400 mg TID	Neuropathic
Valproic acid	250 mg daily	1000 mg BID	Neuropathic
Gabapentin	100 mg TID	3200 mg daily	Neuropathic
Lamotrigine	50 mg daily	600 mg daily	Neuropathic
Mexiletine	150 mg BID	1200 mg daily	Neuropathic
Calcitonin	50-100 IV subcutaneous daily	8 IV/kg subcutaneous q6hr	Bone
Pamidronate	60-90 mg every 3-4 wks	-	Bone
Zoledronate	4 mg every 4 wks	-	Bone
Ketamine	25 mg PO q6hr & titrate	-	Neuropathic

BID, 2 times/day; *QID,* 3 times/day; *HS,* at bedtime; *TID,* 3 times/day; *IU,* international unit; *PO,* by mouth.

the treatment of diabetic neuropathy, acquired immunodeficiency syndrome (AIDS)–associated polyneuropathy, central mediated pain from a CVA, and trigeminal neuralgia. Side effects to lamotrigine are similar to those of other antiseizure medications and include ataxia, impaired coordination, blurred vision, and diplopia.

Local Anesthetics. Mexiletine, an oral congener of lidocaine, has been reported to improve pain from diabetic neuropathy and CVA pain (see Table 10-3). Neuropathic pain that has not responded to trials of a tricyclic antidepressant or antiseizure medications may respond to mexiletine. Mexiletine, an antidysrhythmic, should not be used in patients with second- or third-degree heart block or in patients with a prolonged QTc interval. Common side effects to mexiletine include nausea, vomiting, dizziness, tremor, irritability, nervousness, and headaches (Guay, 2001). An alternative to systemic "local" anesthetics is a lidocaine patch for a mononeuropathy or localized neuropathic pain. The lidocaine patch will not produce systemic levels of lidocaine and as a result has minimal side effects.

Bisphosphonates and Calcitonin. Bisphosphonates, such as pamidronate and zolendronate as well as calcitonin, have been used to treat cancer-associated hypercalcemia and bony complications (Body, 1999, 2003; Kellihan & Mangino, 1992; Pavilakis & Stockler, 2002). Bisphosphonates reduce or delay cancer-associated bone complications and thus indirectly reduce pain. Bisphosphonates will also relieve bone pain associated with metastases over a period of months if used consistently over time. Zolendronate in particular has been found to reduce pain associated with solid tumors other than breast cancer that have metastasized to bone (prostate cancer) (see Table 10-3). Bisphosphonates can produce arthralgias and myalgias in a minority of patients, along with electrolyte disturbances such as hypocalcemia, hypokalemia, hypophosphatemia, and hypomagnesemia. Calcitonin is reported to reduce bone pain as well as phantom limb pain. Calcitonin side effects include nausea, vomiting, and local skin reactions. Commercially available calcitonin is derived from salmon, and reactions can occur if the patient is allergic to fish (Guay, 2001).

Miscellaneous Medications. Diazepam improves opioid analgesia by acting as an anxiolytic and a muscle relaxant. Muscle spasms do not respond to opioids but may dramatically respond to diazepam. Paravertebral muscle spasm from painful vertebral metastases responds well to diazepam, and the combination of diazepam with an opioid often reduces the need for opioid titration. Initial diazepam doses are 2 mg every 8 to 12 hours and should be titrated to response (Walsh, 2000).

Anticholinergics such as glycopyrronium reduce intestinal colic associated with mechanical bowel obstruction that will not respond to opioids. Usual doses are 0.1 to 0.2 mg every 6 to 8 hours given either subcutaneous or intravenous. The parenteral maximum dose is 1.2 mg per day. Glycopyrrolate is also available orally at 1 to 2 mg every 6 hours. Glycopyrrolate has a reduced cardiac effect compared with that of other anticholinergics and does not cross the blood-brain barrier, which reduces the risk of causing delirium.

Sublingual nitroglycerin may relieve smooth muscle spasm arising from the esophagus, biliary tree, or pancreatic duct. Usual nitroglycerin doses are 0.4 mg sublingual. Topical nitroglycerin relieves pain from anal fissures (Walsh, 2000).

SUMMARY

Pain is experienced by most cancer patients and requires a methodic assessment and rationale approach to its management. Multiple medications are available and should be prescribed based on principles derived from pharmacology, pathophysiology, and the pattern of the patient's pain experience. The basis of cancer pain management is a practice model that can be applied to all types of chronic nonmalignant patterns of pain, as well as relieve almost all pain associated with malignancy.

Objective Questions

1. Cancer pain:

   a. Has a unique pathophysiology compared with non-cancer pain.

   b. Is the most common symptom cancer patients experience.

Case Study

Mr. G. decided to see his primary care physician because of prolonged lower back pain of a 1-month duration that impaired his activities of daily living. He also complained of diffuse abdominal pain and weight loss. After ingesting food, he experienced a gnawing ache in his epigastrium area. His pain was intensified in a recumbent position and was relieved by a position change from a sitting to a fetal position. He did not realize that he had lost 15 lbs over the past 3 months after being weighed in the office.

As a part of his assessment, a computer tomography (CT) of the abdomen was performed, which revealed a mass in the head of his pancreas. An exploratory laparotomy was then performed that confirmed the diagnosis of pancreatic cancer; unfortunately, multiple liver metastases were not previously seen on CT scan. A choledochojejunostomy was then performed to prevent biliary obstruction, and a celiac plexus block with alcohol was performed for pain control. The postoperative course was uneventful. His residual pain was well controlled with morphine sulfate via parenteral patient-controlled analgesia (PCA). At the time of discharge he was successfully converted to oral sustained-release morphine around the clock and immediate-release morphine prescribed on an as-needed basis.

Mr. G. was started on a palliative gemcitabine dose for 4 weeks following his hospital discharge. Within a few weeks, the quality of his pain changed from a dull, mild ache to a crampy abdominal pain accompanied by nausea that failed to respond to morphine but responded well to glycopyrrolate and haloperidol.

Increasing his opioid doses for his complaints of continuous pain and maintaining his glycopyrrolate dose as an adjuvant analgesic for abdominal colicky pain, he remained comfortable for several weeks, until he suffered a fatal pulmonary embolus and died suddenly.

---

   c. Should be treated with opioids if severe and if prognosis is less than 6 months.

   d. Is responsive to morphine in the majority of patients.

2. Cancer pain:

   a. Is most commonly somatic from bone metastases.

   b. Is rarely mixed (somatic, visceral, or neuropathic).

   c. Arises from most metastases.

   d. Correlates with radiographic findings.

3. Pain at the sacroiliac joint area, worsened by cough and nocturnal in nature:

   a. Should be ignored since this is classic sacral iliac benign pain.

   b. Should be treated empirically with analgesics if pelvic x-ray examination is normal.

   c. May be referred pain from the L1 vertebral body.

   d. Can be managed without further radiographs if plain films of the lumbar spine are normal.

4. Pain in the back radiating to the groin associated with lower extremity swelling:

   a. Should be treated immediately with heparin since this is classic for deep venous thrombosis.

   b. Should be assumed to be from vertebral metastases.

   c. Should be suspected to be cancer-associated lumbar plexus invasion, particularly if pain is improved by hip flexion.

   d. Usually arises from breast cancer or lung cancer.

5. Pain intensity and pain interference:

   a. Are not related.

   b. Are determined by separate tools and are independently related to cancer pain.

c. Require the use of multidimensional pain scales.

d. Are related.

6. Pain diaries:

a. Worsen pain management by constantly reminding patients of their pain.

b. Reduce coping.

c. Improve coping and opioid dosing schedules.

d. Cannot be used in pain trials since these are derived from patients rather than from physicians.

7. Cancer pain treatment:

a. Usually requires several changes at one time (route, dose, or analgesic).

b. Is limited by opioid analgesic ceiling.

c. Is limited by opioid tolerance.

d. Requires continuous (around-the-clock [ATC]) opioid plus provision for rescue doses and co-analgesics in most patients.

8. Opioid toxicity:

a. Requires opioid rotation if myoclonus, hallucination, or confusion occurs even in the absence of pain.

b. Is predictable for all patients.

c. If accompanied by poorly controlled pain, may be managed by opioid-conversion, opioid-rotation, or opioid-sparing strategies.

d. Requires spinal opioids.

9. The choice of adjuvant analgesics is dependent upon:

a. Type of pain.

b. Pain severity.

c. Side effects.

d. All the above.

10. A hostile and complaining patient with severe pain who knows the opioid and dose that previously relieved his pain should:

a. Be assumed to be psychologically addicted.

b. Receive only methadone.

c. Receive his preferred opioid titrated to pain relief, at which time his pain behavior should be reassessed.

d. Be referred to pain management.

REFERENCES

Aaronson, N.K., Ahmedzai, S., Bergman, B., et al. (1993). The European Organization for Research and Treatment of Cancer QLQ-C30: A quality-of-life instrument for use in international clinical trials in oncology. *J Natl Cancer Inst, 85*(5), 365-376.

Agency for Healthcare Research and Quality (AHRQ). (2002). *Management of cancer symptoms: Pain, depression, and fatigue.* Agency for Healthcare Research & Quality. Rockville, Md.: U.S. Department of Health and Human Services.

American Pain Society (APS). (1995). Quality improvement guidelines for the treatment of acute pain and cancer pain. *JAMA, 274,* 1874-1880.

Basbaum, A.I., Clanton, C.H., & Fields, H.L. (1976). Opiate and stimulus-produced analgesia: Functional anatomy of a medullospinal pathway. *Proc Natl Aca Sci USA, 73*(12), 4685-4688.

Basbaum, A.I., & Fields, H.L. (1978). Endogenous pain control mechanisms: Review and hypothesis. *Ann Neurol, 4*(5), 451-462.

Basbaum, A.I., & Fields, H.L. (1984). Endogenous pain control systems: Brainstem spinal pathways and endorphin circuitry. *Annu Rev Neurosci, 7,* 309-338.

Benedetti, C., Brock, C., Cleeland, C., et al. (2000). NCCN practice guidelines for cancer pain. *Oncology, 11A,* 135-150.

Body, J.J. (1999). Bisphosphonates for metastatic bone pain. *Support Care Cancer, 7*(1), 1-3.

Body, J.J. (2003). Zoledronic acid: An advance in tumour bone disease therapy and a new hope for osteoporosis. *Expert Opin Pharmacother, 4*(4), 567-580.

Bonica, J.J. (1980). Cancer Pain. *Res Publ Assoc Res Nerv Ment Dis, 58,* 335-362.

Bowsher, D. (1996). Central pain: Clinical and psychological characteristics. *J Neurol Neurosurg Psychiatry, 61*(1), 62-69.

Bruera, E. (2002). Methadone use in cancer patients with pain: A review. *Palliat Med, 5*(1), 127-138.

Bruera, E., & Lawlor, P. (1997). Cancer pain management. *Acta Anaesthesiol Scand, 41*(1 Pt. 2), 146-153.

Bruera, E., MacMillian, K., Hanson, J., et al. (1989). The Edmonton staging system for cancer pain: Preliminary report. *Pain, 37*(2), 203-209.

Bruera, E., & Watanabe, S. (1994). New developments in the assessment of pain in cancer patients. *Support Care Cancer, 2*(5), 312-318.

Canavero, S., & Conicalzi, V. (1997). Lamotrigine control of trigeminal neuralgia: An expanded study. *J Neurol, 244*(8), 527.

Caraceni, A., Portenoy, R.K. (1999). An international survey of cancer pain characteristics and syndromes. ISAP Task Force on Cancer Pain. International Association for the Study of Pain. PAIN 82(3), 263–274.

Cella, D.F., Tulsky, D.S., Gray, G., et al. (1993). The functional assessment of cancer therapy scale: Development and validation of the general measure. *J Clin Oncol, 11*(3), 570-579.

Chapman, C.R., Casey, K.L., Dubner, R., et al. (1985). Pain measurement: An overview. *Pain, 22*(1), 1-31.

Chuk, P.K. (1999). Vital signs and nurses' choices of titrated dosages of intravenous morphine for relieving pain following cardiac surgery. *J Adv Nurs, 30*(4), 858-865.

Cleeland, C.S., Nakamura, Y., Mendoza, TR., et al. (1996). Dimensions of the impact of cancer pain in a four country sample: New information from multidimensional scaling. *Pain, 67*(2-3), 267-273.

Cleeland, C.S., & Ryan, K.M. (1994). Pain assessment: Global use of the Brief Pain Inventory. *Ann Acad Med Singapore, 23*(2), 129-138.

Daut, R.L., Cleeland, C.S., & Flanery, R.C. (1983). Development of the Wisconsin Brief Pain Questionnaire to assess pain in cancer and other diseases. *Pain, 17*(2), 197-210.

Davis, M.P. (2003). Equianalgesia: Paradox and pitfalls. *J Terminal Oncol, 2*(2), 89.

Davis, M.P., & Nouneh, C. (2000). Modern management of cancer-related intestinal obstruction. *Curr Oncol Rep, 2,* 343-350.

Davis, M., & Walsh, D. (2000). Cancer pain syndromes. *Eur J Palliat Care, 7*(6), 206-209.

Davis, M.P., & Walsh, D. (2001). Methadone for relief of cancer pain: A review of pharmacokinetics, pharmacodynamics, drug interactions and protocols of administration. *Support Care Cancer, 9,* 73-83.

Davis, M.P., Walsh, D., LeGrand, S.B., et al. (2002). Symptom control in cancer patients: The clinical pharmacology and therapeutic role of suppositories and rectal suspensions. *Support Care Cancer, 10,* 117-138.

De Haes, J.C., van Knippenberg, F.C., Neijt, J.P., et al. (1990). Measuring psychological and physical distress in cancer patients: Structure and application of the Rotterdam Symptom Checklist. *Br J Cancer, 62*(6), 1034-1038.

De Stoutz, N.D., Bruera, E., & Suarez-Almazor, M. (1995). Opioid rotation for toxicity reduction in terminal cancer patients. *J Pain Symptom Manage, 19*(5), 378-384.

Devulder, J.E. (2000). Lamotrigine in refractory cancer pain. A case report. *J Clin Anesth, 12*(7), 574-575.

de Wit, R., van Dam, F., Abu-Saad, H.H., et al. (1999). Empirical comparison of commonly used measures to evaluate pain treatment in cancer patients with chronic pain. *J Clin Oncol, 17*(4), 1280.

Dicker, A.P. (2003). Cox-2 inhibitors and cancer therapeutics: Potential roles for inhibitors of Cox-2 in combination with cytotoxic therapy. Reports from a symposium held in conjunction with the Radiation Therapy Oncology Group, June 2001 meeting. *Am J Clin Oncol, 26*(4), S46-47.

Donnelly, S., Davis, M.P., Walsh, D., et al. (2002). Morphine in cancer pain management: A practical guide. *Support Care Cancer, 10,* 13-35.

Eisenberg, E., Alon, N., Ishay, A., et al. (1998). Lamotrigine in the treatment of painful diabetic neuropathy. *Eur J Neurol, 5*(2), 167-173.

Emery, P. (1999). Clinical aspects of Cox-2 inhibitors. *Drugs Today, 35*(4-5), 267-274.

Fallon, M.T., & Hanks, G.W. (1999). Morphine, constipation and performance status in advanced cancer patients. *Palliat Med, 13*(2), 159-160.

Faries, J.E., Mills, D.S., Goldsmith, K.W., et al. (1991). Systematic pain records and their impact on pain control: A pilot study. *Cancer Nurs, 14*(6), 306-313.

Fields, H.L., & Basbaum, A.I. (1978). Brainstem control of spinal pain-transmission neurons. *Annu Rev Physiol, 40,* 217-248.

Fishman, B., Pasternak, S., Wallenstein, S.L., et al. (1987). The Memorial Pain Assessment Card: A valid instrument for the evaluation of cancer pain. *Cancer, 60*(5), 1151-1158.

Galer, B.S., & Dworkin, R.H. (2000). *A clinical guide to neuropathic pain.* Minneapolis: McGraw-Hill Healthcare Information.

Gonzales, G.R. (1995). Central pain: Diagnosis and treatment strategies. *Neurology, 45*(12 Suppl. 9), S11-16.

Graham, C., Bond, S.S., Gerkovich, M.M., et al. (1980). Use of the McGill pain questionnaire in the assessment of cancer pain: Replicability and consistency. *Pain, 8*(3), 377-387.

Grond, S., Zech, D., Diefenbach, C., et al. (1996). Assessment of cancer pain: A prospective evaluation in 2266 cancer patients referred to a pain service. *Pain, 64*(1), 107-114.

Grossman, S.A. (1994). Assessment of cancer pain: A continuous challenge. *Support Care Cancer, 2*(2), 105-110.

Grossman, S.A., Sheidler, V.R., Swedeen, K., et al. (1991). Correlation of patient and caregiver ratings of cancer pain. *J Pain Symptom Manage, 6*(2), 53-57.

Guay, D.R. (2001). Adjunctive agents in the management of chronic pain. *Pharmacotherapy, 21*(9), 1070-1081.

Gutgsell, T., Walsh, D., Zhukovsky, D., et al. (2003). A prospective study of the pathophysiology and clinical characteristics of pain in a palliative medicine population. *Am J Hosp Palliat Care, 20*(2), 140.

Harbison, J., Dennehy, F., & Keating, D. (1997). Lamotrigine for pain in hyperalgesia. *Ir Med J, 90*(2), 56.

Hardy, J.R., Rees, E.A., Gwilliam, B., et al. (2002). A phase II study to establish the efficacy and toxicity of sodium valproate in patients with cancer-related neuropathic pain. *J Pain Symptom Manage, 21*(3), 204-209.

Hefferan, M.P., O'Reilly, D.D., & Loomis, C.W. (2003). Inhibition of spinal prostaglandin synthesis early after L5/L6 nerve ligation prevents the development of prostaglandin-dependent and prostaglandin-independent allodynia in the rat. *Anesthesiology, 99*(5), 1180-1188.

Institute of Medicine (IOM). (2004). *1st annual Crossing the Quality Chasm summit: A focus on communities.* Washington, D.C.: The National Academics.

Jaeckle, K.A. (1991). Nerve plexus metastases. *Neurol Clin, 9*(4), 857-866.

Jaeckle, K.A. (1993). Causes and management of headaches in cancer patients. *Oncology, 7*(4), 27-31.

Jamison, K., Wellisch, D.K., Katz, R.L., et al. (1979). Phantom breast syndrome. *Arch Surg, 114*(1), 93-95.

Jamison, R.N., & Brown, G.K. (1991). Validation of hourly pain intensity profiles with chronic pain patients. *Pain, 45*(2), 123-128.

Joint Commission on Accreditation of Healthcare Organizations (JCAHO). (2003). *Approaches in pain management: An essential guide for clinical leaders, 2003.* Chicago: Joint Commission Resources.

Julius, D., & Basbaum, A.I. (2001). Molecular mechanisms of nociception. *Nature, 413*(6852), 203-210.

Kellihan, M.J., & Mangino, P.D. (1992). Pamidronate. *Ann Pharmacother, 26*(10), 1262-1269.

Khojainova, N., Santiago-Palma, J., Kornick, C., et al. (2002). Olanzapine in the management of cancer pain. *J Pain Symptom Manage, 23*(4), 346-350.

Kochhar, R., LeGrand, S.B., Walsh, D., et al. (2003). Opioids in cancer pain: Common dosing errors. *Oncology, 19*(4), 575-576.

Krech, R.L., & Walsh, D. (1991). Symptoms of pancreatic cancer. *J Pain Symptom Manage, 6*(6), 360-367.

Kwekkeboom, K. (1996). Postmastectomy pain syndromes. *Cancer Nurs, 19*(1), 37-43.

Lanser, P., & Gesell, S. (2001). Pain management: The fifth vital sign. *Healthc Benchmarks, 8*(6), 62, 68-70.

Lashbrook, J.M., Ossipov, M.H., Hunter, J.C., et al. (1999). Synergistic antiallodynic effects of spinal morphine with ketorolac and selective Cox1- and Cox2-inhibitors in nerve-injured rats. *Pain, 82*(1), 65-72.

Levenson, D. (2001). IOM report: Healthcare system short-changes dying cancer patients. *Rep Med Guidel Outcomes Res, 12*(14), 7-9.

Levy, M.H. (1996). Pharmacologic treatment of cancer pain. *N Engl J Med, 335*(15), 1124-1132.

Lipman, A.G. (2003). Symptom-related research from the agency for healthcare research and quality. *J Pain Palliat Care Pharmacother, 17*(1), 39-45.

Lynch, M. (2001). Pain is the fifth vital sign. *J Intraven Nurs, 24*(2), 85-94.

Magni, G. (1991). The use of antidepressants in the treatment of chronic pain: A review of the current evidence. *Drugs, 42*(5), 730-748.

McCleane, G. (2003). Pharmacological management of neuro-pathic pain. *CNS Drugs, 17*(14), 1031-1043.

McCleane, G.J. (2000). Lamotrigine in the management of neuropathic pain: A review of the literature. *Clin J Pain, 16*(4), 321-326.

McCormack, K., & Twycross, R. (2001). Are COX-2 selective inhibitors effective analgesics? *Pain Reviews, 8*, 13-26.

McNicol, E., Horowicz-Mehler, N., Fisk, R.A., et al. (2003). Management of opioid side effects in cancer-related and chronic noncancer pain: A systematic review. *J Pain, 4*(5), 231-256.

Melzack, R., & Wall, P.D. (1965). Pain mechanisms: A new theory. *Science, 150*(699), 971-979.

Merboth, M.K., & Barnason, S. (2000). Managing pain: The fifth vital sign. *Nurs Clin North Am, 35*(2), 375-383.

Mercandante, S. (1997). Malignant bone pain: Pathophysiology and treatment. *Pain, 69*(1-2), 1-18.

Mercandante, S. (1999). Opioid rotation for cancer pain ration-ale and clinical aspects. *Cancer, 86*, 1856-1866.

Mercandante, S., Radbruch, L., Caraceni, A., et al. (2002). Episodic (breakthrough) pain: Consensus conference of an expert working group of the European Association of Palliative Care. *Cancer, 94*(3), 832-839.

Merskey, H. (1979). Pain terms: A list with definitions and notes on usage recommended by the IASP subcommittee on taxonomy. *Pain, 6*, 249-252.

Mukherkji, S.K., Castillo, M., & Wagle, A.G. (1996). The brachial plexus. *Semin Ultrasound CT MR, 17*(6), 519-538.

Nielsen, O.S., Munro, A.J., & Tannock, I.F. (1991). Bone metas-tases: Pathophysiology and management policy. *J Clin Oncol, 9*(3), 509-524.

Nielsen, O.S., & Skovgaard Poulsen, H. (1989). Bone metastasis. *Ugeskr Laeger, 151*(6), 362-365.

Olsen, N.K., Pfieffer, P., Johannsen, L., et al. (1993). Radiation-induced brachial plexopathy: Neurological follow-up in 161 recurrence-free breast cancer patients. *Int J Radiat Oncol Biol Phys, 26*(1), 43-49.

Olson, M.E., Chernik, N.L., & Posner, J.B. (1971). Leptomeningeal metastasis from systemic cancer: A report of 47 cases. *Trans Am Neurol Assoc, 96*, 291-293.

Olson, M.E., Chernik, N.L., & Posner, J.B. (1974). Infiltration of the leptomeninges by systemic cancer: A clinical and patho-logic study. *Arch Neurol, 30*(2), 122-137.

Pavilakis, N., & Stockler, M. (2002). Bisphosphonates for breast cancer. *Cochrane Database Syst Rev,1*, CD003474.

Peng, P.W.H., & Sandler, A.N. (1999). A review of the use of fentanyl analgesia in the management of acute pain in adults. *Anesthesiology, 90*(2), 576-599.

Pereira, J., Lawlor, P., Vigano, A., et al. (2001). Equianalgesic dose ratios for opioids: A critical review and proposals for long-term dosing. *J Pain Symptom Manage, 22*(2), 672-687.

Portenoy, R.K. (1989). Cancer pain: Epidemiology and syndromes. *Cancer, 63*(11 Suppl.), 2298-2307.

Portenoy, R.K. (1992). Cancer pain: Pathophysiology and syndromes. *Lancet, 339*(8800), 1026-1031.

Rigas, B., Kalofonos, H., Lebovics, E., et al. (2003). NO-NSAIDs and cancer: Promising novel agents. *Dig Liver Dis, 35*(Suppl. 2), S27-34.

Ripamonti, C., Ticozzi, C., Zecca, E., et al. (1996). Continuous subcutaneous infusion of ketorolac in cancer neuropathic pain unresponsive to opioid and adjuvant drugs: A case report. *Tumori, 82*(4), 413-415.

Ripamonti, C., Zecca, E., & De Conno, F. (1998). Pharmacological treatment of cancer pain: Alternative routes of opioid admin-istration. *Tumori, 84*, 289-300.

Sandkuhler, J. (2002). Fear the pain. *Lancet, 360*(9331), 426.

Sarhill, N., Walsh, D., & Nelson, K.A. (2001). Hydromorphone: Pharmacology and clinical applications in cancer patients. *Support Care Cancer, 9*, 84-96.

Schipper, H., Clinch, J., McMurray, A., et al. (1984). Measuring the quality of life of cancer patients: The Functional Living Index Cancer: Development and validation. *J Clin Oncol, 2*(5), 472-483.

Serlin, R.C., Mendoza, T.R., Nakamura, Y., et al. (1995). When is cancer pain mild, moderate or severe? Grading pain severity by its interference with function. *Pain, 62*(2), 277-284.

Simmons, J.C. (2001). Pain management: New initiatives arise to provide quality of care. *Qual Letter Healthc Lead, 13*(6), 2-11.

Sloan, J.A., Loprinizi, C.L., Kuross, S.A., et al. (1999). Randomized comparison of four tools measuring overall quality of life in patients with advanced cancer. *J Clin Oncol, 17*(2), 738-740.

Smith, W.B., & Safer, M.A. (1993). Effects of present pain level on recall of chronic pain and medication use. *Pain, 55*(3), 355-361.

Stevens, P.E., Dibble, S.L., & Miaskowski, C. (1995). Prevalence, characteristics, and impact of postmastectomy pain syndrome: An investigation of women's experiences. *Pain, 61*(1), 61-68.

Stjernsward, J., Colleau, S.M., & Ventafridda, V. (1996). The World Health Organization Cancer Pain and Palliative Care Program: Past, present and future. *J Pain Symptom Manage, 12*(2), 65-72.

Stromgren, A.S., Groenvold, M., Pedersen, L., et al. (2001). Does the medical record cover the symptoms experienced by cancer patients receiving palliative care? A comparison of the record and patient self-rating. *J Pain Symptom Manage, 21*(3), 189-196.

Tarnawski, A.S., & Jones, M.K. (2003). Inhibition of angiogenesis by NSAIDs: Molecular mechanisms and clinical implications. *J Mol Med, 81*(10), 627-636.

Turk, D.C. (2002). Remember the distinction between malig-nant and benign pain? Well, forget it. *Clin J Pain, 18*, 75-76.

Twycross, R. (2002). Cancer pain syndromes. In N. Sykes, M. Fallon, & R. Patt (Eds.), *Clinical pain management, cancer pain* (pp. 3-19). London: Arnold Publishers.

Twycross, R., Harcourt, J., & Bergl, S. (1996). A survey of pain in patients with advanced cancer. *J Pain Symptom Manage, 12*(5), 273-282.

Ventafridda, V., & Stjernsward, J. (1995). Pain control and the World Health Organization analgesic ladder. *JAMA, 274*(23), 1870-1873.

Von Roenn, J.H., Cleeland, C.S., Gonin, R., et al. (1993). Physician attitudes and practice in cancer pain management: A survey of the Eastern Cooperative Oncology Group. *Ann Intern Med, 119*(2), 121-126.

Walker, V.A., Hoskin, P.J., Hanks, G.W., et al. (1988). Evaluation of WHO analgesic guidelines for cancer pain in a hospital-based palliative care unit. *J Pain Symptom Manage, 3*(3), 145-149.

Walsh, D. (2000). Pharmacological management of cancer pain. *Semin Oncol, 27*(1), 45-63.

Wantanabe, S., & Bruera, E. (1994). Corticosteroids as adjuvant analgesics. *J Pain Symptom Manage, 9*(7), 442-445.

Wantanabe, S., Periera, J., Hanson, J., et al. (1998). Fentanyl by continuous subcutaneous infusion for the management of cancer pain: A retrospective study. *J Pain Symptom Manage, 16*(5), 323-326.

Watson, C.P., Vernich, L., Chipman, M., et al. (1998). Nortriptyline versus amitriptyline in postherpetic neuralgia: A randomized trial. *Neurology, 51*(4), 1166-1171.

Weber, M., & Huber, C. (1999). Documentation of severe pain, opioid doses, and opioid-related side effects in outpatients with cancer: A retrospective study. *J Pain Symptom Manage, 17*(1), 49-54.

Weinstein, S.M. (1994). Phantom pain. *Oncology, 8*(3), 65-70.

Wilder-Smith, C.H. (2001). Opioids in cancer pain: Which one is best? *Support Care Cancer, 9*, 71-72.

Zech, D.F., Grond, S., Lynch, J., et al. (1995). Validation of World Health Organization guidelines for cancer pain relief: A 10-year prospective study. *Pain, 63*(1), 65-76.

CHAPTER 11

Neurology

Mellar P. Davis
Bushra I. Cheema
David Oliver
Pamela Sue Spencer

OBJECTIVES

After the completion of this chapter, the reader should be able to:

1. Understand the El Escorial diagnostic criteria and their limitations.
2. Discuss the importance of palliative medicine and a multidisciplinary approach to the care of a patient diagnosed with amyotrophic lateral sclerosis (ALS).
3. Identify follow-up care and monitoring criteria for the ALS patient.
4. Describe the clusters of symptoms present in ALS and their management.
5. Explain the diagnosis and management of Huntington's disease (HD).

AMYOTROPHIC LATERAL SCLEROSIS

Introduction

Though several neurologic diseases are encountered in the palliative setting, this chapter focuses primarily on amyotrophic lateral sclerosis (ALS) disease and provides a brief discussion on Huntington's disease (HD). ALS is also known as *Lou Gehrig's disease* in the United States, named after the famous baseball player who died as a result of ALS (Carter, Krivickas, Weydt, et al., 2003). In the United Kingdom, ALS is referred to as *motor neuron disease (MND)*. ALS is one of the three main neurodegenerative disorders (O'Brien, 2001). The others are Parkinson's disease and Alzheimer's disease (Borasio, 2001; Strong, 2001). A cardinal feature that distinguishes ALS is the combination of upper and lower motor neuron degeneration that spares sensory neurons, in particularly bowel and bladder function (Borasio, 2001; O'Brien, 2001). In the United Kingdom, if the clinical presentation is predominantly lower motor neuron loss, the disease is called *progressive muscular atrophy* and if the disease is predominantly upper motor neuron loss, it is termed *primary lateral sclerosis*. However, most patients have mixed disease as the disease progresses. Increasing evidence suggests that other nerves are involved. Diffuse fibrous gliosis in the frontotemporal area may account for dementia seen in a minority of ALS patients (Yoshida, 2004).

Epidemiology

ALS, a relatively rare disease, has a uniform incidence across geographic and cultural boundaries. The unusually high incidence in Guam after World War II has disappeared (Borasio, 2001; Haddock & Chen, 2003). The incidence is 1 per 100,000 and the prevalence is 6 to 8 per 100,000 because of the high death rate from this relentlessly progressive disease (O'Brien, 2001; Strong & Rosenfeld, 2003). Men have a higher incidence, which often occurs before the age of 50 (1.7:1 male to female). After the age of 50, the incidence rises, then plateaus, and then declines after age 70 (Borasio, 2001). Mortality and shortened survival of ALS increase with age (Strong, 2001; Strong & Rosenfeld, 2003). Young men survive longer than do young women. When symptoms occur before the age of 45, the median survival is 55 months, but it is only 25 months if symptoms occur after the age of 45 (Strong, 2001). Smoking may be a risk factor (Armon, 2003). The incidence in veterans of the

Gulf War is reported to be higher than normal, and the risk of ALS has been associated with trauma (Horner, Kamins, Feussner, et al., 2003; Piazza, Siren, & Ehrenreich, 2004).

Clinical Features

In the early stages of disease, the diagnosis is often missed because of the rarity of this disease and its subtle presentation (Strong & Rosenfeld, 2003) (Table 11-1). Patients are frequently referred to other subspecialties before being seen by a neurologist. The patient often presents with a combination of upper and lower motor neuron dysfunction. Patients will have muscle wasting, weakness, and fasciculation (twitching) with loss of lower motor neuron function, whereas upper motor neuron signs include stiffness, spasticity, and hyperreflexia. Patients may complain of problems with limb movement, or they may have difficulties with speech and swallowing (Borasio, 2001; O'Brien, 2001). Patients may have only one extremity affected or may present with bulbar signs and symptoms and limited limb weakness (Borasio, Voltz, & Miller, 2001; O'Brien, 2001). Progressive bulbar palsy can be the only presentation in a minority of patients (Strong & Rosenfeld, 2003). Patients with bulbar involvement will have tongue fasciculations, a poor elevation of the soft palate with phonation, and an exaggerated gag and jaw jerk (Borasio, 2001; Borasio & Miller, 2001; Strong & Rosenfeld, 2003). As the disease progresses, patients will be unable to dress and toilet themselves and will become socially isolated as they lose the ability to speak and walk. Nutritional deficits supervene because of dysphagia. As the disease advances, dyspnea becomes a prominent symptom as the result of the loss of respiratory muscle strength. Dementia is relatively rare, so patients remain aware of their declining health (Strong & Rosenfeld, 2003). Death is usually the result of respiratory failure. The average duration of ALS from diagnosis is 3 years. ALS is a rapidly progressive disease that does not wax and wane and thus significantly differs from multiple sclerosis. It is rare to see remissions (Borasio & Miller, 2001). However, there can be a broad range of survivorship among patients, and a small proportion may actually live for a decade or two (Strong & Rosenfeld, 2003).

Table 11-1   ALS Prognostic Table

Clinical Presentation	Diagnostic Evaluation	Pathophysiology
Age	History	Unknown ? co-morbidity
Short delay in diagnosis	History	More rapid disease course
Female	History	Unknown
Lack of marital partner	History	Lack of social support
Attendance at a general neurology clinic rather than multidisciplinary	—	Failure to use disease-modifying and support care (NIPPV) to maximum benefit
Failure to use riluzole	History	Anti-glutamate therapy delays progression of disease
Bulbar onset	Physical examination	Early onset of nutritional deficiency, risk of aspiration?
Reduced body mass index	Physical examination	Nutritional deficiency and muscle atrophy
Dyspnea, weakness, morning headache, fatigue, daytime sleepiness	FVC, nocturnal oximetry, and performance score by activities of daily living	Hypoventilation from respiratory muscle weakness, peripheral (extremity) muscle atrophy

ALS, Amyotrophic lateral sclerosis; *NIPPV,* noninvasive positive-pressure ventilation; *FVC,* forced vital capacity.
Data from del Aguila, M.A., Longstreth, W.T., McGuire, V., et al. (2003). Prognosis in amyotrophic lateral sclerosis: A population-based study. *Neurology, 60*(5), 813-819; Traynor, B.J., Alexander, M., Corr, B., et al. (2003). An outcome study of riluzole in amyotrophic lateral sclerosis: A population-based study in Ireland, 1996-2000. *J Neurol, 250*(4), 473-479.

Diagnosis

It is important to consider and rule out other neurologic diseases other than ALS, particularly in its early presentation (Box 11-1). Procedures that aid in the diagnosis of ALS are magnetic resonance imaging (MRI) of the brain and spinal cord, electromyography, electroneurography (EMG/ENG), muscle biopsy, lumbar puncture, immunoelectrophoresis, and calcium and thyroid function tests.

The EL Escorial criteria for the diagnosis of ALS were formulated as an inclusion guideline for the purpose of clinical research and should not be used as exclusion criteria when seeking a diagnosis of ALS (Beghi, Balzarini, Boglium, et al., 2002).

Pathology

The anatomic appearance of the spinal cord and brain, at least early in the course of disease, is relatively normal (Festoff, Suo, & Citron, 2003; Strong & Rosenfeld, 2003). Microscopic inspection demonstrates a loss of large motor neuron cell bodies from the anterior horn of the spinal cord and the motor strip in the cerebral cortex, which is associated with astrocyte overgrowth. Inclusion bodies are found within neuron cell bodies. Lipofuscin pigments and neurofilaments are found in the neuronal cell bodies (Strong, 1999; Strong, Leystra-Lantz, & Ge, 2004). Inclusion proteins are ubiquitinated in preparation for destruction by proteasomes (Chung, Joo, Lee, et al., 2003; Strong, Leystra-Lantz, Ge, 2004; Wood, Beayjeux, Shaw, 2003). The neuronal machinery that governs programmed cell death is activated and leads to progressive neuron loss (Przedborski, 2004; Strong, 2001; Takeuchi, Niwa, Hishikawa, et al., 2004).

Etiology. ALS involves the pathways that influence oxidative stress (SOD_1), neuron excitability (glutamate and AMPA), cytoskeleton proteins (neurofilaments), and calcium homeostasis in the mitochondrion (Anderson, Restagno, Stewart, et al., 2004; Anderson, Sims, Xin, et al., 2003; Arisato, Okubo, Arata, et al., 2003; Crow, Ye, Strong, et al., 1997; Jackson, Llado, & Rothstein, 2002; Przedborski, Mitsumoto, & Rowland, 2003; Sato, Yamamoto, Nakanishi, et al., 2004; Strong, 2001). The cause of ALS in the vast majority of patients is unknown. Genetic mutations of the superoxide dismutase gene (SOD_1) account for 20% of familial forms of ALS (Kato, Saeki, Aoki, et al., 2004). The SOD_1 gene defect leads to protein accumulation within motor neurons and predisposes neurons to glutamate neurotoxicity and reduced glutamate cellular transporters (Tortarolo, Crossthwaite, Conforti, et al., 2004). Loss of the regulation of glutamate transport ($EAAT_2$ gene mutations) has been detected in some individuals (Guo, Lai, Butchbach, et al, 2003; Simpson, Yen, & Appel, 2003). The loss of glutamate transport leads to accumulation of glutamate that binds to N-methyl-D-asparate (NMDA) and AMPA receptors and leads to neurotoxicity (Pieri, Gaetti, Spalloni, et al., 2003; Spalloni, Albo, Ferrari, et al., 2004). Activated glutamate receptors increase intracellular calcium, which stimulates neuron apoptosis through the activation of caspases (Iwasaki, Ikeda, & Kinoshita, 2002; Festoff et al., 2003; Kawahara, Ito, Sun, et al., 2004).

Mutations of the neurofilament genes can lead to an accumulation of neurofilaments within the neuron, contributing to the pathology of ALS (Jackson et al., 2002). The motor neuron will ultimately succumb as a result of neurofilament accumulation and mitochondrion dysfunction from oxidative stress (Strong, 2003).

Box 11-1 DIFFERENTIAL DIAGNOSIS TO EARLY ALS

- Spinal disease (disk, spinal conal stenosis, cyst, or tumor)
- Autoimmune neuropathy (GM1 ganglioside autoantibody)
- Paraproteinemia (amyloid)
- Thyrotoxicosis
- Hyperparathyroidism
- Diabetic myotrophy
- GM2 gangliosidosis
- Myopathy (Lambert-Eaton)

ALS, Amyotrophic lateral sclerosis.
Data from Ross, M.A. (1997). Acquired motor neuron disorders. *Neurol Clin, 15*(3), 481-500; Niebroj-Dobosz, I., Janik, P., & Kwiecinski, H. (2004). Serum IgM anti-GM1 ganglioside antibodies in lower motor neuron syndromes. *Eur J Neurol, 11*(1), 13-16.

Clinical and Experimental Drugs That Influence ALS

Multiple medications have been used to treat ALS in hopes of modifying the course of disease (Table 11-2). However, only riluzole has been licensed in the United States for the management of ALS. Riluzole is a glutamate release inhibitor. Riluzole prolongs the time spent within less severe stages of disease (Strong, 2001). Treatment reduces the risk of death or need for ventilation at 18 months compared with patients who do not receive riluzole. In some patients the benefit may be longer compared with untreated controls. Survival is increased on average by 3 months (Lacomblez, Bensimon, Leigh, et al., 1996; Bensimon, Lacomblez, & Meininger, 1994).

Most patients trial riluzole, vitamin E, and creatine to slow the rate of ALS since these interventions are generally well tolerated (Carter et al., 2003; Debove, Zeisser, Salzman, et al., 2001; Demaerschalk & Strong, 2000; Dib, 2003; Festoff et al., 2003; Klivenyi, Kiaei, Gardian, et al., 2004; Strong, 2003; Strong & Pattee, 2000).

Treatment of ALS

General Principles. The treatment of ALS should be based on the guiding principles of palliative medicine: (1) affirming life and regarding the dying process as a natural part of life; (2) neither hastening or postponing dying; (3) providing relief from symptom distress; (4) integrating care in a holistic approach (physical, psychologic, and

Table **11-2**   CLINICAL AND EXPERIMENTAL DRUGS THAT MAY DIRECTLY INFLUENCE ALS

Drug	Benefit
Riluzole	Glutamate release inhibitor that delays death by 3 months on average. Benefits are lost with time. Survival may be more marked with patients who have bulbar disease.[1] Serious side effects from riluzole are rare.[2] There is no beneficial effect on bulbar function or muscle strength; however, progression appears to be delayed.[3-6]
Gabapentin	Alone is ineffective but may potentiate the benefits of riluzole.[7,8] Trials showed little effect but major side effects.
Neurotrophins	Have been disappointing in experimental studies.[9,10]

[1]Traynor, B.J., Alexander, M., Corr, B., et al. (2003). An outcome study of riluzole in amyotrophic lateral sclerosis: A population-based study in Ireland, 1996-2000. *J Neurol, 250*(4), 473-479.

[2]Debove, C., Zeisser, P., Salzman, P.M., et al. (2001). The Rilutek (riluzole) Global Early Access Programme: An open-label safety evaluation in the treatment of amyotrophic lateral sclerosis. *Amyotroph Lateral Scler Other Motor Neuron Disord, 2*(3), 153-158.

[3]Miller, R.G., Mitchell, J.D., & Moore, D.H. (2000). Riluzole for amyotrophic lateral sclerosis (ALS)/motor neuron disease (MND). *Cochrane Database Syst Rev, 2*, CD001447.

[4]Ludolph, A.C. (2000). Treatment of amyotrophic lateral sclerosis: What is the next step? *J Neurol, 247*, 13-18.

[5]Ludolph, A.C., Meyer, T., & Riepe, M.W. (1999). Antiglutamate therapy of ALS: What is the next step? *J Neural Transm Suppl, 55*, 79-95.

[6]Mitsumoto, H. (1997). Riluzole: What is its impact in our treatment and understanding of amyotrophic lateral sclerosis? *Ann Pharmacother, 31*(6), 779-781.

[7]Festoff, B.W., Suo, Z., & Citron, B.A. (2003). Prospects for the pharmacotherapy of amyotrophic lateral sclerosis: Old strategies and new paradigms for the third millennium. *CNS Drugs, 17*(10), 699-717.

[8]Mazzini, L., Mora, G., Balzarini, C., et al. (1998). The natural history and the effects of gabapentin in amyotrophic lateral sclerosis. *J Neurol Sci, 160*(Suppl. 1), S57-63.

[9]Al-Chalabi, A., Scheffler, M.D., Smith, B.N., et al. (2003). Ciliary neurotrophic factor genotype does not influence clinical phenotype in amyotrophic lateral sclerosis. *Ann Neurol, 54*(1), 130-134.

[10]Carter, G.T., Krivickas, L.S., Weydt, P., et al. (2003). Drug therapy for amyotrophic lateral sclerosis: Where are we now? *Idrugs 6*(2), 147-153.

ALS, Amyotrophic lateral sclerosis.

spiritual); and (5) recognizing the family as part of the plan of care and an integral component to the support system of the patient (Oliver, 1996; O'Brien, 2001).

Characteristics of good palliative care include acceptance and affirmation of the individual and his or her individual goals and expectations of care by the clinician. This individualized approach to care helps foster dignity, hope, and honesty (Twycross, 1997). Symptom relief requires a team of disciplines that embrace the principles of palliation. Flexibility and respect for autonomy and choice (within the limitations and trajectory of illness) will instill hope and forestall the sense of being a burden. Communication between members of the team and the patient is of utmost importance to be congruent with patient-centered goals. The final result is the "discovery of creativity, and beauty even in the midst of death and dying" (Twycross, 1997).

The care of the patient with ALS begins with providing adequate information about the disease early in the course of illness. There is an art to providing this type of information to the patient and his or her family. Too much information can overwhelm the patient and family, and if it is given in a non-personal or "cold" manner, hope is deflated and may make the medical management difficult throughout the course of illness (Borasio, Sloan, & Pongratz, 1998; Ross, 1997). Too little or lack of information may increase the patient's anxiety and fears about the future of his or her disease, creating misperceptions about ALS and causing patients to seek information from other (perhaps incorrect) sources (Ross, 1997). ALS patient education resources are available through the Muscular Dystrophy Association and the Amyotrophic Lateral Sclerosis Association (Ross, 1997).

Information should be divulged across several visits rather than all at one time, depending on the patient's need. Information should be balanced between the general discourse about the disease and specific queries the patient may have (Ross, 1997). Patients with predominantly bulbar disease will want to understand dysphagia and its treatment options (e.g., gastrostomy tubes) sooner than patients with predominantly extremity weakness,

who have concerns about physical therapy and walking aids. The name and type of the disease should be described and explained to distinguish it from multiple sclerosis (or myasthenia gravis) or other neuromuscular disorders. Positive aspects about ALS should be emphasized, which include a general absence of severe pain, incontinence, and dementia (Borasio et al., 2001).

A subset of patients will present early and may have a suspected but not confirmed diagnosis according to the El Escorial criteria. This may provoke anxiety in the patient since there is an absence of certainty. It would be important to screen these individuals for other diagnoses but even more important to follow them closely in a supportive way and to be available to see them if other manifestations should occur between visits.

Discussions about gastrostomy feeding and ventilatory support as well as advance directives should follow the discussion related to the trajectory of illness (Borasio et al., 1998). If these issues are discussed too early, it may be taken as an indicator of rapidly progressive disease and result in a negative reaction. If these matters are discussed too late, the clinician may be perceived as being dishonest and uncaring.

Physician-Assisted Suicide Issues. In societies where it is permitted, it is relatively common for those in this patient population to seek euthanasia and physician-assisted suicide (Reagan, Hurst, Cook, et al., 2003; Zylicz, 2000, Zylicz & Findlay, 1999). The five main reasons patients request physician-assisted suicide are (Ganzini, Johnston, & Hoffman, 1999; Ganzini, Johnston, MacFarland, et al., 1998; Ganzini, Silveira, & Johnston, 2002; Zylicz, 2000; Zylicz & Findlay, 1999):

1. Fear of choking or pain
2. Burnout from relentless progressive disability and exhaustion
3. Lack of control (progressive dependence)
4. Depression
5. Pain

The demographic profile of those who seek to end their life include (1) male, (2) higher education, (3) lack of religious affiliation, (4) hopelessness, and (5) perceived poor quality of life (Ganzini et al., 1998; Plahuta, McCullough, Kasarskis, et al., 2002).

The provision for optimal supportive palliative therapy is instrumental when helping relieve patient fears and circumventing requests for physician-assisted suicide. Patients informed about the clinical course of ALS on invasive ventilation (including the "locked in" syndrome) will frequently avoid invasive ventilation as a means of support and often document this in their advance directives (Borasio et al., 2001).

Advance Directives. The information in Box 11-2 will help when establishing advance directives (AD) for the ALS patient. Medical decision making for this patient should include issues that surround (Borasio & Voltz, 2000):

- Trials of disease-modifying therapy (on or off study)
- Noninvasive ventilation
- Percutaneous gastrostomy for nutritional support

Box 11-2   ADVANCE DIRECTIVES

1. The physician should initiate discussion of advance directives (ADs).
2. Discussion should proceed after establishing a therapeutic relationship and long-standing communication.
3. Discussion should occur before the terminal phase of illness—ideally, before dyspnea.
4. AD should clearly state the patient's preference for gastrostomy and ventilation support.
5. Family and the primary physician should be involved and informed about the specific decisions within the AD.
6. Cultural background should play a role in decision making and must be recognized and respected.
7. If a health care proxy is involved, a written directive should be provided (and signed, depending on the regional law and regulations).
8. Copies of the AD should accompany the patient to the local physician and hospital.
9. Nurses and hospice staff should be informed about the AD particulars.
10. ADs should be periodically revised if the patient has had a change of heart.

- Cardiopulmonary resuscitation
- Tracheotomy
- Invasive ventilation
- Antibiotics
- Hydration
- Emergency treatment for acute dyspnea and/or pain

Symptom Management

Patients with ALS initially experience focal weakness, but over time this progresses with the development of multiple symptoms including muscle fasciculations, spasticity, dysarthria, dysphagia, constipation, gastroesophageal reflux, drooling, sleep disturbances, pathologic crying and laughing, depression, dyspnea, symptoms of hypoventilation, and pain. Each symptom has to be assessed and managed appropriately to reduce the symptom burden that accompanies advanced ALS (Lyall, Moxham, & Leigh, 2000; Mandler, Anderson, Miller, et al., 2001; Miller, Rosenberg, Gelinas, et al., 1999; Oliver, 1996).

Weakness. Weakness is primarily the presenting symptom of ALS and can be successfully managed by walking aids or ankle/foot orthoses (AFO braces) (Ross, 1997). Patients who are in a state of denial about their weakness may continue to walk despite the risk of falls or fractures. ALS patients need to learn to be "dependently independent." To remain mobile they will need assistance, either mechanical or personal (Ross, 1997). A wheelchair should be obtained before the loss of ambulatory capacity in order to remain socially active and mobile within the home (Ross, 1997). A raised toilet seat, bedside commode, grab bars, banisters in the halls, shower seats, and hand-held shower devices can simplify toileting (and give patients some independence that they would not have had otherwise). Velcro, rather than buttons and shoestrings, and modified utensils will assist in dressing and eating (Borasio et al., 2001). A Hoyer lift in advanced ALS may help in positioning the patient and changing the bed linens. The stamina of an ALS patient will fluctuate to a greater extent than normal. A period of low energy and weakness does not necessarily mean rapidly progressive disease, and counter-wise, a good day does not mean remission (Borasio et al., 2001).

Physical therapy is important to forestall deconditioning, maintain joint mobility, and prevent contractures and adhesive capsulitis. Physical therapy may reduce pain that is associated with immobility. Another advantage to physical therapy is the warmth of human touch. Massage can also be used to help reduce pain and increase joint mobility and provide the opportunity for reminiscing and psychosocial support (Borasio & Miller, 2001; Borasio & Oliver, 2000; Borasio et al., 2001; Ross, 1997).

Physical therapists should oversee rehabilitation by educating both the families and patients about the proper use of assistive devices, measuring the patients for appropriate fit, and observing the patients who are using those devices appropriately.

The secondary benefits to maintaining mobility are reduced risk of constipation (which worsens with inactivity), reduced boredom, and reduced edema, as well as avoidance of decubitus ulcers (though decubitus ulcers in ALS are rare). Lymphedema of the lower extremities can also occur from the lack of using the muscular pump (found with leg movement) against the small lymphatic vessels (Borasio et al., 2001).

Acetylcholinesterase inhibitors such as pyridostigmine may provide short-term benefit to weakness but do not alter the course of disease (Borasio et al., 2001).

Fasciculation, Spasticity, and Pain. Fasciculation occurs with weakness and arises from degeneration of intramuscular motor neurons. Fasciculation can cause muscular cramps (Borasio et al, 2001). Spasticity arises from degeneration of the upper motor neurons and can be quite severe and painful (Borasio et al., 2001; Ross, 1997). There are multiple medications that may reduce fasciculation and spasticity (Table 11-3).

Benzodiazepines may reduce spasticity but often create sedation. Dantrolene is not as helpful and may worsen weakness (Borasio et al., 2001; Ross, 1997). Antispasticity drugs should be titrated to symptom response and not objective reduction in fasciculation since moderate degrees of spasticity help maintain mobility (Borasio et al., 2001).

Immobility and joint contractures are a major cause of pain for ALS patients. Some patients

Table **11-3** TREATMENT OF FASCICULATIONS AND SPASTICITY

Drug	Dosage
Lioresal	10 mg three times daily
Carbamazepine	200 mg twice daily
Phenytoin	100 mg three times daily
Quinine sulfate	200 mg twice daily
Magnesium	5 mmol three times daily
Vitamin E	400 International Units twice daily
Verapamil	120 mg daily
Tizanidine	6-24 mg daily
Memantine	10-60 mg daily

Data from Borasio, G.D., Voltz R., & Miller, R.G. (2001). Palliative care in amyotrophic lateral sclerosis. *Neurol Clin, 19*(4), 829-847; Borasio, G.D., & Oliver, D. (2000). The control of other symptoms. In D. Oliver, G.D. Borasio, & D. Walsh (Eds.), *Palliative care in amyotrophic lateral sclerosis* (Chapter 4, pp. 72-81). New York: Oxford University Press.

(fortunately a small minority) will have severe pain from ALS. Massage may reduce muscular pain, and frequent repositioning and passive range of motion are nonpharmacologic approaches to pain reduction (Ross, 1997). The World Health Organization's analgesic ladder should govern pain management. Nonsteroidal antiinflammatory drugs are used initially; if these are insufficient to control the pain, opioids should be considered and the dose titrated to optimally control pain (Borasio et al., 2001). Laxatives should be started at the onset of opioids.

Dysarthria and Dysphagia. The progressive loss of communication and inarticulate phonation can cause social isolation and embarrassment. Communication takes longer and is more exhausting and hence limited or not attempted at all. Physicians and family may mistake dysfunctional communication for dementia. Simple alphabet charts can be helpful (Borasio et al., 2001). Computer technology is an alternative while the patient has voluntary muscle movement. Eventually, particularly if invasive respiratory support is initiated, the patient will become "locked in" and may be left with eye movement as the only means of communication (Borasio et al., 2001; Borasio & Miller, 2001). The speech and language therapist/pathologist should be included—to help in assessment and management.

Dysphagia can be treated with a modified diet consisting of thickened liquids and soft foods. Learning to tuck the chin while swallowing can facilitate eating (Ross, 1997). A percutaneous endoscopic gastrostomy (PEG) tube (or radiographically placed gastrostomy tube) should be considered before the forced vital capacity (FVC) is less than 50% or there is a body weight loss of more than 10% (Wagner-Sonnatag, Allison, Oliver, Prosiegel, et al., 2000). Nutritional failure resulting from caloric deprivation can lead to secondary weakness (Ross, 1997). Choking and aspiration of food are indications of ineffective oral nutrition and also indications for the placement of a percutaneous endoscopic gastrostomy (PEG) tube. A PEG tube placement does not prevent aspiration and can lead to pneumonia due to gastroesophageal reflux, gastric insufflation from the PEG tube placement, and/or overfeeding. Lack of nutrition increases the risk of death sevenfold to eightfold (Desport, Preux, Truong, et al., 1999).

Noninvasive positive-pressure ventilation (NIPPV) can be used safely during PEG tube placement to support the patient (Box 11-3) (Boitano, Jordan, & Benditt, 2001; Chio, Finocchiaro, Meineri, et al., 1999; Gregory, Siderowf, Golaszewski, et al., 2002; Mitsumoto, Davidson, Moore, et al., 2003).

Drooling. Drooling is associated with bulbar dysfunction and not an overproduction of saliva. Sialorrhea (drooling) can be an embarrassment to individuals with ALS. Amitriptyline 25 mg at

bedtime, by virtue of having anticholinergic properties, will reduce sialorrhea and is preferred over secondary tricyclic antidepressants, desipramine, and nortriptyline. Amitriptyline, however, can worsen gastroesophageal reflux and cause gastroparesis and worsen constipation (Ross, 1997). Glycopyrrolate, a quaternary scopolamine, reduces drooling and minimizes the risk of cognitive failure that can occur with tertiary amine anticholinergics. The usual dose is 1 to 2 mg twice to three times a day (Ross, 1997). In case of refractory sialorrhea, a combination of amitriptyline and glycopyrrolate may be helpful. Transdermal scopolamine is an alternative that improves compliance and minimizes the "pill" burden patients with advanced ALS often experience. Other options include (1) salivary gland irradiation, (2) transtympanic neurectomy, or (3) injections of botulinum toxin A into the salivary glands (Borasio et al., 2001; Giess, Naumann, Werner, et al., 2000).

Insomnia, Pathologic Emotions, and Depression. Sleep disorders occur as a direct or indirect result of having ALS. Patients are unable to change their position during sleep, resulting in pain from immobility. Fasciculation and cramps may waken the patient from sleep. Dysphagia with aspiration or reflux is more prominent at night. Respiratory insufficiency and hypoventilation occur initially at night, leading to repeated wakening episodes (Borasio et al., 2001). Indirect causes that worsen both pain and insomnia are anxiety and depression. Assessment for nocturnal oxygen desaturation is key when both insomnia and daytime sleepiness are observed. Nocturnal oximetry or polysomnography is done to detect nocturnal desaturation (discussed later). NIPPV should be initiated for nocturnal desaturation rather than sedation or oxygen (Borasio et al., 2001). Sedatives should be used sparingly. Chloral hydrate 250 to 1000 mg or flurazepam or temazepam 15 to 30 mg could be used if nocturnal saturation is not a factor; however, short-acting benzodiazepines are preferred. Diphenhydramine, though popular as a sleeping medication, has the risk of delirium. Alternatively, if depression is a major reason for insomnia, amitriptyline 25 mg at night titrated to benefit or mirtazapine 15 to 30 mg (which is an

---

BOX 11-3   INDICATIONS FOR NONINVASIVE POSITIVE-PRESSURE VENTILATION

- Hypercapnia
- FVC <50% of predicted
- MIP <−60 cm H_2O
- Symptoms of nocturnal hypoventilation

FVC, Forced vital capacity; *MIP,* maximum inspiratory pressure.

antidepressant and sleep aid) is a reasonable choice. Citalopram or selective serotonin reuptake inhibitors (SSRIs) are alternatives, depending on patient or physician preference.

Pathologic crying and laughing need to be differentiated from depression. This pseudobulbar effect is a state of uncontrolled laughing alternating with crying (Borasio & Miller, 2001) and occurs in half of ALS patients. This process appears to be related to progressive frontal lobe dysfunction and can be associated with some selective cognitive impairment (Abrahams, Goldstein, Al-Chalabi, et al., 1997; Abrahams, Goldstein, Kew, et al., 1996; McCullagh, Moore, Gawel, et al., 1999). This is not a mood disturbance and is seldom volunteered (Borasio & Miller, 2001). Treatment is with amitriptyline 10 to 50 mg at night. Other alternatives are fluvoxamine, lithium carbonate, or levodopa (L-Dopa) (Borasio et al., 2001; Borasio & Miller, 2001).

Dyspnea and Hypoventilation. Respiratory failure is the most common cause of death in ALS and is a result of progressive respiratory muscle dysfunction. Respiratory failure rarely presents early (Melo, Homma, Iturriaga, et al., 1999). Patients with ALS will usually have limb weakness before respiratory failure. Because of immobility, patients cannot exert themselves to the point of dyspnea, and as a result, dyspnea appears late in the course of illness (Lechtzin, Rothstein, Clawson, et al., 2002). Respiratory symptoms poorly correspond to the degree of diaphragmatic and accessory respiratory muscle impairment (Lechtzin et al., 2002). However, the presence of dyspnea, orthopnea, sleep disturbances, daytime sleepiness, or morning headaches should alert clinicians that severe respiratory muscle weakness is present and there is probably a significant degree of hypoventilation (Lechtzin et al., 2002). Other signs that may indirectly indicate respiratory muscle weakness include lethargy, fatigue, and poor concentration and appetite (Bourke, Bullock, Williams, et al., 2003).

Serial pulmonary function tests are useful when evaluating a decline in respiratory function. These evaluations include a forced expiratory volume (FEV) in one second, a forced vital capacity (FVC), and maximum voluntary ventilation (MVV). Spirometry (FEV_1/FVC) should be repeated in 3-month intervals (Lechtzin et al., 2002; Melo et al., 1999). The average decrease in FEV_1/FVC is 3.5% per month. Secondary tests include: a maximum inspiratory pressure (MIP), which measures diaphragmatic function; and a maximum expiratory pressure (MEP), which measures abdominal and intercostal muscle strength (Melo et al., 1999; Ross, 1997). The degree of dyspnea actually correlates better with MEP and MIP than with FEV_1/FVC (Melo et al., 1999). The MEP also predicts the ability to generate an effective cough. A decrease in the MEP (less than 270 cubic millimeters of water per minute) usually indicates that the patient is unlikely to generate an effective cough and remove secretions (Oppenheimer, 2003; Ross, 1997).

Serum chloride can drop below normal as respiratory function fails and is an indicator of respiratory acidosis (and elevated CO_2) (Melo et al., 1999). Patients with bulbar weakness may have a falsely low FVC as a result of the inability to couple their lips to the cannula of a spirometer or hold the mouthpiece properly (Lechtzin et al., 2002). A normal vital capacity in the face of symptoms does not exclude significant muscle weakness, and further evaluation of the MIP and MEP should follow. Daytime hypercapnia is rare, at least initially, in asymptomatic patients; therefore, blood gases are not helpful and may falsely reassure clinicians. Pulse oximetry alone, like arterial blood gases, should not be relied on as the only test for hypoventilation. Nocturnal desaturation initially occurs during rapid eye movement (REM) sleep (Oppenheimer, 2003). Nocturnal blood gas monitoring may be necessary to determine if hypoventilation is present (Lechtzin et al., 2002). Nocturnal oximetry is useful as a measure of respiratory muscle dysfunction for those patients with bulbar ALS who are unable to perform spirometry (Lechtzin et al., 2002). Oxygen desaturation below 88% for 5 minutes can be a positive indication for NIPPV.

The treatment of dyspnea and respiratory failure in ALS differs from that for cancer. Oxygen should be used sparingly since this may worsen hypoventilation. The problem with ALS patients is not gas exchange but muscle weakness. High-flow oxygen further blunts the respiratory drive and can lead to increasing hypercapnia.

The use of NIPPV should be instituted relatively early in the course of hypoventilation to achieve its full benefit. The early use of NIPPV improves survival (Lechtzin et al., 2002; Oppenheimer, 2003). Continuous positive airway pressure (CPAP), a type of NIPPV, supports the airways but does not offer inspiratory respiratory support and should be avoided (Lechtzin et al., 2002). The most commonly used NIPPV is bilevel positive airway pressure (BIPAP), which initially is used intermittently or during sleep. Usual settings are 6 to 10 cm of water for expiratory pressures and 3 to 5 cm of water for inspiratory pressures. Inspiratory pressures are then titrated by 2 to 3 cm of water pressure based on symptoms and tolerability (Butz, Wollinsky, Wiedemuth-Catrinescu, et al., 2003; Kleopa, Sherman, Neal, et al., 1999; Melo et al., 1999).

Education and experience with an NIPPV before overt respiratory failure can increase acceptance and reduce anxiety. A trial of NIPPV in an elective setting allows the patient to make an informed choice about the benefits of BIPAP (Oppenheimer, 2003).

Patients and families need increasing support and information to make informed choices about ventilation in ALS (Oliver, 2004). Patients on invasive ventilation eventually become "locked in" with no means of communication. Advance directives that clearly direct care, in particular about instituting or withdrawing invasive ventilation, should be completed by patients before becoming dependent on invasive ventilation or before being placed on a ventilator in an emergency room situation (Oliver, 2004).

Lorazepam may break the cycle of dyspnea-anxiety-dyspnea (Borasio et al., 2001; Oppenheimer, 2003). Theophylline has been used to improve inspiratory muscle function (as measured by MIP and peak inspiratory flow rates) but has been reported in only a small group of patients. Side effects to theophylline may limit its efficacy, and further trials are needed to judge its value in this patient population (Lechtzin et al., 2002).

Tracheostomy and invasive ventilation are used in only a small minority of ALS patients (4%-6%) (Gelinas, 2000). The prospects of long-term (life-long) requirements for mechanical support combined with an evolution to the "locked in" syndrome (complete immobility) deter most patients from this choice (Lechtzin et al., 2002). The burden of caregivers who manage relatives at home on invasive ventilation is enormous and can lead to poor caregiver health and quality of life. Most interesting, though, is that patients who receive invasive respiratory support rate their quality of life as acceptable (Gelinas, O'Connor, & Miller, 1998; Kaub-Wittemer, Steinbuchel, Wasner, et al., 2003; Lechtzin et al., 2002).

Progressive respiratory muscle weakness leads to an ineffective cough. Bulbar impairment predisposes to aspiration, which further weakens cough as well as worsens nutritional intake. Cough requires the ability to take a deep breath; intact bulbar function, which coordinates glottic opening; and a forceful peak expiratory muscle contraction (Oppenheimer, 2003). Respiratory secretions if problematic can be managed with chest percussion and/or postural drainage early in the course of illness, but the benefits diminish as the patient weakens. The removal of secretions will facilitate NIPPV (Lechtzin et al., 2002). Mechanical insufflation/exsufflation improves cough and expiratory flow rates by clearing secretions in those with a weak cough (Mustfa, Aiello, Lyall, et al., 2003; Sancho, Servera, Diaz, et al., 2004). These devices may also improve tolerance to BIPAP or can be used alone in patients with problems with mobilizing secretions who elect not to undergo NIPPV or do not tolerate BIPAP (Bach, 1993; Bach, 2002; Gomez-Merino, Sancho, Marin, et al., 2002; Hanayama, Ishikawa, Bach, 1997; Lahrmann, Wild, Zdrahal, et al., 2003; Lechtzin et al., 2002).

Patients who elect to discontinue noninvasive or invasive ventilation are made comfortable with the use of either intermittent or continuous parenteral morphine plus either a benzodiazepine or chlorpromazine for respiratory panic. For those on invasive ventilation there is little reason to wean the ventilator, the tracheostomy can be converted to a tracheotomy collar and the ventilator discontinued (Lechtzin et al., 2002).

Hospices who accept ALS patients should be skilled in managing NIPPV since this is both palliative and more effective than drug management for respiratory symptoms. Many patients will wish to try NIPPV, and they should not be denied care by hospices if they elect BIPAP therapy Oppenheimer, 2003).

The Dying ALS Patient

Common symptoms that occur during the last month of life include difficulties with communication, dyspnea, insomnia, and discomfort other than pain (Ganzini, Johnston, & Silveira, 2002). Frequent symptoms that occur in the last 24 hours of life are dyspnea, cough, anxiety, and restlessness (Neudert, Oliver, Wasner, et al., 2001). Most patients will have a PEG tube, which facilitates drug administration in terminal care. Many patients will be on noninvasive ventilation and elect to be withdrawn. Most will be on morphine and benzodiazepines to palliate dyspnea, cough, and anxiety (Neudert et al., 2001). One half of the patients will be on oxygen (Mandler et al., 2001). The majority (88%) of patients have advance directives and often die peacefully (90%) (Ganzini, Johnston, Silveira, 2002; Mandler et al., 2001; Neudert et al., 2001). In the United States, two thirds of the patients are enrolled in hospice. Hospice patients are associated with dying in their preferred location, dying outside the hospital, and using morphine for dyspnea (Ganzini, Johnston, & Silveira, 2002). Many hospices are involved only in the terminal phase of ALS or provide respite care.

For a minority of patients, symptoms will not be satisfactorily relieved. This can be caused by mucus plugging and airway congestion, restlessness, anxiety, or painful cramps (Neudert et al., 2001). These symptoms should be anticipated and emergency medications (morphine, lorazepam, chlorpromazine) available at home. In general, families regard the PEG, NIPPV, morphine, and benzodiazepines as helpful in the last days and believe that these measures improve the quality of dying. Before the dying process, both the patient and family should be informed that death is not a result of "choking to death." This may have to be reinforced during the terminal phase (Neudert et al., 2001).

Death can occur suddenly, usually at night, due to worsening nocturnal hypoventilation (Sykes, 2001).

As the patient enters the terminal phase, personal autonomy decreases, dependence increases, and suffering intensifies. Such suffering should not be medicalized as each patient needs to progress to a resolution and closure. Closure includes resolution of personal conflicts, spiritual practices in the form of traditional rituals, or personalized spiritual exercises for those individuals not associated with traditional religions can give meaning to existence. Confession and last rites are a conduit for reconciliation and an incarnate sign of readiness to move on into the next life.

HUNTINGTON'S DISEASE
Introduction

Huntington's disease is a progressive, non-curable, inherited neurologic illness that can affect patients for a number of years before death. The natural course of Huntington's disease (HD) is quite variable, with the duration from diagnosis to death at approximately 15 years for an adult and 8 to 10 years for the juvenile form. Currently, no cure is available and palliative care assumes priority throughout the disease trajectory. The importance of integrating palliative interventions lies in the ability of reducing symptoms and improving the patient's quality of life. Huntington's disease affects people of all races and ethnic groups around the world, with a prevalence rate of about 5 per 100,000 population (Emerich, 2001.)

In 1072 George Huntington published a paper on "Huntington's Chorea," providing a graphic account of this disease based on observations of patients that both his father and grandfather collected during the course of their medical practice. He noted that when Huntington's chorea progressed, it caused involuntary movements of the body. These involuntary movements that became more pronounced over a period of years became the hallmark of this disease and were termed *chorea*. The word *chorea* is derived from the Greek word meaning "dance" and refers to involuntary arrhythmic repetitions of forceful, rapid, jerky-type movements. In later years the medical diagnosis of Huntington's chorea was adapted to Huntington's *disease* with chorea identified as one of the manifestations of the disease. Two other components of Huntington's disease are cognitive deterioration and various psychiatric symptoms.

Epidemiology

Before the discovery of the Huntington's disease gene in 1993 (Huntington Disease Collaborative Research Group, 1993), the diagnosis of HD was made in the presence of characteristic neurologic signs and symptoms coupled with a familial history of HD. Therefore, patients with an atypical clinical presentation without an established family history of HD were likely misdiagnosed or underdiagnosed. The advent of the direct gene mutation test is useful to correctly identify patients with HD. A recent study by Almqvist, Elterman, MacLeod, et al. (2001) found striking evidence that a high occurrence (24.1%) of symptomatic patients were lacking a family history of HD and a cytosine-adenine-guanine (CAG) expansion greater than 36. Thus the discovery of the genetic mutation for HD allows, for the first time, the examination of relationships between the etiology of the disease and its clinical presentation (Brandt, Bylsma, Gross, et al., 1996).

Clinical Features

The clinical presentation of Huntington's disease has devastating involvement physically, cognitively, emotionally, and socially. HD symptoms vary widely from person to person, even within the same family (International Huntington Association [IHA] & World Federation of Neurology [WFN], 1994). Clinically, HD varies in presentation between adult onset and juvenile onset. Juvenile HD is defined as onset before the age of 21 years and occurs in 7% of HD cases. Characteristics include more severe neuropathologic involvement, including rigidity and seizures (Gilroy, 2000; Higgins, 2001). Approximately one third of these individuals experience recurrent seizures. Research has shown that the juvenile form of HD has a rapidly progressive nature. Children

diagnosed with HD most often inherit the disease from their fathers with HD and have a large number of CAG and thymine (Higgins, 2001). Adult-onset HD is differentiated from juvenile onset in that adults experience slower disease progression.

Early signs and symptoms in adult-onset include abnormality of movement that is initially insidious and involves the hands and face; the patient may be considered fidgety, restless, or "nervous." Slowness of movement in the fingers and hands, a reduced rate of finger tapping, and difficulty in performing a sequence of hand movements are evident (Adams, Victor, & Ropper, 1997). Other early signs and symptoms include loss of intellectual facilities, anxiety, irritability, and depression. Depression is perhaps the most prominent initial symptom, presenting itself long before the diagnosis of HD is made. Patients may also become less communicative and socially withdrawn throughout the course of the disease. Hypotonia, facial twitching, bradykinesia, impaired odor recognition, impulsiveness, hostility, agitation, and abnormal eye movements are common features of HD in the early stages (Adams et al., 1997). Studies of motor onset in the Lake Maracibo, Venezuela, community in which HD is endemic revealed that patients first develop subtle changes in volitional eye movement and clumsiness before they show frank motor changes caused by the disease (Penney, Young, Shoulson, et al., 1990).

Juvenile HD signs and symptoms are often subtle and are difficult to distinguish from normal patterns of "growing pains" children can experience in the early years of development. These include clumsiness, being less coordinated, and subtle personality changes. Another common sign of HD in a younger individual is a rapid decline in school performance with handwriting and delays in problem solving.

Late signs and symptoms for Juvenile HD include tremors, rigidity, stiffness of muscles, speech difficulties, difficulty in swallowing, and seizures. Generally, children with HD diagnosed at an earlier age are less likely to experience chorea. Chorea seems to present itself through the disease trajectory in individuals approximately 15 to 18 years old. Variable signs and symptoms include weight loss, accompanied with swallowing difficulties, aggressiveness, mania, hallucinations, and paranoia (Higgins, 2001).

Signs and symptoms of advanced adult-onset HD include dysphagia, dysarthria, bladder and bowel incontinence, gait disturbance, postural instability, hyperkinesias, dementia, rigidity, hypertonia, clonus primitive reflexes, loss of the ability to communicate, and chorea (Adams et al., 1997). In the late stage of HD, or approximately 10 to 15 years after diagnosis, most patients deteriorate to a vegetative state (Adams et al., 1997). Britton and colleagues (1995) reported exceptional cases in which the movement disorder existed for 10 to 30 years without the presence of mental changes in patients (Britton, Urti, & Ahlskog, 1995).

Diagnosis

It is imperative that clinicians perform a complete comprehensive examination, including a series of neurologic and psychologic examinations, and a detailed history of injuries, habits, and family illnesses when evaluating for HD. Huntington's disease can mimic other disorders such as Parkinson's disease or alcoholism; thus it is recommended that these patients are referred to a neurologist who specializes in these disease processes, for appropriate diagnosis and treatment.

Diagnostic testing should include a computed tomography (CT) or an MRI of the brain, with and without contrast, which evaluates for cerebral atrophy and atrophy of the basal ganglia. Positron emission tomography (PET) scanning will also help identify a loss of glucose uptake in the caudate nuclei that may be a valuable indication of affection in the pre-synaptomatic space (Hayden, 1986).

A major consequence of decline in individuals with HD is loss of autonomy, both physically and cognitively. Therefore the progression of HD is divided into fives stages defined by the patient's score on the Total Functional Capacity (TFC) scale, which details the level of function in the domains of workplace, finance, domestic chores, activities of daily living, and requirements for unskilled or skilled care (Bamford, Caine, Kido, et al., 1995). The TFC scale is used as an index of illness progression, which

has been significantly helpful in planning long-term care of HD patients.

Direct genetic testing may be beneficial because this test can confirm a diagnosis of HD in an individual who is exhibiting HD-like symptoms. This genetic test analyzes deoxyribonucleic acid (DNA) for the HD mutation by identifying the number of CAG repeats in the HD region. The DNA contains the "trinucleotide repeats." Nucleotides are the building blocks of DNA and are represented by the letters, C, A, G, and T (cytosine, adenine, guanine, and thymine). Individuals who do not have HD usually have 28 or fewer CAG repeats. Individuals diagnosed with HD usually have 40 or more repeats. A small percentage, however, have a number of repeats that fall within a borderline region (Maat-Kievit, Losekoot, Van Den Boer-Van Den Berg, et al., 2001).

Pathology

Huntington's disease was first mapped to the tip of the short arm of chromosome 4 by Gusella and colleagues (Gusella, Wexler, Conneally, et al., 1983). In 1993 the Huntington gene was isolated and associated with a cytosine-adenine-guanine (CAG) trinucleotide repeat expansion in a large gene on the short arm of chromosome 4. The gene encodes the protein "Huntingtin," which selectively accumulates in clumps within the brain cells. These cells appear sensitive to damage by the aggregated toxic levels of huntingtin (Sobel & Cowan, 2000). Multiple transmitters are also affected in patients with HD. These neurotransmitters include diminished GABA, substance P, en-kephalin, central dopamine, choline acetyltransferase, and increased glutamate activity. Somatostatin, neuropeptide Y, and nitric oxide appear resistant in Huntington's disease (Myers, Marans, & Macdonald, 1998).

HD is a familial disease, passed on from one generation to the next by the transmission from parent to child of a "mutated" (altered) gene. Males and females have an equal chance of inheriting the gene from the affected parent. Each child of an HD parent has a 50-50 chance of inheriting the HD gene. If a child does not inherit the HD gene, he or she will not develop the disease and cannot pass it to subsequent generations (IHDA & WFN, 1994).

The usual age of onset ranges between 30 and 50 years; however, HD can strike young children (juvenile form) and the elderly (IHDA & WFN, 1994).

Gross bilateral atrophy of the head of the caudate nucleus and putamen is the characteristic abnormality. This is usually accompanied by a moderate degree of gyral atrophy in the frontal and temporal regions in the brain. The caudatal atrophy alters the configuration of the frontal horns of the lateral ventricles; the inferolateral borders do not show the usual bulge formed by the head of the caudate nucleus; in addition, the ventricles are diffusely enlarged. In CT scans, the bicaudate-cranial ratio is increased in the majority of patients. This finding corroborates the clinical diagnosis in the moderately advanced case (Adams et al., 1997). Other pathologic findings include micro loss of small neurons of striatum with fibrillary gliosis in the ventrolateral thalamic nucleus. In addition, other pathologic findings include electron microscopy of membranous whorl and increased numbers of dense synaptic vesicles in pre-synaptic nerve terminals (Higgins, 2001). Also affected is the brain's outer surface, or cortex, which controls thought, perception, and memory (Higgins, 2001).

Symptom Management

There is no cure for Huntington's disease and currently no treatments available that will reverse or halt the progression of this illness. Treatment is aimed at reducing symptoms, preventing complications, and maximizing the individual's ability to function as long as possible throughout the disease trajectory.

Treatment recommendations used specifically for juvenile HD include anticonvulsant medications to help prevent and control seizures. Patients respond more favorably with the use of valproic acid and benzodiazepines, such as clonazepam, than with other medications for non-HD seizures. Adams and colleagues (1997) have recommended anti-parkinsonian medications as beneficial for treatment of the juvenile form (e.g., dopamine agonists).

Treatment recommendations for adult-onset HD include SSRIs or the tricyclic antidepressants for the management of anxiety and depression. Depression and suicide are common in individuals diagnosed with HD. Thus it is important for family members, caregivers, and health care providers to frequently monitor for these symptoms. Lithium may be prescribed to combat pathologic excitement and severe mood swings.

Drugs that block dopamine receptors, such as reserpine, clonazepam, and tetrabenazine, can be used to suppress and control chorea movements. Clonazepam can be initiated at 0.5 mg at bedtime, increasing the dose over several months to a maximum of 9 mg a day in divided doses. Reserpine is started at 0.1 mg/day and is increased at 7- to 10-day intervals to a maximum of 3 mg/day. Tetrabenazine is started at 12.5 mg/day and can be increased by 12.5 mg every 7 days to 25 mg QID dosing maximum (Adams et al., 1997).

The dopamine antagonist haloperidol, in daily doses of 2 to 10 mg, can be used to control dyskinesias. Haloperidol may also help alleviate abnormalities of behavior or emotional lability; however, it does not alter disease progression (Adams et al., 1997). Lioresal can be used in the management of rigidity. Lioresal is initiated at 10 mg/day and then is increased slowly to 120 mg maximum in divided doses. Lioresal may be administered with clonazepam if symptom management dictates.

Huntington's disease is a progressive condition that causes substantial disability; therefore, it is extremely important that individuals with both juvenile and adult forms maintain physical fitness as their condition permits. A daily regimen of exercise can help promote optimal physical and emotional balance. Both physical and aqua therapy are recommended because these activities help ease the symptoms of rigidity and prevent muscle atrophy. As HD advances, coordination and ambulation become significantly affected; thus patients become more vulnerable to accidents, falls, and injuries. Ultimately, patients completely depend on their caregivers for all aspects of daily living.

In addition, it is essential to maintain adequate fluid and nutrition individuals with HD require an unusually higher number of calories to maintain their body weight. Many times, individuals with HD may expend 5000 calories a day without gaining weight. Integrating a nutritionist can be an essential member of the palliative care team for both short- and long-term management of HD. In later stages of disease, feeding tubes are recommended for adequate nutritional supplementation as the ability to swallow becomes significantly impaired.

The Dying HD Patient

Death usually occurs within 10 to 20 years after diagnosis, although suicide is more prevalent in those with early-onset HD. Aspiration and inanition result from severe dysphagia, as well as from an apparent increased metabolic demand (Caselli & Boeve, 1999). HD, as with other neurologic disorders, poses many challenges related to appropriate long-term care. Implementing palliative care at disease onset can help facilitate patient and family conferences to define and address the goals of care and assist in the development of advance directives.

SUMMARY

ALS is a progressive illness that rarely waxes and wanes. Only a minority of patients will have familial ALS. This disease requires ongoing monitoring—in particular, respiratory function with a forced vital capacity. Advance directives should be addressed early and before dyspnea. Disease-modifying therapy has a limited effect on the overall course of disease. Noninvasive positive-pressure ventilation extends survival, may relieve symptoms, and is preferred over oxygen and sedatives alone. Most patients will die peacefully if managed properly.

Individuals at risk for HD have an intensely difficult decision to make when it comes to determining if genetic testing is appropriate for them. Ethical and psychologic questions are challenged in the minds of those at risk. Individually, risks and benefits of genetic testing must be examined.

Many individuals prefer the choice of living with this uncertainty rather than taking a genetic test, because the unknowing provides them with an opportunity for hope. For others, genetic testing answers the uncertainty for their future and thus is deemed necessary. In the final decision, if genetic testing is chosen, pre-test counseling is recommended on an individual basis. Pre-test counseling encompasses relevant up-to-date information of clinical and psychologic implications, reproductive options, and risks and benefits of testing. Palliative interventions can support the progressive and disabling factors associated with these neurologic diseases.

Objective Questions

1. T.W. is a 52-year-old male who presents with weakness and mild fasciculation involving his right lower extremity. Initial studies include a normal lumbar spine radiograph and normal MRI of his spine and brain. Blood studies including a normal thyroid function test. Two months later he is seen as an outpatient on a routine visit. He complains of slurred speech and on further examination is noted to have tongue fasciculation. Based on the El Escorial criteria, this patient has:

   a. Suspected ALS.
   b. Probable ALS.
   c. Clinically probable ALS.
   d. Clinically definitive ALS.

2. ALS:

   a. Waxes and wanes in severity similar to multiple sclerosis.
   b. Is almost always familial.
   c. Has a rather uniform prevalence across culture and geography.
   d. Is associated with incontinence.

3. The El Escorial criteria for ALS:

   a. Are exclusive and developed for clinical use.
   b. Are inclusive for research purposes.
   c. Are valid in only some countries.
   d. Do not include familial ALS.

4. In following a patient with ALS:

   a. Oximetry should be obtained with each visit and spirometry (FEV_1/FVC) only with symptoms of dyspnea or hypoventilation.
   b. An FEV_1/FVC should be obtained initially and then at the onset of symptoms.
   c. An FEV_1/FVC should be obtained every 3 months.

Case Study

Mr. Burke is a 48-year-old male who was diagnosed with Huntington's disease (HD) 7 years ago. Both his grandfather and father suffered the long-term effects of HD. Over the past 9 months, Mr. Burke had been experiencing increased intermittent episodes of forceful involuntary movements (chorea). These disturbing movements have affected his balance, causing gait abnormalities and risk for falls. In fact, he has fallen several times in the past month and was placed on clonazepam 1 mg every 8 hours, which has controlled his chorea relatively well.

Until recently, Mr. Burke had been using the treadmill daily to maintain his muscle strength and tone and help support his balance. However, lack of coordination and postural instability has significantly worsened, preventing him from safely using the treadmill.

Mr. Burke's progressive decline has caused a loss in cognitive functioning, including memory, reasoning, problem solving, and the successful completion of intellectual tasks. In addition, his ability to communicate has deteriorated and his speech has become slurred. His inability to communicate with others has created social withdrawal. The onset of all these symptoms has brought on depression. Mr. Burke's wife and son provide most of his care and recently requested a neurology consultation. His neurologist initiated low-dose fluoxetine to address his emotional lability. During the visit with the neurologist, his family was provided education on the progressive debilitating nature of his disease. It was suggested that Mr. Burke would require frequent reevaluations for his symptoms and their

management because his medications may require adjusting accordingly.

Mr. Burke's family noticed a significant improvement in his mood with an improvement in his nutritional intake. He is eating six small meals a day to include a total of approximately 5000 calories. Though he had lost 15 pounds over the past few months, he is able to maintain his weight at 140 pounds. Mr. Burke is also being evaluated by a speech therapist both to assess his speaking abilities and to assist in promoting his swallowing ability to prevent choking while eating and drinking fluids. An assigned social worker and nutritionist provide ongoing evaluations and supportive interventions at home. Gradually, Mr. Burke experienced a progressive decline in his physical, emotional, and cognitive abilities—creating a need for closer supervision and assistance in all aspects of his daily living.

HD expands a disease trajectory of many years, and the family experiences caregiver burden in maintaining basic needs. Caregiver stress is often superimposed by other responsibilities such as their careers, and their own family obligations. Though Mr. Burke's family continues to care for him daily, the social worker recently encouraged them to incorporate the assistance of an in-home health aide three evenings a week to help reduce the burden of physical care that his family is encountering. Mr. Burke wishes to remain in his home for as long as he is able, and his family is willing to take all the steps possible to ensure that Mr. Burke receives the best care possible through the utilization of his palliative care team. This will enable him to remain in his comfortable and familiar surroundings.

d. A forced expiratory volume in 1 second (FEV_1) should be obtained since obstructive airway disease is common with ALS.

5. Physical therapy and walking aids:

    a. Should be used only when absolutely necessary since walking devices foster dependence.

    b. Are a minor part in the rehabilitation of ALS.

c. Should be instituted early with the disability of ALS, and an attitude of "dependently independence" should be encouraged.

d. Passive range of motion and massage have little role in the management of ALS.

6. Spasticity and muscle fasciculation:

    a. Should be treated aggressively with benzodiazepines based on clinical findings rather than on symptom severity.

b. Should be treated with spinal baclofen early in the course of disease.

c. Should be treated with dantrolene as initial treatment.

d. Should be managed based on symptom severity with baclofen, quinine, carbamazepine, phenytoin, magnesium, or verapamil.

7. Enteral nutrition:

a. Should be instituted once there is a 10% loss of body weight.

b. Should be instituted with a PEG tube, which should be placed once the FVC is less than 50% of predicted.

c. Is an important part of the management of ALS and may improve strength in a nutritionally depleted individual, particularly true for bulbar forms of ALS.

d. Once started should never be discontinued for ethical reasons since nutrition is not a medical therapy.

8. Secretions should be managed by all of the following except:

a. Glycopyrrolate.

b. Tonsillar suction.

c. Mechanical insufflation/exsufflation.

d. Chest physiotherapy.

e. Diuretic therapy.

9. Noninvasive positive-pressure ventilation (NIPPV):

a. Should be instituted only after oxygen therapy.

b. Should include continuous positive airway pressure (CPAP).

c. Excludes the use of mechanical insufflation/exsufflation.

d. Most commonly involves bilevel positive airway pressure (BIPAP), which changes pressures during inspiration and expiration.

10. The use of morphine in ALS:

a. Is contraindicated because of the risk of respiratory suppression.

b. Should be used only with intractable symptoms.

c. Can reduce dyspnea and cough.

d. Should be used for anxiety in the terminal phase of illness.

e. Can be used only with NIPPV.

REFERENCES

Abrahams, S., Goldstein, L.H., Al-Chalabi, A., et al. (1997). Relation between cognitive dysfunction and pseudobulbar palsy in amyotrophic lateral sclerosis. *J Neurol Neurosurg Psychiatry, 62*(5), 464-472.

Abrahams, S., Goldstein, L.H., Kew, J.J., et al. (1996). Frontal lobe dysfunction in amyotrophic lateral sclerosis: A PET study. *Brain, 119*(Pt. 6), 2105-2120.

Adams, R.D., Victor, M.V., & Ropper, A.H. (1997). *Principles of neurology* (6th ed., pp. 1060-1064). New York: McGraw-Hill.

Al-Chalabi, A., Scheffler, M.D., Smith, B.N., et al. (2003). Ciliary neurotrophic factor genotype does not influence clinical phenotype in amyotrophic lateral sclerosis. *Ann Neurol, 54*(1), 130-134.

Almqvist, E.W., Elterman, D.S., MacLeod, P.M., et al. (2001). High incidence rate and absent family histories in one quarter of patients newly diagnosed with Huntington's disease in British Columbia. *Clin Genet, 60*(3), 198-205.

Anderson, P.M., Restagno, G., Stewart, H.G., et al. (2004). Disease penetrance in amyotrophic lateral sclerosis associated with mutations in the SOD1 gene. *Ann Neurol, 55*(2), 298-299.

Anderson, P.M., Sims, K.B., Xin, W.W., et al. (2003). Sixteen novel mutations in the Cu/Zn superoxide dismutase gene in amyotrophic lateral sclerosis: A decade of discoveries, defects and disputes. *Amyotroph Lateral Scler Other Motor Neuron Disord, 4*(2), 62-73.

Arisato, T., Okubo, R., Arata, H., et al. (2003). Clinical pathological studies of familial amyotrophic lateral sclerosis (FALS) with SOD1 H46R mutation in large Japanese families. *Acta Neuropathol (Berl), 100*(6), 561-568.

Armon, C. (2003). An evidence-based medicine approach to the evaluation of the role of exogenous risk factors in sporadic amyotrophic lateral sclerosis. *Neuroepidemiology, 22*(4), 217-228.

Bach, J.R. (1993). Mechanical insufflation-exsufflation. Comparison of peak expiratory flows with manually assisted and unassisted coughing techniques. *Chest, 104*(5), 1553-1562.

Bach, J.R. (2002). Amyotrophic lateral sclerosis: Prolongation of life by noninvasive respiratory AIDS. *Chest, 122*(1), 92-98.

Bamford, K.A., Caine, E.D., Kido, D.K., et al. (1995). A prospective evaluation of cognitive decline in early Huntington's disease: Functional and radiographic correlates. *Neurology, 45*, 1867-1873.

Beghi, E., Balzarini, C., Boglium, G., et al. (2002). Reliability of the El Escorial diagnostic criteria for amyotrophic lateral sclerosis. *Neuroepidemiology, 21*(6), 265-270.

Boitano, L.J., Jordan, T., & Benditt, J.O. (2001). Noninvasive ventilation allows gastrostomy tube placement in patients with advanced ALS. *Neurology, 56*(3), 413-414.

Borasio, G.D. (2001). Palliative care in ALS: Searching for the evidence base. *Amyotroph Lateral Scler Other Motor Neuron Disord, 2*(Suppl. 1), S31-35.

Borasio, G.D., & Miller, R.G. (2001). Clinical characteristics and management of ALS. *Semin Neurol, 21*(2), 155-166.

Borasio, G.D., & Oliver, D. (2000). The control of other symptoms. In D. Oliver, G.D. Borasio, & D. Walsh (Eds.), *Palliative care in amyotrophic lateral sclerosis* (Chapter 4, pp. 72-81). New York: Oxford University Press.

Borasio, G.D., Sloan, R., & Pongratz, D.E. (1998). Breaking the news in amyotrophic lateral sclerosis. *J Neurol Sci, 160* (Suppl.1), S127-133.

Borasio, G.D., & Voltz, R. (2000). Advance directives. In D. Oliver, G.D. Borasio, & D. Walsh (Eds.), *Palliative care in amyotrophic lateral sclerosis* (Appendix, p. 36). New York: Oxford University Press.

Borasio, G.D., Voltz, R., & Miller, R.G. (2001). Palliative care in amyotrophic lateral sclerosis. *Neurol Clin, 19*(4), 829-847.

Bourke, S.C., Bullock, R.E., Williams, T.L., et al. (2003). Noninvasive ventilation in ALS: Indications and effect on quality of life. *Neurology, 61*(2), 171-177.

Brandt, J., Bylsma, F.W., Gross, R., et al. (1996). Trinucleotide repeat length and clinical progression in Huntington's Disease. *Neurology, 46,* 527-531.

Britton, J.W., Urti, R.J., & Ahlskog, J.E. (1995). Hereditary late-onset chorea without significant dementia. *Neurology, 45,* 443.

Butz, M., Wollinsky, K.H., Wiedemuth-Catrinescu, U., et al. (2003). Longitudinal effects of noninvasive positive-pressure ventilation in patients with amyotrophic lateral sclerosis. *Am J Phys Med Rehabil, 82*(8), 597-604.

Carter, G.T., Krivickas, L.S., Weydt, P., et al. (2003). Drug therapy for amyotrophic lateral sclerosis: Where are we now? *Idrugs 6*(2), 147-153.

Caselli, R.J., & Boeve, B.F. (1999). The degenerative dementias. In C.G. Goetz & E.J. Pappert, *Textbook of clinical neurology* (pp.629-653). Philadelphia: Saunders.

Chio, A., Finocchiaro, E., Meineri, P., et al. (1999). Safety and factors related to survival after percutaneous endoscopic gastrostomy in ALS. ALS Percutaneous Endoscopic Gastrostomy Study Group. *Neurology, 53*(5), 1123-1125.

Chung, Y.H., Joo, K.M., Lee, Y.J., et al. (2003). Immuno-histochemical study on the aggregation of ubiquitin in the central nervous system of the transgenic mice expressing a human Cu/Zn SOD mutation. *Neurol Res, 25*(4), 395-400.

Crow, J.P., Ye, Y.Z., Strong, M., et al. (1997). Superoxide dismutase catalyzes nitration of tyrosines by peroxynitrite in the rod and head domains of neurofilament-L. *J Neurochem, 69*(5), 1945-1953.

Debove, C., Zeisser, P., Salzman, P.M., et al. (2001). The Rilutek (riluzole) Global Early Access Programme: An open-label safety evaluation in the treatment of amyotrophic lateral sclerosis. *Amyotroph Lateral Scler Other Motor Neuron Disord, 2*(3), 153-158.

Demaerschalk, B.M., & Strong, M.J. (2000). Amyotrophic lateral sclerosis. *Curr Treat Options Neurol, 2*(1), 13-22.

Desport, J.C., Preux, P.M., Truong, T.C., et al. (1999). Nutritional status is a prognostic factor for survival in ALS patients. *Neurology, 53*(5), 1059-1063.

Dib, M. (2003). Amyotrophic lateral sclerosis: Progress and prospects for treatment. *Drugs, 63*(3), 289-310.

Emerich, D. (2001). Neuroprotective possibilities for Huntington's disease. *Expert Opin Biolog Theory,* 1:467.

Festoff, B.W., Suo, Z., & Citron, B.A. (2003). Prospects for the pharmacotherapy of amyotrophic lateral sclerosis: Old strategies and new paradigms for the third millennium. *CNS Drugs, 17*(10), 699-717.

Ganzini, L., Johnston, W.S., & Hoffman, W.F. (1999). Correlates of suffering in amyotrophic lateral sclerosis. *Neurology, 52*(7), 1434-1440.

Ganzini, L., Johnston, W.S., McFarland, B.H., et al. (1998). Attitudes of patients with amyotrophic lateral sclerosis and their care givers toward assisted suicide. *N Engl J Med, 339*(14), 967-973.

Ganzini, L., Johnston, W.S., & Silveira, M.J. (2002). The final month of life in patients with ALS. *Neurology, 59*(3), 428-431.

Ganzini, L., Silveira, M.J., & Johnston, W.S. (2002). Predictors and correlates of interest in assisted suicide in the final month of life among ALS patients in Oregon and Washington. *J Pain Symptom Manage, 24*(3), 312-317.

Gelinas, D. (2000). Amyotrophic lateral sclerosis and invasive ventilation. In D. Oliver, G.D. Borasio, & D. Walsh (Eds.), *Palliative care in amyotrophic lateral sclerosis* (Appendix, pp. 56-62). New York: Oxford University Press.

Gelinas, D.F., O'Connor, P., & Miller, R.G. (1998). Quality of life for ventilator-dependent ALS patients and their caregivers. *J Neurol Sci, 160*(Suppl. 1), S134-136.

Giess, R., Naumann, M., Werner, E., et al. (2000). Injections of botulinum toxin A into the salivary glands improve sialorrhea in amyotrophic lateral sclerosis. *J Neurol Neurosurg Psychiatry, 69,* 121-123.

Gilroy, J.B. (2000). *Basic neurology* (3rd ed.). New York: McGraw-Hill.

Gomez-Merino, E., Sancho, J., Marin, J., et al. (2002). Mechanical insufflation-exsufflation: Pressure, volume, and flow relationships and the adequacy of the manufacturer's guidelines. *Am J Phys Med Rehabil, 81*(8), 579-583.

Gregory, S., Siderowf, A., Golaszewski, A.L., et al. (2002). Gastrostomy insertion in ALS patients with low vital capacity: Respiratory support and survival. *Neurology, 58*(3), 485-487.

Guo, H., Lai, L., Butchbach, M.E., et al. (2003). Increased expression of the glial glutamate transporter EAAT2 modulates excitotoxicity and delays the onset but not the outcome of ALS in mice. *Hum Mol Genet, 12*(19), 2519-2532.

Gusella, J.F., Wexler, N.S., Conneally, P.M., et al. (1983). A polymorphic DNA marker genetically linked to Huntington's disease. *Nature, 306,* 234-238.

Haddock, R.L., & Chen, K.M. (2003). Amyotrophic lateral sclerosis and diabetes on Guam: Changing patterns of chronic disease in an island community. *Southeast Asian J Trop Med Public Health, 34*(3), 659-661.

Hanayama, K., Ishikawa, Y., & Bach, J.R. (1997). Amyotrophic lateral sclerosis: Successful treatment of mucous plugging by mechanical insufflation-exsufflation. *Am J Phys Med Rehabil, 76*(4), 338-339.

Hayden, M.R. (1986). *Huntington's chorea.* Berlin: Springer-Verlag.

Higgins, D.S. (2001). Chorea and its disorders. *Neurol Clin, 19*(3), 707-722.

Horner, R.D., Kamins, K.G., Feussner, J.R., et al. (2003). Occurrence of amyotrophic lateral sclerosis among Gulf War veterans. *Neurology, 61*(6), 742-749.

Huntington's Disease Collaborative Research Group. (1993). A novel gene containing a trinucleotide repeat that is expanded and unstable on Huntington's disease chromosomes. *Cell, 72,* 971-983.

International Huntington Association (IHDA), & World Federation of Neurology (WFN) Research Group on Huntington's Chorea. (1994). Guidelines for the molecular genetics predictive test in Huntington's disease. *J Med Genet, 31*(7), 555-559.

Iwasaki, Y., Ikeda, K., & Kinoshita, M. (2002). Molecular and cellular mechanism of glutamate receptors in relation to amyotrophic lateral sclerosis. *Curr Drug Targets CNS Neurol Disord, 1*(5), 511-518.

Jackson, M., Llado, J., & Rothstein, J.D. (2002). Therapeutic developments in the treatment of amyotrophic lateral sclerosis. *Exp Opin Investig Drugs, 11*(10), 1343-1364.

Kato, S., Saeki, Y., Aoki, M., et al. (2004). Histological evidence of redox system breakdown caused by superoxide dismutase 1 (SOD1) aggregation is common to SOD1-mutated motor neurons in humans and animal models. *Acta Neuropathol (Berl), 107*(2), 149-158.

Kaub-Wittemer, D., Steinbuchel, N., Wasner, M., et al. (2003). Quality of life and psychosocial issues in ventilated patients with amyotrophic lateral sclerosis and their caregivers. *J Pain Symptom Manage, 26*(4), 890-896.

Kawahara, Y., Ito, K., Sun, H., et al. (2004). Glutamate receptors: RNA editing and death of motor neurons. *Nature, 427* (6977), 801.

Kleopa, K.A., Sherman, M., Neal, B., et al. (1999). Bipap improves survival and rate of pulmonary function decline in patients with ALS. *J Neurol Sci, 164*(1), 82-88.

Lacomblez, L., Bensimon, G., Leigh, P.N., et al. (1996). A confirmatory dose-ranging study of riluzole in ALS/Riluzole Study Group-II. *Neurology, 47*(6 Suppl. 4), S242-250.

Lahrmann, H., Wild, M., Zdrahal, F., et al. (2003). Expiratory muscle weakness and assisted cough in ALS. *Amyotroph Lateral Scler Other Motor Neuron Disord, 4*, 49-51.

Lechtzin, N., Rothstein, J., Clawson, L., et al. (2002). Amyotrophic lateral sclerosis: Evaluation and treatment of respiratory impairment. *Amyotroph Lateral Scler Other Motor Neuron Disord, 3*(1), 5-13.

Ludolph, A.C. (2000). Treatment of amyotrophic lateral sclerosis: What is the next step? *J Neurol, 247*, 13-18.

Ludolph, A.C., Meyer, T., & Riepe, M.W. (1999). Antiglutamate therapy of ALS: What is the next step? *J Neural Transm Suppl, 55*, 79-95.

Lyall, R., Moxham, J., & Leigh, N. (2000). Dyspnoea. In D. Oliver, G.D. Borasio, & D. Walsh (Eds.), *Palliative care in amyotrophic lateral sclerosis* (pp. 55-56). New York: Oxford University Press.

Maat-Kievit, A., Losekoot, M., Van Den Boer-Van Den Berg, H., et al. (2001). New problems in testing for Huntington's disease. The issue of intermediate and reduced penetrance alleles. *J Med Genet, 38*(4), E12.

Mandler, R.N., Anderson, F.A. Jr., Miller, R.G., et al. (2001). The ALS patient care database: Insights into end-of-life care in ALS. *Amyotroph Lateral Scler Other Motor Neuron Disord, 2*(4), 203-208.

Mazzini, L., Mora, G., Balzarini, C., et al. (1998). The natural history and the effects of gabapentin in amyotrophic lateral sclerosis. *J Neurol Sci, 160*(Suppl. 1), S57-63.

McCullagh, S., Moore, M., Gawel, M., et al. (1999). Pathological laughing and crying in amyotrophic lateral sclerosis: An association with prefrontal cognitive dysfunction. *J Neurol Sci, 169*(1-2), 43-48.

Melo, J., Homma, A., Iturriaga, E., et al. (1999). Pulmonary evaluation and prevalence of non-invasive ventilation in patients with amyotrophic lateral sclerosis: A multicenter survey and proposal of a pulmonary protocol. *J Neurol Sci, 169*(1-2), 114-117.

Miller, R.G., Mitchell, J.D., & Moore, D.H. (2000). Riluzole for amyotrophic lateral sclerosis (ALS)/motor neuron disease (MND). *Cochrane Database Syst Rev, 2*, CD001447.

Miller, R.G., Rosenberg, J.A., Gelinas, D.F., et al. (1999). Practice parameter: The care of the patient with amyotrophic lateral sclerosis (an evidence-based review): Report of the Quality Standards Subcommittee of the American Academy of Neurology: ALS practice parameters task force. *Neurology, 52*(7), 1311-1323.

Mitsumoto, H. (1997). Riluzole: What is its impact in our treatment and understanding of amyotrophic lateral sclerosis? *Ann Pharmacother, 31*(6), 779-781.

Mitsumoto, H., Davidson, M., Moore, D., et al. (2003). Percutaneous endoscopic gastrostomy (PEG) in patients with ALS and bulbar dysfunction. *Amyotroph Lateral Scler Other Motor Neuron Disord, 4*(3), 177-185.

Mustfa, N., Aiello, M., Lyall, R.A., et al. (2003). Cough augmentation in amyotrophic lateral sclerosis. *Neurology, 61*(9), 1285-1287.

Myers, R.H., Marans, K.S., & MacDonald, M.E. (1998). Huntington's disease. In W.D. Wells & S.T. Warren (Eds.), *Genetic instabilities and hereditary neurological diseases* (pp. 301-323). California: Academic Press.

Neudert, C., Oliver, D., Wasner, M., et al. (2001). The course of the terminal phase in patients with amyotrophic lateral sclerosis. *Neurology, 248*(7), 612-616.

Niebroj-Dobosz, I., Janik, P., & Kwiecinski, H. (2004). Serum IgM anti-GM1 ganglioside antibodies in lower motor neuron syndromes. *Eur J Neurol, 11*(1), 13-16.

O'Brien, T. (2001). Neurodegenerative disease. In J. Addington-Hall & I. Higginson (Eds.), *Palliative care for non-cancer patients* (Chapter 4, pp. 44-45). Oxford: Oxford University Press.

Oliver, D. (1996). The quality of care and symptom control: The effects on the terminal phase of ALS/MND. *J Neurol Sci, 139*(Suppl.), 134-136.

Oliver, D. (1998). Opioid medication in the palliative care of motor neurone disease. *Palliat Med, 12*, 113-115.

Oliver, D. (2004). Ventilation in motor neuron disease: Difficult decisions in difficult circumstances. *Amyotroph Lateral Scler Other Motor Neuron Disord, 5*, 6-8.

Oliver, D., & Webb, S. (2000). The involvement of specialist palliative care in the care of people with motor neurone disease. *Palliat Med, 14*, 427-428.

Oppenheimer, E.A. (2003). Treating respiratory failure in ALS: The details are becoming clearer. *J Neurol Sci, 209*, 1-4.

Penney, J.B. Jr., Young, A.B., Shoulson, I., et al. (1990). Huntington's disease in Venezuela; 7 years of follow-up on symptomatic and asymptomatic individuals. *Mov Disord, 5*(2), 93-99.

Piazza, O., Siren, A.L., & Ehrenreich, H. (2004). Soccer, neurotrauma and amyotrophic lateral sclerosis: Is there a connection? *Curr Med Res Opin, 20*(4), 505-508.

Pieri, M., Gaetti, C., Spalloni, A., et al. (2003). Alpha-amino-3-hydroxy-5-methyl-isoxazole-4-propionate receptors in spinal cord motor neurons are altered in transgenic mice overexpressing human Cu, ZN superoxide dismutase (Gly93→Ala) mutation. *Neuroscience, 122*(1), 47-58.

Plahuta, J.M., McCulloch, B.J., Kasarskis, E.J., et al. (2002). Amyotrophic lateral sclerosis and hopelessness: Psychosocial factors. *Soc Sci Med, 55*(12), 2131-2140.

Przedborski, S. (2004). Programmed cell death in amyotrophic lateral sclerosis: A mechanism of pathogenic and therapeutic importance. *Neurologist, 10*(1), 1-7.

Przedborski, S., Mitsumoto, H., & Rowland, L.P. (2003). Recent advances in amyotrophic lateral sclerosis research. *Curr Neurol Neurosci Rep, 3*(1), 70-77.

Reagan, P., Hurst, R., Cook, L., et al. (2003). Physician-assisted death: Dying with dignity? *Lancet, 2*(10), 637-643.

Ross, M.A. (1997). Acquired motor neuron disorders. *Neurol Clin, 15*(3), 481-500.

Sancho, J., Servera, E., Diaz, J., et al. (2004). Efficacy of mechanical insufflation-exsufflation in medically stable patients with amyotrophic lateral sclerosis. *Chest, 125*(4), 1400-1405.

Sato, T., Yamamoto, Y., Nakanishi, T., et al. (2004). Identification of two novel mutations in the Cu/Zn superoxide dismutase gene with familial amyotrophic lateral sclerosis: Mass spectrometric and genomic analyses. *J Neurol Sci, 218*(1-2), 79-83.

Simpson, E.P., Yen, A.A., & Appel, S.H. (2003). Oxidative stress: A common denominator in the pathogenesis of amyotrophic lateral sclerosis. *Curr Opin Rheumatol, 15*(6), 730-736.

Sobel, S.K., & Cowan, D.B. (2000). Impact of genetic testing for Huntington disease on the family system. *Am J Med Genet, 90*(1), 49-59.

Spalloni, A., Albo, F., Ferrari, F., et al. (2004). Cu/Zn-superoxide dismutase (GLY93—ALA) mutation alters AMPA receptor subunit expression and function and potentiates kainate-mediated toxicity in motor neurons in culture. *Neurobiol Dis, 15*(2), 340-350.

Strong, M.J. (1999). Neurofilament metabolism in sporadic amyotrophic lateral sclerosis. *J Neurol Sci, 169*(1-2), 170-177.

Strong, M.J. (2001). Progress in clinical neurosciences: The evidence for ALS as a multisystems disorder of limited phenotypic expression. *Can J Neurol Sci, 28*(4), 283-298.

Strong, M.J. (2003). The basic aspects of therapeutics in amyotrophic lateral sclerosis. *Pharmacol Ther, 98*(3), 379-414.

Strong, M.J., Leystra-Lantz, C., & Ge, W.W. (2004). Intermediate filament steady-state mRNA levels in amyotrophic lateral sclerosis. *Biochem Biophys Res Commun, 316*(2), 317-322.

Strong, M.J., & Pattee, G.L. (2000). Creatine and coenzyme Q10 in the treatment of ALS. *Amyotroph Lateral Scler Other Motor Neuron Disord, 1*(Suppl. 4), 17-20.

Strong, M.J., & Rosenfeld, J. (2003). Amyotrophic lateral sclerosis: A review of current concepts. *Amyotroph Lateral Scler Other Motor Neuron Disord, 4*(3), 136-143.

Sykes, N. (2000). End of life care in ALS. In D. Oliver, G.D. Borasio, & D. Walsh (Eds.), *Palliative care in amyotrophic lateral sclerosis* (Chapter 8). New York: Oxford University Press.

Takeuchi, H., Niwa, J., Hishikawa, N., et al (2004). Dorfin prevents cell death by reducing mitochondrial localizing mutant superoxide dismutase 1 in a neuronal cell model of familial amyotrophic lateral sclerosis. *J Neurochem, 89*(1), 64-72.

Tortarolo, M., Crossthwaite, A.J., Conforti, L., et al. (2004). Expression of SOD1 G93A or wild-type SOD1 in primary cultures of astrocytes down-regulates the glutamate transporter GLT-1: Lack of involvement of oxidative stress. *J Neurochem, 88*(2), 481-493.

Traynor, B.J., Alexander, M., Corr, B., et al. (2003). An outcome study of riluzole in amyotrophic lateral sclerosis: A population-based study in Ireland, 1996-2000. *J Neurol, 250*(4), 473-479.

Twycross, R. (1997). Palliative care: The joy of death. *Lancet, 350*(Suppl. 3), SIII20.

Wagner-Sonntag, A.S., Oliver, D., Prosiegel, M., et al. (2000). Dysphagia. In D. Oliver, G.D. Borasio, & D. Walsh (Eds.), *Palliative care in amyotrophic lateral sclerosis* (Chapter 4, pp. 62-72). New York: Oxford University Press.

Wood, J.D., Beaujeux, T.P., & Shaw, P.J. (2003). Protein aggregation in motor neuron disorders. *Neuropathol Appl Neurobiol, 29*(6), 529-545.

Yoshida, M. (2004). Amyotrophic lateral sclerosis with dementia: The clinicopathological spectrum. *Neuropathology, 24*(1), 87-102.

Zylicz, Z. (2000). Ethical considerations in the treatment of pain in a hospice environment. *Patient Educ Couns, 41*(1), 47-53.

Zylicz, Z., & Finlay, I.G. (1999). Euthanasia and palliative care: Reflections from The Netherlands and the UK. *J R Soc Med, 92*(7), 370-373.

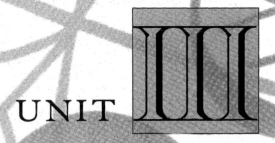

UNIT III

The Dying Process, Grief, and Bereavement

12 *Ethical Issues*

Tom Tomlinson

OBJECTIVES

After the completion of this chapter, the reader should be able to:

1. Examine the limits to the obligation to prolong life.
2. Identify the standards for limiting life-prolonging treatment.
3. Understand informed patient decision making.
4. Describe the roles of family members in the decision-making process.
5. Understand the use of advance directives.
6. Describe the role of "futility" judgments.
7. State the Doctrine of Double Effect.
8. List permissible methods for limiting or withdrawing treatment.
9. Examine the use of high-dose narcotics and terminal sedation.
10. Discuss ethical aspects of pain management.

INTRODUCTION

Palliative care is an option that can appropriately be considered in virtually any phase of illness. Patients may suffer the effects of illness at any time, not just at the end of life, in a variety of ways—not only from pain or other physical symptoms. Therefore it is misleading to identify palliative care solely with end-of-life care. In fact, such identification can be pernicious, discouraging patients and families from exploring palliative options when they do not yet feel ready to accept that cure is not a possibility.

In current practice, palliative care most often is provided for those patients who are terminally ill. This reality is accommodated in the present discussion by addressing palliative care primarily in the context of terminal illness. This allows for some

reasonable bounds to be placed on a topic that otherwise would be an impossible project for a single chapter. Nevertheless, at times, certain issues are addressed that can transcend the end-of-life context.

This chapter is divided into two sections. In the first, some key ethical questions that arise in the *transition to* a palliative care plan will be reviewed. Specific topics include:

- Questions about the nature of the health professionals' obligation to save life
- Informed patient/family decision making
- Standards used in deciding when and how to limit life-sustaining treatment and the role of the family in the application of those standards
- Use of advance directives
- The proper role of "futility judgments"

In the second section, central issues that may complicate palliative care decisions considered and made by the patient and/or family are discussed. These issues include a variety of questions surrounding:

- Limitations on life-prolonging treatments and the ethical relationship between euthanasia and/or assisted suicide
- Use of high dosages of narcotics or sedatives to relieve pain or agitation
- Controversies surrounding the practice of terminal sedation

ETHICAL ISSUES IN THE TRANSITION TO PALLIATIVE CARE

The Duty to Prolong Life

Most people would agree that once there is nothing more to be done to prolong a patient's life, "care" rather than "cure" should be offered. But when is there nothing more to be done? The conventional answer to this question looks to the patient's wishes and values, either as they are directly expressed by the patient, represented in an advance directive, or communicated by the family. The move from "cure" to "care" should occur when the patient says so. The provider's duty to prolong life is just a species of the duty to serve the patient's interests, as defined by the patient. Once the patient no longer has an interest in prolonging life, the provider no longer has a duty to do so.

Actual practice may be at odds with this ethical model. The landmark Study to Understand Prognoses and Preferences for Outcomes and Risks of Treatment (SUPPORT) study investigators systematically gathered information about critically ill patients' preferences for care at the end of life and provided that information to their attending physicians (The SUPPORT Principal Investigators, 1995). This information had no discernible effect on the intensity of life-prolonging treatment that these patients received. One explanation of this result is that physicians typically turn attention to the patient's values and wishes only after the physician has reached the conclusion that there is nothing more that can or should be done to further extend the patient's life. The sometimes ironic upshot is that a patient's desire to refuse further life-prolonging treatment is recognized only when no further life-prolonging treatment is possible.

Part of what is at work here is the idea that the health professional has an obligation to prolong the patient's life that (1) operates without knowledge of any particular patient's wishes; and (2) presumes that it is a good thing, within some limits, to prolong life whenever possible. Indeed, health care professionals should feel bound by some such obligation. When a person presents at the emergency room with a life-threatening condition, it is not an open question whether treatment should be given. It is expected. It is what physicians' and nurses' training and everyday experience inculcate in them. Striving to pull a patient out of harm's way is and should be an habitual way of thinking and acting for health care professionals. Problems arise, however, when the momentum of that habit leads the provider to continue traveling down every avenue of treatment,

even long after this pursuit no longer serves the patient's interests.

So, how can the limits of this obligation be identified, slowing the curative momentum enough to change focus toward a more palliative goal? One option would be to develop a set of clinical parameters defining when continued treatment would no longer be considered medically beneficial for the patient, after which it would be appropriate to inquire as to the patient's wishes regarding more palliative options. Outside of the scope of genuinely "futile" treatments (discussion follows), this is not a promising strategy. Any such set of parameters would have to be either exceedingly general or impossibly detailed to account for the variety of factors affecting prognosis in critical illness. It would, moreover, be driven by providers' readiness to concede that the prognosis is grim. It is the providers' reluctance to do this that is the source of the problem. For example, Quill (2000) suggests that end-of-life discussions should be initiated when "Patients [are] suffering out of proportion to prognosis" (p. 2504). For the reasons explained earlier, it is unrealistic to expect most clinicians to recognize on their own that this boundary has been crossed. Christakis and Lamont (2000) provide evidence that physicians typically overestimate survival time more than fivefold and frequently misrepresent their own estimates to patients. Clinical parameters alone will not be adequate for appropriately limiting the natural impulse to treat.

A better option starts with the recognition that the normally laudable obligation to prevent death is limited by the patient's right to refuse treatment. Once the provider is giving treatment that the patient might refuse if offered adequate information about its risk, benefits, and alternatives, the provider risks violating the patient's right to informed consent, even if the patient has not yet explicitly refused that particular treatment. Although not acting *against* the patient's will, the provider risks acting in a way that is *contrary to* the patient's values and preferences, and so against the patient's interests, as those would be understood by the patient.

Thus the provider should initiate conversations about the possibility of limiting life-prolonging treatment and suggest palliative care options whenever there is reason to believe that the patient *might* wish to limit care. Palliative care options should also be discussed when treatment options offered will not change the outcome or positively influence the quality of life. Some obvious signs include the patient's talking about wanting to die or inquiring about hospice options (Quill, 2000). More generally, the clinician should inquire about limiting life-prolonging treatment in circumstances where other patients or families have, with any frequency, wanted to limit such care. This includes, for example, cases of repeated hospitalizations for progressive illnesses, situations of limited life expectancy (especially when accompanied by high iatrogenic risk), and circumstances dominated by poor quality of life. The clinician should ask, "Would I be surprised to have a patient decide to limit care under these conditions?" If the answer is "no," the clinician should ascertain the patient's and family's goals and preferences regarding life-sustaining care.

The key ethical question is not "When is it in my patient's interest to shift toward a palliative care plan?" Rather it is, "How can I best avoid frustrating my patient's values and goals?" The second question does not require the clinician to abandon the therapeutic imperative that rightly shapes so much of the interactions with patients. All it requires is to be alert to when this imperative risks colliding with the individual goals of patients. A provider's own estimate of when a palliative care plan would be best does not have to change as long as he or she is willing to allow that the patient or family reach that decision sooner. This requires the provider to be alert to the signs that the patient's or family's view of the situation is diverging from his or her own.

Involving Patients and Families in Decision Making

This approach puts a premium on effective and early communication with patients and families. However, this often happens too little and too late for many patients. There are a number of reasons for this, some already alluded to. There are, in addition, two perceived ethical impediments to these conversations that need some discussion.

One is that disclosing the truth about prognosis or the failure of treatment will strip the patient of any hope. This ancient line of reasoning is still thriving, as reflected in contemporary studies of the reasons for physician reluctance to engage in open discussion with terminally ill patients. One study surveying the attitudes of physicians caring for acquired immunodeficiency syndrome (AIDS) patients reported that for 35% of the patient subjects, physicians reported that discussion was limited because "I worry that discussing end-of-life care with (patient name) will take away his/her hope." This was the highest-scoring item of any of the physician-identified barriers to communication about end-of-life care surveyed in the study (Curtis, Patrick, Caldwell, et al., 2000b).

This is an ethical miscalculation for two reasons. The first is that disclosure will strip the patient of all hope only if the patient's sole hope is for cure. To suppose that even patients in advanced stages of terminal illness cling to this belief imputes a power of self-deception that in fact few patients possess. Even if their physician has not yet verbally told them that they are likely to die from their illness, they themselves will likely be contemplating that possibility. Contemplating it gives rise to other concerns that they may hope will be met: hope that they will not be abandoned, that they will not suffer while dying, that they will be able to put affairs in order, that they will be able to say goodbyes and make amends, and many others. Even if the hope for cure is no longer realistic, many other hopes and dreams are achievable with the help of faith, spirituality, family, friends, the physician, and other providers.

The other miscalculation lies in ignoring the harms caused by hiding the truth. Fallowfield, Jenkins, and Beveridge (2002) review a number of these. Without the truth and left to speculation, patients often imagine matters to be worse than they are, precipitating increased anxiety and fear. The conspiracy of silence inhibits open discussion of patients' and families' fears and curtails the realistic reassurances that could help calm them. Acting on false assumptions about prognosis invites patients to pursue treatment options that will only make their deaths more unbearable or to put off goodbyes until it is too late. The pretense affects families as well, locking them into banal and stilted conversations with their loved one.

The second ethical impediment to early and honest discussion is the idea that patients themselves do not want to know too much. Because patients, as an exercise of their autonomy, have the right to control what sort of information they are given, physicians are justified in limiting the disclosure of bad news. There are undoubtedly patients who do not want to know the full truth about their condition and prognosis, but evidence indicates that they are in the minority. Reporting on a large sample of cancer patients, Fallowfield et al. (2002) report that 84.9% of patients with palliative care plans and 89% of other patients "want as much information as possible, good and bad."

In any event, recognition of the importance of total disclosure of the truth to the patient does not require brutal honesty that ignores sensitivity and the patient's readiness to hear it. What it does require is that the offer of truth be reiterated sincerely and often. Making the offer, rather than dumping the truth on the patient, communicates that the information is important to the patient's well-being while leaving the amount and timing of the information that patients receive in their control (Freedman, 1993).

Despite the gloomy findings of the SUPPORT study, more recent evidence is that timely discussions about options with terminally ill patients or their families have a positive effect on care at the end of life. This is especially true when these options are deliberately incorporated into the decision-making process. These options may include reduction in the use of intensive care services and earlier access to palliative care (Lilly, DeMeo, Sonna, et al., 2000), along with decreased length of hospitalization and earlier decisions to limit non-beneficial treatments such as cardiopulmonary resuscitation (CPR) (Campbell & Guzman, 2003).

Uses and Limits of Advance Directives

As previously argued, decisions to begin limiting life-prolonging treatments in favor of palliative ones should be shaped primarily by the patient's values and preferences. While still competent, the patient can be consulted directly about these choices.

Not infrequently, however, patients at the end of their terminal illness will no longer be competent to make their own decisions. In these circumstances, one must rely on one of two mechanisms for determining what the patient would prefer: (1) written advance directives, or (2) consultation with family members or others with intimate knowledge of the patient.

Advance directives are completed when the patient is still competent to express informed medical treatment preferences. These treatment preferences are intended to guide decisions at some future time when patient competency has been lost. Advance directives typically take two forms. One is a living will, in which the patient says *what* medical treatment is to be done or not done. The other is a durable power of attorney for health care (DPOAHC), in which the patient indicates *who* should be making decisions on his or her behalf. This would ideally be someone the patient trusts to make decisions consistent with the patient's values. Each of these forms has its particular strengths and weaknesses (a discussion of which is beyond the scope of this chapter), and they can be combined into a single document. All states recognize one or another form of advance directive but vary in the requirements for its proper execution and in the limits placed on its use. From the point of view of its function, an "advance directive" need not be a legal document but could be a direct communication from the patient in conversation with family or health care providers.

Advance directives provide evidence for "substituted judgment," a decision that represents what a patient would want if competent to express his or her wishes. It is misleading, however, to think of advance directives as simple extensions of the competent patient's right to informed refusal of treatment. This can sometimes be the case when the patient is in a position to accurately anticipate the illness trajectory and the character of the treatment choices that will present when the patient is no longer competent. This may be possible for patients with chronic progressive illness when they have had prior experience with the treatments that might be implemented. For example, a person with chronic obstructive pulmonary disease (COPD) might be in a good position to make an informed refusal of a ventilator "in advance" and expect that it is likely to be directly relevant to future care.

More often, however, such specific predictions are impossible. Those who must interpret the advance directive then have the task of translating the patient's wishes and desires to determine how it might be relevant to the situation at hand. Typically, prior expressions of wishes are left vague in the effort to cover as many of the contingencies as possible. Such terms as "reasonable chance," "terminal illness," "irreversibly ill," "heroic treatment," and even "resuscitation" have no precise and universally accepted meaning. What the patient meant and what the family and providers understand by these terms may be two different things. This is most obviously a problem with living wills, which are static expressions of the patient's literal words. It is thought by some that one of the advantages of DPOAHCs is that since they do not rely on the written word, they avoid problems of interpretation. This is a mistake. The person appointed as the patient's agent under the DPOAHC will be guided, it is hoped, by what the patient said. What patients say, even more than what they write, is often vague or ambiguous, requiring interpretation. This interpretive leap may account for the fact that persons with intimate knowledge of patients, even those who have had discussions with the patient about end-of-life matters, are only 60% to 70% accurate in representing what the patient would want regarding treatment for critical illness (Hare, Pratt, & Nelson, 1992; Tomlinson, Howe, Notman, et al., 1990).

If interpretations are so often necessary, by what standard should they be made? Not just any interpretation will do, because some interpretations may not be clearly in the patient's best interests as those interests are judged from the values widely accepted by others. Such interpretations will be less plausible, on the assumption that the patient most likely shares the common values rather than deviates from them. The implementation of these perceived wishes would be more objectionable, since this may involve harming the patient in the absence of any countervailing reason based in respect for patient autonomy. For example, in the mid-1980s, the Associated Press wire service reported the case of an intensive care unit (ICU) nurse who had

"No CPR" tattooed on her chest. Imagine that she suffers an electric shock, and on arrival the emergency medical services (EMS) team finds her in ventricular fibrillation. Should they attempt to defibrillate her? It is not impossible that she meant to include just such a scenario within the meaning of "No CPR." But given what is at stake (she is not suffering the co-morbidities of terminal illness, and the chances of successful defibrillation and return to normal life may be quite high), it would be better to discount this interpretation in favor of the view that she had something quite different in mind when she got her tattoo.

It is the standard of the patient's best interest, then, that provides the framework within which the patient's wishes are interpreted. This standard establishes the acceptable level of evidence regarding a patient's wishes not to have treatment. To see this, imagine two patients:

- Mrs. Randall, 72, has throat cancer metastatic to the brain. Her condition rapidly deteriorates, and she is placed on a ventilator. Her husband (with DPOAHC) insists that she would not want CPR if her heart stops.
- Mr. Clark, 72, previously in good health, presented to the emergency room with unilateral face and hand tingling. His neurologic condition rapidly deteriorated, and he is now incompetent. A thorough diagnostic workup confirms a diagnosis of thrombotic thrombocytic purpura, treatable by plasmapheresis. His wife (with DPOAHC) refuses consent to treatment.

Although hardly anyone would challenge Mr. Randall's representation of his wife's wishes, many health professionals would be reluctant to follow Mrs. Clark's insistence that treatment not be provided, unless considerably more evidence was presented supporting the claim that this indeed would be what the patient wanted. This suggests a sliding scale relating judgments of best interest with the standard of evidence required of the patient's wishes. As the stakes for the patient of limiting treatment rise, so too should the standard of evidence for the patient's preferences.

There is no single standard of evidence governing the interpretation of patients' advance directives. It can be a matter of controversy what standard of evidence should be applied in select cases, particularly when there is disagreement about the quality of the life that might be prolonged by continued treatment. Examples are two recent controversial cases concerning conscious patients with severely impaired cognitive functions who were being maintained primarily by artificial feeding. The courts (in Michigan and California) took the position that in these circumstances, the stakes for the patient were so high that they required "clear and convincing" evidence that the patient would have wanted treatment terminated (Nelson & Cranford, 1999).

Despite the limitations and controversies, advance directives can be of great value in terminal care. At present, they are used surprisingly little, even among patients presumably ready to enter into a discussion of advance care planning who are in a good position to make informed judgments. One typical study, for example, found that only 27% of critically ill patients at a tertiary cancer center had advance directives (Kish, Martin, & Price, 2000).

Discussion and completion of advance directives can have a number of beneficial effects. Directives help make patients partners in shaping the plan of care, giving them a sense of control from which to manage the inevitable uncertainty and anxiety occasioned by their diagnoses. Knowing that their wishes regarding treatment limitations will be respected may make patients more willing to consider experimental or other trials of treatments that might be helpful. Greater clarity about the patient's own views regarding the acceptable goals of care lifts the burden of decision making from the shoulders of family and providers, who otherwise may feel driven to "err on the side of life."

Families as Decision Makers

At the end of life, patients are frequently unable to make their own decisions and most have not left explicit advance directives. Health care professionals must often rely on families or friends to make decisions about moving toward a palliative plan of care. This traditional reliance on family members has a number of ethical justifications, recently reviewed by Arnold and Kellum (2003). The first, and most central, is that the family is best able to represent the patient's own values and preferences.

Of all those present in the caregiving context, the family is usually most intimately acquainted with the patient. They may be able to recall specific expressions of preferences and concerns made by the patient that directly bear on the health care decisions needing to be made. Even where no such specific declarations were made, the family may best know the patient "as a person," understanding what the patient would likely want if able to speak.

A second justification argues that the family has the greatest degree of loving concern for the welfare of the patient and so are the most highly motivated to make a decision that is in the patient's best interest. This stands in contrast to strangers, such as health professionals, who at best will be acting out of their perceived duty to the patient and who may be caught in the grip of conflicting duties (e.g., duties to other patients, personal beliefs and values), which may make them less single-minded in pursuing this particular person's best interest.

The third is that, next to the patient, family members have the most at stake in the decisions made. Their interests can be affected in any number of ways. They may have to bear the burden of a home-care plan, they may be suffering emotionally and physically from the strains of the patient's long illness, or they may have to live with a bad memory of their loved one's dying process that may dominate their recollection of the patient's life.

There are two sorts of limitations to these justifications. The first is that the justifications rely on presumptions that may not be true or may not be equally true of all families. Some families have much better knowledge of the patient's express wishes than others, since many families do not have conversations about end-of-life issues at all. Not all families are equally loving; some are in fact malevolent and cannot be counted on to aim only at what is best for the patient. The second is that the three justifications are not entirely congruent with one another. The third in particular can pull against the other two. Even among families that are well motivated, their own needs may undermine their ability to reliably represent what the patient would want. Most often, this leads to over-treatment, not abandonment. Families may insist that treatment continue, perhaps as a symbolic compensation for their perceived failure to take proper care of a parent or as a way to avoid later guilty regrets over having "pulled the plug." Still, so long as these limitations are kept in mind, the three together support several important ethical guidelines in having families serve as decision makers.

First, families should be explicitly asked what the patient would want done rather than what they think should be done. There is evidence that when this question is asked, families in fact come closer to accurately representing the patient's preferences (Tomlinson et al., 1990). Such a question symbolically puts the burden of a momentous decision on the patient's shoulders, reducing the potential for guilty regret that can arise if the family is made to feel that the decision is entirely their responsibility.

Second, family needs and burdens that may be affected by a medical decision should be openly acknowledged and discussed. They are not per se ethically irrelevant, insofar as they do not lead to decisions blatantly at odds with the patient's preferences or interests. It is important to recognize that among the patient's values will often be concern about what happens to loved ones. "I don't want to be a burden to my family" is a sentiment patients often express. Families can be asked to consider how the patient would want family burdens considered. This allows the family to reconceptualize their concerns as something that may be more worthy than simple "selfishness."

Third, several guidelines emerge for the selection of particular family members to serve as primary decision makers. Family members who demonstrate specific knowledge of the patient's previously expressed preferences and values are to be preferred, as are those whose history shows a pattern of loving concern for the welfare of the patient. The mere existence of a potential conflict of interest or secondary gain (e.g., an inheritance or continuing Social Security payment) does not disqualify a family member from assuming this role.

These criteria do not always map onto degrees of kinship. The patient's spouse may be a less ethically appropriate decision maker than the granddaughter. The patient's friend may be in a better position to represent the patient's wishes than the brother. The application of these criteria may lead to ethical conflict with the statutes found in some states that mandate a particular hierarchy of decision makers.

Futile Treatments

A final ethical controversy that may complicate the transition into palliative care concerns judgments of futility. The idea that some medical interventions may be "futile" and therefore should not be provided by the responsible physician is a traditional one. The rise of principles respecting patient autonomy and authority over treatment in the late 1960s, however, for some time eclipsed this "paternalistic" perspective. Only in the past decade has the concept of futile treatment and the physician authority that it implies seen resurgence as a legitimate ethical perspective (Council on Ethical and Judicial Affairs, 1991; Schneiderman, Jecker, & Jonsen, 1990; Tomlinson & Brody, 1990).

Nearly all of this modern discussion has focused on the use of CPR. This is understandable, since CPR has stood as the only intervention requiring an order not to provide. Until very recently, this was a decision always requiring the patient's or surrogate's consent, at least in the United States. Physicians had to ask the patient/family about their wishes regarding CPR, even when they were sure of its uselessness. This possibly precipitated the creation of conflicts between the demands of patients or families for CPR and the physician's (or staff's) reluctance to provide it.

Two sorts of arguments have been given on behalf of the physician's authority to say "no" to family or patient demands for futile CPR. The first, and most central, starts from the claim that patients' "rights of autonomy," by now well established in law and ethics, are negative rights, not positive ones. They are rights to refuse a recommended treatment or to choose among those treatment options offered. There can be no general positive right of patients to demand whatever intervention they might choose, since this would make it impossible for health professionals to practice with integrity. They would be forced to provide, with their own hands and skills, interventions that would violate the most fundamental duty defining the character of the medical profession—in particular, the duty to help rather than hurt. This right of professional integrity is reflected in everyday medical practice. It is not the cardiac patient, for example, who decides whether he is a candidate for by-pass. It is the surgeon, who must consider the moral weight of the possibility that the patient's death might be by his or her hands.

The second argument is concerned with how to properly enable the exercise of patient autonomy. Making choices is important when real alternatives are at stake, that is, when what is chosen will significantly affect one's interests. The "autonomy" that is offered to the patient or his surrogate is a bogus one when a useless intervention is one of the options. The offer of it is inherently duplicitous as well and so corrodes informed, autonomous decisions. On one hand, the offer of the intervention by a person who is duty-bound to help rather than hurt implies that the intervention offers some benefit. On the other hand, in the spirit of informed consent, the provider must explain that nothing of the sort is true. The message that patients and families receive often in a time of crisis can be a hopelessly mixed and confusing one.

The most frequent and powerful objection to the use of futility judgments focuses on the fact that these always rely on some set of values. The extreme version of the argument asserts that since only patients should have authority over value-laden choices, no futility judgments can be warranted (Truog, Brett, & Frader, 1992). But one need not go this far to be worried about the threat that a policy permitting futility judgments can pose to patient autonomy. Futility judgments privilege the physician's professional values over the patient's individual values. The danger is that the scope of those professional values will expand in ways that appropriate decisions, particularly about quality of life, that properly belong in the hands of the patient and family. A challenge for any futility policy is how to prevent this slide back into an objectionable physician paternalism (Tomlinson & Czlonka, 1995).

The ultimate legitimacy of futility judgments remains controversial, and this is not the place to settle the matter. There seem to be two possible benefits of framing certain treatment interventions to patients and families in terms of futility. First, as

just argued, it avoids sending the mixed message inherent in a treatment choice that is framed as a matter of informed consent. Patients and families facing the end of life are already struggling with uncertain and difficult choices. Being told that some intervention (particularly resuscitation) should not be employed because it could only make matters worse can relieve an unwanted burden. There is some evidence that patients are more likely than not to agree with a well-explained judgment that a futile treatment should not be tried (Curtis, Patrick, Caldwell, et al., 2000a).

Second, making it clear that some things will not be done because they violate the provider's duty to serve the patient's best interest can open a chink in the armor of denial in which some families operate (to the ultimate detriment of their loved one). Although there are no systematic studies on this phenomenon, clinical experience indicates that families who had initially resisted the physician's decision not to attempt resuscitation came to accept it after several days of intensive family discussion and soul searching. Once this boundary had been crossed, they were then open to discussion of other treatment limitation decisions that had formerly been unacceptable.

ETHICAL ISSUES WITHIN PALLIATIVE CARE

Once a decision has been made to forego or cease life-prolonging efforts and move to a palliative plan of care, another set of ethical issues arises. Because the conventional approach to many of these employs the Doctrine of Double Effect (DDE), it will be useful to explain that doctrine before discussing the more specific contexts in which it is applied.

The Doctrine of Double Effect

The DDE has a long history in Jewish and Roman Catholic moral theology, and history has seen a variety of formulations of the doctrine (Marquis, 1991). Although the differences among these can significantly affect the application of the doctrine, for the purposes of this chapter the most common formulation is used: It is permissible to perform an action that has both a good and a bad effect so

long as (Marquis, 1991):
• The act in itself is not evil or impermissible
• The good effect, and not the bad one, is the effect intended (even though the bad effect is a foreseen consequence)
• The bad effect is not the means used for achieving the good effect (e.g., the good effect outweighs the bad effect)

The heart of the doctrine is the second condition. The first and the last conditions set moral boundaries that are independent of the agent's intentions, ensuring that the act is not objectionable on either deontologic or utilitarian grounds. The third condition is merely a criterion for assessing whether the bad effect is not also intended, employing the idea that one cannot intend the effect without also intending the means.

The distinction between intended and merely foreseen consequences has most often been used in medical ethics to identify those deaths for which the physician is not morally culpable. One application, for example, concerns the use of pain medication. The physician who administers morphine in doses large enough to hasten a patient's death is not culpable so long as the intention is to relieve pain and not to bring about a quicker death (Pellegrino, 1998). (A discussion of this issue follows.)

There are a number of grounds on which the DDE itself, or a particular application of it, might be challenged (Quill, Dresser, & Brock, 1997). First, it relies on an assumption about what effects can be ethically intended. Traditionally, the pertinent assumption has been that it is not permissible to intend to cause the death of an innocent person. But that assumption requires some justification, about which people may disagree. To the extent that they do, they will also disagree on the verdict of the DDE. If someone thinks that killing a suffering person at that person's request is not a fundamental wrong, he or she will believe that the DDE exonerates his or her action, rather than prohibits it. Second, it requires that one can sharply distinguish between those effects of an action that are intended and those that are not. In some cases this may be straightforward; in others it will not be, since people's intentions are often complex and not fully transparent, even to them. Third, the use of

the DDE requires a claim about which unintended effects are acceptable. "I didn't mean to" is not an all-purpose excuse for negligence or indifference. The DDE includes the requirement of proportionality to rule out some unintended effects as unacceptable. The action is not justified by the DDE if the evil unintended effect is disproportionately greater than the intended good effect. But, of course, there may be disagreement about the value (or disvalue) of the intended effect, the unintended effect, or both. An examination of some of the palliative care contexts in which the DDE is employed follows.

Issues Regarding Withdrawal of Treatment

The DDE is traditionally one of the principles used to distinguish the ethics of withdrawing life-prolonging treatments from the ethics of assisted suicide or active euthanasia. Because in the latter cases, the professed intention (by the patient, the caregiver, or both) is to end the patient's suffering by ending his life, such "mercy killing" is ethically impermissible. In withdrawing life-prolonging treatment, however, it is possible to aim only at stopping the suffering and indignity caused by the treatment itself. The death that results is not intended, but only foreseen. Although the death remains an evil, the end of a terminal illness is a lesser evil than the additional suffering that would be caused by extending it. Even though withdrawal of a ventilator and a lethal injection might both be equally likely to result in death and both might be equally consented to by the patient, only the withdrawal of treatment meets the requirements of the DDE.

However, this is only a limited defense of withdrawing treatment. Its application will depend on the intentions enmeshed in the context. What, for example, would the DDE say about withdrawal of food and fluids from a patient in a persistent vegetative state? One cannot plausibly claim that the withdrawal of the treatment is to reduce the suffering it causes, since, according to the Multi-Society Task Force on Persistent Vegetative State (1994), such a patient is beyond suffering. What intention can one have, then, except to hasten death—the intention one is forbidden to have. For some commentators, this withdrawal of treatment is ethically akin to active euthanasia and so is morally troubling (Meilaender, 1984).

Terminal Weaning. An attempt not to violate the strictures of the DDE leads some physicians to advocate terminal weaning as the method of withdrawing support from ventilator-dependent patients (Gilligan & Raffin, 1996). Because this maximizes whatever chances there may be for the patient to survive for a time off the ventilator, caregivers and families can distance themselves from the charge that the patient's earlier death was their primary objective in withdrawing support.

There are several ethical difficulties with this thinking. First and foremost, the patient's earlier death may be exactly what the patient might have hoped for. At the very least, the prospect of lingering for some time longer off the ventilator, more functionally impaired than when on it, would often be the outcome the patient most feared. Thus caregivers and families may secure their own ethical comfort at the price of compromising the patient's values and goals. Second, the prolonged dying process that may result from removal of the ventilator exposes the patient to more suffering and indignity rather than less. The DDE cannot justify the method if in addition to causing the presumed evil of the patient's earlier demise, the prolonged terminal weaning also causes more suffering for the patient. Finally, even if more rapid methods (e.g., extubation) made the patient's death a certainty, this would not necessarily matter for application of the DDE. What matters is that the death is merely foreseen and that its occurrence is warranted by the intended good effect (reduction of suffering).

One problem of applying the DDE is the difficulty in clearly distinguishing the agent's intentions. To the extent that the good and evil effects are causally separable, so that one can readily imagine the one occurring without the other, the more plausible it is to claim that only one of the effects is intended. When the two go hand in glove, it may be impossible for anyone other than the agent himself to say whether only the good effect is intended. One is forced into relying on the agent's report of his or her own intentions, so that the ethics of these decisions become entirely subjective.

To the extent, then, that more rapid methods of discontinuing ventilation make the patient's immediate death more certain, the ethics of such methods remain murky if the DDE is our primary ethical principle. The result, however, is to encourage the use of more cautious methods that threaten both the welfare and the rights of patients.

An alternative framework starts with recognition that patients (and the families representing them) have the right to stop treatment. Any method that runs contrary to the interests, goals, and values of the patient violate the patient's right to bodily integrity. This is an evil to be avoided. If avoiding it leads to another evil (causing the death of the patient), then some judgment must be made of the relative weight of these evils. In the context of terminal illness, this is a judgment that will almost always favor a decision respecting the patient's values. It does not matter, either, whether both "evils" are intended or only one. Even if intending the patient's death is an evil, the alternative of intentionally violating the patient's rights is also an evil. Where there is no avoiding evil intentions, the distinction between foreseen and intended effects, and with it the DDE, becomes irrelevant for justifying a course of action.

Thus the ethics of discontinuing ventilation need have nothing to do with the DDE. Rather, these decisions should aim both to comport as fully as possible with the patient's values and goals and to minimize discomfort. It does not matter how certain the patient's death becomes except insofar as that is an issue of concern to the patient. In most circumstances, although perhaps not all, these twin objectives can be best achieved using the methods advocated by Gilligan and Raffin (1996; Brody, Campbell, Faber-Langendoen, et al., 1997). Rapid ventilator setting reductions minimize the chances of prolonged dying, or undesirable survival off the ventilator, while minimizing the chances of discomfort as a result of loss of the airway.

A similar analysis applies to situations in which the patient is under the effect of a paralyzing drug. Kirkland (1994) presents the case of a 68-year-old man with advanced emphysema who was placed on mechanical ventilation when his condition began to deteriorate. With his family's support, he made it clear that if his condition did not improve within 5 days, he wanted the ventilator withdrawn. During the course of his treatment, he was heavily sedated and given a paralyzing agent to relax the chest wall and increase the volume of respiration. Despite this and other measures, his level of oxygenation continued to decline and his kidneys began to fail. At this point, the patient was no longer conscious and clearly dying despite aggressive measures. His family then reiterated his request and asked that the ventilator be withdrawn.

Respect for the patient's values and goals implies the necessity of withdrawing the ventilator as expeditiously as possible, even if (or perhaps because) death is certain. On the other hand, the patient's death is ensured in part because of a drug that the physician had provided. Even though the drug had first been given for therapeutic reasons, a further decision not to wait until its effects had subsided might be interpreted to imply that its deadly effect was welcomed, not merely tolerated. And so, the prompt discontinuation of the ventilator under these conditions would violate the DDE.

Again, however, the choice is not whether one intends the good effect rather than the evil one. It is a choice between two evils, and the question is which evil is the greater one under the circumstances. It is a choice to be settled by weighing the moral consequences, not by discerning what the agent's intentions are. In the setting of imminent death, the evil of violating the patient's right to bodily integrity is the greater evil.

This does not mean that the presence of a paralyzing agent is ethically irrelevant. If it is possible to reverse the effects of the agent in a timely way, it would be preferable to do so to avoid any concern among staff and family about complicity in the patient's death. In addition, it may also be difficult to adequately monitor and treat pain and distress in a paralyzed person who has been stripped of the ability to communicate or otherwise reveal signs of distress. These reasons favor the use of short-acting and easily reversible paralytic medications when possible. They do not add up to an argument against ever withdrawing ventilatory support from paralyzed patients.

Withdrawing Food and Fluids and Administering Terminal Sedation. There are clearly circumstances in which limiting administration of fluids and nutrition is warranted by concern for minimizing suffering in the dying patient. It is common for patients to lose their appetites and limit their consumption of food and water in the terminal phases of illness. Both concern for patient comfort and respect for patient autonomy argue against aggressive measures to maintain levels of fluids and nutrition under these circumstances. There is little evidence that tube feeding substantially prolongs life, and it carries additional risks that usually will only add an additional burden of discomfort for dying patients (Finucane, Christmas, & Travis, 1999). Even if limiting fluids and nutrition shortened remaining life, it would be permissible under the DDE so long as it was aimed at avoiding the additional suffering caused by continuing to eat and drink.

But what about the patient who, while terminally ill, is not actively dying? For such a person, food and fluids may not cause any additional suffering. Yet, in the absence of other effective means, some seriously ill patients choose to stop eating and drinking to hasten death (Eddy, 1994; Quill, Lo, & Brock, 1997). When their intention is primarily to cause their death, this is a choice that would be condemned by the DDE. It is a suicide, even if it is judged as a rational one, and contemplating it is a serious ethical matter for the patient.

The question is whether the provider's support for it is a form of assisted suicide or euthanasia. The answer is similar to the one given regarding terminal weaning. When the patient is exercising the right to bodily integrity in refusing the forceful administration of fluids and nutrition, the provider who respects this refusal is only doing what must be done. To do otherwise would be an evil, and even if the provider thinks that the patient's intention to end one's life is also an evil, the question is which evil is the lesser one. Again, in cases of terminal illness when extended survival is likely to involve considerable suffering, causing the patient's earlier demise is usually the lesser evil. Once this judgment has been made, the provider has a further obligation to relieve distressful symptoms associated with the patient's fast. To refuse to do so would compound the evil being caused.

This same approach applies when the withdrawal of food and fluids is combined with terminal sedation. Terminal sedation is the practice of administering large doses of sedatives so that the patient is rendered unconscious, and it is used as a last resort when less extreme measures are not adequate for preventing suffering (Quill & Byock, 2000). Because the patient is now unconscious and so beyond any experience of suffering, some commentators argue that the withdrawal of food and fluids can have only one purpose—the patient's death—and so this practice is ethically indistinguishable from active euthanasia (Orentlicher, 1997). But regardless of intentions, it is distinguishable by one key feature: the patient's right to bodily integrity. The physician who continues to administer treatments the patient did or would refuse risks committing an assault, as Quill and Byock (2000) point out. By contrast, the refusal to serve the patient's intentions in cases of assisted suicide or active euthanasia does not wrong the patient in so fundamental a way. (This is not to say that these patients might be wronged in some other way, nor is this an argument that patients should not have assisted suicide or euthanasia available to them. It only assumes that the argument in favor of these options will have some other ethical basis.)

Ethical Aspects of Pain Management

We know from a variety of studies that pain is not managed well in terminally ill patients, even for cancer patients in the last 3 days of life (McCarthy, Phillips, Zhong, et al., 2000). On the face of it, this appears ethically intolerable. The obligation to relieve pain and the suffering and disability that it causes seems fundamental. Pain is something that might be tolerated in the pursuit of some larger purpose. Patients from some religious traditions, for example, may see pain serving a redemptive purpose. Where pain serves no purpose, it is an unmitigated evil. Failing to relieve it, as Pellegrino (1998) puts it, verges on "moral and legal malpractice" (p. 1521). Indeed, as reported by LaDuke

(2002), the under-treatment of pain has resulted in substantial malpractice judgments.

In light of this, why is pain too often under-treated? There are a number of explanations. Physicians and others may not well understand the phenomenon of pain or the expression of pain and therefore underestimate its severity. Or they may be poorly informed about the options for pain treatment and therefore do a poor job of matching the treatment to the need. These are misunderstandings of a factual nature, which are addressed in other chapters of this book.

But there are also ethical roots to the poor management of pain. First among these is concern that high doses of morphine may accelerate death and therefore become a form of active euthanasia. This concern has traditionally been addressed with the DDE, as mentioned. So long as the intention is only to relieve pain, rather than to hasten death, the theory is that the physician can order—and the nurse can administer—whatever dosage is required by the patient's pain, even if hastened death is a foreseen, even certain, side effect (Pellegrino, 1998).

In the context of terminal illness, however, this application of the DDE is only theoretically satisfying. This is because at the same time that the patient's pain is being managed, decisions to limit life-prolonging treatment are also being made. The patient's earlier death is not just acceptable; it may actually be desired by the patient, the family, and often members of the health care team. The sooner death comes, the better. The use of the DDE to justify high doses of narcotics requires the provider to disavow any such hope and to say instead that he or she would be just as happy if the narcotics relieved the patient's pain while the patient lingered indefinitely. This would be a highly unusual set of motivations.

The DDE can provide an ethical comfort zone for using narcotics—even high doses of them—for patients who are not terminally ill and for whom decisions to limit life-prolonging treatment are not being made, such as patients suffering from chronic pain. But it does not provide a comfort zone for the treatment of the terminally ill. How can that comfort zone be created? One often-employed strategy is to retain the DDE and to argue that, in fact, high doses of narcotics rarely shorten life (Sykes & Thorns, 2003). As important as this message is, it will not have a serious effect so long as physicians retain their prerogative to make such clinical judgments on a case-by-case basis.

A more radical strategy is to abandon the DDE framework. The patient's earlier death, caused by decisions to limit treatment, is a consequence that is not merely accepted but hoped for. Although the patient's death is an evil (it would be better if the patient could miraculously be saved), under the inevitable circumstances his lingering death is an even worse evil. A worse evil than that would be a lingering death marked by unrelieved pain and suffering. If high doses of narcotics are required to relieve the patient's pain, and are likely to hasten death, it is not an argument against their use if the hope is that the patient's death will come more quickly. Even if the premise of the DDE is accepted and it is an evil to intend the patient's quicker death, the alternative of not treating the patient's pain in order not to hasten death results in the greater evil under the circumstances.

Another potential ethical barrier to adequate pain management is concern with avoiding addiction. This can be a concern not just among providers but among patients as well (Weiss, Emanuel, Fairclough, et al., 2001). Most evidence indicates that addiction among terminally ill patients being treated with narcotics is rare, and it is important to distinguish between addiction and tolerance. Even if this is granted, however, it may have little effect on acceptance of even an extremely low risk of addiction if addiction itself is thought to be a very great evil.

Addiction is plausibly a great evil outside of the context of terminal illness. The reasons are important. Compulsions are undesirable when they limit freedom of action in ways that are not in people's interests. They may do that by tying individuals to the pursuit of trivial or unworthy goals or by preventing them from achieving other goals important for a productive and worthy life, or both. Heroin addiction is often (not always) destructive of people's lives in these ways.

But how are these reasons relevant to the terminally ill patient in pain? Even if addicted to pain medication, it is an addiction most likely to serve a patient's interests rather than undermine them. Using narcotics for pain relief is a worthy goal, not a trivial one; and the freedom from pain may permit the patient to pursue activities and interests that would otherwise be difficult. In the context of terminal illness, addiction may not be an evil at all, or at least not a very great one. Unlike for the heroin addict, quality of life for the terminally ill person is more likely enhanced by the use of pain-relieving drugs rather than diminished by it.

The importance of pain control for the protection of the patient's interest and the preservation of capacities for autonomy of action suggests that decisions about pain management for terminally ill patients should be made on the model of shared decision making (Jansen, 2001). Shared decision making assumes that the patient is the best source of knowledge about the experienced effects of illness and its treatment. It also assumes that, ultimately, the patient's values should mediate trade-offs between risks and benefits. This can seem like a radical suggestion in the paternalistic health care world. If physicians were asked to name those treatments over which they should retain absolute control, pain medications would be on almost everyone's list. Outside the terminal care setting, this may have some justification. For example, when pain medications have a high potential for abuse, diversion, and significant harm to the patient or others, it is appropriate that the physician exercise caution in meeting patients' demands for drugs.

As discussed, in terminal illness the threat of harm from the use of narcotics is substantially less significant, both in its likelihood and in its relative ethical importance. This means, among other things, that the physician can take patients' own reports of their pain as authoritative to an extent that might not always be wise when treating chronic pain. The physician can afford to prescribe more liberally and let the patient determine what risks from high doses of pain medication are acceptable. It is only when terminally ill patients are given control of their pain management that they can expect their pain to be adequately treated. The ethical risks of doing so are minimal and acceptable.

SUMMARY

The provision of palliative care to terminally ill patients presents a number of ethical questions. The answers that providers give to these inquiries will have a profound effect on the quality of care that patients and families receive. It is especially important that ethical misperceptions not drive decisions about movement toward a palliative plan of care, about withdrawals of life-prolonging treatment, or about adequate provision of pain management. The Doctrine of Double Effect is an especially potent source of such misperceptions that requires caution in thinking through the ethics of palliative care. Clinicians should be prepared to consider and use alternative ethical frameworks that may better serve the interests and rights of patients.

Case Study

Mrs. J. was a 38-year-old white female with advanced cystic fibrosis and frequent hospitalizations. Over the previous 4 years, her illness had progressively worsened. During the last year of her life, Mrs. J. was dependent on continuous supplemental oxygen and received a high level of medical support at home in addition to her daily medication requirement, which included maintenance oral and aerosolized antibiotics. On this regimen, she enjoyed a remarkably good status for approximately 6 months but was then hospitalized with high fevers and an infectious exacerbation of her bronchiectasis related to cystic fibrosis.

In the course of her hospital stay, Mrs. J. initially improved but relapsed repeatedly. As her condition deteriorated, she was approached regarding the likelihood that intubation might soon be necessary. She could not make a firm decision, often wavering between a wish to be intubated and a refusal of the same. Over the final week, Mrs. J. told her husband that she would permit intubation but that she expected to be permitted to die if there was no hope for recovery. This decision was reached after numerous consultations with her pastor. In a final effort to improve her status, Mrs. J. agreed to undergo lung lavage to physically remove copious mucus that was resistant to antimicrobial therapy. After the anesthesia, however, her carbon dioxide level remained high and she continued on her declining path.

This culminated in high fevers, with increasing hypoxia requiring intubation and mechanical ventilation. During her short stay in intensive care, Mrs. J. made no progress in weaning from the ventilator, required persistently high oxygen concentrations near 100%, and developed a need for presser support for her blood pressure. Her initial sluggish response to verbal communication ceased. The family, now including the husband, parents, and a sister, were in regular attendance and in communication with the physician.

During a family meeting on the last hospital day, the family expressed gratitude for the medical efforts on behalf of the patient but indicated their desire to withdraw the ventilator. By coincidence, that day was an anniversary of the death of a previous child and because the father was ridden with guilt at his inability to attend that earlier death, it was determined that the entire family be present for the patient's death. They spoke of this fatalistically and often in religious terms. They once again asked the physician whether her status was likely to improve and were told that recovery was very unlikely.

The family then proceeded to the patient's bedside, where they recited prayers and Bible passages, and attempted unsuccessfully to communicate with Mrs. J. After some moments of prayer, the husband asked how he might disconnect the ventilator, and the power switch was pointed out to him by the respiratory therapist in attendance. The nurse in charge of Mrs. J. expressed her concern that Mrs. J. was on a paralyzing agent and that this would mean her certain death. The family asserted that they were requesting no aid or assistance from her, the respiratory therapist, or any other staff member. The husband then turned off the ventilator, and the entire family remained with Mrs. J. until her cardiac monitor showed no cardiac activity. The respiratory therapist removed the endotracheal tube, and the family was permitted some additional time with Mrs. J.'s remains.

Objective Questions

1. The percentage of patients diagnosed with terminal cancer who have advance directives is:

   a. Almost 90%.
   b. About 50%.
   c. Less than 30%.
   d. Less than 10%.

2. Evidence indicates that advance directives or other information about a patient's wishes regarding end-of-life care will have an effect on the treatment they receive:

   a. Almost never.
   b. Whenever the information is included in the medical record.
   c. Almost always.
   d. When there is a defined mechanism for incorporating them into the clinical decision-making process.

3. Mr. Blankenship is dying from widely metastasized liver cancer and is no longer oriented to his surroundings because of metastasis to the brain. A former agent in the Drug Enforcement Agency, he was virulently opposed to the use of psychoactive drugs of all kinds, especially opiates. His opposition to them extended to his own use of them for pain. Ten years previously, when he broke his leg in a skiing accident, he refused repeated offers of morphine, and even Tylenol #3. Included in his living will is the following: "Psychoactive or mood-altering drugs are not to be administered under any circumstances, even for the relief of pain."

   The pain caused by his cancer is increasing in severity and becoming more difficult to control. In your judgment, morphine is the drug of choice for relieving his pain. Mr. Blankenship's wife, well aware of his living will and previous attitudes toward drugs, is nevertheless begging you to "do something" to keep him out of pain. In deciding what course of action to take, you should:

   a. Rely on his wife for decision making, since she is acting sensibly.
   b. Follow the terms of the living will as literally as possible, since it is clear evidence of what the patient would want.
   c. Ignore this clause of his living will, since it is very unlikely that he was anticipating a situation as dire as this one when he wrote it.
   d. Further explore with the patient's wife the reasons for his antipathy to drug use, to see whether morphine might be administered in a form or manner that minimizes unwanted psychotropic effects.

4. When a patient's terminal diagnosis is not openly disclosed and discussed, which of the following is most likely?

   a. The patient will not lose hope.
   b. Families will be more at ease relating to the patient.
   c. Patients will continue to pursue aggressive attempts at cure.
   d. The patient's need for pain medication will be met in a timely way.

5. Families are more likely to accurately represent the patient's wishes about terminal care if they are asked to choose what:

   a. Would make the family most comfortable.
   b. They think the patient would want done.
   c. They think would be best for the patient.
   d. The physician recommends.

6. Which of the following is least reliable as a guideline for selecting a person to serve as a decision maker for an incompetent patient?

   a. The person has nothing to gain from the patient's death (e.g., an inheritance).
   b. The person has good knowledge of the sort of person the patient is.
   c. The person shows deep concern for the patient's welfare and visits often.
   d. The person is named as the patient's surrogate decision maker in a durable power of attorney.

7. When patients or families are told that an intervention like CPR should not be performed

because it will be futile, they are most likely to:

a. Contact their lawyer.
b. Demand other aggressive life-prolonging treatment.
c. Agree with the decision.
d. Transfer the patient's care to another provider.

8. Under the Doctrine of Double Effect, which of the following statements is false?

a. Withdrawal of treatment with the patient's consent is never ethically objectionable.
b. Pain medication can be provided even at doses that may hasten death.
c. Active euthanasia is wrong even with the patient's agreement.
d. It is wrong to intentionally cause someone's death.

9. The most serious ethical problem with using extubation as a method for discontinuing mechanical ventilation is that:

a. It makes the patient's death more certain.
b. It makes the patient's impaired survival more likely.
c. It makes it too easy for the family to distance themselves from the charge that they "let the patient die."
d. The sudden loss of airway may cause more suffering for the patient.

10. One important difference between terminal sedation (TS), combined with the withdrawal of artificial food and fluids, and voluntary active euthanasia (VAE) is that:

a. TS can be used only with patients who are actively dying.
b. The patient's right to TS can be based on the right to bodily integrity.
c. Only VAE deliberately intends to end the patient's life.
d. Only VAE could be employed against the patient's wishes.

11. In the context of terminal illness, the Doctrine of Double Effect (DDE) may not clearly justify high doses of pain medication because:

a. High doses of pain medication often hasten death in the terminally ill.
b. Long courses of pain medication lead to addiction.
c. Patients, families, and providers may often want death to come more quickly.
d. Under the DDE, death is a worse evil than unrelieved pain.

REFERENCES

Arnold, R.M., & Kellum, J. (2003). Moral justifications for surrogate decision-making in the intensive care unit: Implications and limitations. *Crit Care Med, 31*(5), S347-353.

Brody, H., Campbell, M.L., Faber-Langendoen, K., et al. (1997). Withdrawing intensive life-sustaining treatment: Recommendations for compassionate clinical management. *N Engl J Med, 336*(9), 652-657.

Campbell, M.L., & Guzman, J.A. (2003). Impact of a proactive approach to improve end-of-life care in a medical ICU. *Chest, 123,* 266-271.

Christakis, N.A., & Lamont, E.B. (2000). Extent and determinants of error in doctors' prognoses in terminally ill patients: Prospective cohort study. *Br Med J, 320,* 469-473.

Council on Ethical and Judicial Affairs. (1991). Guidelines for the appropriate Use of do-not-resuscitate orders. *J Amer Med Assoc, 265*(14), 1868-1871.

Curtis, J.R., Patrick, D.L., Caldwell, E.S., et al. (2000a). The attitudes of patients with advanced AIDS toward use of the medical futility rationale in decisions to forgo mechanical ventilation. *Arch Intern Med, 160*(11), 1597-1601.

Curtis, J.R., Patrick, D.L., Caldwell, E.S., et al. (2000b). Why don't patients and physicians talk about end-of-life care? Barriers to communication for patients with acquired immunodeficiency syndrome and their primary care clinicians. *Arch Intern Med, 160,* 1690-1696.

Eddy, D.M. (1994). A conversation with my mother. *J Amer Med Assoc, 272,* 179-181.

Fallowfield, J.L., Jenkins, V.A., & Beveridge, H.A. (2002). Truth may hurt but deceit hurts more: Communication in palliative care. *Palliat Med, 16*(4), 297-303.

Finucane, T.E., Christmas, C., & Travis, K. (1999). Tube feeding in patients with advanced dementia: A review of the evidence. *J Amer Med Assoc, 282*(14), 1365-1370.

Freedman, B. (1993). Offering truth: One ethical approach to the uninformed cancer patient. *Arch Intern Med, 153*(5), 572-576.

Gilligan, T., & Raffin, T.A. (1996). Withdrawing life support: Extubation and prolonged terminal weans are inappropriate. *Crit Care Med, 24*(2), 352-353.

Hare, J., Pratt, C., & Nelson, C. (1992). Agreement between patients and their self-selected surrogates on difficult medical decisions. *Arch Intern Med, 152*(5), 1049-1054.

Jansen, L.A. (2001). Deliberative decision-making and the treatment of pain. *J Palliat Med, 4*(1), 23-30.

Kirkland, L. (1994). Neuromuscular paralysis and withdrawal of mechanical ventilation. *J Clin Ethics, 5*(1), 38-39.

Kish, S.K., Martin, C.G., & Price, K.J. (2000). Advance directives in critically ill cancer patients. *Crit Care Nurs Clin North Am, 12*(3), 373-383.

LaDuke, S. (2002). Ethical issues in pain management. *Crit Care Nurs Clin North Am, 14,* 165-170.

Lamont, E.B., & Christakis, N.A. (2000). Prognostic disclosure to patients with cancer near the end of life. *Ann Intern Med, 134*(12), 1096-1105.

Lilly, C.M., DeMeo, D.L., Sonna, L.A., et al. (2000). An intensive communication intervention for the critically ill. *Am J Med, 109,* 469-475.

Marquis, D.B. (1991). Four versions of double effect. *J Med Philos, 16,* 515-544.

McCarthy, E.P., Phillips, R.S., Zhong, Z., et al. (2000). Dying with cancer: Patients' function, symptoms, and care preferences as death approaches. *J Am Geriatr Soc, 48*(5 Suppl.), S110-121.

Meilaender, G. (1984). On removing food and water: Against the stream. *Hastings Cent Rep, 14*(6), 11-13.

The Multi-Society Task Force on Persistent Vegetative State (PVS). (1994). Medical aspects of the persistent vegetative state. *N Engl J Med, 330*(21), 1499-1508.

Nelson, L.J., & Cranford, R.E. (1999). Michael Martin and Robert Wendland: Beyond the vegetative state. *J Contemp Health Law Policy, 15,* 427-453.

Orentlicher, D. (1997). The Supreme Court and physician-assisted suicide: Rejecting assisted suicide but embracing euthanasia. *N Engl J Med, 337*(17), 1236-1239.

Pellegrino, E.D. (1998). Emerging ethical issues in palliative care. *J Amer Med Assoc, 279*(19), 1521-1522.

Quill, T.E. (2000). Initiating end-of-life discussions with seriously ill patients: Addressing the "elephant in the room." *J Amer Med Assoc, 284*(19), 2502-2507.

Quill, T.E., & Byock, I.R. (2000). Responding to intractable terminal suffering: The role of terminal sedation and voluntary refusal of food and fluids. *Ann Intern Med, 132*(5), 408-414.

Quill, T.E., Dresser, R., & Brock, D.W. (1997). The rule of double effect: A critique of its role in end-of-life decision-making. *N Engl J Med, 337*(24), 1768-1771.

Quill, T.E., Lo, B., & Brock, D.W. (1997). Palliative options of last resort: A comparison of voluntarily stopping eating and drinking, terminal sedation, physician-assisted suicide, and voluntary active euthanasia. *J Amer Med Assoc, 278*(23), 2099-2104.

Schneiderman, L.J., Jecker, N.S., & Jonsen, A.R. (1990). Medical futility: Its meaning and ethical implications. *Ann Intern Med, 112,* 949-954.

The SUPPORT Principal Investigators. (1995). A controlled trial to improve care for seriously ill hospitalized patients: The Study to Understand Prognoses and Preferences for Outcomes and Risks of Treatments (SUPPORT). *J Amer Med Assoc, 274,* 1591-1598.

Sykes, N., & Thorns, A. (2003). Sedative use in the last week of life and the implications for end-of-life decision-making. *Arch Intern Med, 163,* 341-344.

Tomlinson, T., & Brody, H. (1990). Futility and the ethics of resuscitation. *J Amer Med Assoc, 264,* 1276-1280.

Tomlinson, T., & Czlonka, D. (1995). Futility and hospital policy. *Hastings Cent Rep, 25*(3), 28-35.

Tomlinson, T., Howe, K., Notman, M., et al. (1990). An empirical study of proxy consent for elderly persons. *Gerontologist, 30*(1), 54-64.

Truog, R.D., Brett, A.S., & Frader J. (1992). The problem with futility. *N Engl J Med, 326,* 1560-1564.

Weiss, S.C., Emanuel, L.L., Fairclough, D.L., et al. (2001). Understanding the experience of pain in terminally ill patients. *Lancet, 357*(9265), 1311-1315.

CHAPTER

13

Cultural and Spiritual Issues

Diane B. Loseth
Crystal Dea Moore
John A. Mulder
Chad S. Peterson

OBJECTIVES

After the completion of this chapter, the reader should be able to:

1. Understand the importance of cultural and spiritual issues in high quality, individualized palliative care.
2. Understand basic cultural themes in the context of palliative care for the following five groups: African-American, Asian-American, Hispanic, Native American, and Muslim.
3. Comprehend the concepts of spiritual needs, well-being, distress, and suffering as they relate to treating patients with advanced illness.
4. Assess the importance of cultural values and spiritual issues in the lives of patients who are receiving palliative care.

INTRODUCTION

Negotiating the process of dying and death is an intensely personal experience. An individual person facing the reality of a terminal illness or imminent death will draw upon the resources that have been accumulated through a lifetime of experiences. Influences from firsthand exposure to illness, physicians, hospitals, death, funeral homes, and grief (from a variety of losses) all influence the way in which one copes with end-of-life issues. Although there is indeed individual uniqueness in facing death and dying, culture and spirituality play large roles in an individual's response to advanced illness and the dying process.

This chapter provides an introduction to cultural and spiritual influences on patients' adjustment to advanced illness and palliative care. It is not intended to be an exhaustive treatment of either culture or spirituality; the purpose is to enhance palliative care professionals' spiritual and cultural sensitivity, competence, and assessment skills and provide resources for further professional development in these areas. Although culture and spirituality are inextricably linked, particularly spirituality as expressed through religious practices, spirituality is more encompassing than religion and is discussed in more global terms apart from specific American cultural groups. Thus the chapter is divided into two sections. The first section discusses the concept of culture and provides basic information about five cultural groups in the context of palliative and end-of-life care (African-American, Asian-American, Hispanic, Native American, and Muslim). The second section covers broad spiritual concerns and addresses spiritual needs, well-being, distress, assessment, and suffering as they pertain to working with patients and families at the end of life.

CULTURAL IMPACTS ON PALLIATIVE CARE

One's cultural background and heritage establish the framework upon which an end-of-life experience will be manifest, modified by individual, family, and community influences. Health care providers must therefore develop cultural sensitivity, cultural competence, appropriate attitudes, and skills that facilitate high quality, individualized palliative and end-of-life care (Crawley, Marshall, Lo, et al., 2002; Tervalon & Murray-Garcia, 1998). Cultural sensitivity is characterized by awareness and acknowledgment of the central role that culture plays in molding patients' worldviews and values, made apparent by a nonjudgmental attitude when encountering belief systems and customs that vary from one's own. To facilitate this openness, an understanding of one's own cultural beliefs and biases is also central. Cultural competence involves developing a knowledge base about patients' cultural values, beliefs, and behaviors, which can empower health care professionals to communicate with patients and families in an appropriate and respectful manner (Crawley et al., 2002). It is important that providers avoid applying generalized, generic assumptions about various groups and likewise avoid common stereotypes. Failing to take patients cultural values seriously is ethnocentric and compromises rapport, trust, and the working relationships among patients and health care professionals.

Culture, broadly defined, is "the totality of socially transmitted behavior, patterns, arts, beliefs, institutions, and all products of human work and thought typical of a population or community at a given time" (Webster's II New College Dictionary, 1999). A specific culture is often believed to include a group of people who share the same racial background and language, religious/spiritual practices, approaches to family and community life, and worldview. Although culture is often associated with ethnicity, the term also applies to specific religious and spiritual groups, institutions, regional groups, and lifestyle/interest groups (Braun, Pietsch, & Blanchette, 2000). In other words, culture is an encompassing term that can transcend ethnicity or race; it can be thought of as the norms, behaviors, values, and general worldview of a specific interconnected group of people.

The United States can be considered a pluralistic society in which diverse groups maintain their own traditional culture in the context of a shared society. Within this shared society a dominant culture operates, one that is characterized by such values as individual autonomy, democracy, activity, and freedom (Braun et al., 2000). These values are relatively more or less important to other cultural groups in the United States (i.e., subcultures) that participate in the common society, and the relative degree to which dominant and subcultural values and customs are adopted varies considerably among individuals. Braun et al. (2000) suggest that when discussing subcultures, one should consider "the categorization of a person as traditional (functioning well within the subculture but not well within

the dominant culture), bicultural (functioning equally well in both the subculture and the dominant culture), or acculturated (having given up practices of the subculture in favor of the dominant culture)" (p. 4). In the context of palliative and end-of-life care, the values, norms, roles, and expected behaviors that characterize Western medicine and health care organizations interact with the traditions of the dominant culture and its subcultures. Finally, individuals have personal values and beliefs that may or may not correspond to larger cultural systems. Numerous cultural forces simultaneously influence the attitudes, emotions, thoughts, and behaviors of patients with advanced illness or who may be imminently dying. These forces ultimately influence treatment and end-of-life decision making. Figure 13-1 captures these multiple influences on decision-making behaviors.

Although one's coping style when facing advanced illness and end-of-life issues is uniquely personal, general philosophic perspectives exist among various ethnic and cultural groups. Identification of these is not intended to foster generalizations or stereotypes but rather to provide a broader framework that will allow the practitioner to better understand certain practices and behaviors. The importance of assessment of individual perspectives cannot be overemphasized. Kagawa-Singer and Blackhall (2001) quote an insightful patient in their discussion of negotiating cross-cultural boundaries: "You got to find out the identity of the person to even get to know them. Because if you don't know a person, you got to find out his identity...and he's got to open up and tell you these things" (p. 2993). They go on to say, "[Providers] can use knowledge about particular cultural beliefs, values, and practices to respectfully recognize a person's identity and to assess the degree to which an individual patient or family might adhere to their cultural background" (p. 2999).

Each patient's unique life history, family system and social supports, and socioeconomic status provide the context for interpreting the impact of cultural beliefs and traditions on palliative and end-of-life care (Koenig & Gates-Williams, 1995). Table 13-1 provides an assessment format to help clinicians ascertain the level of cultural influence

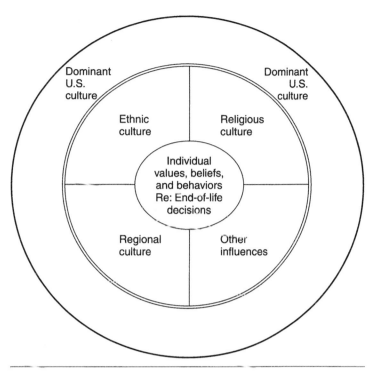

FIGURE **13-1** Multiple influences on end-of-life decision-making behavior. (From Braun, K., Pietsch, J., & Blanchette, P. [2000]. An introduction to culture and its influence on end-of-life decision making. In K. Braun, J. Pietsch, & P. Blanchette [Eds.], *Cultural issues in end-of-life decision making.* Thousand Oaks, Calif.: Sage Publications.)

Table **13-1**   ASSESS ABCDEs TO ASCERTAIN LEVEL OF CULTURAL INFLUENCE

	Relevant Information	Questions and Strategies
Attitudes of patients and families	What attitudes do this ethnic group in general, and the patient and family in particular, have toward truth telling about diagnosis and prognosis? What is their general attitude toward discussions of death and dying? How reflective are their practices of traditional beliefs and practices?	Educate yourself about attitudes common to the ethnic groups most frequently seen in your practice. Determine attitudes of your patient and their family. For example, what is the symbolic meaning of the particular disease?
Beliefs	What are the patient's and family's religious and spiritual beliefs, especially those relating to the meaning of death, the afterlife, the possibility of miracles?	See Box 13-1.

Continued

Table **13-1**   ASSESS ABCDES TO ASCERTAIN LEVEL OF CULTURAL INFLUENCE—CONT'D

	Relevant Information	Questions and Strategies
Context	Questions about the historical and political context of their lives, including place of birth, refugee or immigrations status, poverty, experience with discrimination or lack of access to care, languages spoken, and degree of integration within their ethnic community.	Religious and community organizations may be able to provide general information about the relevant group (see below, "Environment"). Ascertain specific information by asking the following: "Where were you born and raised?" "When did you immigrate to the United States, and what has been your experience coming to a new country? How has your life changed?" "What language would you feel most comfortable speaking to discuss your health concerns?" Life history assessment: "What were other important times in your life, and how might these experiences help us understand your situation?"
Decision-making style	What decision-making styles are held by the group in general and by the patient and family in particular? Is the emphasis on the individual patient making his or her own decisions, or is the approach family-centered?	Learn about the dominant ethnic groups in your practice: How are decisions made in this cultural group? Who is the head of the household? Does this family adhere to traditional cultural guidelines, or do they adhere more to the Western mode?
Environment	What resources are available to aid the effort to interpret the significance of cultural dimensions of a case, including translators, health care workers from the same community, community religious leaders, and family members?	Identify religious and community organizations associated with the ethnic groups common in your practice (hospital social workers and chaplains may be able to help you in this effort).

From Braun, K., Pietsch, J., & Blanchette, P. (2000). An introduction to culture and its influence on end-of-life decision making. In K. Braun, J. Pietsch, & P. Blanchette (Eds.), *Cultural issues in end-of-life decision making.* Thousand Oaks, Calif.: Sage Publications.

experienced by patients and their families. The following general information about end-of-life practices and attitudes can help professionals offer culturally sensitive care, but application of such knowledge without information about the individual leads to stereotyping and can harm working relationships.

African-Americans

As a group, African-Americans are heterogenous; some are descendants of slaves, and others have immigrated from the Caribbean basin or recently from the African continent with no slavery in their backgrounds (Mouton, 2000). According to the 2000 U.S. census, African-Americans make up about

Box 13-1 RESOURCES

CULTURAL

Braun, K., Pietsh, J., & Blanchette, P. (Eds.). (2000). *Cultural issues in end-of-life decision making.* Thousand Oaks, Calif.: Sage Publications.
> An excellent handbook on a variety of cultural issues that pertain to the palliative care setting.

The Cross Cultural Health Care Program.
www.xculture.org
> The CCHCP provides links to numerous resources that address broad cultural issues that have an impact on the health of individuals and families in ethnic minority communities.

Lipson, J., Dibble, S., & Minarik, P. (Eds.). (1996). *Culture and nursing care:* A pocket guide. San Francisco: UCSF Nursing Press.
> A comprehensive guide to various cultural traditions, themes, and mores presented for use in the health care context.

The Office of Minority Health.
www.omhrc.gov
> The mission of the Office of Minority Health (OMH) is to improve and protect the health of racial and ethnic minority populations through the development of health policies and programs that will eliminate health disparities. The website provides many links and resources to support this mission.

Supportive Care of the Dying: A Coalition for Compassionate Care.
www.careofdying.org
> This group has many tools, one of which is a self-assessment of cross-cultural end-of-life care. This tool is for organizations and systems to assess their supportive structures related to culture and spiritual care against standards.

SPIRITUAL

American Academy of Hospice and Palliative Medicine (AAHPM). (2003). **UNIPAC 2:** *Alleviating psychological and spiritual pain in the terminally ill* (2nd ed.). Larchmont, NY: Mary Ann Liebert, Inc. Self-study guide book for physicians.

Ferrell, B.R. (Ed.). (1996). *Suffering.* Boston: Jones & Bartlett.
> Chapters cover multiple aspects of suffering including suffering in the first person, professional studies, and the impact of suffering on family members, clergy, and caregivers.

Gallup, H. (1997). *Spiritual beliefs and the dying process:* A report on a national survey conducted for the Nathan Cummings Foundation and Fetzer Institute. The George H. Gallup International Institute.
> Report of a survey of 1200 persons across the United States related to spirituality and dying. Asks about advance directives, worries, spiritual support, and more.

The George Washington Institute for Spirituality and Health.
www.gwish.org
> A university-based organization dedicated to recognizing the spiritual dimension of health and suffering, to addressing the spiritual needs of patients, and to educating health care professionals about the role of spirituality.

International Working Group on Death, Dying and Bereavement. (1990). Assumptions and principles of spiritual care. *Death Stud, 14,* 75-81.
> Covers definitions of spiritual care, general assumptions, and principles for the individual patient, the family, and the (health) caregivers, plus community coordination and education and research.

The Education for Physicians on End-of-life Care (EPEC). (1999). *Curriculum module #3: Whole person assessment.* The EPEC Project.
> A section of this module covers spiritual assessment and rituals.

National Hospice and Palliative Care Organization. (2001). *Guidelines for spiritual care in hospice.*
> Geared toward chaplains but has some general guidelines applicable to any health care professional.

Continued

Box **13-1**   RESOURCES—CONT'D

RELIGIOUS

Assemblies of God
www.ag.org

B'ahai
www.bcca.org

Baptist
www.sbc.net
www.baptist.org

Buddhism
www.tricycle.com
www.tibet.com

Catholic
www.catholic.net
www.vatican.va

Christian Scientists
www.tfccs.com

Disciples of Christ
www.disciples.org

Episcopal
www.ecusa.org

Greek Orthodox
www.goarch.org

Hinduism
www.hindunet.org

Islam
www.islam.org

Jehovah's Witnesses
www.watchtower.org

Judaism
www.clickonjudaism.org

Lutheran Church-MS
www.lcms.org

Lutheran, Evangelical
www.elca.org

Methodist
www.umc.org

Mormon
www.lds.org

Presbyterian
www.pcusa.org
www.pcanet.org

United Church of Christ
www.ucc.org

12% of the United States population and European-Americans make up 75% of the population. As users of palliative care and hospice services, African-Americans are underrepresented. Whites comprise 83% of the population of patients who participate in hospice care, whereas only 8% of hospice users are African-American. Understanding some of the reasons for this discrepancy can help the clinician who is dealing with African-American patients better assess their attitudes toward dying and palliative care.

The African-American perspective on death and dying has been informed by a unique history: slavery, continued oppression and discrimination, a disproportionate incidence of illness and disease, and differential access to health care all contribute to the general stance of African-Americans that death is something to be overcome (Brant, Ishida, Itano, et al., 2000). The act of dying can therefore be seen as one last expression of the determination that has brought African-Americans social and economic gains in the face of individual and institutional racism. Despite these gains, however, recent studies have documented decreased use of cardiac procedures (Gillum, Mussolino, & Madans, 1997; Johnson, Lee, Cook, et al., 1993; Peterson, Shaw,

DeLong, et al., 1997; Peterson, Wright, Daley, et al., 1994) and renal dialysis (Barker-Cummings, McClellan, Soucie, et al., 1995) for African-American patients with coronary artery disease and end-stage renal disease, respectively, compared with European-American patients. Similar inequalities were found for medical issues as disparate as access to mammograms and renal transplantation and incidence of pneumonia and congestive heart disease. Other studies have demonstrated poorer overall health of African-American patients, shorter life expectancy, and higher incidence of diabetes mellitus, hypertension, end-stage renal disease, cardiovascular disease, stroke, tuberculosis, and acquired immunodeficiency disease (AIDS) (Krakauer, Crenner, & Fox, 2002). Inadequate access to health care, lack of health insurance coverage, and overall mistrust of medical institutions all contribute to these health-related inequities.

These differences between African-Americans and European-Americans regarding health care utilization and access and overall health status are realities that medical professionals working with the African-American community must face. Whether these differences engender a lack of trust by African-Americans toward the medical community as a whole is controversial (Blackhall, Frank, Murphy, et al., 1999; Kao, Green, Zaslavsky, et al., 1998; Krakauer & Truog, 1997; McKinley, Garrett, Evans, et al., 1996). It should be remembered that a member of any minority population might look upon a discussion of do-not-resuscitate (DNR)/do-not-intubate (DNI) as a way to deny care, and this could foster a greater sensitivity when talking about end-of-life issues with these patients. Appreciating the historical context of such possible mistrust, namely slavery, abuses in medical research (e.g., Tuskegee syphilis study), and institutional racism, is helpful in understanding the suspicions of African-Americans.

Other studies have consistently shown ethnic disparities in access to health care. In the Study to Understand Prognoses and Preferences for Outcomes and Risks of Treatment (SUPPORT), researchers found that use of resources for seriously ill African-American patients was lower than for other patients, even after controlling for illness severity and demographics (Borum, Lynn, & Zhong, 2000; Phillips, Hamel, Teno, et al., 1996). Findings from other studies indicate that lower levels of analgesia are used for minority patients with cancer and trauma in a variety of settings, from emergency departments to nursing homes (Bernabei, Gambassi, Lapane, et al., 1998; Cleeland, Gonin, Baez, et al., 1997; Engle, Fox-Hill, & Graney, 1998; Todd, Lee, & Hoffman, 2000). Developing a better understanding of a patient's relationship to his or her pain will foster greater efficacy in ameliorating suffering.

The religious view that pain is a test from God, something to be endured rather than ameliorated, is one that may be held by any patient, but one that might manifest more among African-Americans (Garrett, Harris, Norburn, et al., 1993; Kumasaka & Miles, 1996; Low, 1997). Although on its surface this belief seems to be at odds with the goals of palliative care, the disparity resolves somewhat when the focus is shifted from pain to suffering. All patients should be assessed as individuals, and if a patient chooses to endure a higher level of pain than may be acceptable to the clinician, that clinician can still provide a valuable service to the patient by standing as witness to the dignity with

which that patient faced the pain. This can be accomplished by engaging in a nonjudgmental discussion about what a trial of this kind might mean to the individual who chooses it.

In considering the approach to providing care for the African-American patient at the end of life, certain preferences have been consistently documented in the literature, especially pertaining to use of life-sustaining technologies and advance directives. A study of 800 patients ages 65 years and older who were African-American, Korean-American, Mexican-American, or European-American showed that African-American patients were the most likely to want to be kept alive on life support (Blackhall et al., 1999). Ethnographic interviews conducted as part of that same study suggested that religiosity and barriers to access to health care were important factors in the thinking of many of the African-American participants. Financial resources were also noted to figure prominently in their attitudes toward life-sustaining treatments and toward the physicians who provide them; many participants indicated the expectation that physicians will withdraw life support more quickly if a patient or patient's family has insufficient insurance or is poor. Similar conclusions about the attitude of African Americans toward aggressive life support were drawn by Garrett et al. (1993) and Gramelspacher, Zhou, Hanna, et al. (1997) in studies comparing preferences of African-American patients with those of whites. These data are consistent with other findings that African-Americans are less likely than other ethnic groups to endorse DNR orders for themselves (Murphy, Palmer, Azen, et al., 1996; Phillips, Wenger, Teno, et al., 1996; Shepardson, Gordon, Ibrahim, et al., 1999).

Blackhall, Murphy, Frank, et al. (1995) also found that African-American participants were the most likely of all groups studied to believe that a patient should be told of a diagnosis of metastatic cancer. These participants were also more likely than either Korean-American or Mexican-American subjects to believe that the patient, not the family, should make decisions about the use of life-sustaining technologies. African-American patients are similar to other ethnic groups in their general desire to die at home. It is customary for family members to provide care to the dying patient, possibly explaining in part the findings of Reese, Ahern, Nair, et al. (1999) that African-Americans endorsed a significantly lower interest in hospice care than European-Americans. It is also possible that lack of knowledge about hospice services could contribute to this finding, as could barriers to access to services faced by African-Americans.

Asian-American

The Asian cultures are some of the oldest, and there is considerable variability among the cultural groups classified as Asian/Pacific Islanders (Yeo & Hikoyeda, 2000). Individuals with backgrounds from more than 30 countries and cultures, each with its own language and customs, are classified as Asian-American/Pacific Islanders. Thus this heterogeneous population is enormously complex; an exhaustive recitation of beliefs and norms of all constituents is beyond the scope of this chapter, yet some of the relatively more common and overarching beliefs can be described that can assist palliative care professionals in providing culturally sensitive care to this group.

Asian-Americans tend to endorse a more group-centered attitude toward medical decision making than do European-Americans and African-Americans (Nishimoto & Foley, 2001). The fundamental social unit of the Asian population is the family, and often there is a great deal of interdependence among members. Families are often patriarchal, with age, sex, and generational status important determinants of individual family roles (Balgopal, 1995). Filial piety, the expectation that offspring will unquestioningly care for their parents in gratitude for their parent's love and care, is an important value (Kagawa-Singer & Blackhall, 2001). This has implications for referring Asian-American patients to such services as hospice, where outsiders can play large caregiving roles. The guiding principle of Western medicine, patient autonomy, may produce conflicting expectations for Asian families who have a member with an advanced illness. Yeo and Hikoyeda (2000) provide the example, "Even if an older patient clearly is competent to make decisions...one or more family members might feel that it is their duty to protect

their elder by assuming the decision-making role" (p. 103).

Another Western medical value, truth telling, may run contrary to some Asian-American values vis-à-vis medical diagnoses and prognostication. The direct discussion of death and advanced illness is discouraged in some Asian cultures. For example, 53% of Korean-Americans in one study believed a patient with metastatic cancer should not be told of the diagnosis, and 65% believed a patient should not be informed of a terminal prognosis (Blackhall et al., 1995). This compared with 37% of African-Americans and 31% of European-Americans in the same study who also thought a terminal prognosis should not be shared with the patient. Related to these facts are the findings that Korean-Americans strive to protect their loved ones from the knowledge of a terminal illness while doing everything to keep that loved one alive. It has been shown that even if the eldest son, who usually makes the decisions in these cases, knows that the personal wish of his mother or father is to eschew life-sustaining measures, he will feel bound by filial duty to accept such measures if offered by a physician (Blackhall et al., 1999).

The Asian-American patient's attitude toward fidelity and direct discussion about death and dying needs to be assessed on an individual basis. Yeo and Hikoyeda (2000) cite conflicting evidence in regard to Asian-Americans' willingness to discuss such issues. Depending on the study's methodology, the level of acculturation of the participants, and the Asian group that was studied, preferences varied. In terms of truth telling, some Asian patients may want to know the truth indirectly, euphemistically, or through nonverbal cues (Kagawa-Singer & Blackhall, 2001). *Zhih Yi* is the Chinese term that denotes nonverbal communication, "just knowing what the other thinks and feels," and the Japanese term *inshin denshin* denotes a similar concept of knowing without being told. The Korean word *nunchi* denotes understanding through social, nonverbal cues. The purpose of indirect communication in these cultures is to "preserve the 'face' of the other" (Kagawa-Singer & Blackhall, 2001, pp. 2997-2998). It is important that providers assess the information preferences of each individual patient, asking directly, "How much information about your illness do you want to know? Is there a person in the family that should be given specific details about your illness?" This can help the health care professional communicate with the patient and family in the most sensitive way.

An examination of Korean-American attitudes toward dying and death gleaned from research provides an interesting and illustrative paradox (Blackhall et al., 1995). Studies show that this group is most likely to endorse the use of life-sustaining technologies for other people but also are most likely to reject these interventions for themselves. The explanation for the difference between general and personal views held by Korean-American participants was explained by the tendency of Koreans to focus on the family as the decision-making unit. So, although an individual might believe that life-sustaining technologies are acceptable in the abstract, he or she would leave the decision about use of such interventions in his or her particular case up to the family or a single designated decision maker (usually the eldest male) within the immediate family.

Similar to other Asian-American groups, Japanese-Americans tend to adopt a strongly group-centered approach to decision making. They may feel that conversations about DNR/DNI issues will hasten the death of the patient, but they may nod their heads in seeming agreement when approached about such discussions. As with every ethnic group, certain cultural beliefs may have a direct impact on patient care at the end of life. For example, placing the patient with his or her head facing north or with his or her feet facing the door might be a source of stress to the Japanese-American patient (or family) who believes that those positions are used only for the dead (Nishimoto & Foley, 2001). Another important cultural concept, honor, is well accounted for in the palliative care literature (Shiba & Oka, 1996). It is a point of honor, for example, to be present at the bedside of a family member at the time of death. Adults typically are not expected to produce great shows of sorrow upon the death of a loved one, although crying is permissible. Contrary to European-Americans, Japanese-Americans are more likely to show support

for the bereaved through silence than through touching. The typical color of mourning is black (in contrast, for example, to that of Chinese mourners, who generally wear white) (Nishimoto & Foley, 2001).

In terms of the diversity among Asian-Americans related to grief, Cambodian-Americans believe that excessive grieving is detrimental and can lead to *pruit chiit/kiit chraen,* a condition in which one experiences headaches and dizziness from thinking too much about a deceased family member (Yeo & Hikoyeda, 2000). The Buddhist tradition, on the other hand, encourages ritualistic, continued contact with the deceased for decades after death. Neither of these extremes is commonly considered typical by Western psychiatric standards, but interventions aimed at changing either of these attitudes would be seen as inappropriate at best by the respective grievers. Clearly, an open and flexible stance is most helpful when discussing issues of this nature.

The question of degree of acculturation and its influence on beliefs about and needs during the dying process is one that can (and arguably should) be asked of every individual regardless of cultural background. In a fascinating study comparing Japanese-Americans with their Japanese counterparts, Matsumura, Bito, Liu, et al. (2002) found that the degree of acculturation of the patient predicted a shift toward more traditionally Western ways of approaching care at the end of life where disclosure, willingness to forego care, and attitudes toward advance care planning were concerned. In contrast, they found that the desire for group-based decision making was relatively preserved. This study has implications not only for the care of the patient but also for formulating an approach to dealing with the entire family system in which different generations exhibit different degrees of acculturation. It can be anticipated that family and/or couples therapy might be a useful approach to bridging different viewpoints within a given family system (Mohr, Moran, Kohn, et al., 2003).

The issue of language must also be considered when working with anyone from a different culture. This is especially true in Asian cultures, where words with very similar pronunciations can have completely different meanings. Neither Taiwanese-American nor Japanese-Americans are generally comfortable when the number *four* is part of the room number; the pronunciation of the numeral is similar or identical to that for death in both languages. As another example, the pronunciation of the word *clock* in Chinese is the same as that for the word *ending*; clearly it could be distressing for a Chinese patient to receive a clock when he or she is sick or dying. It would not be practical to list all the homonymous intricacies that exist when dealing with patients from different linguistic backgrounds, but being mindful of such complications can help the health care team better understand the needs of these populations.

Hispanic-Americans (Latinos)

The Hispanic culture comprises numerous subcultures that are often lumped together by non-Hispanics. These groups share the common language of Spanish yet may have different countries of origin. Some of these subgroups include Mexican-Americans, Cubans, Puerto Ricans, Central Americans, and South Americans. The experiences in their countries of origin, with immigration or colonization, influence each group's own cultural perspective (Talamantes, Gomez, & Braun, 2000). Hispanics can come from any racial group (e.g., Asian, Caucasian, Negroid) and, as with other cultural groups, differ in respect to their level of acculturation and adherence to cultural norms and mores.

Although considerable cultural diversity exists among the Hispanic subcultures, there are some common cultural themes or "Pan-Hispanic values" (Talamantes et al., 2000, p. 85). Religion plays a large role in the lives of Hispanic-Americans, with most identifying as Christian, particularly Roman Catholic (Sandoval, 2003; Talamantes et al., 2000). In an examination of the Hispanic-American culture in the context of providing medical support to patients with human immunodeficiency virus (HIV)/AIDS, Sandoval (2003) discusses the works of Bastida, Cuellar, and Ferris, identifying six broad cultural themes:

- Familismo: emphasis on the welfare of the family over individual welfare

- Personalismo: trust that is built over time manifested by expressions of mutual respect
- Jerarquismo: respect for hierarchy
- Presentismo: time orientation that emphasizes the present, not the past or future
- Espiritismo: the belief that spirits, both good and evil, can influence health and overall well-being
- Fatalismo: the belief that fate is an inescapable determinant of life outcomes, including one's health status

These values manifest themselves in many Hispanics' attitudes toward end-of-life and palliative care issues.

In consideration of these values, Talamantes et al. (2000) indicate that health care professionals should include family members in medical discussions when working with Hispanic patients. Providers should also be aware that presentismo may make advance care planning difficult, but advance care planning that culminates from a clinical relationship based on mutual respect, trust, and rapport is possible. Latinos' tendency to defer to authority makes it important to ensure that patients are not agreeing with the provider out of respect. Finally, learning about various spiritual beliefs and their relationships to preferences about autopsy and organ donation is vital to providing culturally sensitive palliative care.

Although Mexican-Americans represent only one segment of the rapidly growing Latino population in America, they are the largest subgroup (Talamantes et al., 2000), and consideration of their experiences at the end of life illustrates the difficulties involved in delivering care to such a differentially acculturated demographic. The Mexican-American view of death is informed by centuries of ritual surrounding death and the afterlife, as well as by beliefs of Catholicism. Given the diversity of beliefs found in Mexico itself, it is not surprising that there is broad variability in perceptions of Mexican-Americans. In Mexico, children are exposed to death at an early age. They are present at rituals such as the Day of the Dead and are present during mourning for the deceased (Munet-Vilaro, 1998). The family is also commonly intimately involved in care of sick and dying members.

It is thought that this exposure to death at an early age may decrease anxiety about the dying process.

In America, the family structure tends to be more fragmented than it is in Mexico, raising the possibility that support for dying family members may be diminished. Indeed, studies suggest that social forces such as immigration and acculturation have impaired the family's ability to care for its ill members. One study in the mid-1990s reported that 30% of Mexican-Americans believed they would no longer have a caregiver if they became debilitated by illness (Talamantes et al., 1996). The cultural expectation that the family take care of its ill members may lead to a reluctance of Mexican-American families to seek hospice care. Data from the National Hospice and Palliative Care Organization (2001) show a decrease in the percent of hospice patients of Hispanic descent from 4% in 1995 to 2.3% in 2000. Understanding the reasons for this trend might help to better facilitate outreach to those Hispanic patients who might benefit from hospice care but who experience barriers to access. This tendency to avoid hospice care, combined with the difficulties of providing such care at home within the context of fragmented families and economic realities, may result in many Mexican-Americans receiving inadequate care (Gelfand, Balcazar, Parzuchowski, et al., 2001).

In a study that examined attitudes of European-Americans, Mexican-Americans, Korean Americans, and African-Americans, Mexican-Americans were the most likely to support the use of life-sustaining technologies both in general and for themselves personally (Blackhall et al., 1999). This desire may in part explain why one large survey showed that more Mexican-Americans than other ethnic groups died in the hospital (Iwashyna & Chang, 2002). Mexican-Americans tend to believe that the patient should not be informed of a terminal diagnosis; however, they strongly believe that the patient's family should be informed. This is consistent with their more family-centered approach to medical decision making as compared with European-Americans and is more similar to the approach endorsed by Korean-Americans (Blackhall et al., 1995). In fact, a recent study (Gelfand et al., 2001) showed that patient discussions with family

members about dying were discouraged. Instead, it was found that shielding the patient from a terminal diagnosis and "encouraging" him or her (i.e., providing hope of recovery) were deemed more valuable. Consistent with the desire of the family to protect the patient from a terminal diagnosis was the finding that, although prayer was considered to be useful, having a priest visit the dying patient was not generally acceptable since this was a sure sign that the patient was in fact dying.

Native Americans

There are approximately 2 million Native Americans in the United States, constituting more than 300 federally recognized tribes. As the original inhabitants of North America, they have been subjected to a history of systematic annihilation and subjugation by the European settlers and U.S. Government. In providing an overview of the Native American relationship with the U.S. Government, Van Winkle (2000) indicates during the westward expansion, when European-Americans were often clashing with the indigenous peoples, government policies pushed assimilation (e.g., The Dawes General Allotment Act of 1887). This resulted in the loss of Native American life and land. In 1934, the Indian Reorganization Act allowed tribes to self-govern and granted control to the tribes over certain matters, yet the government still controlled many of the tribes' affairs (e.g., financial matters, natural resources). After the tumultuous 1960s, the federal government began to shift its policy emphasis toward more tribal autonomy with such pieces of legislation as the Indian Self-Determination and Education Assistance Act of 1975 and the Indian Health Care Improvement Act of 1976. More legislation was passed over the next 2 decades, and many tribes have contracts with the federal government to provide social services including education and health care. It is not surprising that many Native Americans distrust the government and other institutions associated with the dominant culture.

Native American tribes have discrete languages and lifestyles, as well as unique cultures in art, music, dance, and life-cycle rituals, belief systems, social organization, coping strategies, and instruction for their young (Parillo, 1997). Although there are many obvious differences, some similarities exist among the various tribal groups. In general, Native American culture rests primarily on the value of living in harmony with nature. Overall, the beliefs that all things are interdependent and the world is interconnected structure Native American community practices, religious beliefs, and family values. Customarily, Native American tribes find individual and family relationships very important and they value the maintenance of extended family networks. Through these networks, there is generally a strong collective sense of family solidarity. Decisions usually are made by group and family consensus, rather than on an individual basis. Many Native Americans value silence and are not outspoken about their needs, especially with strangers. They tend to avoid confrontation and have a strong affiliation with both their church and community (Van Winkle, 2000).

Native American religions include Christianity, pan–Native American religions, and the Native American Church. Many of the Native American practices include believing in supernatural phenomena and spiritual forces. There is also a focus on Native American and Christian spiritual beings (e.g., the Great Spirit, saints, Christ), as well as reverence for ancestors and nature. An evident connection between spirituality and health care attitudes is among these groups. Many Native Americans tend to view disease as a problem that is caused by spiritual force rather than being of biologic origin. Life and death are viewed as part of a circular pattern, rather than in a linear Western view (Van Winkle, 2000). Some groups see the harmony of the endless circle of creation and re-creation manifested by the life-death cycle: "interred bodies return nourishment to the earth; the earth makes plants grow; the plants feed the animals; the animals feed humanity" (Lombardi & Lombardi, 1982, p. 36 as cited by Van Winkle, 2000). Given this spiritual vantage point, Native Americans view death as a natural and acceptable part of life, although tribal groups do vary with respect to their customs related to death and dying. For example, it is taboo for the Navajo to touch the body of the deceased to prohibit the spirit of the dead person from contaminating them (Van Winkle, 2000).

The historical context of the European-American settlement of the United States and the common spiritual and cultural themes has an impact on the Native American perspective on health care. Native Americans are eligible for health care sponsored by the U.S. Government, and many members of these cultural groups view Western health care on the whole as undesirable, especially at end of life. Although funding for Native American health care services has never been adequate, Van Winkle (2000) reports Indian Health Services statistics that demonstrate a decrease in maternal and infant mortality and an increase in the life expectancy among Native American peoples from the early 1970s compared with the early 1990s, corresponding with increases in funding.

Although there is little research on end-of-life decision making among Native-American groups, based on their historical context as well as the extant literature that does exist, Van Winkle (2000) offers these suggestions for those providing palliative and end-of-life care to this population:

- Health care professionals need to understand that there is great diversity in beliefs, customs, and values among various tribes, and this variation is further complicated by an individual's level of acculturation.
- An understanding of specific tribal customs is important, as is the assessment of individual patient's adherence to those traditions and values.
- Patient autonomy in the context of consensus and cooperation among extended family and tribe members can be a guiding principle in negotiating the many treatment decisions that accompany the end of life. The patient should be asked to define who is considered family.
- Many Native Americans prefer to have family members stay with a hospitalized patient to help in the recovery process. Institutional policy should allow for this continued, around-the-clock social support of hospitalized patients.
- Language issues should be considered. Do the patient and/or family need an interpreter? If family members are used as interpreters, are they able to adequately present the medical information that needs to be communicated?

- Communication styles among Native American patients and their Western medical professionals may conflict. For example, direct eye contact is not appropriate for some tribes, and many members of these groups value silence and take time to respond during conversations. Health care professionals need to become comfortable with silence when interacting with these patients.
- Some Native American patients may prefer indirect communication. For example, a discussion of a patient's perspective as to how a loved one or friend was medically managed could be a way of communicating about that patient's treatment preferences.
- Advance care planning may be difficult with some Native American patients. For example, the Navajo believe that language can shape reality, so discussions about death can have deadly consequences (Caresse & Rhodes, 1995). Given their history of broken treaties and oppression in the dominant culture, Native Americans may be reticent to put their end-of-life wishes in writing and sign forms that can limit care. For some members of this group, advance care planning may be best done verbally with the family actively participating in the process.
- Western medical professionals can work with traditional healers identified by the patient to provide palliative care that is truly holistic to Native American patients.
- Again, attitudes toward death and dying vary among tribes; thus some are accepting of death and others view dying people and death with fear (Lewis, 1990). Therefore some Native Americans want their family members to die at home, others prefer a hospital setting, and others will stay away from places where a person has died (Kramer, 1996).

Muslims

Although Muslims are a cultural group defined by religious belief and practices and not an ethnicity or nationality, the growth of the Muslim movement in the United States underscores the importance of understanding Islamic attitudes toward dying and death. The literature on this topic is limited, however. A recent review of the topic provides an excellent introduction into the rich complexities of Islamic faith and highlights important points about death and dying (Sarhill, LeGrand, Islambouli, et al., 2001). Muslims believe in God (Allah) and all other Semitic prophets, although they do not worship the prophets as they do Allah. The word *Islam* means submission to the will of Allah. This definition dictates many of the beliefs and behaviors one observes when working with the dying Muslim. God's last prophet is Mohammed, whose traditions shape the practices of Muslims to a large degree. Muslims practice prayer five times a day and observe fasting from sunrise to sunset every day during the month of Ramadan.

The Koran (the Islamic Holy Book) describes death as a transition from one segment of life to another; however, one must experience a day of judgment before passing on. The Islamic definition of death according to the Koran is only loosely defined by the standards of Western medicine. For example, death is defined as the soul's departure from the body, but clear physical signs of death are not elucidated in the Koran. Therefore brain death is not defined as true death because some bodily functions persist in this state (Sheikh, 1998). This stance is consistent with the Muslim belief that life is a sacred gift from Allah (suicide is strictly and specifically prohibited in Islamic law, which may in part explain the low incidence of suicide among Muslims).

A Muslim patient should optimally be attended by doctors and nurses of the same sex if at all possible. Some Muslim patients will in fact refuse to be attended by a provider of the opposite sex. Muslim women will wish to remain clothed from head to toe and should be asked permission before uncovering an arm for invasive procedures such as blood draws. Consumption of certain foods is restricted in the Muslim tradition. Therefore, patients should be asked specifically about this upon admission to the hospital. By Islamic law, alcohol may not be consumed, so patients should be informed when they are receiving formulations of drugs that use alcohol. Other Muslim practices include prayer five times daily. Significant anxiety may arise if this need is not met by positioning bed-bound patients toward Mecca. It must also be kept in mind that Muslims cannot pray until they have washed properly. This ritual involves washing face, ears, forehead, arms, hands, and feet in running water. The nose, mouth, and genitals must also be washed. This procedure might be difficult to fully accommodate in a hospital or hospice setting, but effort should be made to provide appropriate access to water.

Because Muslims hold such strong feelings about the sanctity of life, euthanasia is not acceptable in the Islamic faith (Gatrad, 1994). However, because Muslims view the material life as continuous with the afterlife, prolongation of life using ventilators is not generally acceptable. Hospital or hospice staff should work closely with the patient to formulate a DNR order that respects these complex beliefs.

Muslims share the almost universal desire to die at home. If a Muslim dies in the hospital, family members need to be allowed to perform certain important rituals on the deceased. After death, the face is turned toward Mecca. The arms and legs are straightened and the toes bound together by string. The mouth and eyes are closed and a ritual body wash is performed by a family member of the same sex. The body is then wrapped in a simple white cloth, which may have been prepared especially for this use by the deceased during his or her lifetime. Muslims are always buried, and they are resistant to autopsy. In many circumstances, the standard practice of engaging a funeral home for embalming and burial is eschewed in favor of involvement of members of the faith community, who will typically prepare and bury the body within 24 hours. Strong, voluble displays of grief are generally not encouraged, although grief is shared and processed by the family. The extent of grief resolution by the family should be evaluated before counseling is discussed.

Conclusion: Cultural Influences

Facing one's own mortality is a disorganizing and frequently overwhelming experience (Yalom, 1980). As can be seen from the preceding discussion, different cultures have developed similar but unique ways of coping with some of the feelings of isolation and disorientation brought about by a life-limiting illness. The preceding section focuses primarily on the actions or rituals used in different cultures to orient the patient and provide him or her with a sense of identity, community, and support during what is arguably the most trying time in a person's life. This information can provide a very basic level of knowledge related to these groups. However, to provide individualized, culturally sensitive palliative care, health care professionals must assess individual patients' levels of acculturation and attitudes toward cultural values and traditions. Approaching each patient as a unique person allows the treatment team to explore an individual's concerns about his or her death from the broadest possible perspective. Such a holistic approach guards against generalizations and stereotypes that present barriers to alleviation of the total suffering of the palliative care patient, allowing for a richer experience for patient and clinicians alike (Block, 2001).

SPIRITUAL ISSUES IN PALLIATIVE CARE

As patients approach the end of their lives, it is often a time of life review and a search for meaning and purpose. Spirituality encompasses one's search for meaning, for transcendence. For some, the search may begin at the time of diagnosis and continues throughout the illness. For others, it becomes paramount in the dying phase of life and may be the ultimate crisis of their lives. The origin of spirituality is spirit, the Latin *spiritus*—breath. It can be thought of as that which gives the patient breath, a life force. But often spirituality is confused with religion. Spirituality is more encompassing than religion. Religion is a formal set of beliefs, tenets, and practices of a particular faith. It is only one way that patients express their spirituality.

In medicine and nursing, health care providers have traditionally addressed the physical, emotional, and social aspects of care. Great strides have been made in caring for the physical needs of patients at the end of life, and emotional and social needs are now beginning to be addressed, but spiritual needs of patients need more attention. In recent years, interest in this dimension of patient care has steadily increased. Traditionally, the spiritual dimension has been thought of as exclusively the domain of clergy, but if care is to focus on the whole person, health care providers must become sensitive to this dimension, learning ways to assess and care for the spiritual needs of patients.

Spiritual Needs

Several authors have addressed spirituality in terms of needs. Highfield and Cason (1983) identified four needs: the need for meaning and purpose in life, the need to receive love, the need to give love, and the need for hope and creativity. They then identified signs of spiritual problems and signs of spiritual health within each need. For instance, the patient might express despair or feeling no reason to live, as a sign of a spiritual problem under the need for meaning. The patient may worry about a loss of faith in God or express feelings of guilt, as a sign of a need to receive love. As a sign of spiritual problems, within the need to give love, the patient might worry about financial issues, worry about separation, and/or have difficulty expressing love. The last need, the need for hope and creativity, is where the patient might express fears of loss of control or deny the reality of the illness. Even though some of these needs may appear to have only a psychosocial dimension, the authors contend that different interventions are necessary when a problem is identified as a psychosocial versus a spiritual need. For example, if a problem is identified in the psychologic domain but is truly of a spiritual nature, a pastoral care referral might have been missed.

Clinebell (1988), a noted pastoral care expert, identified nine basic spiritual needs. Two of the needs are specifically related to God in terms of a relationship with God and having an awareness of God's love. The rest are more spiritual in the global sense. They have to do with developing a philosophy of life, values to guide life, and a higher sense of self or "soul as the center of their whole being" (p.110). The rest of the needs are for maintaining hope in the midst of losses, belonging to a caring community, discovering ways to move toward reconciliation of forgiveness, and having regular moments of transcendence.

Moadel, Morgan, Fatone, et al. (1999) investigated the spiritual and existential needs of 248 cancer patients in an outpatient clinic. Almost 60% were patients who had recurrent disease, and it was not specified if any were approaching the end of life. Patients indicated that they wanted help in overcoming fears, finding hope, finding meaning in their lives now, and finding spiritual resources. They also indicated a desire to talk with someone about finding peace of mind, the meaning of life, and issues concerning death and dying. Another study described five domains that cancer patients found important (Singer, Martin, & Kelner, 1999). Patients reported that they want adequate symptom control, not to be a burden, not to prolong the dying process, to strengthen relationships with loved ones, and to achieve a sense of spiritual peace. It is easy to put these domains into the perspective of needs, for example, that patients have a need not to be a burden or have a need for spiritual peace.

Hermann (2001) conducted semi-structured interviews with hospice patients, and he expressed the themes in terms of spiritual needs. His two interview questions were: "What does the word *spiritual* means to you personally?" and "What needs can you identify related to your spirituality as you described it?" Analysis yielded six major themes: the need for religion, for companionship, for involvement and control, for a positive outlook, to experience nature, and to finish business. Another qualitative study by Murray, Kendall, Boyd, et al. (2004) involved interviews with patients dying of heart failure or lung cancer. Their findings revealed that patients do experience significant spiritual needs. The aspects of spiritual need with which they analyzed the interviews were expressions of despair, fear, isolation, relationship issues, losing control, and knowing where to fit in, trying to make sense of the illness. Byock (2004), a noted palliative care physician, identifies four needs that may touch on the spiritual: the need to ask for forgiveness, to offer forgiveness, to say thank you, and to say goodbye. Being able to do these four things before one dies can be a transforming experience—even a spiritual experience. He identified these needs through his life's experience as a physician in the emergency room and then as a hospice and palliative care physician. Even though he writes of these in the context of dying, he admits that they are applicable any time.

Kellehear (2000) explains spiritual need as multidimensional, comprising three distinct dimensions of needs. The first dimension is situational needs, those needs that include purpose, meaning and affirmation, hope, connectedness, social presence, and mutuality. These needs come from the immediacy of the illness. The second dimension, moral and biographic needs, have to do with peace and reconciliation, reunion with others, forgiveness, moral and social analysis, prayer, and closure. The final dimension is one of religious need. This dimension includes religious reconciliation, divine forgiveness and support, visits by clergy, religious rites/sacraments, religious literature, and discussion about God, eschatology, eternal life, and hope. He believes that these different aspects of spirituality do not compete with each other but are part of the human need to find meaning in illness and suffering. This ability to make meaning can contribute to one's spiritual well-being.

Spiritual Well-being

Another way spirituality has been conceptualized is through spiritual well-being. David Moberg, a sociologist and research pioneer in this area, developed the concept of vertical and horizontal dimensions of spiritual well-being (Moberg & Bruseck, 1978). The vertical dimension describes one's relationship with God. The horizontal dimension describes one's perception of life's purpose and satisfaction. It was from this framework with Paloutzian and Ellison (1982) that a 20-item instrument was developed—the Spiritual Well-Being Scale, which includes religious well-being (RWB) and existential well-being (EWB). The ten RWB questions all refer to God and can be problematic for the patient whose sense of spirituality does not include a monotheistic deity. In these earlier years, most of the research on spirituality and health has been related to a particular faith tradition or religiosity and its effect on coping and mental health, on disease states such as cancer and heart disease, and on mortality and morbidity (Larson, 1993; Matthews & Larson, 1995; Matthews,

Larson, & Barry, 1993; Matthews & Saunders, 1997).

In the first decade after Moberg and Brusek began to develop the concepts of spiritual well-being in research, only three studies investigated the spirituality of patients at the end of life. Yates, Chalmer, St. James, et al. (1981) studied 71 patients with cancer with a prognosis of 3 to 12 months. They noted that higher levels of well-being were associated with greater religious activity and connections and with lower pain levels. It is interesting to note that those patients with a higher level of spiritual well-being did not live longer. O'Brien (1982) investigated patients with end-stage renal disease who were on hemodialysis. Her purpose was to observe changes in religious faith and the impact of these changes on adjustment to this disease, specifically the correlation between religious affiliation, religious participation and social functioning, religion, and sick-role behavior. The sick-role behavior was indicated by compliance with the treatment regimen. The most compliant and least alienated patients were also those whose perceived religious faith was associated with acceptance of their condition and its treatment. For those patients whom she was able to interview 3 years later, 27% changed from a negative to positive attitude or had increased the degree of religious importance. Finally, Reed (1986, 1987) conducted two studies, with the second an extension of the first, using her Spiritual Perspective Scale. Demographic variables were accounted for by matching age, gender, education, and religious background in three groups of 100 patients each. The participants were terminally ill and hospitalized, non-terminally ill and hospitalized, or healthy and non-hospitalized. The terminally ill patients showed the greatest spiritual perspective when compared with the other groups.

More recently, a study of cancer and AIDS patients with a life expectancy of 6 months or less investigated the impact of spirituality and religiosity on depressive symptom severity (Nelson, Rosenfeld, Breitbart, et al., 2002). The AIDS patients and the cancer patients were analyzed separately because of major demographic differences. Overall, the results showed that patients who had a lower score of meaning/peace were more likely to be depressed. It is interesting to note that the relationship between the faith and depression was not significant. McClain, Rosenfeld, and Breitbart (2003) also investigated hope and mood but added desire for hastened death into their research as well. They found lower levels of spiritual well-being to be associated with hopelessness, desire for hastened death, and suicidal ideation in patients who were terminally ill. Hopelessness had the highest negative correlation to spiritual well-being. In addition, those with high scores on the spiritual well-being scale and high scores on the depression scale were not correlated with a desire for hastened death. This was in contrast with those patients who had a low sense of spirituality and high depression who were more likely to have a desire for hastened death. Similar to Nelson et al. (2002), the meaning/peace aspect of spirituality had stronger correlations with hopelessness, desire for hastened death, and suicidal ideation than did faith. Their overall conclusion was that spiritual well-being may offer some sort of protection against hopelessness and desire for hastened death.

Several studies were conducted in patients with life-threatening illnesses, but it was not clear if any of these patients were at the end of life or dying. One study (Fehring, Miller, & Shaw, 1997) addressed mood, hope, and spirituality. Higher sense of spirituality was correlated with hope and positive mood states, and lower spirituality scores were associated with depression in these elderly cancer patients. In a study that investigated enjoyment of life related to spirituality but also included symptoms experienced by the participants, cancer and AIDS patients were able to still enjoy life, even with symptoms such as pain or fatigue, if they also had a higher sense of meaning and peace or a greater sense of faith (Brady, Peterman, Fitchett, et al., 1999). Only a small percentage of those with high levels of symptoms and low levels of meaning and peace were able to experience significant enjoyment of life. Chibnall, Videen, Duckro, et al. (2002) studied patients with life-threatening illness and examined death distress and spirituality. The patients in this research had a wide variety of diseases, and physical, psychosocial, spiritual, and other factors were analyzed in relation to death distress. The authors

found lower spiritual well-being was associated with higher death distress.

Some of the spiritual well-being work has been done through the development of instruments for research, including the Spiritual Well-Being Scale and the Spiritual Perspective Scale that were mentioned earlier. Over the years, as the view of spirituality has become less God-focused, researchers have developed spiritual well-being tools that are less religiously oriented and incorporate wider definitions of spirituality. Some of these tools were designed as quality-of-life tools, having included a spiritual dimension. Others are stand-alone spiritual well-being instruments. The McGill Quality of Life Questionnaire (Cohen, Mount, Tomas, et al., 1996) was validated in cancer patients in all stages of the disease including those without evidence of disease. It has four subscales addressing the physical, psychologic, and support systems and existential concerns.

The Functional Assessment of Chronic Illness Therapy–Spiritual Well-Being Scale (FACIT–Sp) (Brady et al., 1999; Peterman, Fitchett, Brady, et al., 2002) is a subscale of a functional assessment scale for those with a chronic illness but does not exclude those with a life-threatening illness. It covers meaning and purpose in addition to the faith factor: the strength and comfort of one's faith or beliefs. The System of Belief Inventory (SBI) (Holland, Kash, Passik, et al., 1998), developed at a cancer center, was originally studied in patients with a life-threatening illness. It stands alone and is not part of a larger quality-of-life tool. It addresses the patients' spirituality in terms of beliefs and practices and social support from a faith community.

Although these tools do not exclude patients at the end of life, only one was designed specifically for dying patients. The Missoula-VITAS Quality of Life Index (Byock, 1998) inquires about patients' symptoms, function, interpersonal relationships, well-being, and the transcendent. The transcendent questions concern being at peace and having meaning and connectedness. The most recent tool is the QUAL-E or Quality of Life at the End of Life developed by Steinhauser, Bosworth, Clipp, et al. (2002). Through in-depth interviews and focus groups with patients, families, and health care providers, they identify five domains as important to the quality of life in dying patients: physical symptoms, relationships with the health care system, worries and fears, social support, and completion. The completion aspect involves finding meaning and purpose or a sense of peace. Patients who struggle with completion and meaning can experience spiritual distress.

Spiritual Distress

Another way to think about spirituality is from the perspective of spiritual distress. The struggle of the search for meaning can be identified as spiritual distress or distress of the human spirit. It is defined in terms of a disruption in the life principle that infuses the patient with a variety of characteristics that are both religiously oriented and existentially oriented. Some of the characteristics could be viewed either from a psychologic perspective or a spiritual perspective. For instance, the patient who engages in self-blame or experiences nightmares could be seen as having a psychologic problem or a spiritual problem (Kim, McFarland, & McLane, 1987). Milton Hay, a chaplain, describes spiritual distress in terms of spiritual diagnoses and problems. He identified four spiritual diagnoses, each with a statement of the problem, a definition, defining characteristics, assessments, goals/expected outcomes, and interventions. His four diagnoses are religious request, belief system problem, inner resource deficiency, and spiritual suffering (Hay, 1989).

Other nurse authors conceptualized spiritual distress of dying patients in terms of Kübler-Ross' stages at the end of life (1969) with stages of spiritual development (Stepnick & Perry, 1992). And finally, the National Comprehensive Cancer Network developed practice guidelines entitled "Distress." They integrated psychologic, social, and spiritual areas of distress into one document. The guidelines define distress as "an unpleasant emotional experience of a psychological (cognitive, behavioral, emotional), social, and/or spiritual nature that may interfere with the ability to cope effectively with cancer and its treatment" (National Comprehensive Cancer Network [NCCN], 2003). The areas identified as specifically spiritual are pastoral services, isolation from religious community, guilt, conflict between religious beliefs and recommended treatments, hopelessness, and ritual need. Each area has an algorithm outlining the steps a clinician might take in addressing spiritual distress. NCCN also published practice guidelines for palliative care (NCCN, 2004) wherein psychosocial issues, goals, hopes, expectations, concerns, and the religious/spiritual dimension are addressed briefly. These tools encourage the clinician to be aware of this dimension, offering support to the patient.

Spiritual Assessment

Over the same period, the idea of spiritual assessment has also developed. Much of the earlier work has been in the area of research as just noted in the "Spiritual Needs" and "Spiritual Well-being" sections. Many of those tools are cumbersome for patients and may be especially burdensome for patients at the end of life when energy levels are often minimal. Ruth Stoll (1979), a nurse, developed one of the earliest tools and in 1979 offered guidelines for spiritual assessment. She assessed four distinct areas of spirituality: the patient's (1) concept of a deity, (2) source of strength and hope, (3) significance of religious practices and rituals, and (4) perceived relationship between spiritual beliefs and health. Each of these four areas had specific questions to ask the patient.

Carpenito (1997) took the nursing diagnosis of *Spiritual Distress* and applied it to clinical practice. She offers several spiritual assessment questions that ask about the importance of religion or source of strength and the effect of the illness. Two other questions are more religiously focused, asking about religious leaders and religious materials that are important, and, finally, how the nurse might help the patient maintain the patient's spiritual strength. Farran, Fitchett, Quiring-Emblen, et al., a group of nurses and chaplains, developed the 7×7 Model (1989). Their model actually includes medical, psychologic, psychosocial, family systems, ethnic and cultural, and societal dimensions of assessment, in addition to the spiritual dimension. Within the spiritual dimension are then seven areas of assessment: beliefs and meaning, vocation and consequences, experience and emotions, courage and growth, ritual and practice, community, and, finally, authority and guidance (Fitchett, 1993). In its totality, this assessment would be too cumbersome for the busy clinician and burdensome for the patient, especially the patient at the end of life.

Another guide for spiritual assessment, specifically designed for nursing, has to do more with assisting the provider with finding spiritual resources for the patient and family (Highfield, 1993, 2000). The nurse is asked to give the patient *Permission* to talk about spiritual issues, to give the patient/family *Limited* or brief information on how to contact clergy, to *Activate* resources for the patient/family, and to provide *Non-Nursing* functions such as obtaining assistance from clergy when the spiritual issues are beyond the scope of the nurse. The assessment's acronym is *PLAN*. Although PLAN was developed for nurses, any health care provider can complete this model of assessment, but it does lack guidelines for spiritual areas to explore with the patient.

Another assessment tool is the set of HOPE questions (Anandarajah & Hight, 2001). These physician authors developed this tool to help teach medical students, residents, and practicing physicians to incorporate spiritual assessment into their practice with their patients. The following explains the acronym of *HOPE. H:* sources of hope, meaning, peace, strength; *O:* organized religion, its importance and support; *P:* personal spirituality and practices; and *E:* effects on medical and end-of-life issues.

The last assessment instrument is the *FICA.* Pulchalski and Romer (2000) formulated this acronym. The first dimension, *Faith* or beliefs, simply assesses for the presence of faith or belief. It is more unusual for the patient to report none, but that can be followed up with inquiring about what gives meaning or purpose to the individual. *Importance* and *Influence* are those things that the patient considers important in life, how these beliefs influence coping with dying or making end-of-life decisions. *Community,* the third dimension, asks if the patient participates in or is part of a religious or spiritual community and the degree to which this community is currently supportive. Finally, *Address* or *Application* refers to how the patient wants the clinician to help him or her

address the identified concerns. Although Pulchaski believes that clinicians should be assessing spirituality at any point in the patient's life, it is in the care of the dying that the spiritual dimension becomes increasingly important. These assessment tools are not validated but come from the research studies on spiritual needs, well-being, and distress.

These formal tools are guides to use. In addition to these spiritual assessment tools, there are simple cues for the clinician to notice and to respond to:

- Has the patient spoken of fate, hope, faith, or prayers or made "gallows humor" remarks or comments about life review?
- What do you notice in the patient's environment (facility or home)? Are there articles of a particular faith, reading materials, cards, clothing, items on the walls?
- Have you ever observed any spiritual behaviors (e.g., praying, meditating, reading spiritual materials)?

And there are simple questions: "It takes a lot of strength to go through this illness. Where do you get the strength?" Health care professionals should not hesitate to ask patients about their particular faith or practice. This lets them know that the provider wishes to better understand who they are and helps identify ways to support them. The clinician should perform an initial assessment of the spiritual dimension and encourage the conversation, but when the spiritual issues brought up seem beyond the medical professional's scope, a referral to chaplaincy is very appropriate.

Suffering

A primary role of clinicians is to relieve suffering, yet many patients suffer at the end of life, including physical, emotional, and spiritual suffering. Again, there are established ways to alleviate the physical symptoms at the end of life and ways to comfort and support patients emotionally, but health care professionals often struggle to help patients with spiritual suffering or spiritual pain. Suffering is an intensely personal experience for each patient. But what is suffering? Viktor Frankl, a psychotherapist and survivor of the World War II concentration camps, wrote a book entitled *Man's Search for Meaning.* He described his time in the camp and developed a form of psychotherapy to aid others in their search for meaning. He stated that "to live is to suffer, to suffer is to find meaning in the suffering" (Frankl, 1962). Suffering and finding meaning are inextricably linked.

Travelbee (1971) describes suffering in terms of degrees of anguish in any domain, even to "those places beyond anguish." Another author, Cassell (1991), speaks about suffering related to the intactness of the patient; that the patient has multiple dimensions, such as the physical, emotional, social, and spiritual dimensions; that the patient has beliefs and values, memories, dreams, aspirations, and even unconscious realms. He defines suffering as "a state of severe distress associated with events that threaten the intactness of the person" (Cassell, 1991). Although suffering can come from any of the dimensions he describes, he does discuss symptoms in particular. Suffering takes place if a symptom is out of control or overwhelming or feels never-ending or the source is unknown (Cassell, 1991). Cherny, Coyle, and Foley (1994) discuss suffering in the patient with advanced cancer. They group the dimensions of distress or suffering into the physical, psychologic, social, and existential. Other authors are addressing suffering in terms of looking at dignity (Chochinov, 2002; Chochinov, Hack, Hassard, et al., 2002), at demoralization (Kissane, Clarke, & Street, 2001), and at reframing hope through meaning-centered therapy groups (Breitbart, 2002; Breitbart & Heller, 2003).

Suffering is also a part of many faith traditions, recognizing it as a part of being human. Some believe that there is redemptive value in the suffering. For instance, in the Buddhist faith, suffering comes from the attachment to things of this world. For Christians, suffering is also part of being human. It can be seen as a test of moral fiber or even as a punishment. Acknowledging or working through the suffering may enhance the patient's sense of the transcendent. Culture can also have an influence on suffering. In some cultures an outward expression of the suffering is quite acceptable, and in other cultures it is not. Even if the suffering does not have religious or cultural components, finding meaning in the suffering can be transforming and an opportunity for growth.

There are many aspects to suffering at the end of life. The potential list is endless. Box 13-2 offers some aspects of suffering for the clinician to consider. Health care professionals should consider the unit of care as the patient and family. Suffering on the part of the family may have some similarities to that of the patient but may also be very different. There may be specifics that can help alleviate suffering. For instance, if the patient is especially worried about finances and the social worker can assess and address the issues, needs, and resources, the patient may be comforted and have less distress. What are the sources of suffering for this dying patient? What are the sources of meaning? For the patient who cannot easily identify the sources of suffering (other than physical suffering), it may be helpful to state that some patients in their situation worry about these things (e.g., dyspnea, anxiety). This takes the burden of initiating/expressing a concern off the patient and allows the patient to only have to agree with the clinician. From there, further exploration can occur and explanations of how the worry or concern will be addressed can be given to the patient.

Box 13-2   Aspects of Suffering

Physical	Pain, dyspnea, strength/fatigue, sleep/rest, nausea, appetite, constipation, loss of control over body
Psychologic	Anxiety, depression, cognition difficulties, body image, enjoyment of life, symptoms invalidated by family or clinicians, regrets, guilt, fears, loss of control, unfinished business
Social	Changed roles, family issues for the patient, loss of legacy, family exhaustion, isolation, unfinished business
Spiritual	Culture and/or faith traditions, meaning in the illness, despair, meaning of the symptoms, uncertainty, the unknown
Other	Conflicting goals of care

Clinicians understand the dying trajectory of the patient's disease and can anticipate some of the aspects of suffering the patient might experience. The young mother dying of ovarian cancer will have different symptom issues, physically and psychologically, from those of the elder man dying with emphysema. In contrast, the spiritual issues and the suffering component may be quite similar. In addition, certain diseases may be stigmatizing and therefore contribute to the patient's suffering. At the same time, health care professionals can anticipate how the dying experience might be for a particular patient. The first responsibility is to acknowledge the individuality of the patient and perform a complete assessment of the patient's condition—the physical, psychologic, social, and spiritual needs. Ideally, multiple needs or issues can be addressed at the same time. In reality, aggressively managing the patient's physical needs may be the over-riding issue initially. It is quite difficult to jump into spiritual assessment and interventions when the patient is in excruciating pain. Once the physical symptoms are controlled, then these other concerns can be addressed.

Caring for the dying is accomplished best when many disciplines can give input. At the same time, one has to be sensitive to patients—not be burdensome and not have every caregiver who enters their room discussing their suffering and spiritual pain at every visit. Patients develop relationships with different members of the team and will share more with one clinician than another and that needs to be acceptable to all team members. Further, dying patients do not want to discuss or deal with these issues at every waking moment. Palliative care is about helping the patient live as fully as possible, and times of focusing on the living and not the dying need to be facilitated.

It is interesting that the word *compassion* is from the Latin root that means "to suffer with." This is the essence of the clinician's responsibility in responding to the patient's and/or family's suffering. Providers must be present, with compassion, to listen attentively to the suffering, to witness the journey at the end of life. Cultural or spiritual influences must be acknowledged and supported. It is essential that patients are assisted to find meaning in their suffering and find new meaning or re-define meaning in the context of their living and dying. This journey of dying is a deeply personal one, even an intimate one. Even though spiritual suffering cannot be completely relieved, patients can be reassured that they will not be abandoned, that their health care professionals will be compassionately present with them during their journeys through advanced illness.

SUMMARY

Providing palliative care to patients involves addressing the physical, emotional, practical, and spiritual domains of patients' lives. Patients are much more than a collection of physical symptoms. They are unique individuals with a history of life experiences and a future in which the remainder of their life will unfold. To provide high quality, individualized palliative care, health care professionals must be sensitive to and understand different cultural and spiritual perspectives. See Table 13-2 for a summary of the domains of culture. Of paramount importance is the degree to which patients adopt various cultural values and traditions; hence, assessment of each patient is vital. Applying cultural descriptions to individual patients leads to stereotyping, which can harm clinical relationships. Spirituality often becomes increasingly important for patients at the end of life, and like cultural issues, individual patients should be assessed for spiritual well-being and distress. Health care professionals are in a unique position not only to alleviate physical suffering but also to assist patients who are struggling to make meaning at a very trying time in their lives. Palliative care professionals who attend to cultural and spiritual issues are demonstrating respect and compassion, honoring their patients' humanity as they transition from this life.

Objective Questions

1. An individual patient's end-of-life decision making is influenced:

   a. Predominantly by ethnic cultural influences.
   b. By Western medicine's culture.

Table **13-2**   SUMMARY OF THE DOMAINS OF CULTURE

Domain	Description
Ethnic history	Country of origin, ethnicity/culture with which the group identifies, current residence, reasons for migration, degree of acculturation/assimilation, and level of cultural pride
Communication	Dominant language and any dialects, usual volume/tone of speech, willingness to share thoughts/feelings/ideas, meaning of touch, use of eye contact, control of expressions and emotions, spokesperson/decision maker in family
Time and space	Past, present, or future time orientation; preference for personal space/distance
Social organization	Family structure; head of household; gender roles; status/role of elderly; roles of child, adolescents, husband/wife, mother/father, extended family; influences on the decision-making process; importance of social organization and network
Workforce issues	Primary wage earner, impact of illness on work, transportation to clinic visits, health insurance, financial impact, importance of work
Health beliefs, practices, and practitioners	Meaning/cause of illness/health, living with life-threatening illness, expectations and use of Western treatment and health care team, religious/spiritual beliefs and practices, use of traditional healers/practitioners, expectations of practitioners, loss of body part/body image, acceptance of blood transfusions/organ donations, sick role and health-seeking behaviors
Nutrition	Meaning of food and mealtimes, preferences and preparation of food, taboos/rituals, religious influences on food preferences and preparation
Biologic variations	Skin/mucous membrane color, physical variations, drug metabolism, laboratory data, and genetic variations—specific risk factors and differences in incidence/survival/mortality of specific diseases
Sexuality and reproductive fears	Beliefs about sexuality and reproductive/childbearing activities, taboos, privacy issues, interaction of diagnosis/treatments with beliefs about sexuality
Religion and spirituality	Dominant religion; religious beliefs, rituals, and ceremonies; use of prayer, meditation, or other symbolic activities; meaning of life; sources of strength
Death and dying	Meaning of dying, death, and the afterlife; belief in fatalism; rituals, expectations and mourning/bereavement practices

From: Brant, J., Ishida, D., Itano, J., et al. (2000). *Oncology Nursing Society multicultural outcomes: Guidelines for cultural competence* (p. 5). Oncology Nursing Press.

c. By numerous factors including individual values.

d. Solely by the dominant U.S. culture.

2. African-Americans' purported distrust of the American health care system stems from:

a. A lack of education.

b. A history of oppression and discrimination by the dominant culture.

c. Unique attitudes toward health care in general.

d. Their religious beliefs.

3. According to research, which of the following cultural groups are *least* likely to believe that a patient should be told of a diagnosis of metastatic cancer?

a. African-Americans.

b. Korean-Americans.

c. Cuban-Americans.

d. European-Americans.

4. Which of the following Pan-Hispanic values refers to trust built over time that is manifested by expression of mutual respect?

    a. Familismo.

    b. Personalismo.

    c. Jerarquismo.

    d. Repectismo.

5. As a group, Native Americans:

    a. Value the maintenance of extended family networks.

    b. Universally share a fear of dead bodies.

    c. Welcome confrontation with non–Native Americans.

    d. Adhere to traditional Native American religious perspectives.

6. The Koran (the Islamic Holy Book):

    a. Clearly defines death in terms of specific physical signs.

    b. Endorses suicide.

    c. Defines death as final.

    d. Describes death as a transition from one segment of life to another.

7. Spiritual needs tend to be:

    a. Unidimensional.

    b. Agreed upon by researchers.

    c. Multidimensional.

    d. Antithetical to spiritual well-being.

8. According to research discussed in the chapter, which of the following is *not* associated with a sense of spiritual well-being?

    a. Longer life expectancy.

    b. Lower pain levels.

    c. Lower levels of depression.

    d. Lower levels of hopelessness.

9. Spiritual assessment tools:

    a. Typically measure only one aspect of spirituality.

    b. Can be burdensome to administer to patients at the end of life.

    c. Do not address religious issues.

    d. Should be administered only by chaplains.

10. Suffering:

    a. Is linked to humans' search for meaning.

    b. Is alleviated with good symptom control.

    c. Should always be avoided by patients.

    d. Has no cultural value.

REFERENCES

Anandarajah, G., & Hight, E. (2001) Spirituality and medical practice: Using the HOPE questions as a practical tool for spiritual assessment. *Am Fam Physician, 63* (1), 81-88.

Balgopal, P. (1995). Asian American overview. *Encyclopedia of social work* (19th ed., pp. 231-237). Washington, D.C.: NASW Press.

Barker-Cummings, C., McClellan, W., Soucie, J.M., et al. (1995). Ethnic differences in the use of peritoneal dialysis as initial treatment for end-stage renal disease. *J Amer Med Assoc, 274*(3), 1858-1862.

Bernabei, R., Gambassi, G., Lapane, K., et al. (1998). Management of pain in elderly patients with cancer. *J Amer Med Assoc, 279,* 1877-1882. Erratum (1999). *J Amer Med Assoc, 281,* 136.

Blackhall, L.J., Frank, G., Murphy, S.T., et al. (1999). Ethnicity and attitudes towards life sustaining technology. *Soc Sci Med, 48,* 1779-1789.

Blackhall, L.J., Murphy, S.T., Frank, G., et al. (1995). Ethnicity and attitudes toward patient autonomy. *J Amer Med Assoc, 274*(10), 820-825.

Block, S.D. (2001). Psychological considerations, growth, and transcendence at the end of life: The art of the possible. *J Amer Med Assoc, 285*(22), 2898-2905.

Borum, M.L., Lynn, J., & Zhong, Z. (2000). The effects of patient race on outcomes in seriously ill patients in SUPPORT: An overview of economic impact, medical intervention, and end-of-life decisions. *J Am Geriatr Soc, 48,* 5194-5198.

Brady, M.J., Peterman, A.H., Fitchett, G., et al. (1999) A case for including spirituality in quality of life measurement in oncology. *Psychooncology, 8*(5), 417-428.

Brant, J., Ishida, D., Itano, J., et al. (2000). *Oncology Nursing Society multicultural outcomes: Guidelines for cultural competence* (p. 5). Oncology Nursing Press.

Braun, K., Pietsch, J., & Blanchette, P. (2000) An introduction to culture and its influence on end-of-life decision making. In K. Braun, J. Pietsch, & P. Blanchette (Eds.), *Cultural issues in end-of-life decision making* (pp. 1-12). Thousand Oaks, Calif.: Sage Publications.

Breitbart, W. (2002) Spirituality and meaning in supportive care: Spirituality- and meaning-centered group psychotherapy interventions in advanced cancer. *Support Care Cancer, 10*(4), 272-280.

Breitbart, W., & Heller, K.S. (2003). Reframing hope: Meaning-centered care for patients near the end of life. *J Palliat Care, 6*(6), 979-988.

Byock, I. (2004). *The four things that matter most.* New York: Free Press.

Byock, I.R., & Merriman, M.P. (1998). Measuring quality of life for patients with terminal illness: The Missoula-VITAS Quality of Life Index. *Palliat Med, 12,* 231-244.

Caresse, J.A., & Rhodes, L.A. (1995). Western bioethics on the Navajo reservation: Benefit or harm? *J Amer Med Assoc, 274,* 826-829.

Carpenito, L.J. (1997). *Nursing diagnosis: Application to clinical practice* (7th ed.). Philadelphia: Lippincott.

Cassell, E.J. (1991). *The nature of suffering and the goals of medicine.* New York: Oxford University Press.

Cherny, N.I., Coyle, N., & Foley, K.M. (1994). Suffering in the advanced cancer patient: A definition and taxonomy. *J Palliat Care, 10*(2), 57-70.

Chibnall, J.T., Videen, S.D., Duckro, P.N., et al. (2002). Psychosocial-spiritual correlates of death distress in patients with life-threatening medical conditions. *Palliat Med, 16*(4), 331-338

Chochinov, H.M. (2002). Dignity-conserving care: A new model for palliative care. *JAMA, 287,* 2253-2260.

Chochinov, H.M., Hack, T., Hassard, T., et al. (2002). Dignity in the terminally ill. *Lancet, 360,* 2026-2030.

Cleeland, C.S., Gonin, R., Baez, L., et al. (1997). Pain and treatment of pain in minority patients with cancer. *Ann Intern Med, 127*(9), 813-816.

Clinebell, H. (1988). *Basic types of pastoral care and counseling* (p. 110). Nashville, Tenn.: Abingdon Press.

Cohen, S.R. Mount, B.M. Tomas, J.J., et al. (1996). Existential well-being is an important determinant of quality of Life. Evidence from the McGill Quality of Life Questionnaire. *Cancer, 77*(3), 576-586.

Crawley, L.M., Marshall, P., Lo, B., et al. (2002). Strategies for culturally effective end-of-life care. *Ann Intern Med, 136*(9), 673-679.

Engle, V.F., Fox-Hill, E., & Graney, M.J. (1998). The experience of living-dying in a nursing home: Self-reports of black and white older adults. *J Am Geriatr Soc, 46,* 1091-1096.

Farran, C.J., Fitchett, G., Quiring-Emblen, J.D., et al. (1989). Development of a model of spiritual assessment and intervention. *J Relig Health, 28*(3), 185-194.

Fehring, R.J., Miller. J.F., & Shaw, C. (1997). Spiritual well-being, religiosity, hope, depression, and other mood states in elderly people coping with cancer. *Oncol Nurs Forum, 24*(4), 663-671.

Fitchett, G. (1993). *Assessing spiritual needs: A guide for caregivers.* Minneapolis: Augsburg Press.

Frankl V. (1962). *Man's search for meaning.* Boston: Beacon Press.

Garrett, J.M., Harris, R.P., Norburn, J.K., et al. (1993). Life-sustaining treatments during terminal illness: Who wants what? *J Gen Intern Med, 8*(7), 361-368.

Gatrad, A.R. (1994). Muslim customs surrounding death, bereavement, postmortem examination, and organ transplantation. *Br Med J, 309*(6953), 521-523.

Gelfand, D.E., Balcazar, H., Parzuchowski, J., et al. (2001). Mexicans and care for the terminally ill: Family, hospice, and the church. *Am J Hosp Palliat Care, 18*(6), 391-396.

Gillum, R.F., Mussolino, M.E., & Madans, J.H. (1997). Coronary artery disease incidence and survival in African-American men and women. *Ann Intern Med, 127,* 111-118.

Gramelspacher, G.P., Zhou, X.H., Hanna, M.P., et al. (1997). Preferences of physicians and their patients for end-of-life care. *J Gen Intern Med, 12*(6), 346-351.

Hay, M.W. (1989). Principles in building spiritual assessment tools. *Am J Hosp Care, 6*(5), 25-31.

Hermann, C.P. (2001). Spiritual needs of dying patients: A qualitative study. *Oncol Nurs Forum, 28*(1), 67-72.

Highfield, M.E. (1993). PLAN: A spiritual care model for every nurse. In M.Z. Cohen & M.B. Whedon (Eds.), *Quality of Life: A Nursing Challenge Monographs, 2*(3), 80-84.

Highfield, M.E. (2000) Providing spiritual care to patients with cancer. *Clin J Oncol Nurs, 4*(3), 115-120.

Highfield, M.F., & Cason, C. (1983). Spiritual needs of cancer patients: Are they recognized? *Cancer Nurs, 6, 187-192.*

Holland, J.C., Kash, K.M., Passik, S., et al. (1998). A brief spiritual beliefs inventory for use in quality of life research in life-threatening illness. *Psychooncology, 7*(6), 460-469.

Iwashyna, T.J., & Chang, V.W. (2002). Racial and ethnic differences in place of death: United States, 1993. *J Am Geriatr Soc, 50,* 1113-1117.

Johnson, P.A., Lee, T.H., Cook, E.F., et al. (1993). Effect of race on the presentation and management of patients with acute chest pain. *Ann Intern Med, 118*(8), 593-601.

Kagawa-Singer, M., & Blackhall, L. (2001). Negotiating cross-cultural issues at the end of life: "You got to go where he lives." *J Amer Med Assoc, 286,* 2993-3001.

Kao, A.C., Green, D.C., Zaslavsky, A.M., et al. (1998). The relationship between method of physician payment and patient trust. *J Amer Med Assoc, 280*(19), 1708-1714.

Kellehear, A. (2000). Spirituality and palliative care: A model of needs. *Palliat Med, 14,* 149-155.

Kim, M.J., McFarland, G.K., & McLane, A.M. (1987). *Pocket guide to nursing diagnosis.* St. Louis: Mosby.

Kissane, D.W., Clarke, D.M., & Street, A.F. (2001). Demoralization syndrome: A relevant psychiatric diagnosis for palliative care. *J Palliat Care, 17,* 12-21.

Koenig, H.G., & Gates-Williams, J. (1995). Understanding cultural difference in caring for dying patients. *West J Med, 156,* 2240-2248.

Krakauer, E.L., Crenner, C., & Fox, K. (2002). Barriers to optimum end-of-life care for minority patients. *J Am Geriatr Soc, 50,* 182-190.

Krakauer, E.L., & Truog, R.D. (1997). Case study: Mistrust, racism, and end-of-life treatment. *Hastings Cent Rep, 27,* 23-25.

Kramer, J. (1996). American Indians. In J. Lipson, S. Dibble, & P. Minarik (Eds.), *Culture and nursing care* (pp. 7-10). San Francisco, Calif.: UCSF Nursing Press.

Kübler-Ross, E. (1969). *On death and dying.* New York: Macmillan Publishing.

Kumasaka, L., & Miles, A. (1996). "My pain is God's will." *Am J Nurs, 96,* 45-47.

Larson, D.B. (1993). *The faith factor: An annotated bibliography of systematic reviews and clinical research on spiritual subjects* (Vol. II). National Institute for Healthcare Research.

Lewis, R. (1990). Death and dying among the American Indians. In J. Parry (Ed.), *Social work with the terminally ill: A transcultural perspective* (pp. 32-33). Springfield, Ill.: Charles C. Thomas.

Low, J.F. (1997). Religious orientation and pain management. *Am J Occup Ther, 51,* 215-219.

Matsumura, S., Bito, S., Liu, H., et al. (2002). Acculturation of attitudes toward end of life care: A cross-cultural survey of Japanese Americans and Japanese. *J Gen Intern Med, 17,* 531-539.

Matthews, D.A., & Larson, D.B. (1995) *The faith factor: An annotated bibliography of clinical research on spiritual subjects* (Vol. III: Enhancing life satisfaction). National Institute for Healthcare Research.

Matthews, D.A., Larson, D.B., & Barry, C.P. (1993). *The faith factor: An annotated bibliography of clinical research on spiritual subjects.* National Institute for Healthcare Research.

Matthews, D.A., & Saunders, D.M. (1997). *The faith factor: An annotated bibliography of clinical research on spiritual subjects* (Vol. IV: Prevention and treatment of illness, addictions and delinquency). National Institute for Healthcare Research.

McClain, C.S., Rosenfeld, B., & Breitbart, W. (2003). Effect of spiritual well-being on end-of-life despair in terminally-ill cancer patients. *Lancet, 361,* 1603-1607.

McKinley, E.D., Garrett, J.M., Evans, A.T., et al. (1996). Differences in end-of-life decision making among black and white ambulatory care patients. *J Gen Intern Med, 11,* 651-656.

Moadel, A., Morgan, C., Fatone, A., et al. (1999). Seeking meaning and hope: Self-reported spiritual and existential needs among an ethnically-diverse cancer patient population. *Psychooncology, 8*(5), 378-385.

Moberg, D.O., & Brusek, P.M. (1978). Spiritual well-being: A neglected subject in quality of life research. *Soc Indic Res, 5,* 303-323.

Mohr, D.C., Moran, P.J., Kohn, C., et al. (2003). Couples therapy at end of life. *Psychooncology, 12*(6), 620-637.

Mouton, C. (2000). Cultural and religious issues for African-Americans. In K. Braun, J. Pietsch, & P. Blanchette (Eds.), *Cultural issues in end-of-life decision making* (pp. 71-82). Thousand Oaks, Calif.: Sage Publications.

Munet-Vilaro, F. (1998). Grieving and death rituals of Latinos. *Oncol Nurs Forum, 25*(10), 1761-1763.

Murphy, S.T., Palmer, J.M., Azen, S., et al. (1996). Ethnicity and advance directives. *J Law Med Ethics, 24*(2), 108-117.

Murray, S.A., Kendall, M., Boyd, K., et al. (2004). Exploring the spiritual needs of people dying of lung cancer or heart failure: A prospective qualitative interview study of patients and their carers. *Palliat Med, 18,* 39-45.

National Comprehensive Cancer Network (NCCN). (2004). *NCCN clinical practice guidelines in oncology: Distress management, 1,* DIS-19-DIS-25.

National Comprehensive Cancer Network (NCCN) (2003). *NCCN clinical practice guidelines in oncology: Palliative care, 1,* PAL-17.

National Hospice and Palliative Care Organization. (2001). Available at: www.nhpco.org/files/public/NDS_National 2000.pdf.

Nelson, C.J., Rosenfeld, B., Breitbart, W., et al. (2002). Spirituality, religion, and depression in the terminally ill. *Psychosomatics, 43*(3), 213-220.

Nishimoto, P.W., & Foley, J. (2001). Cultural beliefs of Asian Americans associated with terminal illness and death. *Semin Oncol Nurs, 17*(3), 179-189.

O'Brien, M.E. (1982). Religious faith and adjustment to long term hemodialysis. *J Relig Health, 21,* 68-80.

Paloutzian, R., & Ellison, C. (1982). Loneliness, spiritual well-being and the quality of life. In D. Perlman & L. Peplau (Eds.), *Loneliness: A sourcebook of current theory, research and therapy* (pp. 224-237). New York: J. Wiley & Sons.

Parillo, V. (1997). The Native Americans. In V. Parillo (Ed.), *Strangers to these shores* (pp. 219-262). Boston: Allyn & Bacon Publishers.

Peterman, A.H, Fitchett, G., Brady, M.J., et al. (2002). Measuring spiritual well-being in people with cancer: The functional assessment of chronic illness therapy: Spiritual well-being scale. *Ann Behav Med, 24*(1), 49-58.

Peterson, E.D., Shaw, L.K., DeLong, E.R., et al. (1997). Racial variation in the use of coronary-revascularization procedures. *New Engl J Med, 336,* 480-486.

Peterson, E.D., Wright, S.M., Daley, J., et al. (1994). Racial variation in cardiac procedure use and survival following acute myocardial infarction in the department of Veterans Affairs, *J Amer Med Assoc, 271*(15), 1175-1180.

Phillips, R.S., Hamel, M.B., Teno, J.M., et al. (1996). Race, resource use, and survival in seriously hospitalized adults. The SUPPORT Investigators. *J Gen Intern Med, 11*(7), 387-396.

Phillips, R.S., Wenger, N.S., Teno, J., et al. (1996). Choices of seriously ill patients about cardiopulmonary resuscitation: Correlates and outcomes. *Am J Med, 100,* 128-137.

Puchalski, C., & Romer, A.L. (2000). Taking a spiritual history allows clinicians to understand patients more fully. *J Palliat Med, 3*(1), 129-137.

Reed, P.G. (1986). Religiousness among terminally ill and healthy adults. *Res Nurs Health, 9,* 35-41.

Reed, P.G. (1987). Spirituality and well-being in terminally ill hospitalized adults. *Res Nurs Health, 10,* 335-344.

Reese, D.J., Ahern, R.E., Nair, S., et al. (1999). Hospice access and use by African-Americans: Addressing cultural and institutional barriers through participatory action research. *Soc Work, 44*(6), 549-559.

Sandoval, C. (2003). *Culture and care. A clinical guide to supportive and palliative care for HIV/AIDS* (2003 edition). Available at: http://hab.hsra.gov/tools/palliative/chap14.html.

Sarhill, N., LeGrand, S., Islambouli, R., et al. (2001). The terminally ill Muslim: Death and dying from the Muslim perspective. *Am J Hosp Palliat Care, 18*(4), 251-255.

Sheikh, A. (1998). Death and dying: A Muslim perspective. *J R Soc Med, 91*(3), 138-140.

Shepardson, L.B., Gordon, H.S., Ibrahim, S.A., et al. (1999). Racial variation in the use of do-not-resuscitate orders. *J Gen Intern Med, 14*(1), 15-20.

Shiba, G., & Oka, R. (1996). Japanese Americans. In J.G. Lipson, S.L. Dibble, & P.A. Minarik (Eds.), *Culture and nursing care: A pocket guide* (pp.180-190). San Francisco, UCSF Nursing Press.

Singer, P.A., Martin, D.K., & Kelner, M. (1999). Quality end of life care: Patients' perspectives. *JAMA, 281,* 163-168.

Steinhauser, K.E., Bosworth, H.B., Clipp, E.C., et al. (2002). Initial assessment of a new instrument to measure quality of life at the end of life. *J Palliat Med, 5,* 829-841.

Stepnick, A., & Perry, T. (1992). Preventing spiritual distress in the dying client. *J Psychosoc Nurs Ment Health Serv, 30*(1), 17-24.

Stoll, R.I. (1979). Guidelines for spiritual assessment. *Am J Nurs, 79,* 1574-1577.

Talamantes, M., Cornell, J., Espino, D., et al. (1996). SES and ethnic differences in perceived caregiver availability among young-old Mexican Americans and non-Hispanic whites. *Gerontologist, 36*(1), 88-99.

Talamantes, M., Gomez, C., & Braun, K. (2000). Advance directives and end-of-life care: The Hispanic perspectives. In K. Braun, J. Pietsch, & P. Blanchette (Eds.), *Cultural issues in end-of-life decision making* (pp. 83-100). Thousand Oaks, Calif.: Sage Publications.

Tervalon, M., & Murray-Garcia, J. (1998). Cultural humility versus cultural competence: A critical distinction in defining physician training outcomes in multicultural education. *J Health Care Poor Underserved, 9*(2), 117-125.

Todd, K.H., Lee, T., & Hoffman, J.R. (2000). Ethnicity and analgesic practice. *Ann Emerg Med, 35*(1), 11-16.

Travelbee, J. (1971). *Interpersonal aspects of nursing* (2nd ed., p. 62). Philadelphia: F.A. Davis.

Van Winkle, N. (2000). End-of-life decision making in American Indian and Alaska Native cultures. In K. Braun,

J. Pietsch, & P. Blanchette (Eds.), *Cultural issues in end-of-life decision making* (pp. 101-126). Thousand Oaks, Calif.: Sage Publications.

Webster's II New College Dictionary. (1999). New York: Houghton Mifflin.

Yalom, I. (1980). *Existential psychotherapy.* U.S.A.: Basic Books.

Yates, J.W., Chalmer, B.J., St. James, P., et al. (1981). Religion in patients with advanced cancer. *Med Pediatr Oncol, 9,* 121-128.

Yeo, G., & Hikoyeda, N. (2000). Cultural issues in end-of-life decision making among Asians and Pacific Islanders in the United States (pp. 101-125). In K.L. Braun, J.H. Pietsch, & P. Blanchette (Eds.), *Cultural issues in end-of-life decision making.* Thousand Oaks, Calif.: Sage Publications.

CHAPTER 14

The Dying Process

Catherine Vena

Kim Kuebler

Sandra E. Schrader

OBJECTIVES

After the completion of this chapter, the reader should be able to:

1. Be familiar with common theoretic perspectives on death and dying.
2. Understand the multidimensional aspects of dying.
3. Distinguish currently recognized trajectories to death and their impact on end-of-life care.
4. Recognize barriers to providing quality end-of-life care.
5. Identify interdisciplinary approaches for end-of-life care.

"The concept of time is an incredible fascination for me. Understanding or maybe just appreciating the idea of aging within this human dimension is a process that we learn living throughout a lifetime. When suddenly we stand facing the ultimate mystery of life ... the transition between what we have always known from the comfort of living within the boundaries of skin and bones toward the spiritual domains of faith and love. None of us are prepared to pass through the door of the unknown despite its inevitable demands.

Do not be afraid dear woman; death will not sneak up on you in the middle of the night. It will come gently and will take place when you are ready to say your last good-byes. You are given the opportunity to teach your family how to dance upon the stage of disease in a healthy and loving way as you begin to let go of the earth's pull"

(Letter to Isabel, 2003).

INTRODUCTION

Monday morning reports from the medical oncology group in a busy academic setting recite the weekend death occurrences with the same nonchalance it tallies admissions for the management of neutropenia. Yet, each individual who died over the weekend met face to face with the inevitability ...of dying. In a moment, disease, trauma, or accident can block the body from performing life-sustaining rhythm and, in the aftermath, detach the afflicted from the arms of those they love. Health care providers often become insensitive to the needs of the dying and their loved ones. Caught up in the demands of performance and production, it is rare to find symptom management and supportive dying as priorities in the plan of care. However, the palliative care practitioner can help bridge the gap in traditional medical practice by providing multidimensional care for the dying. The bedside practitioner, skilled in palliative practice, can provide coordinated, competent, and compassionate care in the last days and hours of life.

DYING IN AMERICA

The demands of an aging society present a challenge for practitioners to provide care for the dying patient. In 7 years, the oldest of the baby boomers will become 65 years of age. For the first time in history, it is predicted that by the year 2030, the old will outnumber the young (Centers for Disease Control & Prevention [CDC], 2002). To further heighten this challenge, Americans are now living longer with chronic illness. Currently, the leading causes of death in the United States include heart disease, cancer, stroke, chronic obstructive pulmonary disease (COPD) and dementia (von Gunten, Ferris, D'Antuono, et al., 2002). Whereas diseases such as cancer have a relatively predictable course, patients diagnosed with congestive heart failure (CHF) and COPD live with chronic illness for many years before death. At a median age of 77 years, the vast majority of Americans often experience a slow, progressive, debilitating, chronic disease trajectory of 2 to 3 years before death (Brumley, 2002).

Contrary to the desires of dying at home, the majority of adults in the United States die within institutional care settings (51.8% in acute care hospitals and 24.1% in nursing homes) (Last Acts, 2002; Teno, Fisher, Hamel, et al., 2002). Dying patients who receive care in these settings experience mediocre or inadequate care during the last days and hours of life (Last Acts, 2002; Pan, Morrison, Meier, et al., 2001; Teno, Fisher, Hamel, et al., 2002). By the year 2020, it is predicted that 40% of Americans will die in the nursing home setting (Cronin, 2001). The constantly increasing numbers of elderly people and their attendant burdens of chronic illness present clinicians with the challenge of reducing the incidence of crisis care that arises out of unmanaged symptoms in a fragmented health care delivery system.

THEORIES ON DEATH AND DYING
Stage Theory

Throughout the past 3 decades, several theories have been advanced to give structure and meaning to the process of death and dying (Table 14-1). Most notably, Elisabeth Kübler-Ross's (1975) stage theory of dying helped lay the initial groundwork in the United States to identify the psychologic stages that patients and their families transition through before death. Kübler-Ross (1975) postulated that the shocked patient and family, receiving the news of a poor prognosis, were often in denial, which, in turn, granted them permission to refuse the bad news. Denial was followed by anger and bargaining such as praying or bartering for an extended life. When it becomes clear that death will ensue, Kübler-Ross identifies depression as the next sequential stage, and finally, time permitting, the patient can reach the last stage of death acceptance (Copp, 1998).

Another stage theory identified by Buckman (1998) is described as the *three-stage model* modified from Kübler-Ross's *five-stage model.* He theorizes that when patients are confronted with impending death, they react in ways that are consistent with their personality (Buckman, 1998). Buckman argued against the sequential stages that Kübler-Ross identified and sought a more individualized reaction to death and dying that included multiple emotions resembling the patient's character. Buckman (1998) identified (1) the initial stage (facing the threat), which contains descriptors of eleven emotions, (2) the chronic stage (being ill), and (3) the final stage (acceptance). In the third and final stage the patient is identified with having less emotional intensity and therefore has accepted his or her own death. The differences between these two stage theories is that Buckman identifies the patient's individualized emotions and reactions to death and dying versus Kübler-Ross's prescriptive stage-bound theory (Copp, 1998).

The Context of Awareness Theory

The *context of awareness theory* was one of the earliest death and dying theories, identified by Glaser and Strauss in 1965. This sociologic theory was developed in the context of dying in the hospital setting and the interactions with health care professionals (Glaser & Strauss, 1965). Observations and interviews of staff and patients revealed four contexts of awareness:

- Closed
- Suspicion
- Mutual pretence
- Open

These theorists believed that the patients' initial awareness of death and dying changed over time and they could move from suspicion awareness (patient begins to suspect a serious condition) to a full awareness of accepting a poor prognosis and/or death (Copp, 1998).

Dying Trajectories

Glaser and Strauss further developed the theory of dying trajectories as a result of their earlier work (Glaser & Strauss, 1968). They believe that a relationship exists between the phases of dying with the trajectory of death. The four trajectories identified are predicted death at a predicted time,

Table **14-1** THEORIES ON DEATH AND DYING

Theory	Theorist	Brief Description
The Five-Stage Model of Dying	E. Kübler-Ross, 1969	Identified five psychologic stages that occur in serial transition through the process of death and dying. denial, anger, bargaining, depression, and acceptance.
The Three-Stage Model of Dying	R. Buckman, 1998	Buckman believes that it is important to individualize the reaction to death and dying based on the patient's character and not the stage of dying. Buckman identifies an initial stage, a chronic stage, and a final stage. Several emotions are identified in each of these stages, and based on the patient's personality, he or she may enter into the final stage of acceptance with less emotional intensity.
The Context of Awareness Theory	B. Glaser & A. Strauss, 1965	Uses a sociologic approach to evaluate the context of dying in an acute care setting. Four contexts of awareness between hospital staff and patients are: Closed Suspicion Mutual pretence Open
Dying Trajectories	B. Glaser & A. Strauss, 1968	Identified a relationship between the phases of dying and the patient's death expectations. The trajectories include: (1) certain death at a known time, (2) certain death at an unknown time, (3) uncertain death but a known time, and (4) uncertain death and an unknown time. The elements of time shapes and influence the duration and form of the dying trajectory.
The Living-Dying Interval Phase Theory of Dying	E. Pattison, 1977	Defines the living-dying interval as occurring between the crisis of knowing death and the point of death. Identifies three clinical phases as acute, crisis, and chronic or terminal. This model combines psychodynamic and humanistic frameworks. It attempts to integrate dying into the pace of living.
Task-Based Approach to Coping With Dying	C. Corr, 1992	Proposed a task-based approach to coping with dying as a paradigm to understand the work of those who are dying and those who care for the dying. Four task areas of coping with dying are physical, psychologic, social, and spiritual.
Readiness to Die Theory	Copp 1996, 1997	Primary focus on the patients' construction and management of their experiences in confronting death through a nursing perspective

Data from Copp, G. (1998). A review of current theories of death and dying. *J Adv Nursing, 28*(2), 382-390.

predicted death at an unknown time, unpredicted death with a known time, and unpredicted death with an unknown time. The dying trajectories are further described in terms of time such as rapid, slow, or having a plateau. Glaser and Strauss (1968) identified conflicts and tensions in the interpersonal relationships with the patient, family, and health care community with expected changes in the death trajectory (Copp, 1998).

The Living-Dying Interval Phase Theory of Dying

Building from Glaser and Strauss's (1965, 1968) two theories, Pattison (1977) developed the living-dying interval theory for the dying patient. He describes the living-dying interval as the time between the crises of learning about death and the death event (Pattison, 1977). He identified three clinical phases of dying as acute, chronic, and terminal. The patients' feelings and reactions as they move through each phase determine their dying process. For example, the acute phase includes the anxiety associated with the news of a terminal prognosis and, as the patient becomes better prepared to live with and die from disease, he or she can then move into the chronic and eventually terminal phases (Copp, 1998).

Task-Based Approach to Coping With Dying

Corr proposes a task-based approach to dying, which identifies four primary task areas associated with coping and dying from terminal illness (Corr, 1992). This multidimensional approach of satisfying and balancing the physical, psychologic, social, and spiritual domains is significant for the patient and family at the end of life. Corr asserts that there is no right way to cope with dying (Corr, 1992). A central theme in Corr's theory is that dying not only is related to the patient but also is extended to all family, friends, and health care providers who are involved in the patient's dying experience (Copp, 1998).

Readiness to Die Theory

Copp (1997, 1998) proposed a recent theory on death and dying from a nursing perspective. The primary focus is on the patients' construction and management of their own experiences of confronting death and how these experiences interface with the experiences of the nurses who care for them during the dying process (Copp, 1997, 1998). This theory is based on the premise that living with the knowledge of impending death can disrupt the patient's routine and life expectations and can stimulate dramatic introspection and reevaluations of the self (Copp, 1998).

Though these are vague overviews of some of the theoretic concepts associated with death and dying, they provide the reader with a basis for understanding the complex experience of the dying

process for the patient, the family, and the health care team.

DIMENSIONS OF DYING

Death is a multidimensional human passage (Benner, 2001; Steinhauser, Christakis, Clipp, et al., 2000) in which everyone participates at some time and at some level. Death encompasses the physiologic, psychosocial, and spiritual aspects of our humanity and occurs not in isolation but in community. Our first brush with death may come in the social order with the death of a family member or loved one. Health care providers will encounter the death of their patients. Eventually, everyone will experience the inevitable end that all humans face. The dying process can be a time of great loss and suffering not only for the patient but also for family members and health care providers. Our reaction to these losses manifests itself in relation to our past, personality, values, outlook on life, perceived sense of threat to self, religious faith and practice, and cultural history (Rousseau, 2000b). Effective care of people who are dying demands understanding how the physical, psychosocial, and spiritual dimensions affect patients and families.

Sulmasy (2002) has proposed a model for understanding the multidimensional and communal aspects of serious illness that leads to death. The model centers on the idea of relationship. Human existence is a composite of *intrapersonal* and *extrapersonal* relationships. Illness disturbs these relationships. It disrupts homeostatic relationships in physiologic variables and organ systems and fractures emotions and coping strategies. Illness challenges people's understanding of who they are and disrupts family and social connections. Illness causes individuals to be placed in unfamiliar and threatening environments. It challenges the meanings assigned to life. As Figure 14-1 illustrates, the two aspects to intrapersonal relationships are (1) relationships between and among physiologic and biochemical processes and organ systems, and (2) the relationship between mind and body. Extrapersonally, relationships are threefold: (1) the relationship between the person and the environment, (2) the relationship between the individual

I. Intrapersonal:

▶ Physical relationships of body parts, organs, physiological, and biochemical processes

▶ Mind-body relationships—multiple relationships between and among symptoms, moods, cognitive understandings, meanings, and the person's physical state

II. Extrapersonal:

1. Relationship with the physical environment

2. Relationship with the interpersonal environment – family, friends, communities, political order

3. Relationship with the transcendent

FIGURE **14-1** Illness and the manifold of relationships of the patient as a human person. (From Sulmasy, D.P. [2002]. A biopsychosocial-spiritual model for the care of patients at the end of life. *Gerontologist, 42*[SIII], 24-33.)

and his or her family and society, and (3) the relationship between the individual and the transcendent. These manifold internal and external relationships are conceptually overlapping and interactive. Disturbance in one set of relationships ultimately leads to disturbance in others. Inasmuch as serious illness, trauma, or aging is the precipitator of death, the model provides a backdrop for examining the physiologic, psychosocial, and spiritual dimensions of dying. Furthermore, the model reminds us of the impact of setting on the dying process and the dying experience.

Physiologic Dimension

The physiologic dimension of the dying process is a reflection of disrupted relationships between biophysiologic variables and organ systems (Engelberg, 1997). As a multicellular organism, human survival relies on properly functioning neural and hormonal information streams and functioning effector organs. When the wear and tear of age or the ravages of disease or trauma compromise these agents, the intricate relationships that maintain a multitude of biochemical and physiologic variables at relatively constant

levels are disturbed. Medicine performs the task of maintaining troubled systems and restoring some toward functional adequacy. When medical efforts are not successful, the system unravels and the human organism irrevocably travels on a path toward death. In many situations, it is common to hear of multiple system organ failure—physiologically a zero state (Wax & Ray, 2002). With neither a functioning communication system nor effector organs, the organism becomes a collection of cells in anarchy. Lacking the basic coordination of activities necessary for joint survival, the cells soon die.

Physical death is individual to the person and depends on the circumstances of internal and external derangement including the number and types of pathologic processes, host factors such as age and baseline health status, and choices in treatment. A discussion of the experience of dying in disease-specific groups can be found in Chapters 6-11. However, regardless of diagnosis, some common symptoms are encountered in imminently dying persons. Some observable physical changes are listed in Box 14-1. In addition, for more than a decade, studies of dying patients have described pain, dyspnea, restlessness or agitation, confusion, and

Box 14-1   Observable Changes as Death Approaches

DEATH LIKELY WITHIN WEEKS OR DAYS

- Profound progressive weakness
- Bed-bound state
- Sleeping much of the time
- Indifference to food and fluid
- Difficulty swallowing
- Disorientation to time with increasingly short attention span
- Low or lower blood pressure not related to hypovolemia
- Urinary incontinence or retention caused by weakness
- Loss of ability to close eyes
- Oliguria
- Vivid dreams or nightmares
- Reports by patient of seeing previously deceased individuals important to the patient
- References to going home or talk of travel

DEATH LIKELY WITHIN HOURS

- Changes in respiratory rate and pattern (Cheyne-stokes, apneas)
- Noisy breathing, airway secretions
- Mottling and coolness of skin from vasomotor instability with venous pooling, particularly in the tibial region
- Dropping blood pressure with rising, weak pulse
- Mental status changes (delirium, restlessness, agitation, coma)

Data from Dunn, G.P., & Milch, R.A. (2002). Is this a bad day or one of the last days? How to recognize and respond to approaching demise. *J Am Coll Surg, 195*(6), 879-887.

neuromuscular irritability in last days of life (Claessens, Lynn, Zhong, et al., 2000; Edmonds, Karlsen, Khan, et al., 2001; Hall, Schroder, & Weaver, 2002; Levenson, McCarthy, Lynn, et al., 2000; Lichter & Hunt, 1990; McCarthy, Phillips, Zhong, et al., 2000; Somogyi-Zalud, Azhong, Lynn, et al., 2000; Turner, Chye, Aggarwal, et al., 1996). These symptoms require persistent assessment and treatment in the last days of life and are identified in the disease specific chapters. The pathophysiology and management of symptoms are addressed elsewhere in this text. However, issues surrounding dehydration, delirium, and sedation therapy in the last days of life deserve special attention in regard to the dying process.

Dehydration. As death approaches, the dying patient, either because of functional disability or lack of desire, gradually decreases and finally ceases intake of oral fluids (Huang & Ahronheim, 2000; Huffman & Dunn, 2002). Given the current practice imperative to be aggressive in the correction of fluid and electrolyte imbalance, the appropriateness of fluid replacement in the last days of life is debated. Common rhetoric concerning the benefits of dehydration includes (Huffman & Dunn, 2002; Zerwekh, 1997):

- Decreased stress on the pulmonary system
- Decreased brain swelling and discomfort related to headaches and confusion
- Reduction in cardiopulmonary problems (congestive heart failure, pulmonary edema)
- Decreased airway secretions
- Reduction in urinary incontinence with decreased urine output
- Decrease in pain from the potential release of endorphins

Some palliative care providers have challenged the idea that dehydration is universally beneficial in dying patients (Fainsinger & Bruera, 1997; Steiner & Bruera, 1998). The potential burdens of terminal dehydration include (Fainsinger & Bruera, 1997; Huffman & Dunn, 2002):

- Precipitation of confusion, restlessness, or neuromuscular irritability from buildup of toxins and metabolites
- Confusion and syncope when dehydration is rapid (diarrhea, paracentesis)
- Discomforting symptoms such as thirst; dry mouth; cracked, parched, or painful oral mucosa
- The lay perspective of dehydration as contributing to an uncomfortable death

The science of hydration/dehydration in terminally ill patients lacks evidence gleaned from randomized controlled trials. The benefits versus the risks of dehydration and the associated effects on symptom management and quality and quantity of life are not well documented. In their absence, current opinion on the benefits and risks of terminal dehydration rests primarily on clinical observation and descriptive studies conducted in the past decade. These studies involved primarily patients with late-stage, terminal cancer, and therefore findings may not be pertinent to other populations. They do, however, provide beginning insight into the experience of dehydration. For example, the distress experienced by dehydrated patients appears to be minimal (Ellershaw, Sutcliffe, & Saunders, 1995; McCann, Hall, & Groth-Juncker, 1994; Vullo-Navich, Smith, Andrews, et al., 1998). Other studies have shown that patients who are clinically dehydrated may have normal laboratory parameters (Ellershaw et al., 1995; Vullo Navich et al., 1998). Although the experience of thirst and dry mouth appears to be common in dying patients, there is little relationship between fluid status or fluid therapy (Burge, 1993; Ellershaw et al., 1995; McCann et al., 1994). On the other hand, dehydration may contribute to neurotoxicity (restlessness, delirium, myoclonus) when it leads to renal failure and accumulation of metabolites and toxins (Lawlor, Gagnon, Mancini, et al., 2000; Morita, You, Tsunoda, et al., 2001). Because dehydration most likely has an interactive effect on development of delirium, rehydration may or may not affect the course of delirium in the terminal phase (Cerchietti, Navigante, Sauri, et al., 2000; Viola, Wells, & Peterson, 1997).

It is possible that clinicians may provide comfort for dying patients by either avoiding or providing artificial hydration in the dying days. Decisions of hydration should be based on careful patient assessment and the goals of the individual patient and family. The decision to avoid artificial hydration in favor of oral fluids and meticulous oral hygiene may avoid problems such as pulmonary edema and intrusive technology. For patients in distress from neurotoxicity or thirst, a time-limited trial of hydration via carefully monitored intravenous or subcutaneous fluid administration may provide relief and promote comfort (Bruera & MacDonald, 2000; Fainsinger & Bruera, 1997).

The administration of fluids subcutaneously, often referred to as *hypodermoclysis*, has been used in palliative medicine since the late 1980s. For patients unable to take sufficient oral fluids to ease symptoms of dehydration, the technique provides an appropriate alternative to intravenous administration of fluids (Frisoli, de Paula, Feldman, et al., 2000; Slesak, Schnurle, Kinzel, et al., 2003; Steiner & Bruera, 1998). The technique is advantageous for terminally ill and geriatric populations because it does not carry the risks associated with venous access (thrombus formation, phlebitis, septicemia, air embolism), it is the least aggressive and least constraining of the infusion techniques, and it can be safely administered in a variety of settings including acute-care and long-term care facilities and the home (Ferry, Dardaine, & Constans, 1999). Side effects include site infection, pain, or hematoma. These can be avoided by meticulous cleansing of skin site and careful monitoring of infusion at onset. See Box 14-2.

Delirium. Although the pathophysiology and management of delirium are discussed in detail in Chapter 10, delirium as a terminal event deserves some comment here. In one of the earliest studies to document symptoms in the last days of life, Lichter and Hunt (1990) postulated that the theoretic basis for many of the common symptoms experienced near death was delirium or acute cerebral insufficiency. Indeed, up to 88% of patients with advanced cancer have been described as delirious in the last hours or days before death (Lawlor, Fainsinger, & Bruera, 2000; Massie, Holland, & Glass, 1983). The literature describes two roads to dying (Emanuel, von Gunten, & Ferris, 1999). Both of these roads are reflective of types of delirium (hypoactive vs. hyperactive). The high road, which progresses from a normal level of consciousness through stages of sleepiness, lethargy, obtundation, and finally coma before death, corresponds to manifestations of hypoactive delirium. The low road, characterized by increasing neurologic irritability manifested by restlessness and progressing through states of confusion, tremulousness, hallucinations, agitation, myoclonus, seizure, and finally coma, bears the hallmarks of hyperactive delirium. In the terminally ill patient who develops delirium in the last days, the management is unique and presents a number of dilemmas.

Some clinicians argue that delirium, especially when it is manifested in hypoactive form, is a

Box 14-2   SUBCUTANEOUS AND RECTAL
ADMINISTRATION OF FLUIDS

Equipment needed:
- Infusion tubing
- 21- to 25-gauge butterfly needle inserted at 45-degree angle into subcutaneous tissue
- Transparent dressing
- Electrolyte-containing solutions
- Saline (0.33% to 0.9%)
- Glucose solution in saline (i.e. 5% glucose in normal saline)

Perfusion sites:
- Upper thighs
- Abdominal wall
- Subclavicular regions of the thorax

Infusion parameters:
- May administer up to 1.5 liters per day per site. Start slowly and increase as tolerated (may give up to 75 ml/hr).
- Hyaluronidase, 150 units per liter of fluid, may improve absorption of fluids if the patient has difficulty. In most cases this will not be necessary.

Data from Bruera, E., Neumann, C.M., Pituskin, E., et al. (1999). A randomized controlled trial of local injections of hyaluronidase versus placebo in cancer patients receiving subcutaneous hydration. *Ann Oncol, 10*(10), 1255-1258; Ferry, M., Dardaine, V., & Constans, T. (1999). Subcutaneous infusion or hypodermoclysis: A practical approach. *J Am Geriatr Soc, 47*(1), 93-95; Kuebler, K.K., & McKinnon, S. (2002). Dehydration. In K.K. Kuebler, P.H. Berry, & D.E. Heidrich (Eds.), *End of life care: Clinical practice guidelines* (pp. 243-251). Philadelphia: Saunders.

natural part of the dying process that should not be treated (Breitbart & Strout, 2000; Portenoy, 1997). However, research has shown that supportive treatment (fluids, medication withdrawal or rotation) and pharmacotherapy (neuroleptics, benzodiazepines) can palliate symptoms of delirium in a significant number of terminal patients (Lawlor, Gagnon, Mancini, et al., 2000). Morita et al. (2001) found that in cancer patients near death, medication- and hypercalcemic-induced delirium were especially amenable to remission with treatment. On the other hand, etiologies related to progressive underlying disease (hepatic failure, dehydration, hypoxia, disseminated intravascular coagulation) were not. Agitated delirium requiring sedation was most associated with hepatic failure, opioids, and steroid use.

The dilemma in approaching treatment of delirium in the terminally ill involves the risk of adopting either an unduly fatalistic or an inappropriately aggressive perspective (Breitbart & Strout, 2000; Portenoy, 1997). If death is indeed imminent, treatment aimed at controlling distressing symptoms without seeking underlying causes may be appropriate. However, if the clinician assumes that death is imminent and does not seek to identify and treat reversible causes that are indeed present, death may be inappropriately hastened (Lawlor, Fainsinger, & Bruera, 2000). The second challenging aspect of terminal delirium is the management of persistent or recurrent symptoms of hyperactive delirium (Breitbart & Strout, 2000). Symptoms such as paranoid delusions, sleep-wake disturbances, confusion, emotional lability, and severe agitation are extremely distressing to patients and families and preclude a peaceful death. Clinicians need to aggressively assess and treat these symptoms. Unfortunately, even with aggressive treatment, a small number of patients exhibit symptoms that are refractory to standard treatments. Such cases may require sedation to the point of a significantly decreased level of consciousness.

Terminal Sedation. In the literature, terms for use of sedative agents to control refractory symptoms in dying patients include sedation, palliative sedation therapy, total pharmacologic sedation, and sedation for intractable distress of a dying patient (SIDDPat) (Chater, Viola, Paterson, et al., 1998; Fainsinger, De Moissac, Mancini, et al., 2000; Krakauer, Penson, Truog, et al., 2000; Morita, Tsuneto, & Shima, 2002; Peruselli, Di Giulio, Toscani, et al., 1999; Quill & Byock, 2000). Unfortunately, the definitions and parameters of this practice are not always agreed upon by palliative care practitioners (Chater et al., 1998). Sedative agents are used in a variety of ways, including the degree of sedation (mild vs. deep), the duration of sedation (intermittent vs. continuous), and the pharmacologic property of medications used (primary vs. secondary)

(Morita et al., 2002). Sykes and Thorns (2003), in a review of the literature, found that most physicians use sedatives in a proportional manner. That is, the sedative dose is titrated against the distress response to specific symptoms, much as opioid doses are titrated against a pain response with the intent of producing symptom relief. In this sense, sedation is considered as adequate if distress is relieved and the patient remains conscious (Sykes & Thorns, 2003). In the classifications just noted, this might be considered mild, intermittent sedation using agents with either primary or secondary sedating characteristics. At the other end of the spectrum, there is the concept of sedation that includes the two core factors of (1) the presence of severe symptoms that are refractory to standard treatment and (2) the use of sedative medication with the primary intent of reducing consciousness (Table 14-2). This type of sedation is appropriately classified as *primary, deep,* and *continuous.*

Table 14-2   PALLIATIVE SEDATION: TERMINOLOGY AND DEFINITIONS

Terminology	Definition
Total pharmacologic sedation[1]	Administration of drugs to obtain total loss of consciousness.
Sedation[2]	Treatment of intractable symptoms by decreasing the patient to an unresponsive condition.
Sedation for intractable distress of a dying patient (SIDDPat)[3]	Use of sedating medications to relieve severe symptoms that cannot be controlled adequately despite aggressive efforts without sedation.
Terminal sedation[4]	A last-resort clinical response to extreme, unrelieved physical suffering. Terminal sedation is the explicit decision to render the patient unconscious to prevent or respond to otherwise unrelievable physical symptoms.
Terminal sedation[5]	Terminal sedation involves (1) a patient with advanced incurable illness; (2) death expected in hours or days; (3) acute or refractory symptoms; (4) symptoms that have not responded to conventional management, or the severity of the symptoms and trajectory of the illness require prompt intervention to relieve distress; (5) sedation is chemically induced using a non-opioid drug; (6) causing death is not the intent.
Palliative sedation therapy[6]	Use of sedative medications to relieve intolerable and refractory distress by reduction of patient consciousness.

[1]Peruselli, C., Di Giulio, P., Toscani, F., et al. (1999). Home palliative care for terminal cancer patients: A survey on the final week of life. *Palliat Med, 13*(3), 233-241.

[2]Fainsinger, R.L., De Moissac, D., Mancini, I., et al. (2000). Sedation for delirium and other symptoms in terminally ill patients in Edmonton. *J Palliat Care, 16*(2), 5-10.

[3]Krakauer, E.R., Penson, R.T., Truog, R.D., et al. (2000). Sedation for intractable distress of a dying patient: Adult palliative care and the principle of double effect. *Oncologist, 5*(1), 53-62.

[4]Quill, T.E., & Byock, I.R. (2000). Responding to intractable terminal suffering: The role of terminal sedation and voluntary refusal of food and fluids. *Ann Intern Med, 132*(5), 408-414.

[5]Cowan, J.D., & Walsh, D. (2001). Terminal sedation in palliative medicine: Definition and review of the literature. *Support Care Cancer, 9*, 403-407.

[6]Morita, T., Tsuneto, S., & Shima, Y. (2002). Definition of sedation for symptom relief: A systematic literature review and a proposal of operational criteria. *J Pain Symptom Manage, 24*(4), 447-453.

There has been significant debate about the ethical validity of sedation for symptom management. Ethical principles most evoked in relation to sedation therapy are double effect, proportionality, and autonomy (Morita, Tei, & Inoue, 2003; Quill, Dresser, & Brock, 1997; Rousseau, 2000a). The principle of double effect emphasizes four key elements (Beauchamp & Childress, 2001). The first element pertains to the nature of the act, which must be good or morally neutral. The second element pertains to the intent of the agent, which must be good. Any bad effect of the act must be unintended but may be foreseen, tolerated, and permitted. The third condition pertains to the boundary between means and effects. That is, the bad effect must not be the means to the good effect. The fourth element pertains to proportionality, where the good effect must outweigh the bad effect. Although proportionality is seen as one element of double effect, it is also often applied separately (Morita et al., 2003; Quill, Lo, & Brock, 1997). Balancing the moral imperative to do good and not harm, the health care practitioner is obligated to act in the patient's best interest and to avoid causing net harm. Finally, autonomy intertwines with double effect and proportionality and affirms the patient's right to make decisions regarding treatment according to his or her own beliefs, personal values, and cultural system. However, the right of a patient with intact decisional capacity to make decisions encompasses two different notions that are particularly relevant to decisions of sedation therapy (Loewy, 2001). The first is the right to reject any and all forms of therapy for themselves. The second notion, one that is more problematic, is that patients are not free to expect that all demands for treatment be met. A particular form of treatment may be denied for a variety of ethical, legal, or technical reasons. What demands are and are not acceptable, who can refuse the demands, and how meeting or not meeting such demands can be justified are significant questions surrounding sedation therapy.

The debate on the ethical validity of palliative sedation is highly centered on the characteristics of the therapy rendered. There is little disagreement that intermittent or continuous sedation that is secondary to titrated medication for symptom palliation (i.e., increased opioids for pain or dyspnea, increased benzodiazepines for anxiety) is justified under the principle of double effect (Hallenbeck, 2000; Jansen & Sulmasy, 2002; Quill, Dresser, & Brock, 1997; Rousseau, 2000a). This type of sedation therapy meets the elements of double effect because:

1. The act is good or morally neutral (treatment of a symptom).
2. The intent of the practitioner is good (symptom control) while the bad effect (sedation or possible hastened death) is possibly foreseen but not intended.
3. The bad effect (sedation or death) is not the means of achieving the good effect (symptom control).
4. The good effect (freedom from intolerable suffering) outweighs the bad effect (sedation or hastened death).

On the other hand, primary deep continuous sedation for management of intractable symptoms in dying patients is much more controversial. Some argue that the practice is supported by the principle of double effect if used in imminently dying patients (Rousseau, 2000a; Wein, 2000). However, both those who agree and those who disagree with the ethical validity of the practice contend that double effect does not authorize primary intentional palliative sedation for several reasons (Jansen & Sulmasy, 2002; Orentlicher, 1997; Quill, Dresser, & Brock, 1997). First, some have voiced concerns that palliative sedation inevitably hastens death and that it is in fact a form of surrogate physician-assisted suicide or euthanasia (Billings & Brock, 1996; Orentlicher, 1997; Quill, Dresser, & Brock, 1997). Within the framework of double effect, this negates the act as good or morally neutral. Second, the idea of intent is problematic. Although the primary intention may be to palliate symptoms, it is possible to also intend to hasten death. Furthermore, if sedation is defined as the bad effect, it is intended and not merely foreseen (Jansen & Sulmasy, 2002; Loewy, 2001; Quill, Lo, & Brock, 1997). Third, the bad effect (sedation or perhaps hastened death) is the means by which the good is achieved.

Although double effect does not support primary deep continuous sedation in dying patients, autonomy and proportionality do provide an ethical basis for determining the morality of its practice (Morita et al., 2003; Quill, Lo, & Brock, 1997). The principle of autonomy underlies the patient's right to make important decisions regarding treatment at end of life. Thus terminal sedation may be supported if the decision to receive the treatment is genuinely autonomous. That being said, the appropriateness of the request for sedation must be determined. Currently, terminal sedation in imminently dying patients is practiced by palliative care practitioners, is tolerated by society, and has been endorsed as appropriate practice by the U.S. Supreme Court (Cowan & Walsh, 2001; Fainsinger, Waller, Bercovici, et al., 2000; Vacco v. Quill, 1997; Washington v. Glucksberg, 1997).

The concept of proportionality requires that the risk of causing harm must bear a direct relationship to the danger or peril of the patient's clinical situation and the expected benefit of the treatment (Beauchamp & Childress, 2001). As death nears, symptoms accumulate that are at times progressively more difficult to manage. When symptoms become refractory to standard medical interventions, the palliative care team must consider extraordinary medical actions. Clearly there is a moral obligation not to abandon patients to refractory suffering. The nature of palliative action should depend on the nature of suffering. As in all health care interventions, the therapy given should be appropriate for the problem presented. The principle of proportionality supports primary deep continuous sedation when it is a method of last resort when standard palliative measures are ineffective (Morita et al., 2003; Quill, Lo, & Brock, 1997).

The literature provides only a moderate account of the use of palliative sedation. Although a number of descriptive studies and case reports are in the literature, results are difficult to interpret and often disparate (Chiu, Hu, Lue, et al., 2001; Fainsinger, Landman, Hoskings, et al., 1998; McIver, Walsh, & Nelson, 1994; Morita, Inoue, & Chihara, 1996; Morita, Tsunoda, Inoue, et al., 1999; Stone, Phillips, Spruyt, et al., 1997; Sykes & Thorns, 2003). This is due in part to variations in definition of sedation, the retrospective nature of most reports, and the inclusion of both proportional and primary deep

sedation in cases presented or reviewed. In most of the reports, the level of sedation aimed for and/or achieved is not described. Many cases were identified by use of sedative agents rather than the intent of therapy. In addition, available data are derived almost exclusively from cancer populations, which provide practitioners with little information on its use in nonmalignant diseases.

Data regarding the use of primary deep continuous sedation therapy are even more limited. Chater et al. (1998), on survey, found that 89% of palliative care experts recognized that "terminal" sedation was sometimes necessary and 77% had used it in the past year. Two groups reported case series in which barbiturates were used to provide primary deep sedation for intractable physical symptoms in cancer patients (Greene & Davis, 1991) and for pain and ventilator withdrawal in terminal patients (Truog, Berde, Mitchell, et al., 1992). Data from three prospective and one retrospective review indicate that prevalence of use ranges from 1% to 60%, with significant variances in practice between settings and cultures (Fainsinger, 1998; Fainsinger, De Moissac, Mancini, et al., 2000; Fainsinger, Waller, Bercovici, et al., 2000; Peruselli et al., 1999). In these studies the symptoms most commonly requiring sedation for control included delirium, dyspnea, pain, and nausea and vomiting. The most frequently used agent was midazolam. Other medications employed included neuroleptics (haloperidol, methotrimeprazine), benzodiazepines (lorazepam, oxazepam, diazepam), phenothiazines (chlorpromazine), and phenobarbitone.

Given the ethical debate and the limited data, primary deep continuous sedation is a procedure fraught with risks (Loewy, 2001; Quill & Byock, 2000; Wein, 2000). Of particular concern are the risks for inappropriate use or a breach of ethics. First, palliative care practitioners agree that deep sedation is a procedure of last resort (Hallenbeck, 2000; Quill & Byock, 2000). Yet the frequency of use varies widely (Fainsinger, Waller, Bercovici, et al., 2000; Peruselli et al., 1999). Although this may be due, in part, to differences in determining the severity of symptoms such as delirium or dyspnea and to cultural variations of coping at the end of life (Fainsinger, Waller, Bercovici, et al., 2000), there may be some cause to urge caution against hasty prescription without adequate evaluation of underlying conditions or symptoms (Rousseau, 2000a). As Fainsinger cautions, the self-fulfilling nature of the use of sedatives cannot be ignored (Fainsinger, Waller, Bercovici, et al., 2000). Clearly, the indiscriminate and arbitrary use of deep sedation violates professional and ethical standards of care. Second, the complexity of dealing with symptom management at the end of life presents practitioners with situations that are rarely black and white. The decision to sedate is appropriate only if the patient and family are informed and consent. However, although respect for autonomy is important, practitioners are not obligated to provide sedation in all circumstances (Hallenbeck, 2000). A careful weighing of the potential risks and benefits is necessary in any decision to provide deliberate sedation. The nature of treatment should depend on the nature of suffering. Not all suffering is appropriately treated with sedation. Furthermore, practitioners should never feel obligated to participate in any process that violates their basic moral precepts (Quill & Byock, 2000).

Clinical guidelines for use of primary deep continuous sedation have been published (Cherny & Portenoy, 1994; Quill & Byock, 2000). The guidelines are intended to protect vulnerable patients from error or abuse and enable practitioners to respond to unrelieved suffering in dying patients. Categories within the guidelines include the following:

1. Palliative care:
   - Excellent palliative care must be available.
   - Severe, unrelieved symptoms (e.g., intractable pain, dyspnea, seizures, delirium) or potential for suffering (sensation of suffocation from discontinuation of mechanical ventilation) is present.
   - Input from the palliative care team and staff involved in the patient's care should be obtained. Staff should be given the opportunity to withdraw from participation.
2. Terminal prognosis:
   - Patient must have a disease that is lethal.
   - Death is expected in hours or days as judged from blood pressure, pulse, respiration, urine output, and level of consciousness.
3. Informed consent:
   - Patient should be competent and fully informed.
   - In an incompetent patient, informed consent of patient's proxy and family members.
   - Input from and consensus of immediate family members are encouraged.
4. Second opinion:
   - A consultant with expertise in palliative care should review the case.
   - A psychiatric consult should be obtained if there is uncertainty regarding depression or mental capacity.

Consideration of primary deep sedation in difficult cases should be marked by intense discussion of the clinical and ethical issues on the part of the palliative care team, the patient, and the family. When the decision to sedate is considered morally acceptable by all parties, sedation can be achieved with several agents (Table 14-3). Midazolam is often the drug of choice. In cases in which midazolam is not effective, phenobarbital or propofol may be substituted (Cheng, Roemer-Becuwe, & Pereira, 2002). Efficacy of these agents appears to be high, but this information is based on descriptive data. No prospective randomized trials have been or will likely be conducted given the nature of the treatment and patient population. Therefore choice of an agent should be made based on availability, routes of administration, patient response, and cost (Cowan & Walsh, 2001). The dose should be rapidly titrated until the patient is adequately sedated and without signs of discomfort (i.e., moaning, grimacing, bracing either spontaneously or with movement) (Hallenbeck, 2000). Once sedation is begun, intense involvement of the palliative care team is necessary for observation, monitoring, and support (Quill & Byock, 2000). Data indicate that average survival after initiation of deep sedation ranges from 1.5 to 3.2 days (Fainsinger, 1998; Fainsinger, De Moissac, Mancini, et al., 2000; Fainsinger, Waller, Bercovici, et al., 2000).

Psychosocial Dimension

Whereas health care professionals tend to focus on the disease or physical dimension of dying, patients and families are more likely to focus on

Table 14-3 MEDICATIONS FOR PRIMARY DEEP SEDATION IN DYING PATIENTS

Medication	Advantages	Disadvantages	Dosing	Reference
Midazolam	Rapid onset Short half-life, easy to titrate Subcutaneous or IV administration	Lack of efficacy in some individuals Potential for tolerance	Bolus: 0.5-2 mg Starting dose: 0.5-6 mg/hr Threshold: 15-20 mg/hr	1-4
Phenobarbital	Rapid onset of action Subcutaneous or IV administration Anticonvulsant action Dissociative effects	Long half-life Potent inducer of hepatic enzymes (high potential for drug interaction) Considerable interindividual variability in pharmacokinetics	Bolus: 100-200 mg IM Starting dose: 600-1200 mg/day Threshold: 2500 mg/day	5-9
Propofol	Ultra-short onset of action and half-life IV administration Safe for use in patients with liver or renal disease Anxiolytic, an iemetic, anticonvulsant, antipyretic, and bronchodilatory effects	Tolerance develops with prolonged use Painful injection Increased risk of infection Potential for hypotension due to negative inotrope and peripheral vasodilator properties Respiratory depression, especially with bolus dosing Special training or anesthesia supervision needed	Bolus: Not recommended Starting dose: 2.5-5 mcg/kg/min (approximately 10 mg/hr). Titrate to effect by increments of 10 mg every 10-20 minutes. Threshold: 200 mg/hr	4, 10-13

[1]Cheng, C., Roemer-Becuwe, C., & Pereira, J.L. (2002). When midazolam fails. *J Pain Symptom Manage, 23*(3), 256-265.
[2]Cowan, J.D., & Walsh, D. (2001). Terminal sedation in palliative medicine: Definition and review of the literature. *Support Care Cancer, 9,* 403-407.
[3]Fainsinger, R.L., Waller, A., Bercovic, M., et al. (2000). A multicentre international study of sedation for uncontrolled symptoms in terminally ill patients. *Palliat Med, 14*(4), 257-265.
[4]Quill, T.E., & Byock, I.R. (2000). Responding to intractable terminal suffering: The role of terminal sedation and voluntary refusal of food and fluids. *Ann Intern Med, 132*(5), 408-414.
[5]Chater, S., Viola, R., Paterson, J., et al. (1998). Sedation for intractable distress in the dying: A survey of experts. *Palliat Med, 12*(4), 255-269.
[6]Cheng, C., Roemer-Becuwe, C., & Pereira, J.L. (2002). When midazolam fails. *J Pain Symptom Manage, 23*(3), 256-265.
[7]Greene, W.R., & Davis, W.H. (1991). Titrated intravenous barbiturates in the control of symptoms in patients with terminal cancer. *South Med J, 84*(3), 332-337.
[8]Stirling, L.C., Kurowska, A., & Tookman, A. (1999). The use of phenobarbitone in the management of agitation and seizures at the end of life. *J Pain Symptom Manage, 17*(5), 363-368.
[9]Truog, R.D., Berde, C.B., Mitchell, C., et al. (1992). Barbiturates in the care of the terminally ill. *N Engl J Med, 327*(23), 1678-1682.
[10]Krakauer, E.R., Penson, R.T., Truog, R.D., et al. (2000). Sedation for intractable distress of a dying patient: Adult palliative care and the principle of double effect. *Oncologist, 5*(1), 53-62.
[11]Mercadante, S., De Conno, F., & Fipamonti, C. (1995). Propofol in terminal care. *J Pain Symptom Manage, 10*(8), 639-642.
[12]Mirenda, J., & Broyles, G. (1995). Propofol as used for sedation in the ICU. *Chest, 108*(2), 539-548.
[13]Moyle, J. (1995). The use of propofol in palliative medicine. *J Pain Symptom Manage, 10*(8), 643-646.
IV, Intravenous; *hr,* hour; *IM,* intramuscular; *mcg,* microgram; *kg,* kilogram; *min,* minute.

psychosocial aspects (Steinhauser, Bosworth, Clipp, et al., 2002). The psychosocial dimension, involving the inner environment, family relationships, and personal dignity, arises from both intrapersonal and extrapersonal relationships (see Fig. 14-1). The intrapersonal relationship between mind and body is evident as a declining physical state precipitates a number of stresses. In addition, humans are social beings, living with other humans in a web of extrapersonal relationships that generate duties, cares, privileges, and responsibilities (Wax & Ray, 2002). Dying disturbs and fractures the relational web (Seale, 1998). Because the self-image is rooted in internal and external relationships, it is no surprise that dying has a major impact on psychosocial issues for patients and families (Wax & Ray, 2002). Dying disturbs the inner environment, disrupts family connections, and threatens personal dignity.

Inner Environment. In spite of the fact that death is a universal human phenomenon, the thoughts, feelings, and sensations of the last moments remain largely unknown. Comprehensive, systematic studies of people in the process of dying are not feasible for methodologic and ethical reasons. However, several sources, including the arts and literature (Edson, 1999; Tolstoy, 1960), biography (Albom, 1997), and descriptive, epidemiologic, and qualitative studies of people experiencing severe life-limiting illnesses (Curtis, Wenrich, Carline, et al., 2002; Heaven & Maguire, 1998; Olson et al., 2000; Singer, Martin, & Kelner, 1999; Steinhauser, Clipp, McNeilly, et al., 2000), provide at least a beginning insight into the thought processes, challenges, and emotions of people facing death. Dying persons are confronted with multiple losses and face the normal, if painful, response to loss—grief. One of the challenges in palliative care is to differentiate the distress of normal grieving from pathologic responses that require intervention (Block, 2001).

The inner environment is profoundly affected by losses of physical abilities and roles. Physical decline can shatter the personal sense of wholeness and integrity necessary for emotional health. Apart from anticipation of further discomfort and disability, physical degeneration and functional decline lead to an inevitable destruction of the personal and social self. Common concerns of dying patients are related to functional losses, particularly being unable to work, handle personal affairs, or enjoy the things they used to enjoy (Heaven & Maguire, 1998). In addition, limited social contacts and physical environment may lead to a death of the social self that precedes death of the physical self (Johnson, Cook, Giacomini, et al., 2000). It is no wonder that a sense of control is important for those with life-limiting illness (Singer et al., 1999). Although in Western culture, control is most often discussed in terms of autonomy in decision-making, control is also, and sometimes more importantly, related to independence. Patients long to be in control of self and not made into a product of the disease (Chen, 2001). Olson, Morse, Smith, et al. (2000) found that patients dying with cancer used two strategies to exert control over their daily lives. Some took direct control by organizing, setting priorities, and deliberately selecting activities that were most enjoyable to them. Others chose a hands-off approach, exerting indirect control by delegating large portions of tasks to others (family or friends). Often these strategies were used in combination. The unfortunate reality that adds burden to the dying person is that disease and aging eventually evade control (Kite, 2002). Patients may be unable to have control or choice in their life because of frailty, the burden of multiple pathologies, or loss of communication (Kafetz, 2002).

Reaction to loss is individual and manifests itself in relation to one's past, personality, values, religious faith, and cultural history (Rousseau, 2000b). Patients are vulnerable to experience many emotions including self-pity, fear, or anger. They may worry over incomplete tasks or experience regret at not reaching life goals (Tierney & McKinley, 2002). Grief over losses may lead to apathy and withdrawal—conditions that may resemble depression (Kafetz, 2002; Olson et al., 2000). Although the number of fears and worries has been associated with the presence of depression and anxiety in hospice patients, several studies have shown that the prevalence of clinical depression and anxiety in patients near death is surprisingly low (Claessens et al., 2000; Heaven & Maguire, 1998; Lo, Woo, Zhoc, et al., 2002).

Family Relationships. Each person is connected to others in significant relationships. These relationships are a mixture of family and friends who are intimately involved with the patient, are concerned and aware of the patient on a regular basis, and who love the patient. For simplicity, these persons will be referred to as the "family." Dying is a severance of human bonds (Seale, 1998) and therefore affects not only the dying person but also the family. The pain of anticipated and actual separation is acutely felt in the family unit. Indeed, dying re-designates the family as a direct participant rather than a mere mediator for the patient.

Some of the most important issues for dying patients and families are related to family relationships. Many dying patients are burdened by concerns for family members. Patients worry about what will happen to loved ones and how the family will cope with their illness and death (Heaven & Maguire, 1998). There is concern over spouses coping with finances and daily responsibilities alone (Tierney & McKinley, 2002). Looming death can leave a sense of emptiness because of the feeling of abandonment of those loved. Many acutely fear being a burden (Holstein, 1997; Steinhauser et al., 2002). For family members, death brings an end to shared needs, promises, and planning. Death leaves a hole in the fabric of their lives.

In the face of such losses and concerns, it is important for patients and family members to find some psychologic comfort in the dying experience. Comfort cannot be found in the creation of hope, treatment goals, or pathways, but in human connection. It is important that family members feel they have not failed the patient, that the best therapeutic efforts have been applied, that the patient will die a "good" death, that the patient's wishes have been fulfilled, and that no moral or ethical wrongs have been committed (Johnson et al., 2000). Because the person is connected to other selves, there is comfort that death is not the zero state considered in the physical dimension, but a translation of being (Wax & Ray, 2002). The deceased live on in the hearts and minds of others. For the patient, it is human connection supported by rituals, routines, and discourse that provides avenues to calm emotions and stress and foster individual value

and dignity (Benner, 2001). Spending time with family and loved ones and having a confidant to share deepest thoughts are related highly to achieving a sense of comfort and completion (Steinhauser et al., 2002).

Personal Dignity. Maintaining dignity in the face of death is an important concern for patients and health care providers. However, it appears that meanings ascribed to "death with dignity" are vague and inconclusive and vary based on the perspectives of the definer. Dignity is rarely defined in the literature and little empiric data can be found to clearly articulate what this term actually means in clinical practice (Street, 2001). Patients, families, and health care providers often have distinctive beliefs and ideas concerning the characteristics of dignity (Seymour, 1999). Dignity from the lay perspective does not always correspond to the perspective espoused in the medical literature. Too often health professionals make assumptions of what they perceive to be indignities, which can differ from what matters most to the patient and family (Coope, 1997; Street, 2001). We will consider dignity within our relational model as arising from social relationships. Dignity evolves from a sense of personal value or worth that each human being has, simply because each is human (Sulmasy, 2001b). Personal value or worth is founded on the belief that others hold us in high regard. This social aspect of dignity suggests why the significant people in the lives of patients affect the way they negotiate death (Holstein, 1997).

In the course of terminal illness or aging, sources of dignity are often robbed. These sources include title, work/profession, appearance, and enjoyment of life's pleasures (Sulmasy, 2001b). However, sources of indignity vary. What may be considered undignified for one person can be acceptable to another, or what was unacceptable to a person at one point may become acceptable after some time has passed. Issues of dignity are a function of the patient's culture and unique value structure and should be reviewed repeatedly, as new challenges and changes occur (Werth, Gordon, & Johnson, 2002). The hope is for patients to achieve a sense of dignity in the face of countless indignities. Toward this end, it is not surprising that dying persons feel the need to be understood as a whole person by those they love and, also important, by health care providers. Being treated like a person and not a disease, case, or number is a primary concern of patients that is not often recognized by health care providers (Wenrich, Curtis, Ambrozy, et al., 2003). Being able to laugh and smile, being touched and hugged, and feeling unique and special are significant aspects of self-respect and dignity for patients (Patrick, Engelberg, & Curtis, 2001). Having an understanding of dignity in the care of the dying patient is important when planning care, evaluating relationships, and determining unfinished business. Varying perspectives on dignity can affect the decisions made by the health care team, the choices that they offer, and the support that they provide patients who make different choices (Street, 2001). This concept is illustrated in the case study at the end of this chapter.

Spiritual Dimension

Death is surrounded by a sense of mystery that is beyond human intervention. The source of this mystery is variously translated as nature, fate, or God (Johnson et al., 2000). Spirituality is that which allows a person to experience transcendent meaning in life. This is often expressed as a relationship with God, but it can also be about nature, art, music, family, community, or whatever beliefs and values give a person a sense of meaning and purpose in life (Puchalski & Romer, 2000). Each person must live and die according to the answer each gives to the question of whether life or death has a meaning that transcends both life and death. Spirituality has been found to be an important concern and main component of quality of life in terminal patients across cultures (Lo et al., 2002; Steinhauser, Christakis, Clipp, et al., 2000). Human beings have a desire to transcend hardship and suffering and to seek a meaning that allows them to make sense of the situation. However, as with the psychosocial dimension, health care providers tend to focus on the physical aspects of dying rather than the spiritual (Steinhauser, Christakis, Clipp, et al., 2000). Focus on the physical has not led us to understand who human beings are or their real needs as persons (Sulmasy, 2002). The main reason for addressing

the spiritual concerns of dying patients is that these concerns have a profound effect on their overall sense of well-being. To ignore these concerns at the end of life is to remove from the patient-provider interaction a significant component of the patient's well-being precisely at the time when standard medical approaches have lost their curative, alleviating, and life-sustaining efficacy (Sulmasy, 2002).

Spirituality is characterized broadly in terms of religious and nonreligious aspects. Both aspects can promote a sense of transcendence. Religious aspects, which encompass religious beliefs, values, commitment, religious practices, and daily spiritual experiences, are often the first associated with spirituality (Hermann, 2001; Sulmasy, 2001a). Spiritual needs related to religion include the need for a belief system, prayer, making peace in one's relationship with God and with others, and readying oneself for the life to come (Hermann, 2001; Koenig, 2002; Steinhauser, Christakis, Clipp, et al., 2000). Spiritual aspects not restricted to religion involve finding purpose and meaning in one's remaining days. Non-religious aspects include what are commonly called the *tasks of dying* and involve peace of mind and human connection. Peace of mind may entail life review, accepting what one has accomplished and become during one's life, preparing for the loss of that physical self, preparing to bring one's life to a close, and making peace with life (Koenig, 2002; Stewart, Teno, Patrick, et al., 1999). For others it may include experiencing nature or maintaining a positive outlook (Hermann, 2001). Human connection is important for life completion in terms of reconciliation and generativity. Reconciliation involves time spent with family and friends, forgiving others and receiving forgiveness, and saying goodbye (Koenig, 2002; Sulmasy, 2001b). Generativity pertains to the sense that one's life extends beyond the physical self into the lives of others as well as into the future (Stewart et al., 1999). Spiritual needs related to generativity include the opportunity to give gifts, contribute to the well-being of others, and pass a legacy on to children and family (Steinhauser, Christakis, Clipp, et al., 2000).

Quality of life for those near death may focus to a greater extent on peace of mind, comfort, and spiritual understanding. For many dying persons, attending to spirituality and transcendence is very important. At the end of life, addressing spiritual issues may provide the only healing possible. Seeking resolution and making peace could substantially contribute to well-being while dying (Stewart et al., 1999). Spiritual or religious beliefs and attitudes as well as rituals and customs affect one's reaction to and ability to cope with stressful life events (Sulmasy, 2001b). However, for some patients, moving through the transition from gravely ill and fighting death to terminally ill and seeking peace is a difficult transition that involves existential angst, the dread of insignificance, and the struggle to avoid annihilation (Finucane, 1999). It is the real and immediate threat to a sense of meaning in the face of death that creates the spiritual distress of the dying (Hinshaw, 2002).

The Multidimensional Aspects of Suffering

When we acknowledge and understand the importance of the physical, psychosocial, and spiritual dimension of dying, we have a truer understanding of suffering at the end of life. As health care providers, we tend to focus on the biomedical perspective. Patients and families in contrast have a much more integrated view of dying in which psychosocial and spiritual issues are as important as physiologic concerns (Steinhauser, Christakis, Clipp, et al., 2000). In fact, psychosocial and spiritual issues related to the inner environment, family relationships, personal dignity, and existential meaning are key components of suffering (Cassell, 1991). Suffering is a more expansive concept than pain or physical discomfort. It encompasses the torment, fears, and despair that dying patients may experience. A dying person with few physical symptoms may suffer greatly in relation to psychosocial and spiritual issues (Field & Cassel, 1997). Consistent evidence of the weightiness of this suffering comes from people who request help in dying faster. Research has shown that patients who requested physician-assisted suicide did so most frequently for psychosocial or spiritual reasons (Emanuel & Emanuel, 1998). The predominant reasons dying individuals used medications prescribed by their physicians to end their lives were loss of autonomy, control, and self-determination; loss of personal dignity; and concerns or fears about being a burden to loved ones (Back, Wallace, Starks, et al., 1996; Chin, Hedberg, Higginson, et al., 1999; Coombs Lee & Werth, 2000; Ganzini, Johnston, McFarland, et al., 1998; Groenewoud, van der Maas, van der Wal, et al., 1997; van der Maas, van der Wal, Haverkate, et al., 1996). These themes were consistent across studies and involved terminally ill patients in the United States, Australia, and the Netherlands. In contrast, these studies revealed that pain and physical suffering were not the primary motivators in seeking physician-assisted suicide or euthanasia. In palliative care, an emphasis on physical pain and symptom management that ignores psychosocial and spiritual aspects is short-sighted and seriously flawed. This is not to say that conscientious, effective palliation of physical symptoms should not be a top priority. Physical pain and discomfort are a sickening, heavy burden for dying patients. However, even with optimal symptom management, patients will struggle against death and, in the process, incur suffering (Finucane, 2002).

DIAGNOSING DYING

Diagnosing dying, or identifying when death is inevitable, is acknowledged as an important clinical skill (Ellershaw & Ward, 2003). Recognition that death is imminent is an important milestone for providing comprehensive terminal care, redefining goals, and redirecting the plan of care (Christakis & Lamont, 2000; Kafetz, 2002). However, the process of diagnosing dying is extremely complex and difficult. Furthermore, given the same clinical scenario, physicians often disagree significantly as to what it means to be terminal (Crippen, Levy, Truog, et al., 2000). Research has shown that physicians typically make prognostic errors. In a cohort of hospice patients, only 20% of prognoses were accurate. Most of the predictions (53%) were optimistic (Christakis & Lamont, 2000). Although the evidence suggested that more experienced physicians and those less familiar with the patient gave more accurate prognoses, exploration of the dynamic processes that physicians use to determine prognoses have only begun (Iwashyna & Christakis, 2001).

Prediction accuracy involves both discrimination (the ability to separate classes) and calibration (the ability to assign meaningful probabilities) (Glare, Virik, Jones, et al. 2003). In the science of prognostication we do not yet have models that aid the physician in accurate calibration (Dunn & Milch, 2002). The Study to Understand Prognoses and Preferences for Outcomes and Risks of Treatment (SUPPORT) investigators, evaluating several models to predict which patients would die in 6 months, found that none were usably accurate (Fox, Landrum-McNiff, Zhong, et al., 1999). Under the most lenient criteria, 70% of patients who were expected to die within 6 months were still alive, whereas 58% of those excluded actually died. Under the strictest criteria, 99% of patients were excluded as being terminal. Of the remaining patients, 53% were still alive at 6 months. Given the numerous individual and social variables that have an impact on the trajectory of an illness and the underdevelopment of the science of prognostication, the idea of accurate prognostication might be expecting too much (Dunn & Milch, 2002; Iwashyna & Christakis, 2001).

Trajectories of Death

Most of what we know of terminal care comes from research in populations with a discrete terminal illness such as cancer (Lunney, Lynn, Foley, et al., 2003). However, only 23% of deaths in the United States are from cancer. Many more will die from acute complications of an otherwise chronic condition, many without a discrete terminal phase. This forces us to look for new models of palliative care and research. Recent, evolving work has provided additional models of dying based on the shape of the trajectory toward death (Field & Cassel, 1997; Lynn, 2001). Four trajectories (Fig. 14-2), each differing in length and slope of functional decline, were able to describe the last phase of life for more than 92% of Medicare beneficiaries (Lunney, Lynn, & Hogan, 2002). Sudden death accounted for 7% of deaths. In this trajectory, death occurred in a brief time, with little advanced warning, and was preceded by normal functioning. A second group died after a distinct terminal phase of illness. This group accounted for 22% of deaths and was most typical of cancer patients. The functional trajectory

was of high function for a considerable time before disease progression, followed by a rapid decline to death over a short period. The third group, accounting for 16% of deaths, consists of serious and eventually fatal organ failure such as chronic lung disease or congestive heart failure. The functional trajectory of this group declines gradually over time and is punctuated by periodic exacerbation of illness. Prognosis for survival is often ambiguous. The fourth and largest group is characterized by advanced frailty of old age and accounts for 47% of deaths. The trajectory of this group follows a steady, slow, progressive decline in function before dying of complications associated with old age, dementia, or stroke. These trajectories provide a useful framework for considering strategies for providing palliative care. The most predominant model for care of the dying in the United States is hospice care. However, given the constraints of this model, it is severely limited in its ability to serve patients dying in trajectories other than the one characterized by terminal illness.

The Experience of Dying With Specific Diseases and in Different Settings

To provide the best care at the end of life, it is important that we consider and understand not only the disease process but also the context in which care is given. We will consider dying with heart failure, lung disease, cancer, and dementia and the context of dying in an acute care facility, in the intensive care unit (ICU), and in long-term care.

Dying With Heart Failure. Heart disease is the leading cause of death in the United States. Half of deaths from heart disease are likely to be sudden, and 90% occur in the elderly (Friesinger & Butler, 2000). Worsening heart failure is not always the result of an "inexorable" progression of underlying pathology but may be related to reversible causes such as pulmonary infection, anemia, dysrhythmia, or inappropriate medications (Ellershaw & Ward, 2003). Typical markers of poor prognosis include severity of symptoms (as measured by a scale such as the New York Heart Association class), ejection fraction, and the response to and intensity of medical therapy. Additional indicators include several admissions to

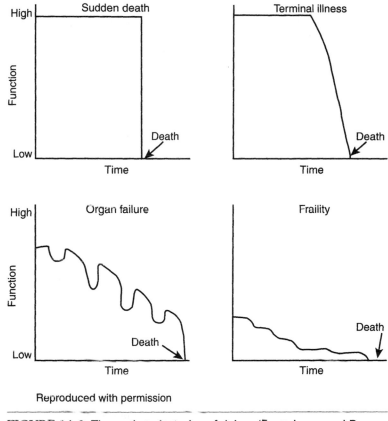

FIGURE 14-2 Theoretic trajectories of dying. (From Lunney, J.R., Lynn J., & Hogan, C. [2002]. Profiles of older Medicare decedents. *J Am Geriatr Soc, 50*[6], 1108-1112.)

an acute care facility for worsening heart failure, increasing edema, lack of a reversible precipitant, receipt of an optimal tolerated drug regimen, deteriorating renal function, and failure to respond within 2 to 3 days to appropriate changes in diuretic or vasodilator drugs (Ellershaw & Ward, 2003; Ward, 2002). However, other factors especially important to the elderly include global subjective elements such as frailty, disability, and patient desires. Disability including mental deterioration is a strong marker for recurrent hospitalizations and death (Friesinger & Butler, 2000). Nevertheless, diagnosing dying in heart failure patients is particularly difficult. Many patients with heart failure never experience a time during which they are clearly dying of their disease. In contrast, the sickest patients are not necessarily the ones who die first (Fox et al., 1999).

It is therefore difficult to determine when terminal care should be considered (Ward, 2002).

The course of heart failure is very unpredictable during the last month of life (Levenson et al., 2000). Up to 58% of patients report good to excellent quality of life in the months before death. However, heart failure patients are also susceptible to a wide range of symptoms that are distressing and often last for more than 6 months (McCarthy, Lay, & Addington-Hall, 1996). The most frequently noted symptoms are pain, dyspnea, depressed mood, and anxiety. These symptoms and functional impairment may increase as death approaches (Levenson et al., 2000).

Dying   With   Chronic   Obstructive Pulmonary Disease. COPD is the fourth leading cause of death in the United States, and age-adjusted death rates from the disease have been increasing (Afessa, Morales, Scanlon, et al., 2002). Patients with advanced lung disease tend to live for variable lengths of time in a continuous state of poor health punctuated by acute exacerbations that benefit from treatment interventions. Although patients who die with COPD are more likely to have mechanical ventilation, tube feeding, and CPR, 75% of mechanically ventilated COPD patients survive to leave the hospital (Claessens et al., 2000). The proximate cause of death is often a sudden and unpredictable event such as sepsis, cardiac failure, pulmonary embolism, or multiple organ failure (Afessa et al., 2002; Fox et al., 1999). Because of these factors, diagnosing dying in this group is very difficult. Several studies have identified predictors of mortality in COPD patients (Abebaw, Baldwin, & Connolly, 2002; Almagro, Calbo, Ochoa de Echaguen, et al., 2002; Oga, Nishimura, Tsukino, et al., 2003; Pistelli, Lange, & Miller, 2003). These include physical disability, long-term oxygen use, multiple exacerbations requiring hospitalization, low body mass index, and cardiac co-morbidity. Nevertheless, the COPD patient maintains a reasonable survival prognosis even when close to death. There is no reliable way to predict which will be the last pneumonia or the last course of mechanical ventilation (Claessens et al., 2000).

As with heart failure, the course of COPD at end of life is very unpredictable without a clearly defined terminal phase. Of 19 major indications for hospice referral, only dementia is associated with a less predictable survival than COPD (Christakis & Escarce, 1996). The most frequent symptoms in the last week of life are dyspnea, weakness, cough, anorexia, and depressed mood (Edmonds et al., 2001). However, these symptoms are also present over the long course of the COPD illness trajectory. These factors probably contribute to the finding that 40% of patients and 48% of family members were not aware that death was imminent (Edmonds et al., 2001).

Dying With Cancer. Approximately 50% of those diagnosed with cancer will die from the disease, making cancer the second leading cause of death in the United States (Ahmedzai & Walsh, 2000). Because the cancer disease trajectory is

characterized by a distinct terminal phase, it is the most studied and therefore the most understood. Although physicians are typically accurate in discriminating those who will die, predictions of time to death (calibration) are not accurate and are often overestimated (Glare et al., 2003). That is, physician predictions of survival to 6 months are reliable because they are highly correlated with actual survival, but probable time to death is inaccurate and diagnosis of dying is often not recognized until the last hours or days (Middlewood, Gardner, & Gardner, 2001; Smith, 2000a). In a review of the literature, Vigano, Dorgan, Buckingham, et al. (2000) found that indicators of poor prognosis in cancer patients included poor performance status and physician clinical prediction along with symptoms of cognitive failure, weight loss, dysphagia, anorexia, and dyspnea (Vigano et al., 2000). However, a meta-analysis of the prognostic literature found that symptoms traditionally recognized as prognostic indicators added little to the accuracy of physician prediction (Glare et al., 2003). This may be because performance status and symptoms are basic contributions to physician judgment. As the science of prognostication evolves, identification of novel prognostic factors such as C-reactive protein, cytokines, and patient-rated health status and quality of life may provide clinicians with tools to improve assigning of probabilities for survival in cancer patients (Mahmoud & Rivera, 2002; Shadbolt, Barresi, & Craft, 2002; Walsh, Mahmoud, & Barna, 2003).

The cancer disease trajectory is characterized by generally high function until the last 4 to 6 weeks of life (Lunney et al., 2002; McCarthy et al., 2000). The terminal phase is characterized by a rapid decrease in functional status requiring increasing dependence in activities of daily living (McCarthy et al., 2000; Teno, Weitzen, Fennell, et al., 2001). In addition, end-stage cancer patients are likely to experience a significant symptom burden. The most prevalent symptoms include pain, weakness, dyspnea, confusion, anorexia, and sleep problems (Walsh, Donnelly, & Rybicki, 2000).

Dying With Dementia. Dementia is the eighth most prevalent disease in the United States and is likely to increase with the aging of the population

(Murray & Lorez, 1997). For each decade after age 60, the number affected with dementia doubles, resulting in a 30% occurrence in the population older than 85 years (Ritchie & Kildea, 1995). Actual mortality rates from the disease are difficult to determine. Although median survival from diagnosis is 4.5 years, death is usually from co-morbid conditions or complications rather than the disease process (Helmer, Joly, Letenneur, et al., 2001; Kammoun, Gold, Bouras, et al., 2000). Patients with dementia often have multiple causes of death, the most common of which are cardiovascular and cerebrovascular diseases, cachexia, dehydration, and respiratory infections (Boersma, Van Den Brink, Deeg, et al., 1999; Helmer et al., 2001; Kammoun et al., 2000). Predicting death in this group is tenuous. As with other chronic conditions, inaccurate prognoses are common. Nearly 30% of those thought to be terminal within 6 months were alive at 3 years (Aguero-Torres, Fratiglioni, Guo, et al., 1998). Commonly identified predictors of mortality in dementia patients include increased age, functional disability, male gender, and the presence of co-morbidity (Aguero-Torres et al., 1998; Jagger, Clarke, & Stone, 1995; Stern, Tang, Albert, et al., 1997).

Dementia is a component of the frail elderly dying trajectory. Patients with progressive dementia are very heterogeneous and may have a very unpredictable course. Debilitation and vulnerability to developing other life-threatening conditions characterize the state of dementia patients before death (Michel, Pautex, Zekry, et al., 2002). At end of life, patients are often bedridden, uncommunicative, hypophagic, incontinent, and institutionalized (Keene, Hope, Fairburn, et al., 2001). Palliative care for patients with dementia is difficult because clinical science in this area is even more limited than it is in other common chronic diseases (Casarett & Karlawish, 1999). Furthermore, cognitive impairment presents a significant barrier to research needed to build our knowledge and to understand and palliate the sources of discomfort and distress in dying patients.

Dying in an Acute Care Facility. The hospital is an institutional and bureaucratic system that molds the dying experience in many ways. The acute care hospital, particularly the intensive care unit, is the setting for the majority of deaths (Last Acts, 2002; Teno et al., 2002). Diagnosing dying and instituting aggressive palliative care plans are particularly difficult in the acute care setting because the culture is focused on cure. Therefore the tendency is to continue with procedures and investigations aimed at this purpose (Ellershaw & Ward, 2003). Unfortunately, although up to 75% of patients who die have documentation of poor prognosis, there is often no systematic plan for palliative treatment (Goodlin, Winzelberg, Teno, et al., 1998; Jacobs, Bonuck, Burton, et al., 2001). Rather, the norm is for ongoing diagnostic testing and treatment that is performed during the last 24 hours of life, including blood tests, transfusions, x-ray examinations, electrocardiograms (ECGs), cardiac monitoring, mechanical ventilation, and even cardiopulmonary resuscitation (Faber-Langendoen, 1996; Jacobs et al., 2001). Thus death in the hospital is rarely well managed (Emanuel & Emanuel, 1998; Smith, 2000b). Research has shown that in the last days of life, a substantial number of patients across all diagnoses have severe pain, dyspnea, restlessness, and other symptoms that are not controlled (Goodlin et al., 1998; Lynn, Teno, Phillips, et al., 1997). Family members report that nearly 70% of patients find it difficult to tolerate physical and emotional symptoms (Lynn, Teno, Phillips, et al., 1997).

Many variables contribute to hospital care that does not acknowledge or plan for death. Palliative care is influenced by the attitudes and interactions among health care providers, the patient, the family, and the institutional culture (Jacobs et al., 2001). Health care providers often give priority to disease processes that can be managed by aggressive treatment while underestimating patient discomfort from symptoms and nearly disregarding the psychosocial and spiritual dimensions of the person (Kaufman, 2002; Rummans, Bostwick, & Clark, 2000; Steinhauser, Christakis, Clipp, et al., 2000). When treatments fail to halt or bring the disease process under control, providers often deal with a sense of failure (Jacobs et al., 2001). At the same time, providers are not comfortable discussing end-of-life issues with patients and families

(Emanuel, von Gunten, & Ferris, 2000; Jacobs et al., 2001). Jacobs et al. (2001) found that nurses and physicians were able to identify patients likely to die in the hospital but did not communicate these prognoses with the patient or family. This lack of communication often leads to a hope-oriented plan of care despite little expectation of its success. Furthermore, the policy- and procedure-laden environment of the hospital, the time pressures on clinicians, and the demands of documentation leave little time spent at the bedside caring for dying patients. Sulmasy (2001a) found that staff visits for seriously ill patients with poor prognoses (cancer, acquired immunodeficiency syndrome [AIDS], heart failure, obstructive lung disease, advanced dementia) were frequent but brief. The mean length of physician visits was 3±3 minutes or less and nurses averaged 2±1 minutes or less per episode. Patients with advanced dementia and minority patients appeared to have less bedside contact. Because family visits averaged only 24±51 minutes or less, most patients spent their time (18 hr, 39 min per day) in the hospital alone (Sulmasy & Rahn, 2001).

For patients, impaired mental status and loss of communication often complicate the course of hospital care. Up to 80% of dying patients do not have decision-making capacity (Faber-Langendoen, 1996; Jacobs et al., 2001; Lynn, Teno, Phillips, et al., 1997). Likewise, a similar percentage of hospital deaths are preceded by a decision to either withhold or withdraw some form of potentially life-sustaining treatment (Faber-Langendoen, 1996). Because patients rarely articulate to their families their desires for treatment, the use of life-prolonging technology, or wishes at the time of death, a heavy burden of decision making is placed on family members (Kaufman, 2002). However, families are the players with the least amount of knowledge about disease processes, the physiology of decline, and hospital culture. Furthermore, family members describe communication with providers, especially physicians, as inadequate. They relate having limited knowledge of the patient's condition, finding it difficult to obtain information, and not receiving sufficient explanations about what staff are doing or why (Jacobs et al., 2001). These types of

conditions support the family perception that death is unexpected and fuel persistent hopes for a recovery that are not supported by the seriousness of the disease. Families often pursue life-prolonging care to provide every option. Even patients and families who realize the seriousness and/or fatal nature of the disease process may be willing to suffer aggressive treatments in the desire to struggle and not give up the fight to live (Finucane, 1999). In both types of circumstances, families are not able to plan for a good death.

Dying in the Intensive Care Unit. The ICU within the acute care hospital presents not only some of the same barriers to good end-of-life care just mentioned but also some unique challenges. Nearly 25% of deaths occur in an ICU, and as many as 90% of these deaths are preceded by limitation of life-sustaining treatments (Faber-Langendoen, 1996; Ferrand, Robert, Ingrand, et al., 2001; Prendergast & Luce, 1997). Intensive care is the preeminent reflection of medicine's preoccupation with the mastery of disease and the eradication of untimely death (Seymour, 2000). For patients in the ICU, diagnosing dying is a particularly difficult task. The majority of patients admitted to the ICU represent those whose illness is critical enough for death to be a possibility but whom physicians and families hope to treat successfully (Baggs, 2002). This hope is often at the crossroads of the path—one fork that leads to recovery and the other that leads to death (Johnson et al., 2000). Clinical experience and a growing body of evidence have shown that it is very difficult to distinguish in which direction the ICU patient is headed (Lynn, Harrell, Cohn, et al., 1997). Whereas some recover or die quickly, others linger with uncertain capacity to recover from injury or illness (Seymour, 2000). The advanced technology and medical care available in the ICU blur the boundaries between living and dying. Death can be highly unpredictable, hard to identify, and without a distinct period of time to shift from cure-oriented to comfort-oriented care (Nelson & Danis, 2001). A major challenge in the ICU is answering the question of how many days should be spent subjecting very sick, dying patients to aggressive, life-sustaining, and usually uncomfortable treatments in order not to lose lives of very sick but potentially surviving patients (Frick, Uehlinger, & Zuercher Zenklusen, 2003).

There is evidence that ICU patients suffer from significant physical and psychologic symptoms (Nelson, Meier, Oei, et al., 2001; Somogyi-Zalud et al., 2000). A high percentage of patients report unrelieved pain, anxiety, sleep disturbance, hunger, thirst, depression, and dyspnea associated with the disease process (Desbiens, Mueller-Rizner, Connors, et al., 1999; Nelson et al., 2001). In addition, common ICU procedures including mechanical ventilation, catheters, nasogastric tubes, indwelling monitoring devices, and endotracheal suctioning induce a substantial level of discomfort (Nelson et al., 2001). Because many ICU patients have impaired communication secondary to unconsciousness, cognitive impairment, mechanical ventilation, and sedation, identifying and managing discomforting symptoms are additionally difficult (Johnson et al., 2000). This also means that family members are again in the position of bearing the weight of difficult decisions about care. The burden of decision making is increased in the ICU by a sense of urgency coupled with uncertainty, a continually changing environment, and higher costs (Cook, 1997). However, as Kaufman (1998) notes, "incommensurability" of the lay and medical worlds adds an additional impediment for families in the throes of dealing with momentous decisions. Health professionals possess detailed knowledge about human physiology and disease processes, the way in which particular treatments and technologies actually work on the body, and hospital rules regarding consent and resuscitation status. This knowledge—and the institutional directives of the hospital culture—are outside the patient/family experience, creating a vast gulf between lay and professional understanding and making families ill-prepared to make the decisions providers require of them (Kaufman, 1998).

The ICU also presents some unique organizational challenges to good end-of-life care. The environment of the ICU is geared toward aggressive life-saving measures. Good palliative care at end of life is associated with family counseling, contact, and rituals (Kirchhoff, Spuhler, Walker, et al., 2000). In the high technology and busy environment, there is a lack of space and privacy to promote family connection and to provide for family members' needs for food, rest, and space to conference (Asch, Shea, Jedrziewski, et al., 1997; Kirchhoff et al., 2000). Although the ICU is a continuous operation, supportive services (social workers, pastoral counselors) often are not available during nights or weekends.

Another organizational challenge pertains to the relationship among the intensivist, other medical consultants, the patient's primary care practitioner, and other members of the health care team. The intensivist often becomes the responsible attending physician but has little history or relationship with the patient and family. Most intensivists adopt a zero-sum approach: aggressive therapy until it is clear that a patient will not survive and then a clean shift to comfort care (Mularski, Bascom, & Osborne, 2001). Conflicting viewpoints are well known between medical specialists who want to offer more treatment options to ameliorate specific disease processes or reverse specific declining functions and generalist physicians and nurses who want to alleviate suffering with palliative measures (Kaufman, 1998). Any team member may have a clear-cut opinion regarding a treatment plan that is in the best interest of the patient. Unfortunately, research has shown that neither perceived benefit nor prognostic estimates are significant determinants for some provider decision making in the ICU. However, practice style on an interventionist/noninterventionist dimension does influence decision making. That is, some physicians tended to prescribe many interventions and others tended not to prescribe (Elstein, Christensen, Cottrell, et al., 1999). Nurses, on the other hand, seem to be more pessimistic regarding long-term outcomes of mortality and quality of life in long-term sick ICU patients. This pessimistic view leads nurses to consider treatment withdrawal more often and earlier than physicians consider it (Frick et al., 2003). Conflicting practice styles and patients and families who demand that "everything" or "nothing" be done create a potential for discontinuity of care and conflicting goals of care among the providers and families. The challenge is to bring varied perspectives together to identify a plan of care that each party and the family believe would serve the patient's needs (Danis, Federman, Fins, et al., 1999).

Dying in a Long-Term Care Facility. Long-term care (LTC) facilities are increasingly becoming a common site of death for many Americans. One in five deaths in persons older than 65 years occurs in a nursing home (National Center for Health Care Statistics, 1993). More than half of the patients admitted to an LTC facility will die during their stay (Zerzan, Stearns, & Hanson, 2000). Although some patients may be transferred to a hospital, up to 80% of deaths will occur on site (Hanson & Henderson, 2000). With increasing longevity and the aging of the population, it is estimated that by the year 2040, 40% of all deaths will occur in a nursing home (Teno, 1998). Although death may be common, the timing is uncertain and diagnosing dying is difficult and imprecise. Older age and frailty characterize nursing home residents. The majority suffer from chronic debilitating illnesses and dementia that have a disease trajectory characterized by low initial function, with repeated episodes of sudden deterioration and recovery until a fatal episode (Keay, 1999; Lunney et al., 2002). These episodes may be "treatable" illnesses such as pneumonia, sepsis, or dehydration, which complicate decisions regarding treatment (Hanson & Henderson, 2000). It is difficult to know when to push for treatment and when to let go (Travis, Bernard, Dixon, et al., 2002). Changes in function or behavior such as refusal of food, social withdrawal, or mental status changes sometimes herald approaching death (Hanson & Henderson, 2000). However, because these signs are recurrent and nonspecific, they are difficult to interpret. Therefore development of a palliative plan of care is often difficult and untimely (Travis et al., 2002).

Residents in nursing homes have a high symptom load in the last days of life. Common physical symptoms of dying nursing home residents include pain, dyspnea, delirium, incontinence, fatigue, dysphagia, nausea, insomnia, and anorexia (Hall et al., 2002; Reynolds, Henderson, Schulman, et al., 2002). In addition, psychosocial issues found to be present include depression, anxiety, fear of dying, and loneliness (Hall et al., 2002; Kayser-Jones, 2002).

Unfortunately, a significant number report unmet needs for treatment of physical symptoms, for psychosocial support for emotional symptoms, and for personal cleanliness (Reynolds et al., 2002). Pain, dyspnea, and delirium have been identified as inadequately assessed and treated (Bernabei, Gambassi, Lapane, et al., 1998; Hall et al., 2002; Reynolds et al., 2002; Stein & Ferrell, 1996). Kayser-Jones (2002) found that dying residents did not have meaningful activities and were often confined to bed or in their room for long periods. In addition, staff rarely had time to offer emotional support, to discuss the impending death, or to explore feelings of grief. In a population that has severe functional limitations, requirement for assistance with personal hygiene is prevalent. Yet, many patients have inadequate bathing, linen changes, and oral hygiene, all of which threaten dignity (Kayser-Jones, 2002). In a recent survey, nurses, aides, and families agreed that residents needed more care to ensure personal cleanliness (Reynolds et al., 2002).

Residents who die are typically in a health care institution that is also their home (Hanson, Henderson, & Menon, 2002). Up to 90% of care in nursing homes is provided by certified nursing assistants (CNAs) (Hanson & Henderson, 2000). These providers have a few weeks of training and may or may not be high school graduates. CNAs are generally supervised by licensed practical nurses (LPNs) with 1 year of nursing training. Registered nurses (RNs) constitute less than 30% of the nursing staff (Hanson & Henderson, 2000). Although they perform some patient care, they are more likely to serve in managerial or administrative roles. Nurses take primary responsibility for plans of care and provide most of the direct communication with the family and physicians concerning resident care. Physicians, who may visit a facility on a weekly or monthly basis or may see a particular resident only at 3-month intervals, maintain responsibility for medical treatment (Hanson & Henderson, 2000). A few nursing homes hire nurse practitioners or physician assistants to provide onsite diagnostic and therapeutic expertise (Hanson et al., 2002). Ideally, nursing home care permits staff to form long-term relationships with residents and family members and provides the potential for personal and individualized care that is unique from other institutions. However, numerous constraints make achieving this ideal difficult. Some nursing homes provide hospice care, comfort care, or palliative care programs, but generally they are not organized, funded, or staffed to provide comprehensive services. Care at the end of life is often delivered by staff caregivers who work from a schedule that is driven by a facility governed by policies, regulations, staff availability, and workload (Mezey, Dubler, Mitty, et al., 2002). CNAs are poorly paid and have an annual turnover rate of 100% or more in most states (Hanson et al., 2002). Staffing is often inadequate and characterized by overtime and high patient loads (Kayser-Jones, 2002). Furthermore, licensed nurses who have considerable input into the plan of care in nursing homes have significant knowledge deficits in areas such as philosophy and principles of palliative practices, pain and symptom management, and psychosocial aspects of end-of-life care (Ersek, Kraybill, & Hansberry, 1999; Raudonis, Kyba, & Kinsey, 2002).

Additional characteristics of the nursing home culture that impede quality end-of-life care include intense regulation with an emphasis on rehabilitation, the burden of negative public image, and the lack of communication (Hanson & Henderson, 2000; Travis et al., 2002). Following the Institute of Medicine's report of the wide variation in quality of nursing home care, the industry has become one of the most regulated (Institute of Medicine, 1986). In 1987, the U.S. Congress passed the Omnibus Budget Reconciliation Act of 1987 (OBRA87), aimed at improving the quality of care for nursing home residents. The act requires uniform assessment of residents and defines the primary goal of care as attaining and maintaining the highest physical, mental, and psychosocial well-being of each resident (Zerzan et al., 2000). Nursing home culture in the wake of OBRA87 emphasizes rehabilitation rather than excellence in end-of-life care (Reynolds et al., 2002). Customary goals of care are to maximize independence and functionality of residents to the highest level of attainment (Mezey et al., 2002). Nursing home surveyors may recommend penalties for functional decline or weight loss they deem avoidable (Zerzan et al., 2000). In the current

regulatory climate, providers fear implementing a palliative plan of care that might not be seen as sufficiently aggressive if a resident declines without an intervention (Meier & Morrison, 1999).

Although rehabilitative care has improved since OBRA87, many dying patients and their families fear and wish to avoid nursing homes. Public reports of abuse, neglect, and poor quality of care fuel distrust in nursing homes (Brunk, 1998; Thompson, 1997). One third of seriously ill adults say they would rather die than live permanently in a nursing home (Mattimore, Wenger, Lynn, et al., 1997). In addition, recently bereaved family members express greater dissatisfaction with nursing homes than with any other aspect of terminal care (Hanson, Danis, & Garrett, 1997).

Open communication among providers, residents, and families is essential for good palliative care and greatly influences the experience of dying in the nursing home (Kayser-Jones, 2002; Travis, Loving, McClanahan, et al., 2001; von Gunten, Ferris, & Emanuel, 2000). In the nursing home setting there are several barriers to good communication. First, nearly two thirds of nursing home residents have dementia (Bradley, Walker, Blechner, et al., 1997). This, coupled with functional and cognitive decline that often accompany chronic illness, means that a large percentage of patients at end of life do not have the ability to express needs and desires. Residents' inability to communicate complicates the process of decision making and delivery of care (Reynolds et al., 2002). As in the ICU, crucial decisions regarding the course of care remains the family's responsibility. Second, many families have difficulty discussing end-of-life issues and care-limiting plans for a loved one (Roberto, 1999). Likewise, providers from physicians to CNAs may also be uncomfortable discussing these issues. Third, time constraints and organizational structure in the nursing home hinder communication and relationship building. Physicians are not present on a regular basis and rarely meet face to face with family members. This leaves the RN with the pivotal role of liaison between the family and physician and in communicating end-of-life issues (Hall et al., 2002). Registered nurses, making up the smallest percentage of the nursing staff, have not received adequate training in palliative care communication and often are burdened with administrative duties (Kayser-Jones, 2002; Raudonis et al., 2002). Although CNAs spend the most time with residents, lack of education and heavy workload often result in little verbal interaction with residents or disrespectful or insensitive communication (Kayser-Jones, 2002). Given these barriers, it is no surprise that family members express a desire for better communication and timely provision of information in the nursing home setting (Kayser-Jones, 2002; Reynolds et al., 2002). One study found that family members were unable to identify the physician or nurse in charge of their relative's care. (Reynolds et al., 2002). This indicates a serious lack of communication and relationship between family members and staff.

What is a Good Death?

One of the goals of palliative and hospice practice is to help patients achieve a "good death." Given our understanding of the multidimensional aspects of dying, multiple dying trajectories, and the influence of disease and setting on the dying process, one may ask, "What does this really mean?" Advances in biomedical technology at the end of the twentieth century have advanced our capabilities to fight against disease. We have seen that the development of the main path of medicine toward the goal of prolonging life translates into the reality that saving lives with technology has a higher priority than aiding in dying. Nevertheless, medicine maintains control over the dying process for the majority of persons, and most people die in institutions under medical care (Connelly, 1998). This trend has evoked a response in the contemporary death and dying literature against the "medicalization" of death and an idealization of a "natural" death (Aries, 1981; Callahan, 1977; Illich, 1976). Within this discourse, a "good" death is equated with the ideal "natural" death, whereas medical-technologic intervention, the epitome of which is the intensive care unit, is emblematic of inhumane and unnatural death (Moskowitz & Nelson, 1995). The modern hospice movement emerged in parallel with this view with a new definition of a "good" death that included awareness, acceptance and closure, control

over events of care, and a comfortable, peaceful death at home surrounded by friends and family (Hopkinson & Hallett, 2002; Steinhauser, Christakis, Clipp, et al., 2000). This model of dying as developed in the United States was especially influenced by the writings of Kübler-Ross (1975) that originated in observations of aware patients with aware relatives, dying of specific, often malignant diseases. In the view of some health care professionals and a segment of the public, the model has become the "gold" standard against which the dying process is measured (Walsh, 2002). Following this model, the authors of the final report from the Debate of the Age Health and Care Study Group in the United Kingdom proposed 12 principles of a good death (Debate of the Age Health and Care Study Group, 1999). The principles rely heavily on the four themes that emerged in the debate: freedom from pain, control, autonomy, and independence (Smith, 2000b). Six of the principles focus on control or choice over aspects of dying including events, place of death, companions, wishes for care, closure, and timing. The remaining principles relate to the type of care received including pain and symptom management, awareness and understanding of the course of disease, access to information and expertise as necessary, access to hospice care, and assurance of dignity and privacy.

The hospice model has been to focus end-of-life care on adequate symptom management, family support, and psychosocial and spiritual issues, however, the model is limited in serving as a gold standard for all deaths for several reasons. First, the model is based on and is most appropriate for persons dying in the terminal illness trajectory. Because fewer than one fourth of deaths follow this trajectory, it may not be possible to achieve principles of awareness and choice regarding dying (McNeil, 1998). The overwhelming majority of deaths follow the trajectory of chronic illness or frailty (Lunney et al., 2002). The person dying in these trajectories may have little control or choice in their life because of the burden of multiple pathology or cognitive impairment (Kafetz, 2002).

Second, the model tends to relate a good death to the home setting (Low & Payne, 1996; Payne, Langley-Evans, & Hillier, 1996; Walsh, 2002).

When offered a choice, patients most likely choose a home death over an institutional death (Higginson & Sen-Gupta, 2000; Hinton, 1994; Last Acts, 2002). The resources necessary to support patients, especially those in the chronic illness and frailty trajectories, may preclude a home death. Such cases are more likely to finally succumb to organ failure or pneumonia in an acute care hospital, ICU, or nursing home. Therefore, notwithstanding their preference, most patients die outside the comfort and care of their home. A classic study by Hinton (1994) revealed that patients and families opting for a home death would often request inpatient care when the patient became too ill to be effectively cared for at home or the burdens of caregiving became too great. Further data have demonstrated that patient and family awareness about a poor prognosis and impending death and their individual coping response are reliable indicators for determining a home death (Hinton, 1994; Seale, Addington-Hall, & McCarthy, 1997). Cantwell, Turco, Bruera, et al. (1998) developed the Home Care Assessment Tool used in the Edmonton Palliative Care Service to determine a realistic home death based on the patient's support system. They found that patients without adequate home support, including two or more caregivers, were at risk for acute hospitalization.

Finally, many patients, even patients in the terminal illness trajectory, may choose not to approach death within the hospice model (Ackerman, 1997; Walsh, 2002). There are some very strong cultural reasons for this. The model rests on expectations of straightforward decision making. In a multicultural society, there are groups with cultural aversions to discussing future events, including death or dying (Krakauer, Crenner, & Fox, 2002). Even in Western cultures, facing death and telling the truth about imminent death are not universal values (Benner, 2001). In practice, desire to take control during serious illness varies widely. Many do not want to plot the course of their deterioration or dying. In fact, the most frequent human response is to avoid death. As Finucane (2002) relates, humans have a pervasive and powerful desire "not to be dead." Personal dignity is often coupled with the will to live and the courage to fight (Curtis et al., 2002).

Patients and families fear "giving up too soon" (Lo, 1995). These factors, coupled with our inability to accurately diagnose dying, encourage many chronically ill people to actively seek burdensome treatment that allows life or the chance of it. When continued survival is possible, even if remotely unlikely, it is often attractive to patients near death (Finucane, 2002; Lo, 1995). Therefore the model, because it is unrealistic for many dying persons, falls short of serving as a gold standard for end-of-life care (Ackerman, 1997; Seale, 1998).

Field and Cassel (1997), in their report for the Institute of Medicine, defined a good death as one that is "free from avoidable distress and suffering for patients, families, and caregivers; in general accord with patients' and families' wishes; and reasonably consistent with clinical, cultural, and ethical standards" (p. 4). Inasmuch as palliative care promotes the individual process of dying, this definition offers more flexibility in guiding end-of-life care yet its vagueness does not provide distinct guidelines for practice. Studies of factors important to patients and professionals for a good death reveal some consistencies in general themes related to a good death. These include symptoms and personal care, preparation for death, decision making and treatment preferences, family relationships, and whole person concerns (Hopkinson & Hallett, 2002; Kirstjanson, McPhee, Pickstock, et al., 2001; Patrick et al., 2001; Steinhauser, Clipp, McNeilly, et al., 2000; Vig, Davenport, & Pearlman, 2002). What is notable in these studies is the wide variation within these themes on the part of both patients and professionals of what constitutes a good death. Preferences within each theme were often found to appear in descriptions of both good and bad deaths. For example, some expressed a preference for a peaceful death in a nice warm bed, surrounded by friends, yet others expressed preference for dying in a hospital without friends or family present (Vig et al., 2002).

There is not a single, precise definition of a good death (Steinhauser, Christakis, Clipp, et al., 2000). Quality of dying is a personal evaluation according to one's expectations and values. People die in character; that is, they come to death with a lifetime of experiences that shape the dying process

(McCormick & Conley, 1995). Each dying person, family member, and loved one may have his or her own sense of what a "good death" would be (Stewart et al., 1999). Likewise, health care professionals vary in their perceptions of what constitutes a good death (Hopkinson & Hallett, 2002; Payne et al., 1996; Steinhauser, Clipp, McNeilly, et al., 2000) and these perceptions may vary widely from their patients' preferences. Health care professionals must be careful not to project their own concept of a good death onto dying patients. Failure to recognize this puts professional caregivers at a disadvantage in guiding patients and families and can limit the choices that they offer and the support that they provide patients (Street, 2001).

APPROACHES TO CARE

How then should palliative care professionals approach end-of-life care? We have seen that the one-size-fits-all model of a good death is neither realistic nor maybe even desirable. Yet current care of dying patients tends to focus on the 25% of patients who are easily recognized as dying. Care pathways or protocols aimed at improving the care for this group may not be totally relevant to the individual approaching death (Kafetz, 2002). Protocols cannot take into account all variations either in dying trajectories or in attitudes and beliefs. A standardized approach to dying within an institution negates patient individuality and limits the choices offered the patient and his or her family (Payne et al., 1996). Proscribed outcomes hide the possibility of a meaningful death taking multiple forms across patients and settings. New routes of attention are needed on how to care for persons with life-threatening chronic illnesses or frailty who are receiving aggressive management of pathologic conditions (Stewart et al., 1999). As Hopkinson and Hallett (2002) assert, the goal of palliative care at the end of life may not be a good death but a negotiated acceptable death. This concept recognizes that both shared and personal values of patients and providers shape understandings of an acceptable death. Therefore we propose that just as our understanding of the multidimensional aspects of dying rests on the idea of relationship, so must the palliative care practitioner's approach to patients and families focus on relationship. The relationships that are the foundation of health care are twofold: the clinician-patient relationship and interdisciplinary team relationships (Brody, 1995). A relationship-centered approach places scientific knowledge and the use of technology in context. Clinicians who value their relationships with their patients will want to make the patient's preferences about future care the cornerstone of care planning. Likewise, clinicians who prize those relationships will make symptom relief a very high priority within the plan of care. Health care professionals who see interdisciplinary relationships as a key to quality health care will make sure that all members of the health care team have optimal input into decisions and communication with patients and family. Cultivating partner relationships with other health care professionals and with patients may be the crucial step in improving end-of-life care, addressing what matters most to patients and families, and in negotiating acceptable and achievable goals.

Investments of time into mutual understanding and trust building have great potential to improve quality of care, decrease stress, and prevent conflict (Karlawish, Quill, & Meier, 1999). The value of the provider-patient relationship cannot be overestimated (Holstein, 1997). A relationship that extends respect for the individual and contributes to understanding the context of patients' lives, values, and preferences is an important therapeutic tool for health care providers (Steinhauser, Christakis, Clipp, et al., 2000). A health care team that values the voices and roles of all disciplines has significant power to influence the process toward a negotiated acceptable death. However, in an economic environment that substantially limits providers' time, developing relationships may seem unrealistic. Physicians are busy coping with medical diagnoses, tests, and physiologic responses; nurses are busy assessing, monitoring, and administering treatments; social workers are busy with resource evaluation and placements—all of which occur in the context of a bureaucratic health care system that places extraordinary procedural and documentation demands on professionals. Good clinicians always find the time to review and evaluate laboratory data and carefully assess medications deemed essential to good care. The same emphasis and value are rarely placed on techniques of building relationships (Levy, 2001). However, when we consider the physical, psychosocial, and spiritual dimensions of death and those themes that are most important to patients, we must conclude that human relationships among health care providers and between providers and patients are pivotal to providing quality care to those who are dying (Kaufman, 2002).

Given the dying trajectory of the majority of deaths, it is not reasonable to think that the process toward a negotiated acceptable death is best addressed only when death is inevitable. Much of this work is ideally addressed upstream from death as discussed in Chapter 2. However, the reality is that this approach is not taken in many cases. Important conversations regarding patient values, perspectives on disease and trajectory, and preferences for care do not take place until an exacerbation or crisis occurs (Curtis et al., 2002; Steinhauser, Clipp, McNeilly, et al., 2000). Decisions about care and goals of treatment must then be made when the patient may be unable to participate, when the emotional reserve of family members is already low, and when clinicians face the most time constraints. This sets the scene for an unacceptable death in the eyes of family members and providers (Steinhauser, Clipp, McNeilly, et al., 2000). Establishing a therapeutic relationship under these circumstances is additionally difficult but no less important. One important way the palliative care team, working together, can move toward cultivating a partner relationship with patients and families is by exercising excellent communication skills.

Communication

Therapeutic communication is discussed in detail in Chapter 2, and therefore we will only briefly review some points that are salient in regard to dying patients and families. We have sufficient evidence that communication with patients and families is one of the most significant but least accomplished factors in quality care at end of life (Curtis et al., 2002; Hanson et al., 1997). The SUPPORT study showed that a flow of information regarding disease, prognosis, and patient preferences did not alter the quality of the experience or enhance communication

for patients or families nor, apparently, did it foster health care team partnerships (Moskowitz & Nelson, 1995; The SUPPORT Investigators, 1995). In the study intervention, specially trained research nurses attempted to facilitate discussions among physicians, patients, and family members by providing detailed information concerning patient prognoses, discussing these prognoses, advance directives, and pain status with patients/families, and reporting patient preferences to physicians. However, when information was handed to physicians or placed in the patient's chart, most physicians reported that they did not review it, act on it, or share it with the patients and families although 41% of the patients who had not discussed resuscitation or prognosis with their physicians indicated a desire to do so.

The question is: How do we maximize communication so that relationships between providers and patients are strengthened? First, physicians must proactively seek to engage in dialogue with patients, families, and team members. Although nurses and social workers have an important role as culture brokers, interpreters, and communication facilitators (Bern-Klug, Gessert, & Forbes, 2001; Buchman, Cassell, Ray, et al., 2002; Sheldon, 2000; Wax & Ray, 2002), physician-initiated discussion is crucial in the current culture. In the real world of medicine, authority and power are usually hierarchic and lie with the physician (Emanuel, 1995). One reason for the failure of the SUPPORT intervention may be that nurses who served to facilitate discussions did not have enough prestige or power with patients or physicians to facilitate discussions. Second, we must engage in better communication skills, both in relaying and receiving important information. Patients and families may not truly understand the information given them. One study found that 54% of family representatives did not understand the patient's diagnosis, prognosis, or treatment plan after a conference with the physician (Azoulay, Chevret, Leleu, et al., 2000). On the other hand, clinicians may focus on delivery of information but neglect to hear the patient's story. Physicians discussing resuscitation status were observed to spend 75% of the time talking. Opportunities to allow patients to discuss their personal values and goals of therapy were not taken or were missed

(Tulsky, Chesney, & Lo, 1995). Thus discussions that focus on the delivery of complex medical information and specific treatment decisions may not satisfy the real needs of dying patients and their families and do not enhance relationship building (Hanson et al., 1997). Communication that enhances the clinician-patient partnership at end of life must focus on developing shared perspectives and must not neglect the psychosocial and spiritual dimensions that are most important to dying patients and families.

When there is no hope for a cure, communication about the dying process and symptom control delivered in a direct, straightforward, and compassionate manner remains a powerful therapeutic tool (Levy, 2001). In addition to delivering information about diagnosis and prognosis and the benefits and burdens of different treatment options, care must be taken to approach and elicit the extent that patients and families understand the information given. Clinicians must not assume the meaning that patients and families assign to terms but, rather, there must be dialogue in which worlds of understanding are shared (Kaufman, 2002). This is especially true of emotionally charged terms such as *starvation, suffering, quality of life, feeding,* and *dying* that are likely to arise in caring for dying patients (Karlawish et al., 1999). Because dialogues with the patient and family are vulnerable to asymmetric power relationships in which scientific, linguistic, and political power privileges the health care team voices over those of the patient and family, good listening skills are essential. Just being heard can help patients and families recover their own personal sense of dignity (Levy, 2001).

With end-of-life conversations, responding to emotions is also important. Patients and families respond to important news in a variety of emotional reactions. They need time to process information and react. Encountering grief, frustration, or anger in a quiet and nonjudgmental manner conveys respect and support (von Gunten et al., 2000). Productive communication that emphasizes a two-way flow of information and does not censure emotional factors facilitates a movement toward shared narrative (Johnson et al., 2000). This sharing of perspectives aids in establishing

and strengthening relationships and developing common goals (Karlawish et al., 1999).

Care of Dying Patients

Although it is impossible to set forth guidelines for the care of dying patients that are appropriate to individual patients, we have seen that some domains that patients and families feel are essential to good end-of-life care. These are symptom management and personal care, whole person issues, family, and preparation for death. Purposefully focusing on these domains is essential for guiding decisions and the plan of care at end of life. Some suggestions for approaching these domains within the context of clinical care are listed in Table 14-4. These domains should not be neglected, whether the patient has chosen to continue fighting the chronic illness or opted for comfort care only. Careful and meticulous attention to patient comfort and optimal management of symptoms are essential to quality end-of-life care. Appropriate therapies for the many symptoms that patients encounter are described throughout this text. In addition, deliberate focus on whole person issues, family relationships, and preparation for death allows the clinician to see the patient in context, a necessary requisite for establishing realistic and meaningful goals of care. Goals that are in alignment with patient/family desires, expectations, and values are important for two reasons. First, uncertainty always surrounds decisions at end of life. Clarification of values and preferences may increase tolerance for some of this uncertainty (Steinhauser, Clipp, McNeilly, et al., 2000). Second, goals of care should drive the use of technology and not vice versa. Without clear goals, it is easy to fall into the habit of automatically prescribing treatments and therapies because they are available (Danis et al., 1999).

Care at the Time of Death

The Pronouncement. Once death has occurred, the necessity of interventions can slow to a different pace. Some practitioners and families may have a sense of urgency to complete the tasks to confirm the death and carry out legal and related practical matters. It will be important to remain aware that there is not one way to perform the pronouncement; cultural, religious, and even family and individual reactions to the death will have an impact on how the identification of the death and postmortem care are performed.

The pronouncement begins the process once the death has been recognized. Much emotion and ritual can be applied to the expectation of the pronouncement, especially if a lengthy chronic illness or distinct terminal illness period has preceded the death. It is not uncommon for tears and even open weeping to accompany the announcement that death has occurred. There may be silence in the room in anticipation as the pronouncement is performed. Death is medically defined as either the cessation of respiratory and cardiovascular function or irreversible cessation of all functions of the entire brain, including brainstem (Menikoff, 2002). A determination of death must be made in accordance with accepted standards. States vary on who can pronounce death, as determined by their death statutes (Menikoff, 2002). A physician is most likely to perform the pronouncement, although some states will allow nurses in certain settings to establish death with the physician's knowledge and approval. Unanticipated deaths will involve the medical examiner for legal purposes.

Documentation Related to the Death. Upon following the steps that indicate death has occurred, documentation of the death will be required. After an identification of the patient through a nametag or name band or conferring with the family or caregivers present, a general appearance of the body may be noted. Pupils are observed for lack of pupillary light reflex. The chest is then auscultated for absence of lung and heart sounds. The documentation should note the time that the call to pronounce was received and time of death. The physical findings should be documented as well as the response of the family to the death. The time of the pronouncement by a physician or time of notification of the physician is the legal time of death. If a nurse pronounces death, the time of this pronouncement is documented as the legal time of death (Berry & Griffie, 2001).

Supportive Care of the Bereaved at Time of Death. Supportive caring for the persons present

at time of death or individuals notified of the death becomes an important adjunct of the pronouncement process. Professional caregivers who have not been faced with the care for patients and families following a death may be unfamiliar with what to say to provide support and demonstrate caring. It is less important what is said as much as the presence of a caregiver who demonstrates empathy. Bereaved families have identified being discomforted by nurses leaving the area without saying anything (Pitorak, 2003). The availability of a caring nurse helps facilitate a more favorable death experience for the family. Families may comment "I don't remember what we talked about in the room that day but I remember you were there." Professional caregivers trained in care after death are more likely to be proactive and comforting than less trained staff who are more likely to perform tasks perfunctorily and not communicate with the family (Main, 2002). An improved comfort and skill level can develop with experience in providing care after death. What not to say can be more relevant to support bereaved families. It is not helpful to spiritualize or minimize loss by stating "He is in a better place." "I'm sorry about your loss" is one of the most powerful and appropriate phrases as well as simply being available to help the family with next steps. Families may also want to review care such as pain medications, the dying process, and the death itself. This time can help provide support if there is doubt about decision making in relation to previously established advance directives or patient-verbalized requests about end-of-life care (Pitorak, 2003).

Postmortem Care. Postmortem care not only is a practical aspect to attend to related to the death but also may serve as a means of demonstrating concern. Family or significant others may want to be a part of the final preparation of the body to facilitate grieving and acknowledgment of the death (Perry & Potter, 2002). Simply asking about preferences may assist the bereaved to maintain a sense of control in the events following the death. Certain cultures and religions require that only particular persons will touch the body following death, and those preferences should be respected. The bereaved may want to touch, hold, or cradle

Table **14-4**   APPROACHES TO CARING FOR DYING PATIENTS

Domains	Therapeutic Interventions	Related Communication or Approach
Symptom management	Always include symptom management into plan of care regardless of patient/family desires for life-sustaining treatment.	How comfortable are you? What makes you the most uncomfortable?
	Elicit expectations for symptom management.	Would you like more treatment for your pain, have the same treatment, or have less treatment?
	Propose realistic goals and how they can be achieved.	I think that by adjusting your medications, we could decrease the amount of nausea you are having each day.
	Address psychologic distress.	How are you coping with what is happening? Do you have worries or fears? Do you feel downhearted or blue?
	Recognize grief reactions.	Can you tell me how things have changed, how things have gone for you? How has this illness most affected you?
Whole person issues	Be available for questions.	Is there anything about your illness that you would like to know? Are those your grandchildren?
	Acknowledge and take interest in those aspects of the patient's life he or she most values.	What about yourself or your life are you most proud? What part of you is strongest right now?
	Advocate for the patient's quality of life and dignity.	I want to take the best possible care of you until the day you die. We ought to care for your mother in a way that makes us confident that after she's gone, we can say she was treated with dignity and respect.
	Treat the patient/family with esteem and respect.	Is there anything in the way you are treated that is not respectful?
	Be genuine. Listen without distraction.	Face patient at eye level. Make eye contact. If appropriate, use physical touch, such as holding a hand.
Family concerns	Explore patient worries about impact of illness on family members.	Do you worry about being a burden to others? What are you biggest concerns for the people you love?
	Acknowledge the importance of family relationship.	Who are the people most important to you? Who is your closest confidante?
	Do not abandon decision making to a family in distress. Be willing to help the patient/family make decisions or present what you would do.	Right now, if your mother stopped breathing or her heart stopped, the hospital staff would perform CPR. That is, they would breathe for her and pump on her chest. In her frail condition, CPR has almost no chance of restoring her heart function or her ability to breathe on her own. In addition, in

		my experience she is likely to suffer from broken ribs from the procedure, as well as discomfort from having a tube inserted down her windpipe and intravenous needles in her arms or neck. The alternative, which I would recommend, is to order that CPR not be done and that we concentrate on keeping her as comfortable as possible.
	Anticipate conflict in decision making. Recognize that guilt or grief motivates behavior. Free the patient's family to do what they need to do, and do not force them to make difficult decisions about care.	Assess family dynamics. Encourage family members to remember conversations with the patient. Conduct family conference. I know we are asking you to make difficult decisions. Together we will do our best to make the best choices. But even more important now is for your wife and mother to feel important and loved. How do you think you can accomplish this?
Preparing for death	Prepare the patient/family for what to expect. Be uncomfortable with the ambiguity. Acknowledge spiritual/existential issues. Allow patient to participate in spiritual or culturally based practices. Communicate frequently with the family.	You are in the final stages of your disease. Are there things you would like to discuss? Your father has an incurable, progressive, and ultimately fatal disease. I can't say for sure when he will die of his lung disease, but given its severity, we shouldn't be surprised when he does. Is there a special source that gives you peace or comfort? What role does faith or spirituality play in your life? Is there a religious or spiritual leader or community that you would like to be connected with? How do you want to be remembered? Is there an event or something you would like to do that would add a great deal of meaning to your life? Even incremental information, while not new, gives the patient/family time to absorb and prepare.

CPR, Cardiopulmonary resuscitation

Data from Chochinov, H.M. (2002). Dignity-conserving care: A new model for palliative care: Helping the patient feel valued. *JAMA*, 287(17), 2253-2260; Emanuel, E.J., & Emanuel, L.L. (1998). The promise of a good death. *Lancet* 351(Suppl. 2), SII21-29; Finucane, T.E. (2002). Care of patients near death: Another view. *J Am Geriatr Soc*, 50, 551-553; Holstein, M. (1997). Reflections on death and dying. *Acad Med*, 72(10), 848-855; Karlawish, J.H., Quill, T., & Meier, D.E. (1999). A consensus-based approach to providing palliative care to patients who lack decision-making capacity. ACP-ASIM End-of-Life Care Consensus Panel. American College of Physicians-American Society of Internal Medicine. *Ann Intern Med*, 130(10), 835-840; Levy, M.M. (2001). End-of-life care in the intensive care unit: Can we do better? *Crit Care Med*, 29(2 Suppl.), N56-61; Steinhauser, K.E., Christakis, N.A., Clipp, E.C., et al (2000). Factors considered important at the end of life by patients, family, physicians, and other care providers. *JAMA*, 284(19), 2476-2482; Wenrich, M.D., Curtis, J.R., Ambrozy, D.M., et al (2003). Dying patients' need for emotional support and personalized care from physicians: Perspectives of patients with terminal illness, families, and health care providers. *J Pain Symptom Manage*, 25(3), 236-246.

the deceased person. The family or others present may want some time of privacy with the body for prayer and reflection. If the body is going to be cremated, this may be the last opportunity the family will have with the deceased. The family or significant other may also need to be prompted in whom to call and about how to prepare for next steps (Perry & Potter, 2002). In some settings, such as deaths occurring at home, it is often the nurse who will perform the postmortem care. Although there is not a right or wrong way to perform the care, facility policy may dictate the care provided. Dignity of the body preparation is maintained when following family personal wishes and cultural or religious customs. Some techniques will ensure that the body is appropriately preserved, especially if the casket will be open at the funeral service.

Begin the preparation of the body by closing the eyes if not already closed. The eyes can be closed by firmly pressing down on the lids. Wash the parts of the body that are soiled by body fluids. The funeral director will perform this task more completely in preparation of the body. The family may request to do this, and the funeral director needs to be notified of this wish. Place a waterproof pad under the body or apply incontinence briefs to prevent leakage as the body's sphincters relax and may release urine or feces. Clean, dry dressings should be applied with paper tape to wounds or other areas of drainage. Remove the IV line. Removal of other tubing will be dictated by facility policy or local health policies. Brush and comb the hair. Families may even request some makeup be applied or certain gowns or other clothing be used to dress the body.

It is not paramount to remove the deceased person immediately from the home or facility setting. Changes in appearance related to bodily function ceasing may be slowed to permit the family more time for visiting or to allow a family member to arrive from out of town. According to Berry and Griffie (2001), the body could be retained at home for up to 24 hours if air-conditioning is available to be turned down to cool the environment. Informing the family members of this option allows them more time to make the decision regarding their private time to say good-byes. Liver mortis begins within 20 minutes and continues for 2 to 4 hours.

This clinical manifestation is a reddish discoloration of the skin caused by a pooling of blood. To ameliorate this condition, elevate the head of the bed 30 degrees to prevent blood from pooling in the lowest part of the body's vasculature (Harvey, 2001). Place the arms naturally at the sides. Do not place one on top of the other. On the stretcher, the head can be placed on two pillows or the funeral director may use a head block for elevation. It is also not necessary to place any dentures in the mouth because they may be lost in transport. The safest way to transport them is to give them to the funeral director in a labeled cup without water. Communicate with the funeral director the patient's cause of death, if the patient has a communicable disease, and if the patient is extremely large and extra help will be needed (Harvey, 2001).

Processing the Death for the Health Care Provider. It is important for the professional caregiver to process the death verbally with the interdisciplinary team if possible or with a colleague. Cumulative grief can occur for the professional caregiver who does not acknowledge his or her feelings related to attending the death. Also, an opportunity may exist to improve care in another death experience at a later date as the delivery of care is discussed and means for improved outcomes are identified (Pitorak, 2003).

SUMMARY

Abundant evidence exists that the dying process is poor, characterized by inadequately treated physical distress, fragmented and bureaucratic care systems, and enormous strains on family caregiver and support systems (Meier & Morrison, 1999). Health care providers face formidable obstacles in providing care at the end of life. Societal barriers, the culture of medicine and health care institutions, and the lack of training of health care professionals handicap the palliative care clinician's ability to deliver and model quality palliative care. Furthermore, some burdens are associated with dying that are not amenable to control even under the best circumstances. All decisions cannot be covered in advance directives, conflicted relationships are rarely resolved or guilt eliminated, symptom control cannot alleviate all suffering, and the

Case Study

J.L., a 54-year-old African-American woman with metastatic breast cancer, was treated by a comprehensive cancer center in the Northeast and relocated to the Southeast to be with her family. She has received multiple rounds of chemotherapy over the past 2 years and has exhausted further radiation options. She was admitted to the medical oncology unit after entering the emergency department, diagnosed with a pleural effusion. During her hospitalization, the covering physician for the medical oncology service informed J.L. and her large extended family that nothing more could be done for her disease and she would be discharged home with hospice care. The patient and family were extremely upset with this physician, who had announced a change in the plan of care before discussing it with them. The patient and her family were convinced that she was going to win the battle over breast cancer. Within a week after J.L. was discharged home to hospice, she was back in the emergency department with complaints of lymphedema, pain, and dyspnea. The patient and family described being unhappy with hospice care because they would not "do" anything for her illness other than provide morphine and lorazepam (Ativan) for her shortness of breath. After the second hospital admission, J.L. was discharged home to skilled care and within 2 days entered the hospice program for the second time. J.L. soon developed acute respiratory distress, and the hospice primary care nurse told her to take additional morphine and lorazepam to relieve her symptoms. The nurse promised to visit at the end of the day. Upset with this directive, J.L. and her family drove to the emergency department. After re-entering the acute care setting for the third time in less than 3 weeks, she was diagnosed with recurrent pleural effusion.

During this admission, the palliative care nurse practitioner was consulted, who determined that J.L.'s idea of care and the care that was being offered to her were philosophically at odds. The patient's hope for a cure was strongly influenced by her family, and anyone who offered a realistic perspective on the extent of her disease was perceived by the family as robbing J.L.'s hope and an indication that aggressive care was being denied her. While in the hospital, she underwent a chest tube placement to drain the pleural effusion and became progressively weaker. J.L. and her family were very angry with the physician and nurses providing care because they believed curative care was not being offered and refused to be discharged home from the hospital with any home care services.

Before her planned discharge, J.L.'s weakness was exacerbated and she was less responsive to her family. Her dyspnea had become more pronounced and was accompanied by excessive secretions. Urine output had decreased and she had not eaten anything by mouth in over 24 hours. Despite her family's reluctance to accept her prognosis, J.L. was actively dying.

Initiating palliative interventions was difficult with a family who were apprehensive about the plan of care and J.L.'s prognosis. They continued to object to the use of opioids and anticholinergics and attempted to arrange for a discharge home. The health care team's efforts to comfort the family by engaging a social worker and the hospital chaplain went without success. The chaplain, however, communicated with the family's local pastor who agreed to come to the hospital in an attempt to calm the family. During this time, the patient had become unresponsive with Cheyne-Stokes breathing, tachycardia, and lower extremity mottling.

After a family conference, the family's pastor was able to convince them that J.L was dying and the health care team could promote comfort during her last hours of life. The family was then approached by the palliative care nurse practitioner and social worker to mutually discuss the plan of care that would best support J.L. during her dying process. The family agreed upon the recommended use of medications to control the patient's symptoms. The patient died peacefully in the presence of her family.

best palliative care may be unable to sanitize all that is hard about dying (Finucane, 2002; von Gunten et al., 2000). Therefore we must not define success too narrowly.

Providers of palliative care often hold to the myth that if the 'right' things are done, a 'good' death can be ensured for all patients in which suffering is alleviated, death is discussed and accepted, all business is finished, good-byes are well-articulated, and the exit is made gracefully. In many cases, however, death is neither good nor graceful. Many problems and issues confronted by dying cannot be fixed (Brenneis, Perry, Read-Paul, et al., 1998, p. 94).

Nevertheless, dying patients and their families have the right to expect best care at end of life, regardless of setting. To accomplish this, palliative care clinicians must continue to encourage all providers not to focus exclusively on the disease process, body systems, and treatment strategies. Although these skills are important, the ability to assist patients and families achieve an acceptable death are related to relationship skills—understanding the patient's story and his or her place in the family, understanding values and preferences, and acknowledging dignity and worth.

Objective Questions

1. Criticism about the stage theories of death and dying include:

    a. Prescriptive in nature.
    b. Influences the practitioner's decision making.
    c. Determined by the extent of pathophysiology.
    d. Influences the quality of care provided the patient and family.

2. Death with dignity is a vague concept because:

    a. It requires dying at home.
    b. It is also associated with physician-assisted suicide.
    c. There are no quality indicators to determine dignity.
    d. There is increased attention to promote death with dignity.

3. Human existence is a composite of intrapersonal and extrapersonal relationships. Illness disturbs these relationships in all of the following ways *except:*

    a. Homeostasis.
    b. Coping skills.
    c. Disruption of important relationships.
    d. Fear of using medications and associated addiction.

4. Common rhetoric concerning the benefits of dehydration does *not* include:

    a. Decreased airway secretions.
    b. Reduction in cardiopulmonary problems.
    c. Dehydration as universally beneficial in dying patients.
    d. Decrease in the pain perception because of the release of endorphins.

5. Hypoactive delirium is described as:

    a. Should not be treated.
    b. Increased neurologic irritability.
    c. Manifested by restlessness and progressing through stages of confusion.
    d. Progresses from a normal level of cognition through stages of sleepiness and lethargy.

6. In the literature, terms used to describe sedative interventions include all of the following *except:*

    a. Terminal sedation.
    b. Physician-assisted suicide.
    c. Palliative sedation therapy.
    d. Total pharmacologic sedation.

7. A key element in terminal sedation is to:

    a. Ensure that the patient remains cognitively alert and aware.
    b. Discontinue all central nervous system–stimulating medications.
    c. Evaluate the patient and family for depressive symptoms.
    d. Titrate the sedative of choice against the distress response of a specific symptom.

8. Sedation therapy that meets the elements of double effect includes all but the following:

   a. Sedation to treat intractable symptoms is good or morally neutral.
   b. The intent of the provider to prescribe medication to sedate is good.
   c. Sedation or hastening of death is not a benefit in the actively dying patient.
   d. Freedom from intractable symptoms in dying patients is a good effect.

9. The largest percentage of deaths in the United States follows which dying trajectory?

   a. Sudden death.
   b. Terminal illness.
   c. Organ failure.
   d. Frailty.

10. Diagnosing dying is difficult because:

   a. Physicians are too emotionally involved with their patients.
   b. Prognostication is not a priority in medical education.
   c. The science of prognostication has not developed accurate models to aid clinicians.
   d. Physicians see death as a failure.

11. Prognosticating the need for palliative interventions for patients living with heart failure is difficult and includes all of the following barriers except:

   a. Typical markers of poor prognosis include severity of symptoms.
   b. The course of heart failure is predictable during the last month of life.
   c. The most frequent symptoms include pain, dyspnea, depressed mood, and anxiety.
   d. Patients with heart failure never experience a time when they are dying from their illness.

12. Dementia, the eighth most prevalent disease in the United States, is difficult to predict

impending death because:

   a. There is a 30% occurrence of disease in patients older than 85 years.
   b. There is not a predictable group of symptoms that accompany this illness.
   c. As with other chronic conditions, an inaccurate prognosis is common.
   d. Nearly 30% of those thought to be terminal within 6 months were alive at 3 years.

13. What barrier contributes to the lack of palliative care in the acute care setting?

   a. The focus of care is on comfort versus curative interventions.
   b. Hospitalized care acknowledges and provides for death planning.
   c. Providers place the priority of care on the disease process versus symptom management.
   d. The institutional culture provides an interdisciplinary team to support the patient and family needs.

REFERENCES

Abebaw, M.Y., Baldwin, R.C., & Connolly, M. (2002). Mortality predictors in disabling chronic obstructive pulmonary disease in old age. Age Ageing, 31, 137-140.

Ackerman, F. (1997). Goldilocks and Mrs. Ilych: A critical look at the "philosophy of hospice." Cambridge Q Healthc Ethics, 6(3), 314-324.

Afessa, B., Morales, I.J., Scanlon, P.D., et al. (2002). Prognostic factors, clinical course, and hospital outcome of patients with chronic obstructive pulmonary disease admitted to an intensive care unit for acute respiratory failure. Crit Care Med, 30(7), 1610-1615.

Aguero-Torres, H., Fratiglioni, L., Guo, Z., et al. (1998). Prognostic factors in very old demented adults: A seven-year follow-up from a population-based survey in Stockholm. J Am Geriatr Soc, 46, 444-452.

Ahmedzai, S.H., & Walsh, D. (2000). Palliative medicine and modern cancer care. Semin Oncol, 27(1), 1-6.

Albom, M. (1997). Tuesdays with Morrie: An old man, a young man, and life's greatest lesson. New York: Doubleday.

Almagro, P., Calbo, E., Ochoa de Echaguen, A., et al. (2002). Mortality after hospitalization for COPD. Chest, 121(5), 1441-1448.

Aries, P. (1981). The hour of our death. London: Allen Lane.

Asch, D.A., Shea, J.A., Jedrziewski, M., et al. (1997). The limits of suffering: Critical care nurses' views of hospital care at the end of life. Soc Sci Med, 45(11), 1661-1668.

Azoulay, E., Chevret, S., Leleu, G., et al. (2000). Half the families of intensive care unit patients experience inadequate communication with physicians. Crit Care Med, 28(8), 3044-3049.

Back, A., Wallace, J.I., Starks, H.E., et al. (1996). Physician-assisted suicide and euthanasia in Washington State: Patient requests and physician responses. *JAMA, 275*(12), 919-925.

Baggs, J.G. (2002). End-of-life care for older adults in ICUs. *Annu Rev Nurs Res, 20,* 181-229.

Beauchamp, T.L., & Childress, J.F. (2001). *Principles of biomedical ethics* (5th ed.). New York: Oxford University Press.

Benner, P. (2001). Death as a human passage: Compassionate care for persons dying in critical care units. *Am J Crit Care, 10*(5), 355-359.

Bern-Klug, M., Gessert, C., & Forbes, S. (2001). The need to revise assumptions about the end of life: Implications for social work practice. *Health Soc Work, 26*(1), 38-48.

Bernabei, R., Gambassi, G., Lapane, K., et al. (1998). Management of pain in elderly patients with cancer. SAGE Study Group. Systematic assessment of geriatric drug use via epidemiology. *JAMA, 279*(23), 1877-1882.

Berry, P., & Griffie, J. (2001). Planning for the actual death. In B.A. Ferrell & N. Coyle (Eds.), *Textbook of palliative nursing* (pp. 382-394). New York: Oxford University Press.

Billings, J.A., & Brock, S.D. (1996). Slow euthanasia. *J Palliat Care, 12*(4), 21-30.

Block, S. (2001). Psychological considerations, growth, and transcendence at the end of life: The art of the possible. *JAMA, 285*(22), 2898-2905.

Boersma, F., Van Den Brink, W., Deeg, D.J., et al. (1999). Survival in a population-based cohort of dementia patients: Predictors and causes of mortality. *Int J Geriatr Psychiatry, 14*(9), 748-753.

Bradley, E., Walker, L., Blechner, B., et al. (1997). Assessing capacity to participate in discussions of advance directives in nursing homes: Findings from a study of the Patient Self Determination Act. *J Am Geriatr Soc, 45*(1), 79-83.

Breitbart, W., & Strout, D. (2000). Delirium in the terminally ill. *Clin Geriatr Med, 16*(2), 357-372.

Brenneis, C., Perry, B., Read-Paul, L., et al. (1998). Common questions (and answers) about palliative care: A nurse's handbook. Edmonton, Alberta Canada: Regional Palliative Care Program Capital Authority.

Brody, H. (1995). The best system in the world. *Hastings Cent Rep, 25*(6), S18-20.

Bruera, E., & MacDonald, N. (2000). To hydrate or not to hydrate: How should it be? *J Clin Oncol, 18*(5), 1156-1158.

Bruera, E., Neumann, C.M., Pituskin, E., et al. (1999). A randomized controlled trial of local injections of hyaluronidase versus placebo in cancer patients receiving subcutaneous hydration. *Ann Oncol, 10*(10), 1255-1258.

Brumley, R.D. (2002). Future of end-of-life care: The managed care organization perspective. *J Palliat Med, 5*(2), 263-270.

Brunk, D. (1998). Why people hate long-term care. What's behind the industry's bad public image and what can providers do to improve it? *Contemp Longterm Care, 21*(1), 38-40.

Buchman, T.G., Cassell, J., Ray, S.E., et al. (2002). Who should manage the dying patient? Rescue, shame, and the surgical ICU dilemma. *J Am Coll Surg, 194*(5), 665-673.

Buckman, R. (1998). Communication in palliative care: A practical guide. In D.D. Hanks & N. MacDonald (Eds.), *The Oxford textbook of palliative medicine* (pp. 141-156). Oxford: Oxford Medical Publications.

Burge, F.I. (1993). Dehydration symptoms of palliative care cancer patients. *J Pain Symptom Manage, 8*(7), 454-464.

Callahan, D. (1977). On defining a "natural death." *Hastings Cent Rep, 7*(3), 32-37.

Cantwell, P., Turco, S., Bruera, E., et al. (1998). Home death assessment tool: A prospective study. *J Palliat Care, 14,* 104.

Casarett, D.A., & Karlawish, J. (1999). Working in the dark: The state of palliative care for patients with severe dementia. *Generations, 23*(1), 18-23.

Cassell, E.J. (1991). *The nature of suffering: And the goals of medicine.* New York: Oxford University Press.

Centers for Disease Control & Prevention (CDC). (2002). National Center for Health Statistics, *National vital statistics report, 50*(15), Sept. 16.

Cerchietti, L., Navigante, A., Sauri, A., et al. (2000). Clinical trial: Hypodermoclysis for control of dehydration in terminal-stage cancer. *Int J Palliat Nurs, 6*(8), 370-374.

Chater, S., Viola, R., Paterson, J., et al. (1998). Sedation for intractable distress in the dying: A survey of experts. *Palliat Med, 12*(4), 255-269.

Chen, D.C. (2001). On being a doctor: It's only 50 cents. *Ann Intern Med, 135*(12), 1087-1088.

Cheng, C., Roemer-Becuwe, C., & Pereira, J.L. (2002). When midazolam fails. *J Pain Symptom Manage, 23*(3), 256-265.

Cherny, N.I., & Portenoy, R.K. (1994). Sedation in the management of refractory symptoms: Guidelines for evaluation and treatment. *J Palliat Care, 10*(2), 31-38.

Chin, A.E., Hedberg, K., Higginson, G.K., et al. (1999). Legalized physician-assisted suicide in Oregon: The first year's experience. *N Engl J Med, 340*(7), 577-583.

Chiu, T., Hu, W., Lue, B., et al. (2001). Sedation for refractory symptoms of terminal cancer patients in Taiwan. *J Pain Symptom Manage, 21*(6), 467-472.

Chochinov, H.M. (2002). Dignity-conserving care: A new model for palliative care: Helping the patient feel valued. *JAMA, 287*(17), 2253-2260.

Christakis, N., & Escarce, J.J. (1996). Survival of Medicare patients after enrollment in hospice programs. *N Engl J Med, 335,* 172-178.

Christakis, N.A., & Lamont, E.B. (2000). Extent and determination of error in doctor's prognoses in terminally ill patients: Prospective cohort study. *BMJ, 320,* 469-472.

Claessens, M.T., Lynn, J., Zhong, Z., et al. (2000). Dying with lung cancer or chronic obstructive pulmonary disease: Insights from SUPPORT. Study to Understand Prognoses and Preferences for Outcomes and Risks of Treatments. *J Am Geriatr Soc, 48*(5 Suppl.), S146-153.

Connelly, R. (1998). The medicalization of dying: A positive turn on a new path. *Omega—J Death Dying, 36*(4), 331-341.

Cook, D.J. (1997). Health professional decision-making in the ICU: A review of the evidence. *New Horiz, 5*(1), 15-19.

Coombs Lee, B., & Werth, J.L. (2000). Observations on the first year of Oregon's Death with Dignity Act. *Psychol Public Policy Law, 6*(2), 268-290.

Coope, C.M. (1997). Death with dignity. *Hastings Cent Rep, 27*(5), 37-38.

Copp, G. (1997). Patients and nurses: Constructions of death and dying in a hospice setting. *J Cancer Nurs, 1*(1), 2-15.

Copp, G. (1998). A review of current theories of death and dying. *J Adv Nurs, 28*(2), 382-390.

Corr, C. (1992). A task-based approach to coping with dying. *Omega—J Death Dying, 24*(2), 81-94.

Cowan, J.D., & Walsh, D. (2001). Terminal sedation in palliative medicine: Definition and review of the literature. *Support Care Cancer, 9,* 403-407.

Crippen, D., Levy, M., Truog, R., et al. (2000). Debate: What constitutes "terminality" and how does it relate to a living will? *Crit Care, 4*(6), 333-338.

Cronin, D. (2001). Other studies of density and growth. *USA Today* (Feb. 22), 11C80.

Curtis, J.R., Wenrich, M.D., Carline, J.D., et al. (2002). Patients' perspectives on physician skill in end-of-life care: Differences between patients with COPD, cancer, and AIDS. *Chest, 122*(1), 356-362.

Danis, M., Federman, D., Fins, J.J., et al. (1999). Incorporating palliative care into critical care education: Principles, challenges, and opportunities. *Crit Care Med, 27*(9), 2005-2013.

Debate of the Age Health and Care Study Group. (1999). *The future of health and care of older people: The best is yet to come.* London: Age Concern.

Desbiens, N.A., Mueller-Rizner, N., Connors, A.F. Jr., et al. (1999). The symptom burden of seriously ill hospitalized patients. *J Pain Symptom Manage, 17,* 248-255.

Dunn, G.P., & Milch, R.A. (2002). Is this a bad day or one of the last days? How to recognize and respond to approaching demise. *J Am Coll Surg, 195*(6), 879-887.

Edmonds, P., Karlsen, S., Khan, S., et al. (2001). A comparison of the palliative care needs of patients dying from chronic respiratory diseases and lung cancer. *Palliat Med, 15*(4), 287-295.

Edson, M. (1999). *Wit: A play.* New York: Faber & Faber.

Ellershaw, J., & Ward, C. (2003). Care of the dying patient: The last hours or days of life. *BMJ, 326*(7379), 30-34.

Ellershaw, J.E., Sutcliffe, J.M., & Saunders, C.M. (1995). Dehydration and the dying patient. *J Pain Symptom Manage, 10*(3), 192-197.

Elstein, A.S., Christensen, C., Cottrell, J.J., et al. (1999). Effects of prognosis, perceived benefit, and decision style on decision making and critical care. *Crit Care Med, 27*(1), 58-65.

Emanuel, E.J., & Emanuel, L.L. (1998). The promise of a good death. *Lancet, 351*(Suppl. 2), SII21-29.

Emanuel, L.L. (1995). Structure deliberation to improve decision making for the seriously ill. *Hastings Cent Rep, 25*(6), S14-18.

Emanuel, L.L., von Gunten, C.F., & Ferris, F.D. (1999). *The education for physicians on end of life care (EPEC).* Chicago: American Medical Association.

Emanuel, L.L., von Gunten, C.F., & Ferris, F.D. (2000). Gaps in end-of-life care. *Arch Fam Med, 9*(10), 1176-1180.

Engelberg, J. (1997). On the dynamics of dying. *Integr Physiol Behav Sci, 32*(2), 143-148.

Ersek, M., Kraybill, B.M., & Hansberry, J. (1999). Investigating the emotional needs of licensed nursing staff and certified nursing assistants in nursing homes regarding end-of-life care. *Am J Hosp Palliat Care, 16,* 573-582.

Faber-Langendoen, K. (1996). A multi-institutional study of care given to patients dying in hospitals: Ethical and practice implications. *Arch Intern Med, 156*(18), 2130-2136.

Fainsinger, R.L. (1998). Use of sedation by a hospital palliative care support team. *J Palliat Care, 14,* 51-54.

Fainsinger, R.L., & Bruera, E. (1997). When to treat dehydration in a terminally ill patient? *Support Care Cancer, 5*(3), 205-211.

Fainsinger, R.L., De Moissac, D., Mancini, I., et al. (2000). Sedation for delirium and other symptoms in terminally ill patients in Edmonton. *J Palliat Care, 16*(2), 5-10.

Fainsinger, R.L., Landman, W., Hoskings, M., et al. (1998). Sedation for uncontrolled symptoms in a South African hospice. *J Pain Symptom Manage, 16*(3), 145-152.

Fainsinger, R.L., Waller, A., Bercovici, M., et al. (2000). A multicentre international study of sedation for uncontrolled symptoms in terminally ill patients. *Palliat Med, 14*(4), 257-265.

Ferrand, E., Robert, R., Ingrand, P., et al. (2001). Withholding and withdrawal of life support in intensive-care units in France: A prospective survey. French LATAREA Group. *Lancet, 357*(9249), 9-14.

Ferry, M., Dardaine, V., & Constans, T. (1999). Subcutaneous infusion or hypodermoclysis: A practical approach. *J Am Geriatr Soc, 47*(1), 93-95.

Field, M.J., & Cassel, C.K. (Eds.). (1997). *Approaching death: Improving care at the end of life.* Washington, D.C.: National Academy Press.

Finucane, T.E. (1999). How gravely ill becomes dying: A key to end-of-life care. *JAMA, 282*(17), 1670-1672.

Finucane, T.E. (2002). Care of patients near death: Another view. *J Am Geriatr Soc, 50,* 551-553.

Fox, E., Landrum-McNiff, K., Zhong, Z., et al. (1999). Evaluation of prognostic criteria for determining hospice eligibility in patients with advanced lung, heart, or liver disease. SUPPORT Investigators. Study to Understand Prognoses and Preferences for Outcomes and Risks of Treatments. *JAMA, 282*(17), 1638-1645.

Frick, S., Uehlinger, D.E., & Zuercher Zenklusen, R.M. (2003). Medical futility: Predicting outcome of intensive care unit patients by nurses and doctors: A prospective comparative study. *Crit Care Med, 31*(2), 456-461.

Friesinger, G.C., & Butler, J. (2000). End-of-life care for elderly patients with heart failure. *Clin Geriatr Med, 16*(3), 663-675.

Frisoli, A. Jr., de Paula, A.P., Feldman, D., et al. (2000). Subcutaneous hydration by hypodermoclysis. A practical and low cost treatment for elderly patients. *Drugs Aging, 16*(4), 313-319.

Ganzini, L., Johnston, W.S., McFarland, B.H., et al. (1998). Attitudes of patients with amyotrophic lateral sclerosis and their care givers toward assisted suicide. *N Engl J Med, 339*(14), 967-973.

Glare, P., Virik, K., Jones, M., et al. (2003). A systematic review of physicians' survival predictions in terminally ill cancer patients. *BMJ, 327,* 195-200.

Glaser, B.G., & Strauss, A.L. (1965). *Awareness of dying.* New York: Aldine Publishing.

Glaser, B.G., & Strauss, A.L. (1968). *Time for dying.* Chicago: Aldine Publishing.

Goodlin, S.J., Winzelberg, G.S., Teno, J.M., et al. (1998). Death in the hospital. *Arch Intern Med, 158*(14), 1570-1572.

Greene, W.R., & Davis, W.H. (1991). Titrated intravenous barbiturates in the control of symptoms in patients with terminal cancer. *South Med J, 84*(3), 332-337.

Groenewoud, J.H., van der Maas, P.J., van der Wal, G., et al. (1997). Physician-assisted death in psychiatric practice in the Netherlands. *N Engl J Med, 336*(25), 1795-1801.

Hall, P., Schroder, C., & Weaver, L. (2002). The last 48 hours of life in long-term care: A focused chart audit. *J Am Geriatr Soc, 50*(3), 501-506.

Hallenbeck, J.L. (2000). Terminal sedation: Ethical implications in different situations. *J Palliat Med, 3*(3), 313-320.

Hanson, L.C., Danis, M., & Garrett, J. (1997). What is wrong with end-of-life care? Opinions of bereaved family members. *J Am Geriatr Soc, 45*(11), 1339-1344.

Hanson, L.C., & Henderson, M. (2000). Care of the dying in long-term care settings. *Clin Geriatr Med, 16*(2), 225-237.

Hanson, L.C., Henderson, M., & Menon, M. (2002). As individual as death itself: A focus group study of terminal care in nursing homes. *J Palliat Med, 5*(1), 117-125.

Harvey, J. (2001). Debunking myths about postmortem care. *Nursing, 31*(7), 44-45.

Heaven, C.M., & Maguire, P. (1998). The relationship between patients' concerns and psychological distress in a hospice setting. *Psychooncology, 7*, 502-507.

Helmer, C., Joly, P., Letenneur, L., et al. (2001). Mortality with dementia: Results from a French prospective community-based cohort. *Am J Epidemiol, 154*(7), 642-648.

Hermann, C.P. (2001). Spiritual needs of dying patients: A qualitative study. *Oncol Nurs Forum, 28*(1), 67-72.

Higginson, I.J., & Sen-Gupta, G.J.A. (2000). Place of care in advanced cancer: A qualitative systematic literature review of patient preferences. *J Palliat Med, 3*(3), 287-300.

Hinshaw, D.B. (2002). The spiritual needs of the dying patient. *J Am Coll Surg, 4*, 565-568.

Hinton, J. (1994). Can home care maintain an acceptable quality of life for patients with terminal cancer and their relatives? *Palliat Med, 8*(3), 183-196.

Holstein, M. (1997). Reflections on death and dying. *Acad Med, 72*(10), 848-855.

Hopkinson, J., & Hallett, C. (2002). Good death? An exploration of newly qualified nurses' understanding of good death. *Int J Palliat Nurs, 8*(11), 532-539.

Huang, Z.B., & Ahronheim, J.C. (2000). Nutrition and hydration in terminally ill patients: An update. *Clin Geriatr Med, 16*(2), 313-325.

Huffman, J.L., & Dunn, G.P. (2002). The paradox of hydration in advanced terminal illness. *J Am Coll Surg, 194*(6), 835-839.

Illich, I. (1976). *Medical nemesis: The expropriation of health.* Harmondsworth: Penguin.

Institute of Medicine. (1986). *Improving the quality of care in nursing homes.* Washington, D.C.: National Academy Press.

Iwashyna, T.J., & Christakis, N.A. (2001). Signs of death. *J Palliat Med, 4*(4), 451-452.

Jacobs, L.G., Bonuck, K., Burton, W., et al. (2001). Hospital care at the end of life: An institutional assessment. *J Pain Symptom Manage, 24*, 291-298.

Jagger, C., Clarke, M., & Stone, A. (1995). Predictors of survival with Alzheimer's disease: A community-based study. *Psychol Med, 25*(1), 171-177.

Jansen, L.A., & Sulmasy, D.P. (2002). Sedation, alimentation, hydration, and equivocation: Careful conversation about care at the end of life. *Ann Intern Med, 136*(11), 845-849.

Johnson, N., Cook, D., Giacomini, M., et al. (2000). Towards a "good" death: End-of-life narratives constructed in an intensive care unit. *Cult Med Psychiatry, 24*, 275-295.

Kafetz, K. (2002). What happens when elderly people die? *J R Soc Med, 95*, 536-538.

Kammoun, S., Gold, G., Bouras, C., et al. (2000). Immediate causes of death of demented and non-demented elderly. *Acta Neurol Scand Suppl, 176*, 96-99.

Karlawish, J.H., Quill, T., & Meier, D.E. (1999). A consensus-based approach to providing palliative care to patients who lack decision-making capacity. ACP-ASIM End-of-Life Care Consensus Panel. American College of Physicians-American Society of Internal Medicine. *Ann Intern Med, 130*(10), 835-840.

Kaufman, S.R. (1998). Intensive care, old age, and the problem of death in America. *Gerontologist, 38*, 715-725.

Kaufman, S.R. (2002). A commentary: Hospital experience and meaning at the end of life. *Gerontologist, 42*(SIII), 34-39.

Kayser-Jones, J. (2002). The experience of dying: An ethnographic nursing home study. *Gerontologist, 42*(SIII), 11-19.

Keay, T.J. (1999). Palliative care in the nursing home. *Gerontologist, 23*(1), 96-98.

Keene, J., Hope, T., Fairburn, C.G., et al. (2001). Death and dementia. *Int J Geriatr Psychiatry, 16*(10), 969-974.

Kirchhoff, K.T., Spuhler, V., Walker, L., et al. (2000). Intensive care nurses' experiences with end-of-life care. *Am J Crit Care, 9*(1), 36-42.

Kirstjanson, L.J., McPhee, I., Pickstock, S., et al. (2001). Palliative care nurses' perceptions of good and bad deaths and care expectations: A qualitative analysis. *Int J Palliat Nurs, 7*(3), 129-139.

Kite, S. (2002). Upstream from death. *J R Soc Med, 95*, 529.

Koenig, H.G. (2002). A commentary: The role of religion and spirituality at the end of life. *Gerontologist, 42*(SIII), 20-23.

Krakauer, E.L., Crenner, C., & Fox, K. (2002). Barriers to optimum end-of-life care for minority patients. *J Am Geriatr Soc, 50*(1), 182-190.

Krakauer, E.R., Penson, R.T., Truog, R.D., et al. (2000). Sedation for intractable distress of a dying patient: Adult palliative care and the principle of double effect. *Oncologist, 5*(1), 53-62.

Kübler-Ross, E. (1975). Death: The final stage of growth. Englewood Cliffs, N.J.: Prentice Hall.

Kuebler, K.K., & McKinnon, S. (2002). Dehydration. In K.K. Kuebler, P.H. Berry, & D.E. Heidrich (Eds.), *End of life care: Clinical practice guidelines* (pp. 243-251). Philadelphia: Saunders.

Last Acts. (2002). *Means to a better end: A report on dying in America.* Washington, D.C.: Last Acts.

Lawlor, P.G., Fainsinger, R.L., & Bruera, E. (2000). Delirium at the end of life: Critical issues in clinical practice and research. *JAMA, 284*(19), 2427-2429.

Lawlor, P.G., Gagnon, B., Mancini, I.L., et al. (2000). Occurrence, causes, and outcome of delirium in patients with advanced cancer: A prospective study. *Arch Intern Med, 160*(6), 786-794.

Levenson, J.W., McCarthy, E.P., Lynn, J., et al. (2000). The last six months of life for patients with congestive heart failure. *J Am Geriatr Soc, 48*(5 Suppl.), S101-109.

Levy, M.M. (2001). End-of-life care in the intensive care unit: Can we do better? *Crit Care Med, 29*(2 Suppl.), N56-61.

Lichter, I., & Hunt, E. (1990). The last 48 hours of life. *J Palliat Care, 6*(4), 7-15.

Lo, B. (1995). End-of-life care after termination of SUPPORT. *Hastings Cent Rep, 25*(6), S6-8.

Lo, R.S.K., Woo, J., Zhoc, K.C.H., et al. (2002). Quality of life of palliative care patients in the last two weeks of life. *J Pain Symptom Manage, 24*(4), 388-397.

Loewy, E.H. (2001). Terminal sedation, self-starvation, and orchestrating the end of life. *Arch Intern Med, 161*(3), 329-332.

Low, J.T.S., & Payne, S. (1996). The good and bad death perceptions of health professionals working in palliative care. *Eur J Cancer Care (Engl), 5*(4), 237-241.

Lunney, J.R., Lynn, J., Foley, D.J., et al. (2003). Patterns of functional decline at end of life. *JAMA, 289*, 2387-2392.

Lunney, J.R., Lynn, J., & Hogan, C. (2002). Profiles of older Medicare decedents. *J Am Geriatr Soc, 50*(6), 1108-1112.

Lynn, J. (2001). Perspectives on care at the close of life: Serving patients who may die soon and their families: The role of hospice and other services. *JAMA, 285*(7), 925-932.

Lynn, J., Harrell, F. Jr., Cohn, F., et al. (1997). Prognoses of seriously ill hospitalized patients on the days before death: Implications for patient care and public policy. *New Horiz, 5*(1), 56-61.

Lynn, J., Teno, J.M., Phillips, R.S., et al. (1997). Perceptions by family members of the dying experience of older and seriously ill patients. SUPPORT Investigators. Study to Understand Prognoses and Preferences for Outcomes and Risks of Treatments. *Ann Intern Med, 126*(2), 97-106.

Mahmoud, F.A., & Rivera, N.I. (2002). The role of C-reactive protein as a prognostic indicator in advanced cancer. *Curr Oncol Rep, 4*(3), 250-255.

Main, J. (2002). Management of relatives of patients who are dying. *J Clin Nurs, 11*(6), 794-801.

Massie, M.J., Holland, J., & Glass, E. (1983). Delirium in terminally ill cancer patients. *Am J Psychiatry, 140*(8), 1048-1050.

Mattimore, T.J., Wenger, N.S., Lynn, J., et al. (1997). Surrogate and physician understanding of patients' preferences for living permanently in a nursing home. *J Am Geriatr Soc, 45,* 818-824.

McCann, R.M., Hall, W.J., & Groth-Juncker, A. (1994). Comfort care for terminally ill patients: The appropriate use of nutrition and hydration. *JAMA, 272*(16), 1263-1266.

McCarthy, E.P., Phillips, R.S., Zhong, Z., et al. (2000). Dying with cancer: Patient's function, symptoms, and care preferences as death approaches. *J Am Geriatr Soc, 48*(5 Suppl.), S110-S121.

McCarthy, M., Lay, M., & Addington-Hall, J. (1996). Dying from heart disease. *J R Coll Physicians Lond, 30*(4), 325-328.

McCormick, T.R., & Conley, B.J. (1995). Patients' perspectives on dying and on the care of dying patients. *West J Med, 163,* 236-243.

McIver, B., Walsh, D., & Nelson, K. (1994). The use of chlorpromazine for symptom control in dying cancer patients. *J Pain Symptom Manage, 9*(5), 341-345.

McNeil, C. (1998). A good death. *J Palliat Care, 14*(1), 5-6.

Meier, D.E., & Morrison, R.S. (1999). Old age and care near the end of life. *Generations, 23*(1), 6-11.

Menikoff, J. (2002). The importance of being dead: Non-heartbeating organ donation. *Issues Law Med, 18*(1), 3-20.

Mercadante, S., De Conno, F., & Ripamonti, C. (1995). Propofol in terminal care. *J Pain Symptom Manage, 10*(8), 639-642.

Mezey, M., Dubler, N.N., Mitty, E., et al. (2002). What impact do setting and transitions have on the quality of life at the end of life and the quality of the dying process? *Gerontologist, 42*(SIII), 54-67.

Michel, J.P., Pautex, S., Zekry, D., et al. (2002). End-of-life care of persons with dementia. *J Gerontol A Biol Sci Med Sci, 57*(10), M640-644.

Middlewood, S., Gardner, G., & Gardner, A. (2001). Dying in hospital: Medical failure or natural outcome? *J Pain Symptom Manage, 22*(6), 1035-1041.

Mirenda, J., & Broyles, G. (1995). Propofol as used for sedation in the ICU. *Chest, 108*(2), 539-548.

Morita, T., Inoue, S., & Chihara, S. (1996). Sedation for symptom control in Japan: The importance of intermittent use and communication with family members. *J Pain Symptom Manage, 12*(1), 32-38.

Morita, T., Tei, Y., & Inoue, S. (2003). Ethical validity of palliative sedation therapy. *J Pain Symptom Manage, 25*(2), 103-105.

Morita, T., Tsuneto, S., & Shima, Y. (2002). Definition of sedation for symptom relief: A systematic literature review and a proposal of operational criteria. *J Pain Symptom Manage, 24*(4), 447-453.

Morita, T., Tsunoda, J., Inoue, S., et al. (1999). Do hospice clinicians sedate patients intending to hasten death? *J Palliat Care, 15,* 30-32.

Morita, T., You, T., Tsunoda, J., et al. (2001). Underlying pathologies and their associations with clinical features in terminal delirium of cancer patients. *J Pain Symptom Manage, 22*(6), 997-1006.

Moskowitz, E.H., & Nelson, J.L. (1995). The best laid plans. *Hastings Cent Rep, 25*(6 Suppl.), 3-5.

Moyle, J. (1995). The use of propofol in palliative medicine. *J Pain Symptom Manage, 10*(8), 643-646.

Mularski, R.A., Bascom, P., & Osborne, M.L. (2001). Educational agendas for interdisciplinary end-of-life curricula. *Crit Care Med, 29*(2 Suppl.), N16-23.

Murray, C.J., & Lorez, A.D. (1997). *The global burden of disease.* Cambridge, Mass.: Harvard University Press.

National Center for Health Care Statistics. (1993). *National mortality follow-back survey.* Atlanta, Ga.: Centers for Disease Control and Prevention.

Nelson, J.E., & Danis, M. (2001). End-of-life care in the intensive care unit: Where are we now? *Crit Care Med, 29* (2 Suppl.), N2-9.

Nelson, J.E., Meier, D.E., Oei, E.J., et al. (2001). Self-reported symptom experience of critically ill cancer patients receiving intensive care. *Crit Care Med, 29*(2), 277-282.

Oga, T., Nishimura, K., Tsukino, M., et al. (2003). Analysis of the factors related to mortality in chronic obstructive pulmonary disease: Role of exercise capacity and health status. *Am J Respir Crit Care Med, 167*(4), 544-549.

Olson, K.L., Morse, J.M., Smith, J.E., et al. (2000). Linking trajectories of illness and dying. *Omega— J Death Dying, 42*(4), 293-308.

Orentlicher, D.O. (1997). The Supreme Court and physician assisted suicide: Rejecting assisted suicide but embracing euthanasia. *N Engl J Med, 337,* 1236-1239.

Pan, C.X., Morrison, R.S., Meier, D.E., et al. (2001). How prevalent are hospital-based palliative care programs? Status report and future directions. *J Palliat Med, 4*(3), 315-324.

Patrick, D.L., Engelberg, R.A., & Curtis, J.R. (2001). Evaluating the quality of dying and death. *J Pain Symptom Manage, 22*(3), 717-726.

Pattison, E.M. (1977). *The experience of dying.* New York: Simon & Schuster.

Payne, S., Langley-Evans, A., & Hillier, R. (1996). Perceptions of a "good death": A comparative study of the views of hospice staff and patients. *Palliat Med, 10,* 301-312.

Perry, A.G., & Potter, P.A. (2002). *Clinical nursing skills and techniques* (5th ed.). St. Louis: Mosby.

Peruselli, C., Di Giulio, P., Toscani, F., et al. (1999). Home palliative care for terminal cancer patients: A survey on the final week of life. *Palliat Med, 13*(3), 233-241.

Pistelli, R., Lange, P., & Miller, D.L. (2003). Determinants of prognosis of COPD in the elderly: Mucus hypersecretion, infections, cardiovascular comorbidity. *Eur Respir J Suppl, 40,* 10s-14s.

Pitorak, E.F. (2003). Care at the time of death: How nurses can make the last hours of life a richer, more comfortable experience. *Am J Nurs, 103*(7), 42-53.

Portenoy, R.K. (1997). Critical issues in the assessment of delirium. In R.K. Portenoy & E. Bruera (Eds.), *Topics in palliative care* (vol. 1, pp. 3-5). New York: Oxford University Press.

Prendergast, T.J., & Luce, J.M. (1997). Increasing incidence of withholding and withdrawal of life support from the critically ill. *Am J Respir Crit Care Med, 155*(1), 15-20.

Puchalski, C., & Romer, A.L. (2000). Taking a spiritual history allows clinicians to understand patients more fully. *J Palliat Med, 3,* 129-137.

Quill, T.E., & Byock, I.R. (2000). Responding to intractable terminal suffering: The role of terminal sedation and voluntary refusal of food and fluids. *Ann Intern Med, 132*(5), 408-414.

Quill, T.E., Dresser, R., & Brock, D.W. (1997). The rule of double effect: A critique of its role in end-of-life decision making. *N Engl J Med, 227*(24), 1768-1771.

Quill, T.E., Lo, B., & Brock, D.W. (1997). Palliative options of last resort: A comparison of voluntarily stopping eating and drinking, terminal sedation, physician-assisted suicide, and voluntary active euthanasia. *JAMA, 278*(23), 2099-2104.

Raudonis, B.M., Kyba, F.C., & Kinsey, T.A. (2002). Long-term care nurses' knowledge of end-of-life care. *Geriatr Nurs, 23*(6), 296-301.

Reynolds, K., Henderson, M., Schulman, A., et al. (2002). Needs of the dying in nursing homes. *J Palliat Med, 5*(6), 895-901.

Ritchie, K., & Kildea, D. (1995). Is senile dementia "age related" or "aging related"? Evidence from a meta-analysis of dementia prevalence in the oldest old. *Lancet, 346,* 931-934.

Roberto, K.A. (1999). Making critical health care decisions for older adults: Consensus among family members. *Fam Relat, 49,* 167-175.

Rousseau, P. (2000a). The ethical validity and clinical experience of palliative sedation. *Mayo Clin Proc, 75*(10), 1064-1069.

Rousseau, P. (2000b). The losses and suffering of terminal illness. *Mayo Clinic Proc, 75*(2), 197-198.

Rummans, T.A., Bostwick, M.J., & Clark, M.M. (2000). Maintaining quality of life at the end of life. *Mayo Clinic Proc, 75*(12), 1305-1310.

Seale, C. (1998). Theories in health care and research: Theories and studying the care of dying people. *BMJ, 317*(7171), 1518-1520.

Seale, C., Addington-Hall, J., & McCarthy, M. (1997). Awareness of dying prevalence, causes and consequences. *Soc Sci Med, 45*(3), 477-484.

Seymour, J.E. (1999). Revisiting medicalisation and "natural" death. *Soc Sci Med, 49*(5), 691-704.

Seymour, J.E. (2000). Negotiating natural death in intensive care. *Soc Sci Med, 51*(8), 1241-1252.

Shadbolt, B., Barresi, J., & Craft, P. (2002). Self-rated health as a predictor of survival among patients with advanced cancer. *J Clin Oncol, 20,* 2514-2519.

Sheldon, F.M. (2000). Dimensions of the role of the social worker in palliative care. *Palliat Med, 14*(6), 491-498.

Singer, P.A., Martin, D.K., & Kelner, M. (1999). Quality end-of-life care: Patients' perspectives. *JAMA, 281*(2), 163-168.

Slesak, G., Schnurle, J.W., Kinzel, E., et al. (2003). Comparison of subcutaneous and intravenous rehydration in geriatric patients: A randomized trial. *J Am Geriatr Soc, 51*(2), 155-160.

Smith, J.L. (2000a). Why do doctors overestimate? *BMJ, 320,* 469-473.

Smith, R. (2000b). A good death: An important aim for health services and for us all. *BMJ, 320*(7228), 129-130.

Somogyi-Zalud, E., Zhong, Z., Lynn, J., et al. (2000). Dying with acute respiratory failure or multiple organ system failure with sepsis. *J Am Geriatr Soc, 48*(5S), S140-S145.

Stein, W.M., & Ferrell, B.A. (1996). Pain in the nursing home. *Clin Geriatr Med 12*(3), 601-613.

Steiner, N., & Bruera, E. (1998). Methods of hydration in palliative care patients. *J Palliat Care, 14*(2), 6-13.

Steinhauser, K.E., Bosworth, H.B., Clipp, E.C., et al. (2002). Initial assessment of a new instrument to measure quality of life at the end of life. *J Palliat Med, 5*(6), 829-841.

Steinhauser, K.E., Christakis, N.A., Clipp, E.C., et al. (2000). Factors considered important at the end of life by patients, family, physicians, and other care providers. *JAMA, 284*(19), 2476-2482.

Steinhauser, K.E., Clipp, E.C., McNeilly, M., et al. (2000). In search of a good death: Observations of patients, families, and providers. *Ann Intern Med, 132*(10), 825-832.

Stern, Y., Tang, M.X., Albert, M.S., et al. (1997). Predicting time to nursing home care and death in individuals with Alzheimer disease. *JAMA, 277*(10), 806-812.

Stewart, A.L., Teno, J.M., Patrick, D.L., et al. (1999). The concept of quality of life of dying persons in the context of health care. *J Pain Symptom Manage, 17*(2), 93-108.

Stirling, L.C., Kurowska, A., & Tookman, A. (1999). The use of phenobarbitone in the management of agitation and seizures at the end of life. *J Pain Symptom Manage, 17*(5), 363-368.

Stone, P., Phillips, C., Spruyt, O., et al. (1997). A comparison of the use of sedatives in a hospital support team and in a hospice. *Palliat Med, 11*(2), 140-144.

Street, A. (2001). Constructions of dignity in end-of-life care. *J Palliat Med, 17*(2), 93-101.

Sulmasy, D.P. (2001a). Best practice. Evidence-based case review. Addressing the religious and spiritual needs of dying patients. *West J Med, 175*(4), 251-254.

Sulmasy, D.P. (2001b). Forgiveness, dignity, and the care of the dying. *J Gen Intern Med, 16,* 335-338.

Sulmasy, D.P. (2002). A biopsychosocial-spiritual model for the care of patients at the end of life. *Gerontologist, 42*(SIII), 24-33.

Sulmasy, D.P., & Rahn, M. (2001). I was sick and you came to visit me: Time spent at the bedside of seriously ill patients with poor prognoses. *Am J Med, 111,* 385-389.

SUPPORT Investigators. (1995). A controlled trial to improve care for seriously ill hospitalized patients. The study to understand prognoses and preferences for outcomes and risks of treatments (SUPPORT). *JAMA, 274*(20), 1591-1598.

Sykes, N., & Thorns, A. (2003). Sedative use in the last week of life and the implications for end-of-life decision making. *Arch Intern Med, 163*(3), 341-344.

Teno, J.M. (1998). Looking beyond the "form" to complex interventions needed to improve end-of-life care. *J Am Geriatr Soc, 46,* 1170-1171.

Teno, J.M., Fisher, E.S., Hamel, M.B., et al. (2002). Medical care inconsistent with patients' treatment goals: Association with 1-year Medicare resource use and survival. *J Am Geriatr Soc, 50*(3), 496-500.

Teno, J.M., Weitzen, S., Fennell, M.L., et al. (2001). Dying trajectory in the last year of life: Does cancer trajectory fit other diseases? *J Palliat Med, 4*(4), 457-464.

Thompson, M. (1997). Fatal neglect. *Time, 150,* 34-39.

Tierney, W.M, & McKinley, E.D. (2002). When the physician-researcher gets cancer: Understanding cancer, its treatment, and quality of life from the patient's perspective. *Med Care, 40*(6), III-20–III-27.

Tolstoy, L. (1960). *The death of Ivan Ilych and other stories.* New York: New American Library.

Travis, S.S., Bernard, M., Dixon, S., et al. (2002). Obstacles to palliation and end-of-life care in a long-term care facility. *Gerontologist, 42*(3), 342-349.

Travis, S.S., Loving, G., McClanahan, L., et al. (2001). Hospitalization patterns and palliation in the last year of life among residents in long-term care. *Gerontologist, 41*(2), 153-160.

Truog, R.D., Berde, C.B., Mitchell, C., et al. (1992). Barbiturates in the care of the terminally ill. *N Engl J Med, 327*(23), 1678-1682.

Tulsky, J.A., Chesney, M.A., & Lo, B. (1995). How do medical residents discuss resuscitation with patients? *J Gen Intern Med, 10*(8), 436-442.

Turner, K., Chye, R., Aggarwal, G., et al. (1996). Dignity in dying: A preliminary study of patients in the last three days of life. *J Palliat Care, 12*(2), 7-13.

Vacco v. Quill. (1997). 521 U.S. 793.

van der Maas, P.J., van der Wal, G., Haverkate, I., et al. (1996). Euthanasia, physician-assisted suicide, and other medical practices involving the end of life in the Netherlands, 1990-1995. *N Engl J Med, 335*(22), 1699-1705.

Vig, E.K., Davenport, N.A., & Pearlman, R.A. (2002). Good deaths, bad deaths, and preferences for the end of life: A qualitative study of geriatric outpatients. *J Am Geriatr Soc, 50,* 1541-1548.

Vigano, A., Dorgan, M., Buckingham, J., et al. (2000). Survival prediction in terminal cancer patients: A systematic review of the medical literature. *Palliat Med, 14,* 363-374.

Viola, R.A., Wells, G.A., & Peterson, J. (1997). The effects of fluid status and fluid therapy on the dying: A systematic review. *J Palliat Care, 13*(4), 41-52.

von Gunten, C.F., Ferris, F.D., D'Antuono, R., et al. (2002). Recommendations to improve end-of-life care through regulatory change in U.S. health care financing. *J Palliat Med, 5*(1), 35-41.

von Gunten, C.F., Ferris, F.D., & Emanuel, L.L. (2000). The patient-physician relationship: Ensuring competency in end-of-life care: Communication and relational skills. *JAMA, 284*(23), 3051-3057.

Vullo-Navich, K., Smith, S., Andrews, M., et al. (1998). Comfort and incidence of abnormal serum sodium, BUN, creatinine and osmolality in dehydration of terminal illness. *Am J Hosp Palliat Care, 15*(2), 77-84.

Walsh, D., Donnelly, S., & Rybicki, L. (2000). The symptoms of advanced cancer: Relationship to age, gender, and performance status in 1,000 patients. *Support Care Cancer, 8*(3), 175-179.

Walsh, D., Mahmoud, F., & Barna, B. (2003). Assessment of nutritional status and prognosis in advanced cancer: Interleukin-6, C-reactive protein, and the prognostic and inflammatory nutritional index. *Support Care Cancer, 11*(1), 60-62.

Walsh, E. (2002). The organization of death and dying in today's society. *Nurs Stand, 16*(25), 33-38.

Ward, C. (2002). The need for palliative care in the management of heart failure. *Heart, 87*(3), 294-298.

Washington v. Glucksberg. (1997). 521 U.S. 702.

Wax, M.L., & Ray, S.E. (2002). Dilemmas within the surgical intensive care unit. *J Am Coll Surg, 195*(5), 721-728.

Wein, S. (2000). Sedation in the imminently dying patient. *Oncology (Huntingt), 14*(4), 585-592.

Wenrich, M.D., Curtis, J.R., Ambrozy, D.M., et al. (2003). Dying patients' need for emotional support and personalized care from physicians: Perspectives of patients with terminal illness, families, and health care providers. *J Pain Symptom Manage, 25*(3), 236-246.

Werth, J.L. Jr., Gordon, J.R., & Johnson, R.R. Jr. (2002). Psychosocial issues near the end of life. *Aging Ment Health, 6*(4), 402-412.

Zerwekh, J.V. (1997). Do dying patients really need IV fluids? *Am J Nurs, 97*(3), *Nurse Pract Extra Ed:* 26-31.

Zerzan, J., Stearns, S., & Hanson, L. (2000). Access to palliative care and hospice in nursing homes. *JAMA, 284*(19), 2489-2494.

15 *Grief and Bereavement*

Helen Kathleen Brophy McHale

OBJECTIVES

After the completion of this chapter, the reader should be able to:

1. Recognize the pervasive attitude toward death and grief in our society.
2. Differentiate between the various forms of grief.
3. Identify reactions that might indicate an unhealthy grief response.
4. Acquire an understanding of factors that affect bereavement and the grieving process.
5. Demonstrate an understanding of interventions that support a healthy grief reaction.
6. Recognize the significant impact that palliative care has on the grief experience.

INTRODUCTION

Bereavement, a journey traveled while grieving, can be full of growth and self-discovery or darkened with loneliness and pain. This is especially true in Western society where adults often avoid the discussion of death and grief. The National Hospice and Palliative Care Organization (NHPCO) reported that Americans who are uncomfortable talking about death would more likely discuss safe sex and drugs with their children than talk with their terminally ill parents about end-of-life choices (National Hospice Foundation [NHF], 1999a). Twenty-five percent of Americans older than 45 years say they would not talk to their parents about death "...even if the parent had a terminal illness and less than six months to live" (NHF, 1999a, p. 1).

Our society withdraws from individuals in mourning to avoid emotional pain, and "...the

assistance they do offer is superficial and full of platitudes" (Silverman, 1974, p. 320). The medical community is no more therapeutic than the general public when they deal with death and grief. If a medical treatment will not cure a patient (and could cause harm, especially late in the disease), the health care professional may continue to offer it under the guise of hope.

Advanced medical technologies, such as pharmaceuticals that mask unpleasant manifestations of disease, provide patients with incurable illness a better quality of life. Symptoms are often hidden, which allows patients and families to disregard disease progression. According to Bales (1997), improved end-of-life care is needed to assist the public as they plan their futures and make crucial choices.

Individuals who suffer the loss of a loved one often experience physical and emotional illness after the death. Bereaved individuals feel waves of ill-defined distress accompanied by feelings of emptiness or emotional distance from others. They experience decreased muscle power, insomnia, hopelessness, or depression (Blank, 1969; Lindemann, 1944/1994). Support that eases the journey through bereavement and lessens suffering from grief is priceless. Resolution of grief relies heavily on support the bereaved receives.

It can be difficult to make a distinction between the terms *grief* and *bereavement*. Saunders (1981) described grief as a psychologic process that includes emotions and memories experienced in response to a loss. "Grief is the normal psychological reaction to loss" (Kaye, 1999, p. 139). It may include losing a person, an object, or any highly valued concept. It also includes the bereaved person's affect and surrounding intrapsychic dynamics. Bereavement is "…the broad, umbrella term that cushioned and gave context to mourning and grief" (Kaye, 1999, p. 319). Simply put, "Bereavement is the reaction to loss of a loved person" (Kaye, 1999, p. 139). Mourning includes actions or feelings of sorrowing, expressing grief; lamentation; specifically, a verbal expression of grief over a death (McKechnie, 1973). Mourning may also be "…the cultural response to grief" (Burge, 1999, p. 280). Wolfelt (1992) defined mourning as publicly expressing personal ideas and feelings about the loved one. Based on these definitions, it is safe to say that grief is the lived experience, whereas bereavement is the personal journey.

Western society's inability to accept and address death and grief can complicate the bereavement journey. Health care professionals who believe avoiding the discussion of death and dying spares individuals emotional pain are really robbing them of a chance to grieve in anticipation of the coming loss. Patients are denied precious time needed to prepare for death and the chance to interact in a new light with family and friends. A longer grieving process adversely affects one physically, emotionally, and financially, while it taxes our society. During the late 1960s and early 1970s, Elisabeth Kübler-Ross struggled with an unprepared health care system as she turned her attention to people's fear of death. She recognized that fear of death was prevalent among physicians, nurses, and other health care professionals, as well as terminally ill patients and families. Kübler-Ross (1969) eloquently described this fear of death as "…universal…. It might be more helpful if people would talk about death and dying as an intrinsic part of life just as they do not hesitate to mention when someone is expecting a baby" (pp. 5 & 141). Although literature suggests that patients and families can benefit from the experience of anticipatory grief (Lindemann, 1944/1994), it often goes unsupported and unacknowledged in health care.

Our society encourages communication that circumvents the reality of "death" and "dying" by using more pleasant statements such as "grave or serious illness," "passed away," and "expired." Euphemisms, by their very nature, deter further communication and prevent open, honest discussion. Health care professionals, who may be unwilling to be candid, may believe "…such information can be detrimental to the dying person. There is, in fact, no reliable evidence that honest communication has detrimental effects, at least not when such communication is responsive to the needs of the dying person and is carried out in a thoughtful and caring way" (Corr, 1993, p. 33). The reticent professional may lose patient and family trust by withholding information, especially when the dying person recognizes the terminal changes in his or her body. Fear of upsetting the patient with "bad news" and little knowledge of how to help can cause professional reluctance. Professionals might also fear that providing frank information would lead to blame. They could be blamed "…when the patient's clinical condition begins to deteriorate" (Buckman, 1993, p. 49). Professionals, who receive little training in palliative care, feel unprepared to treat the incurable patient whose health is deteriorating. An interdisciplinary approach that meets the dying patients' needs for "…relief from distressing symptoms of disease, the security of a caring environment, sustained expert care, and assurance that they and their families will not be abandoned" (Corr, 1993, p. 35) is crucial.

DEATH AND LOSS

Professionals in the field of psychiatry have long studied death and loss. Classic works continue to be referred to and studied as new theories are investigated and developed. Dr. Erich Lindemann (1944/1994) reflected that in 1917 Freud described universal feelings and behaviors associated with grief in his classic work, *Mourning and Melancholia*. Lindemann, who was Instructor of Psychiatry at Harvard Medical School, coined the term *anticipatory grief* in his 1944 presentation, *Symptomatology and Management of Acute Grief*. This work was republished in 1994 and remains helpful today.

Saunders (1981) stated "The death of a loved one has been recognized universally as unequalled in its capacity to give rise to personal pain and suffering" (p. 319). Death is a stressful event, but two characteristics can convert the experience to a crisis situation. First, the loss is so final; the human being is lost forever. He or she can not be replaced; one can only adjust to the loss. Second, death comes infrequently. Individuals have little experience and are forced to create new personal solutions to deal with the situation (Goldberg, 1973).

Grief is powerful; "It can make a stone of your heart" (Youll & Wilson, 1996, p. 40). It can destroy a person physically and mentally. Normal grief reactions include crying, feeling empty, or being intensely preoccupied with the deceased. Words used to describe grief, such as "...'loss' and 'blow' have real physical connotations" (Hasler, 1996, p. 52). Just as physical wounds need to heal, so does grief. "There is no shortcut to the resolution of grief. People learn to live around the painful memories rather than eliminate them" (McKissock & McKissock, 1996, p. 31).

According to Valente and McIntyre (1996), the bereavement process is dynamic and normal. Individuals, families, generations, and cultures have their own "...unique style of grieving. Grief does not occur in a rigid, linear, or uniform pattern. Symptoms of grief wax and wane over time" (p. 10). Personalities, diverse relationships, and individual circumstances affect how humans cope with the death of a loved one (Doka, 2000b).

TYPES OF GRIEF

Normal Grief

Because most individuals experience grief during their lifetime, it is essential that those who work in the psychosocial and spiritual realms understand that grief is not a disease but an emotion. Grief is as natural a reaction as eating when hungry, drinking when thirsty, or sleeping when tired. "Grief is nature's way of healing a broken heart. Grief is love not wanting to let go" (Kleyman, 1996, p. 8). "Recent conceptualizations of grief reflect the tendency to view grief as a normal, dynamic, pervasive, individualized experience" (Jacob, 1996, p. 280).

Lindemann (1944/1994) described physical symptoms often experienced by those who suffered from grief. Individuals were overcome by waves of distress lasting up to an hour. They experienced difficulty with swallowing or breathing, a feeling of emptiness in their abdomen, or weakness in their muscles. Some grieving individuals encountered a

distress they described as *tension*. Others reported a slight sense of unreality, a feeling of increased emotional distance from other people (they appear shadowy or small). Blank (1969) considered the initial physical symptoms experienced after the loss of a loved one to be a normal manifestation of the grief reaction. Grieving individuals felt depression "...characterized by dejection, tearfulness, restlessness or retardation, insomnia, and the expression of feelings of hopelessness, helplessness, emptiness and guilt" (p. 204).

Openness and flexibility related to the duration of mourning permit bereaved individuals more time to adjust to their loss. Time for grieving might be influenced by an individual's culture. The amount of time tolerated for loss readjustment is often related to the "...value *we* place on the lost object, person, or function, and this may differ widely from the value the bereaved attaches to that which is lost" (Speck, 1978, p. 146). Length of time spent in mourning depends on successful "...*grief work*, namely, emancipation from the bondage to the deceased, readjustment to the environment in which the deceased is missing, and formation of new relationships" (Lindemann, 1944/1994, p. 156).

Length and intensity of the grief response depend on dynamics including age, coping capability, support system, and how the bereaved "...perceives the loss and changes in his life" (Wheeler, 1996, p. 26). Survivors can experience feelings of remorse or guilt about their relationship. They can feel angry with God, physicians, or even the deceased (for leaving them behind). To "...avoid blundering in giving advice to the bereaved, or avoid making unrealistic demands on him, it would be safe to assume 1 year to be the minimum duration of mourning" (Blank, 1969, p. 204), with up to 2 years typical.

"Symptoms may recur on significant anniversaries, such as birthdays, holidays, or date of death" (Stoudemire & Blazer, 1985, p. 574). Psychologists and sociologists believe it takes years to accept the loss of a spouse. The bereaved suffer low spots as long as several years after the loss (Doka, 2000a). "It may be around 2 to 5 years before the bereaved person experiences life with something like the sense of meaning and purpose that existed before the death" (McKissock & McKissock, 1996, p. 30). If the bereavement process was not started before death, it may help the bereaved to understand that it is not unusual for a year or more to pass before one feels healing from a loss such as his or hers. "Schuchter and Zisook comment that 'some aspects of grief work may never end for a significant proportion of otherwise normal bereaved individuals'" (Ott, 2003, p. 265).

Even after the initial grief reaction, bereaved individuals continued to feel tearful, empty, or upset. How can bereaved move beyond this great burden and pain? Traditionally, psychiatrists helped individuals struggling to recover from grief, but not all psychiatrists specialize in grief work. Although it has been over 50 years since the concept of anticipatory grief was developed, the focus of most assistance continues to come after the death. Because society strives to escape pain, discussion of death is also avoided. It is avoided before death, during the dying process, and even after death. There are times when practitioners have to change their way of thinking. "The problem is not simple. Is care different today than when Travelbee (1971) proclaimed 'We cling to the glorious delusion that our job is to cure people. We have failed to come to grips with the unpopular fact that most illness we see is incurably" (p. 6) (McHale, 2001, p. 134).

Individuals in mourning feel abandoned, even by friends and family. Much of the support they do receive is "...without any real comprehension of what is needed for successful coping" (Silverman, 1974, p. 320). But the pain experience does not just erode the grieving individual. Through the pain of grief one becomes strong, more able to help others, more able to help himself or herself. "Grief is powerful alchemy. It plunges us into sorrow and forces us to face the finiteness of life, the mightiness of death, and the meaning of our existence on this earth" (Quigley & Schatz, 1999, p. 78).

Anticipatory Grief

When a loved one is lost, an expected period of grief follows. In contrast, anticipatory grief is experienced before the actual loss occurs. Lindemann (1944/1994) described preliminary pain, pain experienced before a loss, as *anticipatory grief.* Norris and Murrell (1987) posited, "...the adaptational requirements of bereavement begin well before the death event" (p. 611). For a chronic illness such as cancer, anticipatory grief can begin at the time of diagnosis. Families of patients with life-limiting illness, poor prognosis, and a predictable death have an opportunity to address their coming loss if they can openly grieve in anticipation of it.

Anticipatory feelings of "...helplessness, guilt, anger, denial, fear, confusion, and rage can be as intense as the emotions a person experiences after his loved one actually dies" (Wheeler, 1996, p. 26). If the patient and family are prepared in anticipation of the loss, "...then they may be enabled to meet the loss in a more constructive way" (Speck, 1978, p. 15). Grief work should be started when the physical, psychologic, or spiritual impact of the impending death is first felt. While the individual prepares for the loss, the reality is gradually absorbed. Grief experienced before the loss empowers the bereaved to face the loss and hastens healing from that loss (Huber & Gibson, 1990; Speck, 1978).

An interactive multidisciplinary approach to care, one that intimately involves the patient and family, provides a process for anticipatory grief work. Although anticipatory grief work may not lessen every survivor's grief, it does have benefits. Those who express feelings of loss before an expected death gradually absorb the reality of the loss over time, finish unfinished business, and change their assumptions about life and their own identity. Anticipatory grief can provide time "...to acknowledge that the patient is dying, to prepare for the death, to adapt to changes... to participate in a review of life, to tend to matters left unsettled, and to resolve conflicts" (Egan & Arnold, 2003, p. 46).

Hospice was originally a place of refuge for travelers, the sick, and the poor (Como, 1990). Today "Hospice is a system of family-centered care designed to assist the terminally ill person to be comfortable and to maintain a satisfactory life style through the phases of dying" (McHale, 1998, p. 1). Many hospice families believe preparatory work, done during hospice care, assisted with their bereavement journey. A funeral director said, "Most hospice families had it all together" during funeral preparation and services (House, 2004). They focus on difficult tasks and make sound decisions without the influence of unreliable emotions. They are prepared, through anticipation, for events that surround death. These families surely suffer from the loss of their loved one, but they are better prepared to face the stark reality.

Hospice has helped millions of patients and families experience a dignified death for over 20 years (NHF, 1999b). Cultural diversity may dictate what constitutes a dignified death; therefore professionals providing end-of-life care should become familiar with various cultural practices. Patient and family needs can vary and "...will depend on how closely they identify with a particular group" (Mazanec & Tyler, 2003, p. 53). In Western culture, a dignified death may be defined as being fully informed, receiving support from family and friends, having symptoms controlled, choosing the place of death, planning post-death events, remaining in control, and following religious rituals. Among Muslims, for example, "The dying [person] may well want to sit or lie with his face turned towards Mecca..." (Neuberger, 1993, p. 509) while family members pray at the bedside. After death, only Muslims should touch the body; if necessary, others should wear gloves. The unwashed body is wrapped in a plain sheet. It will be washed later, at home or a mosque, where camphor is often placed under armpits and in orifices. Limbs are straightened and the head turned toward the right shoulder, because the face must be turned toward Mecca when buried. An autopsy can cause significant distress (Neuberger, 1993). "Muslims are always buried, never cremated, and this is carried out as soon as possible" (Neuberger, 1993, p. 509). The memory of a loved one dying a dignified death may depend on how closely cultural rituals were followed. "We may not understand or accept the religious beliefs of our patients, but we can respect them (Kaye, 1999, p. 266). It would be impossible to know all the rituals of every religion, but it is vital to be interested and ask questions to facilitate respect for the dying and promote healthy grief work among the bereaved.

The goal of anticipatory grief work is to help the individual cope by discussing details of the crisis before it occurs. All those sharing the loss (patient, family, health care professionals) can benefit from anticipatory grief work. The anticipation permits a healthy reaction to the loss, which can lower anxiety and facilitate early mobilization of strength. This allows the actual loss to be met more constructively. Full preparation for a coming loss can never occur, but anticipation can make the event less traumatic (Speck, 1978).

Kübler-Ross (1969) believed anticipatory grief allows patients to face issues surrounding death and live more fully in the time they have left. Kübler-Ross observed depressed patients who were not communicating—that is, until staff discussed their terminal illness with them. These patients began to eat, their depression lessened, and some of them were surprisingly discharged to home and family. Kübler-Ross believed that "...we do more harm avoiding the issue than by using time and timing to sit, listen, and share" (1969, p. 142). She encouraged staff to "...help the patient and family get 'in tune' to each others' needs and come to an acceptance of an unavoidable reality together" (1969, p. 142). Effective use of resources prevents "...unnecessary agony and suffering on the part of the dying and even more so on the part of the family that is left behind" (1969, p. 142).

Transition requires that individuals relinquish many "old assumptions, and then construct a whole new set of assumptions which will enable them to cope with their changed world without their loved one" (Huber & Gibson, 1990, p. 52). Anticipatory grief "cannot and does not exempt survivors from all sadness in advance but it does provide a means of setting in motion a unique process of relinquishing a key person and then filling a void" (Costello, 1996, p. 174). Usually "...the principle that emerges from these studies is that before any crisis or loss occurs it helps if people can worry" (Speck, 1978, p. 20).

Complicated Grief

Complicated grief can be defined as a "...disorder that occurs after the death of a significant other. Symptoms of separation distress are the core of the disorder and amalgamate with bereavement-specific symptoms of being devastated and traumatized by the death" (Jacobs, 1999, p. 24). It can be difficult to differentiate between normal and complicated grief soon after the death. It has been recommended that the earliest that bereaved individuals should be assessed for complicated grief is 6 months after the death (Prigerson, Bierhals, Kasl, et al., 1997). Further emphasizing this difficulty, Horowitz, Siegel, Holen, et al. (1997) suggested a wait of 12 months after the death before grief can be categorized as complicated.

Complicated grief interferes with the individual's ability to carry on a normal life. Although normal grief reactions can interfere with daily life, the intensity of those reactions lessens over time but not so with complicated grief. Crying uncontrollably soon after the loss of a spouse is normal and contributes to the healing process. The same sort of uncontrollable crying month after month, with no change in intensity, is maladaptive and a sign of complicated grief. The bereaved whose grief is complicated may experience symptoms such as severe depression or isolation and unusual or destructive behavior.

Complicated grief can result if an individual has other unresolved significant losses. Grief can be complicated when death is sudden or a child dies. Individuals who face unusually stressful lives and who have poor support systems can experience complicated grief. Complications can also arise when the bereaved has been with a loved one who suffered needlessly at the end of life. Those who suffer from complicated grief should be referred for specialized care. Egan and Arnold (2003) describe five types of complicated grief: chronic, delayed, exaggerated, masked, and disenfranchised.

Chronic Grief. Normal grief is categorized as *chronic grief* when it continues unchanged for an unusually long time. To differentiate between normal and chronic grief, the practitioner should know the survivor and how he or she has adjusted to past losses. Bereaved who define themselves by the experience of their loss, for instance as "Samantha's widower," should be assessed for chronic grief and may need to be referred for professional psychiatric help (Egan & Arnold, 2003).

Delayed Grief. When a survivor deliberately avoids feeling his or her grief, it can be classified as *delayed grief.* The bereaved can delay grief's pain by avoiding persons or circumstances that are reminders of the loss. He might work extra hours or become "…overly concerned with others' problems" (Egan & Arnold, 2003, p. 48). Resolution comes only after the individual takes time to grieve. Often support from a close friend or clergy member may help. A grief support group can provide additional insight and assistance.

Exaggerated Grief. A more serious form of complicated grief is *exaggerated grief.* The survivor is so devastated by the loss that he seeks relief by engaging in "…self-destructive behavior…" (Egan & Arnold, 2003, p. 48). The behaviors may include unsafe sexual practices or drug and alcohol abuse. With exaggerated grief, survivor safety is a concern. A number of these individuals will attempt suicide. The practitioner should review the survivor's intent and inquire about suicide. Individuals experiencing exaggerated grief should be referred for an appropriate mental health evaluation.

Masked Grief. When a survivor's unintentional actions are "…interfering with his ability to function," he could be suffering from *masked grief.* The bereaved may have an unknown fear of further loss. He may unconsciously distance himself from others and reject attempts to help. "In contrast, some survivors become overly dependent…. Either extreme can strain relationships" (Egan & Arnold, 2003, p. 48). Although support groups can help, the initial recognition of masked grief may be the result of insight from loved ones.

Disenfranchised Grief. Individuals who are engaged in "…culturally unacceptable or marginalized…" (Egan & Arnold, 2003, p. 48) relationships can experience *disenfranchised grief.* The social stigma attached to divorced or gay relationships may prevent an open expression of grief. These individuals often suffer sadness or anger in isolation. Disenfranchised grief can also occur when individuals miss the opportunity to formally grieve because of distance or financial hardship. Having someone to share feelings with, either individually or through a group, will facilitate healing from disenfranchised grief.

STAGE THEORIES

Kübler-Ross (1969), pioneer in the field of death and dying in the United States, developed a model for the grieving process, which remains foundational today. The steps of her stage theory are:

- Denial (They must be wrong. This can't happen to me.)
- Anger (Why would this happen to me? What did I do?)
- Bargaining (I'll do everything the doctor says. Please God, I'll listen.)
- Depression (I just can't do this anymore. I don't care if I die.)
- Acceptance (The doctors did all they could. I have things I want to do before I die.)

Stage theories enhance our understanding of grief and bereavement, but clinicians must be flexible. As a grieving individual moves between stages or phases, "...he or she can also experience what seem on the surface to be conflicting emotions" (Hasler, 1996, p. 52). As with other stage theories, each stage may not be evident and might be processed in a changed order, but individuals usually do complete each one.

Completion of several tasks is another way to organize the grief process. By addressing loss-related issues with spouses of terminally ill patients, the first task, accepting the reality of death, can be facilitated (Huber & Gibson, 1990). Bereaved will gain control over their grief when they complete the following tasks (Huber & Gibson, 1990; Lloyd-Richards & Rees, 1996):

- Accept the reality of death.
- Experience the pain of grief.
- Change their environment and adjust to the missing deceased.
- Reinvest their emotional energy into living their life and planning their future.

The families of dying or bereaved individuals often ask about the stages of death and dying. It is more important that they support the individual where they are in the process than it is to identify what stage they are in. Friends and family often need as much assistance and support as the bereaved individual does. Although there is no template for grief, reviewing stage theories facilitates insight into the grief process. According to Burge (1999), ultimately the individual must "...feel the reality of the loss and then find new ways of living without the person who has died" (p. 280).

REACTIONS TO GRIEF

Avoidance

Research shows that most people are uncomfortable with the prospect of death. Findings from a 1995 study of more than 9000 patients in hospitals and nursing homes stunned and shocked researchers (SUPPORT Principal Investigators, 1995). The results indicated that communication among patients, families, and physicians was lacking and end-of-life care was depersonalized, resulting in poor pain and symptom management. The Robert Wood Johnson Foundation funded the study, which shed light on the problem, hence "...the term end-of-life issues came into full vogue" (Harper, 2000, p. 23). These results were serious for health care professionals and facilities that provided end-of-life care. Care as well as communication related to the dying trajectory was reevaluated to identify inadequacies for patients, families, health care professionals, and the community.

Bereaved may try to avoid uncomfortable feelings associated with the emotional expression of grief. According to Lindemann (1944/1994), people learn that visits from family and friends, mention of the deceased, and receipt of sympathy precipitates waves of discomfort. "There is a tendency to avoid the syndrome at any cost, to keep deliberately from thought all references to the deceased" (Lindemann, 1944/1994, pp. 155-156). This explains some of the isolation preferred by many bereaved individuals.

It is healthier to express grief through talking and tears than to suppress the pain. Sharing "facilitates the mastery of these feelings" (Blank, 1969, p. 204). Bereaved individuals complete grief work only by traveling through the pain. Anything that "...allows the person to avoid or suppress the pain can be expected to prolong the course of mourning. [One must] allow bereaved people to experience the full, unmitigated grief of the loss; anything that detracts from this will have to be dealt with later" (Hasler, 1996, p. 53).

Denial

Older women in one study were told that their husbands with cancer had a poor prognosis and less than 6 months to live. Later, only 66% reported that they were told their husbands were dying (Levy, 1991). Levy suggested that one's usual level of emotional adjustment and ability to cope with stress influenced the outcome of anticipatory grief work. Professionals working with dying patients and families should "...exercise caution in attempting to facilitate anticipatory grief" (p. 26). They must be able to recognize those individuals who are not ready to hear bad news. "The person may react with anger or may deny having heard the information and yet become very anxious" (Kaye, 1999, p. 57). An individual's response provides other signs that they are not ready to hear bad news. They may look down or turn away during the conversation. They may interrupt often, change the subject, or fidget. The individual's eyes may widen, indicating that too much information has been provided. It is important to assess the amount and kind of support an individual has. "Adjusting to illness or having an ill family member... can provoke a crisis" (Kaye, 1999, p. 95). An individual who has support can usually develop solutions. Denial is often used when there is more bad news than the individuals can handle. They accept what they can deal with and block out portions they cannot. Accepting bad news takes time. "Loss of control results in a deep inner pain which can be linked to loss of hope" (Urquhart, 1999, p. 36). By listening to patients and families and observing subtle signs, the professional will develop sensitivity to individual needs related to anticipatory grief.

Levy (1991) suggested knowledge of a future loss and an opportunity to grieve did not equal anticipatory grief. "It would seem self-evident that simply having the opportunity to experience anticipatory grief does not ensure that one will. To believe otherwise would be to ignore all that we know about the operation of denial in the face of threat" (p. 4). Engel (1961) discussed denial in his classic work, "Yet the human mind, that wonderful instrument of discovery, has a disconcerting capacity to use denial, to turn away from that which is not easily comprehended or which has awesome

implications" (p. 22). If unable to anticipate their loss, the bereaved will need more help after the death of their loved one.

Illness

Professionals involved in grief work recognize a relationship between suffering a loss and subsequent illness. Bereaved can suffer an exacerbation of a chronic disease or develop an entirely new illness. According to Parkes (1988), patients "...showed a significant depression of lymphocyte (T-cell) function during the early weeks after bereavement" (p. 367). Norris and Murrell (1987) also reported that "...grief following the loss alters immunologic effectiveness and leaves the bereaved less resistant to infection and pathological organisms" (p. 606). Valente and McIntyre (1996) found that grief can affect mental well-being; "10% to 15% of those who seek treatment at mental health clinics have underlying unresolved grief" (p. 11).

THE IMPACT OF GRIEF
Relationships

According to Speck (1978), when we grieve, part of our world is lost. He described grief as a "...deep or violent sorrow...with an implied pining for the world, which is lost, rather than the object itself" (p. 8). Life as it was is lost and significantly changed. "Grief places us outside of our existing social roles while we reclaim and reestablish our place in the social world" (Shapiro, 1996, p. 317). Professionals must be sensitive to grief even though a relationship was less than perfect. A wife who was abused may find it difficult to understand conflicting feelings such as both relief and sadness over the death of her husband. "Painful deeds do not magically evaporate because the person is no longer alive. Death does not abruptly resolve hurtful actions" (Grollman, 2000a, p. 3).

The focus of grief work in our society is on "...individuals rather than relationships and denies the enduring nature of our important attachments" (Shapiro, 1996, p. 314). A lost loved one is not replaceable. Parkes (1988) explained, "Each love relationship is unique ...libido can not be withdrawn from one object in order to become invested in another similar object" (p. 366). The person who died represented a key element in a social system. "The bereaved is surprised to find out how large a part of his customary activity was done in some meaningful relationship to the deceased and [this activity] has now lost its significance" (Lindemann, 1944/1994, pp. 156 & 159). The bereaved will benefit from acceptance, professional interaction, and guidance.

Families

The patient, family, and society are best served when the patient and family are treated as a unit. Wright and Leahey (1994) believe comprehensive care that involves families requires an interactive approach. Through communication, professionals can anticipate family needs and prevent or "…reduce some of the difficulties which occur at a later date" (Chesson & Todd, 1996, p. 18). Families who have problems functioning during an early phase of illness may continue to have problems during bereavement and will need additional follow-up and support (Kristjanson, Sloan, Dudgeon, et al., 1996).

Kübler-Ross (1969) was dedicated to meeting the needs of both patient and family. Professionals cannot " …help the terminally ill patient in a really meaningful way if we do not include his family" (p. 157). She believed family members were more comfortable expressing emotions before their loved one died. Families could work through feelings of "…anger, resentment, and guilt…" and would "…then go through a phase of preparatory grief, just as the dying person does" (p. 169). Grief work done before death would "…bridge the gulf between themselves and the dying one, half the battle would have been won" (p. 162). Couldrick (1992) agreed that family communication was essential. It also allowed the patient "…to share the responsibility for the management of his illness and his death" (p. 1522).

During the terminal phase of an illness, the patient can become detached and less able or willing to communicate. This may be heartbreaking for family members who want to interact and say their good-byes. Kübler-Ross (1969) shared, "Our goal should always be to help the patient and his family face the crisis together in order to achieve

acceptance of this final reality simultaneously" (p. 180). Families should be told that detachment is a normal part of the separation process as the patient gradually leaves this life. The professional providing end-of-life care can anticipate when to share this information by becoming familiar with the pathophysiology of terminal illness. Patients who suffer from end-stage kidney or liver disease and those with brain tumors often demonstrate an inability to communicate earlier than other terminal patients do.

Not everyone treats the knowledge of impending death the same way. Professionals can help family members understand that it is normal to have thoughts that are hard to control and feelings that fluctuate. Individuals who attempt to protect themselves from the reality of an impending death by detaching from the patient need to be encouraged by professionals to interact with their loved one. It may help if they make short, frequent visits rather than long ones. If talking is difficult, they might review family pictures and recall past memories. It is imperative they realize that avoiding interaction may "…make the dying patient feel isolated and alone" (Wheeler, 1996, p. 28). Later, they may regret not spending more time with their loved one.

Although it is important for the patient and family to spend time together, for some a gradual detachment is necessary. "An important part of supporting someone who has experienced anticipatory grief is enabling them to detach emotionally" (Costello, 1996, pp. 173-174). Detachment requires efforts before the death such as offering respite care and providing social support. Family members who spend long periods at home with the ill patient and those who suffer financial hardship may be most vulnerable.

The patient and family can feel a great peace at the time of death when they experience grief through anticipation. This peace provides individuals with the strength they need to go on with the rest of their lives. Encouraging family members to communicate and express their feelings and then listening to those feelings are the most significant help the professional can provide. Gabany (2000) speculated that professionals who help patients plan their end-of-life wishes, while they still can, ensure satisfaction with those choices and ease the bereavement journey for their families.

Spouses

The loss of a spouse involves the loss of a history and a level of investment. It can be more painful than other adult losses. According to Ransford and Smith (1991), so much is shared between spouses that "...the disruption in daily routines, presence of mementos, and overall sense of loss would be far greater" (p. 302). Kurtz, Kurtz, Given, et al. (1997) recognize that this phenomenon, loss of a spouse, can create a severely disturbed social structure. It "...often involves a loss of social or economic status, and may necessitate substantial reorganization of social roles" (p. 60). "When we lose a spouse we lose our present [life]" (Doka, 2000b, p. 1).

To relinquish a familiar role, time and considerable emotional and cognitive work are required. Therapists found that the discussion of death at times touches just the surface and often focuses only on social concerns. Given ample time to discuss feelings and concerns in a safe environment allows adults to develop trust. As a result, subsequent discussion becomes more intimate and emotional (Davis-Berman, Berman, & Faris, 1995). The goals of this grief work are to help the individual travel through bereavement and to allow him or her to face a new reality—a changed life without the spouse.

Older Adults

Bereavement studies often involve older adults because they are "...the age group most commonly bereaved" (Parkes, 1988, p. 371). Jacob (1996) studied widows who had been married about 50 years. The widows' major complaint was loneliness, which caused them great emotional suffering. Some felt nothing could ever take the place of their spouse. One widow described feeling like she was only half there and half of her was gone. Losing a spouse is both an emotional loss and a social loss. The loss requires significant changes in the individual's role as well as his or her lifestyle. Having such critical changes occur during the already stressful grieving process can create illness. The elderly widowed show high "...rates of disabling illness and hospitalization, as well as higher rates of suicide and death from other causes. Death sometimes occurs soon after the loss of the spouse" (Potocky, 1993, p. 288). It is imperative to understand that vulnerable older adults may need more individualized support and bereavement care.

Many in our society consider death a taboo topic, but some older individuals do not treat death as such a dreaded event. Older adults have usually encountered the deaths of several friends and family members. Some of them even consider that they are living on borrowed time. Various losses experienced during a lifetime prepare an individual, somewhat, for the only remaining loss, that of their own life. "Such deprivations may be described as *anticipatory losses,* or 'little deaths'" (Speck, 1978, p. 7). Although these adults expect death and may have experienced it before, experience alone does not protect them from the effects of grief and bereavement.

Children

Issues related to death, grief, and bereavement for children differ somewhat from those of adults. Knowledge about how children, as well as their parents and families, relate to issues surrounding death can aid health care professional as they care for them.

Children's ability to understand death, even their own, parallels the series of developmental stages described by Piaget (Stevens, 1993). Under normal circumstances children develop in an orderly fashion, although children of the same age may be at different places in their development. This same principle holds true for a child's understanding of terminal illness and grief. An inquisitive 4-year-old, wondering what a cemetery is, may respond to his father's answer that "People who died are buried there" by asking "Aren't they hungry?" (Kaye, 1999). Children's comprehension and reaction will depend "...on their experience, intelligence and emotional development, and whether their natural curiosity is encouraged and their questions answered" (Kaye, 1999, p. 69). Stevens reported that although terminally ill children may be aware of their condition, they might not be able to talk about it using adult vocabulary. Also, little difference was found between sick and well children's understanding of death.

According to Stevens (1993), dying children are more aware of the seriousness of their own illness than adults care to admit. Children grieve although it may not be outwardly evident. They may express their feelings through behavior rather than words. They are sensitive to the messages sent by adults such as "we are 'doing good' if we don't cry when someone we love dies." Complicating this, adults often exclude children from conversations and planning related to death. A child's need to express his or her feelings related to death and grief is similar to that of an adult's (Monroe, 1993). Play is an important tool used by children to adapt to new situations. They can effectively communicate through art and music therapy. These tools can also be used to evaluate how children are adapting (Stevens, 1993). Younger children can be helped by presenting appropriate pictures and allowing them to share their feelings. It can take several sessions to help, since during an encounter, a child may be able to share only what he is emotionally prepared for. According to Doyle (1993), parents want "...to be listened to and to be acknowledged as experts in the care of their own children" (p. 630). It is therefore essential that professionals who provide care to children involve parents.

"Death is never so unwelcome nor so incomprehensible as when its victim is a child" (deVeber, Jacobson, Koren, et al., 1993, p. 697). To help parents adjust to their child's terminal illness and ensuing death, health care professionals must become familiar with the parents' "...attitude toward their child's illness, the tasks related to it, and the caregiver burden" (Meleski, 2002, p. 48). Family life with a terminally ill child is dictated by changes caused by the disease. If the child needs hospitalization, parents may have to rearrange their work schedules so one of them can be with the child. With other children in the family, parents must face additional burdens. Those children also need their parents' love and attention. They need someone with the emotional strength to normalize the situation and provide them with relevant information.

Professionals should recognize that although the illness is difficult for both parent and child, it also creates a disturbance in the entire family structure. Health care professionals can assist parents by helping them recognize and utilize their personal support systems. According to Meleski (2002), "...when parents formed a strong support system, they adapted better to the demands of a child's illness" (p. 52). Professionals can help parents plan their time away from home and work by updating them with changes. Parents are usually a comfort to their child and one another at the time of death. The loss of a child is different from any other loss; "...the grief of parents is more intense, more complex, and longer lasting" (Davies & Eng, 1993, p. 726) than other types of grief. Parents may consider themselves victims. They have lost their hopes and dreams and have failed to protect their child from death (Davies & Eng, 1993). Bereaved parents may receive "...compassionate understanding and support..." (Stevens, 1993, p. 714) from a group consisting of other parents who have experienced a similar loss. Professionals who provide care should also provide support group information. The information might be most helpful if provided a few weeks later, when the reality of their child's death is more apparent.

Gender

Although men and women are understood to grieve differently, how these differences affect them during bereavement is not understood. According to Parkes (1988), it was a mystery that widowers were more likely to die after the death of their spouse than widows were. He explained that among the Huli people of New Guinea, the rate of mortality among widowers was higher than the rate among widows. He attributed this "...to the fact that in that society widows grieve but widowers do not. One wonders if Anglo-American society is very different" (Parkes, 1988, p. 369).

In Western culture the expression of grief is often restricted. This restriction may contribute to pathologic grief in our society. Parkes (1988) studied bereaved women from Boston who were younger than 45 years. During the first year of bereavement these widows showed more signs of emotional disturbance than comparable young widowers did. Within 2 to 4 years, despite their initial emotional turmoil, these widows returned to an emotional level equal to married women about the same age. The widowers appeared to continue grieving. According to Shapiro (1996), gender roles, predetermined by society, stipulate what is acceptable bereavement for men and women.

Despite research indicating that the grief exhibited by men was different from that exhibited by women, Quigley and Schatz's (1999) study of older adults revealed conflicting findings. The study discovered comparable emotional experiences for both genders. The older men and women reported similar levels of guilt, anger, despair, denial, sadness, and isolation when grieving the loss of a spouse. As people age, they may ignore social expectations related to grieving. They may also recognize and experience grief differently from when they were younger. Although few men attended a bereavement group, those who did were older than 60 years. These men were willing to share their experience and express their innermost feelings.

Expressing grief openly is often inhibited for both men and women, but professionals should encourage it. Succumbing to and expressing grief's pain is viewed as "...morbid, unhealthy, and demoralizing, and the proper action of a friend is to distract the mourner from his or her grief" (Hasler, 1996, p. 53). Inhibiting the expression of grief causes the bereaved to feel out of control, as if they are losing touch with reality. Subsequent anxiety will be reduced if professionals dismiss this inhibition as a social problem and allow the bereaved to ventilate their feelings (Jalowiec, Murphy, & Powers, 1984) while helping them identify, express, and understand their emotions.

Beliefs

Individuals have diverse beliefs determined by ethnic, racial, religious, or economic influences, which can affect end-of-life issues. Challenges they face and strengths they may draw from can be influenced by these beliefs. Current literature promotes the discussion of terminal illness, but this is inappropriate for patients from a Muslim culture (Habel, 2001). The gender of the health care professional who provides patient care can have a cultural impact. Other factors of cultural

significance that can affect grieving include the use of touch, eye contact, and facial expression. Although cultural groups have identifiable death rituals, professionals providing end-of-life care recognize that these "...may or may not be relevant to all people from a specific cultural group" (Habel, 2001, p. 29).

Rituals, customs, and beliefs can facilitate the grieving process, but they can also complicate it. Bereaved with a deep sense of spirituality can be comforted by the belief that a loved one is in heaven or at peace (Doka, 2000b). Although religion is often mentioned as a way of coping with a difficult death (Maddox, 2001), very religious individuals sometimes become angry with God over the loss of a loved one (Grollman, 2000b). This is devastating since they believe their feelings of rage or anger toward God are sinful. Learning that these feelings are a normal part of grief might help them recover.

Families take memories created during end-of-life care with them into bereavement. The understanding and expression of pain can be defined by culture. In some cultures "...people are socialized to be stoic in the face of pain" (Habel, 2001, p. 29). In others, an open display of pain and frequent requests for medication are common. Some view pain and suffering as deserved, representing past misdeeds, or divine will. Patients can use suffering as a way to control their circumstances and manipulate others (Urquhart, 1999). One must be sensitive to a patient's and family's cultural needs related to symptom control.

The patient may need for sacred items or symbols such as religious beads or dream catchers to stay close to him or her. Many cultures have required rituals for the time of death. These can involve allowing the patient's spirit to leave by taking the body outside, opening a window, or lighting candles (Habel, 2001). Loud wailing and lamenting, even in public, are normal for some people. To support a patient's and family's best use of resources, they are trusted and respected as the authority of their own cultural assessment and coping. After all, it is their grief experience (Shapiro, 1996). Consultation with a transcultural nurse will advance professional understanding of the influence culture has on grief.

Palliative Symptoms

Palliative care specialists utilize advanced skills to manage pain and symptoms while they ensure that patients and families receive quality end-of-life care. Roles and responsibilities are enhanced through awareness of grief's effects and recognition of preventive solutions. It is not death people fear but, rather, the dying process. "How their loved ones will die is a major source of anxiety and presents a major challenge..." (Costello, 1996, p. 173). Patients are afraid of being alone and suffering unrelieved symptoms such as pain and choking. Speck (1978) discovered that patients wondered "what would happen to them and the sensations they might experience" (p. 20). Symptom control and emotional support help a patient feel "...cared for, safe, and more open to expressing his true feelings and emotions" (Wheeler, 1996, p. 29).

Watching a loved one die in pain has negative effects. Genuine reassurance provided by a confident palliative care team relieves the anxiety, panic, and uncertainty experienced by the patient and family. Cameron and Parkes (1983) explained, "Relatives of patients who have suffered severe, unrelieved pain before death are left with intense feelings of anger which disturb their sleep and impair the process of grieving" (p. 76). Sheehan and Schirm (2003) commented that "...many family members do witness a loved one dying in unrelieved pain, dyspnea, or anxiety, and they don't forget providers' inability to attend to these needs" (p. 51). Dame Cicely Saunders, founder of hospice, observed, "'How people die remains in the memories of those who live on'" (Pitorak, 2003, p. 42). Pain is best controlled through a collaborative interdisciplinary approach, making certain that "...patients receive the highest quality of pain control possible with the most efficient use of resources" (Cronin & Ladd, 1997, p. 47). Involving family members in patient care addresses their worries and concerns, optimizes the time they have together, and is vital to successful anticipatory grief work.

PROFESSIONAL RESPONSIBILITIES

Grief has far-reaching effects. If left unrecognized and unresolved, grief can cause somatic symptoms.

Preventing these symptoms and the related depression is a frugal use of health care dollars. Hospital nurses were asked if they discuss bereavement with relatives before a patient dies, and 56% said they do not. Of those same nurses, 72% said they received no training in bereavement (Lloyd-Richards & Rees, 1996). Nursing educators are challenged to incorporate a palliative end-of-life approach, including pain assessment and management, into the nursing curriculum (Ferrell, 1999b).

Assuring a peaceful death for terminally ill patients and families is an extraordinary and fundamental responsibility facing the nursing profession as they affect end-of-life care (Ferrell, 1999a). Practitioners, available in consultative, educative, and supportive ways, assist health care professionals by contributing to protocols and planning end-of-life care (Karrer, 1996; Shuler, Huebscher, & Hallock, 2001). Effective palliative care involves collaboration based on medical and nursing research findings (Steele, 1990).

An interactive approach is the most effective means for rendering care. Travelbee (1966) believed that the more "...skillful a nurse is in the area of interpersonal relationships, the more likely it is that she will be able to meet the nursing needs" (preface). McKissock and McKissock (1996) said that professionals who "...confront personal values and beliefs about death, dying, and bereavement..." (p. 30) will intervene effectively. "'Much of the work ...is about human relationships and helping the patient and family adjust to changes'" (Karrer, 1996, p. 378). Interventions can affect the grieving process "...at three points: before a loss occurs (primary prevention); following a loss, before the grief process becomes dysfunctional (secondary prevention); and after symptoms of morbid grief appear, (tertiary prevention)" (Potocky, 1993, p. 289). Death's closet companion is grief. The aching pain of bereavement can last for years.

Patients and families who experience a terminal illness and the associated grief and bereavement need the support and skills provided by the diverse talents found in an interdisciplinary palliative care team. This team includes the patient and family who will share their reaction to the illness and their ability to cope. One team member is no more important than another as they are working together toward a common goal. Current concerns will dictate which member will guide the team. Members available on any team may differ because of program size and resources. Hospice palliative care teams are composed of physicians, nurses, social workers, chaplains, and volunteers, with dietitians, physical therapists, occupational therapists, and speech therapists available as needed.

The physician's primary responsibility is to control the patient's pain and other physical symptoms. These symptoms must be controlled before any other end-of-life work can begin. The palliative physician must remain informed about the most recent use of medications and treatments for the terminally ill and provide education, guidance, and support to other team members. When deciding whether a treatment will help or harm a patient, the patient's current condition and stage of disease must be considered. This decision is guided by medical expertise. The physician, as well as other team members, treat the whole person and consider both the patient and the family when making decisions.

The nurse's primary responsibility is to help the patient and family cope with the effects of the terminal disease. The nurse's close contact with the patient and family provides an opportunity to know who they are as persons. This relationship allows early recognition of changing symptoms and needs, which promotes timely intervention by other team members. The nurse provides physical care such as bathing, bowel and bladder care, and assistance with administering medication and regular nutrition. Teaching the family how to provide patient care allows them to remain in control. Compassionate nursing care also provides emotional support, which can enhance the benefits available from other disciplines.

A social worker helps the patient and family cope with personal and psychosocial problems caused by or interfering with the terminal condition. They investigate and assist with the patient's and family's understanding and expectations of the illness and prognosis. They provide invaluable services such as referral to needed community resources and assistance with future plans for the bereaved. The social worker also helps investigate emotional status and potential support. His or her findings, including cultural considerations, are shared with team members.

The palliative care chaplain assists the patient and family as they struggle to find meaning and spiritual sense in their lives. Although the chaplain may be of a particular faith, the patient and family are met where they are in their spiritual development. The chaplain can assist with concerns about guilt, regrets, and how their beliefs might help them through stress caused by the illness. The chaplain often addresses ethical issues. Meaningful end-of-life rituals or traditions can provide an additional source of support and encouragement. Spiritual findings are reported to the team members. Patients and families often ask the palliative care chaplain to assist with the funeral or memorial service.

Hospice or palliative care volunteers assist the team to provide quality of life for the patient and family. Because these team members are unpaid, they help preserve valuable health care dollars. Volunteers come from all walks of life. They may have a medical background but often do not. Former hospice family members and caring individuals from the community also make up the volunteer team. Volunteers assist with many functions of the program. A volunteer is matched with a position by considering his or her talents and desires. Volunteers can provide support by helping with administrative duties such as filing charts, organizing bulk mailings, and raising funds. Some volunteers assist by sharing skills such as accountant, computer specialist, or musician. When choosing a volunteer who will provide direct patient and family care, common cultural and social interests are considered. Volunteers are also involved in assisting survivors through bereavement. Because of the serious nature of the work and the vulnerability of the patient and family, volunteers must be chosen carefully. Like any other position that requires specific skills, the program will use particular criteria when choosing potential volunteers.

The team also comprises available members who may not be needed by every patient and family. The dietitian working in palliative care will assess nutritional status and make logical suggestions.

A cancer patient may have cravings for particular foods and distaste for others. The effects of the terminal illness may dictate what the patient can eat. Educating the family and suggesting small, frequent meals of the foods the patient likes often are the solution. The physical therapist will attempt to improve the patient's ability to function despite the deteriorating condition. This might be accomplished by assisting with active and passive range of motion to keep limbs mobile and by teaching the patient and family transfer skills. The occupational therapist will assess the patient's and family's ability to provide self-care. The goal is to help the patient remain independent longer. The patient and family are educated about the use of adaptive devices such as splints to help the patient feed himself or herself. A speech therapist can help the patient who loses the ability to talk but who remains alert and able to communicate. Storyboards and, more recently, specialized computers, can provide a solution for optimal patient communication. The ability to communicate affords the patient a sense of control. Treatment plans are changed as the patient's ability diminishes. Although team members may have different methods and areas of expertise, they all contribute to the patient's and family's sense of well-being as they work through the challenges of advanced illness.

ASSISTANCE

Understandably, a number of grieving individuals will need help, otherwise, they "...may spend long, agonizing months working through their pain and suffering alone" (Greifzu, 1996, p. 22). It is imperative that professionals observe family interaction, especially the type of support the caregiver receives from family members. This may predict the support they will need after the death. While studying Australian widows, Parkes (1988) found that "The strongest single predictor of a poor health outcome was the bereaved person's perception of his family as unhelpful or lacking in understanding. Also interesting is Raphael's finding that this is also the group who benefit most from counseling" (p. 370).

Whereas some individuals ask for assistance, others do not. Requesting assistance cannot be trusted as an indicator of who truly needs it.

"Duke found that 'shyness to ask for help' predicts poor outcome, and this suggests that those who do ask for help may have less need of it than those who are too frightened or depressed to ask" (Parkes, 1988, p. 371). According to Lloyd-Richards and Rees (1996), individuals who understand the grief process should work with the bereaved "...as soon as eminent (sic) death is known, the sooner that bereavement is initiated the easier the process will be to manage" (p. 109).

When an individual loses a loved one, the pain must be felt and experienced. "Comfort alone does not provide adequate assistance.... He will have to express his sorrow and sense of loss" (Lindemann, 1944/1994, p. 159). A supportive environment guides bereaved individuals to complete the two major tasks of grief: (1) accept the death as real, and (2) cope with problems, both emotional and social, that are created by the loss (Rognlie, 1989). Be frank when communicating. "When discussing the loved one with family members, use words like 'dying' and 'dead' rather than 'lost' or 'gone' to help them accept reality" (Wheeler, 1996, p. 29). Anticipation provides some preparation, but the reality of death usually remains a shock. According to Mazanec and Tyler (2003), one of the palliative care team's responsibilities is "Helping the family to understand... that hope can coexist with terminal illness..." (p. 55).

Honest discussion about imminent death allows patients to complete unfinished business. Professionals should suggest that "...it's never too late to bring closure to an unresolved issue" (Wheeler, 1996, p. 27). Ira Byock (1997) offered a formula to facilitate this closure. Byock suggested that families consider "...'the five things of relationship completion' —saying 'I forgive you'; 'Forgive me'; 'Thank you'; 'I love you'; and 'Goodbye'. [These give the patient] a kind of script with which to greet his final days with courage and determination" (p. 140). It is hoped that use of such a script will foster intimate patient and family communication. Gabany (2000) reported that those who help patients and families complete end-of-life tasks ensure satisfaction and ease the bereavement journey.

"Palliative care is the active total care provided to patients living with advanced incurable illness and their families. The focus of care shifts to quality of life and alleviation of distressing symptoms…. Furthermore, it offers a support system to help relatives and friends cope during the patient's illness and bereavement" (National Coalition on Health Care, 2001 as cited in McHale, 2002, p. 193). Complementing palliative care is hospice care, which is available to everyone, regardless of financial status. Hospice care is considered the gold standard for end-of-life care in this country. Hospice uses an interdisciplinary team of health care professionals and trained volunteers to provide pain management, symptom control, psychosocial support, and spiritual care to the dying and their families.

Practitioners from all disciplines can refer a patient and family to hospice for an informational visit. This can empower the patient and family and foster hope. They will understand that they have choices about end-of-life care. Terminally ill hospital patients often express a wish to die at home, yet many of these same patients die in the hospital despite their wishes. In contrast, most hospice patients do die in their own homes.

Box 15-1   COMPLICATED GRIEF

DEFINITION

When a bereaved individual is unable to reinvest his emotional energies into other things after the death of a loved one, he may be suffering from complicated grief.[1] Complicated grief occurs when the grief responses are overwhelming, maladaptive, or unusually prolonged.[2]

SIGNS AND SYMPTOMS

An abbreviated list includes[1]:
- Absence of sadness (failure to grieve)
- Delayed or prolonged grieving
- Avoidance of grief (by avoiding the funeral, grave, etc.)
- Feelings of extreme guilt and self-reproach
- Loss of decisiveness and initiative
- Self-destructive behaviors
- Vague physical distress
- Prolonged searching and overactivity
- A sense that death occurred yesterday, even after considerable time has passed
- Unwillingness to move the possessions of the deceased
- Deterioration in other relationships after the death
- Decreased participation in religious rituals
- Inability to discuss the dead person without intense emotion (p. 283)

RISK FACTORS

Complicated grief can result if[2]:
- A loved one's death is sudden (as in cases of suicide, homicide, or accident).
- The survivor and the deceased were estranged or relations were strained.
- A child dies.
- The survivor has had more than one loss.
- The survivor has unresolved grief from previous losses.
- A loved one suffered greatly at the end of life.
- The survivor lacks adequate support.
- The survivor's grief is so intense that he cannot function as he would normally or accept that the relationship has ended, or both" (p. 48).

[1]Burge, F. (1999). Grief and bereavement. In N. MacDonald (Ed.), *Palliative medicine: A case-based manual* (pp. 278-284). New York: Oxford University Press.
[2]Egan K. A., & Arnold, R. L. (2003). Grief and bereavement care. *American Journal of Nursing, 103* (9), 42-53.

The benefit of hospice care goes beyond the patient. Bereaved individuals who are knowledgeable about the patient's illness, especially knowing that the patient will die from the illness, do better during bereavement. Literature and study for over 50 years has "...suggested a relationship between bereavement progress and length of time with knowledge of an impending death. Anticipatory grief work can only happen if one knows about the coming death, and has enough time to digest and work with the implications. Problems infect all aspects of the dying trajectory related to this knowing" (McHale, 2001, p. 131). Practitioners must be open and honest. They must educate patients and families about their illness and the options that are available for end-of-life care.

Discussion of death may not decrease sadness, but it can decrease fear. "The way the diagnosis of life-threatening illness is first imparted can affect the family's ability to cope" (Kaye, 1999, p. 56). When professionals address death and dying they "...relieve anxiety and allow all those affected by a patient's death to think more clearly, face fear and make decisions...." (Griffie, Nelson-Martin, & Muchka, 2004, pp. 49-50). To meet patient and family needs does not have to be time-consuming. Professionals may find the following basic principles helpful (Kaye, 1999, p. 57):

Box 15-2   RESOURCES

There is a trend in many communities to offer support groups through various agencies including hospice organizations, hospitals, funeral homes, churches, and community mental health services. Books and publications are available through local libraries.

ORGANIZATIONS

The American Association of Retired Persons (AARP): AARP Grief and Loss Programs, 601 E Street, NW, Washington, D.C. 20049; or E-mail griefandloss@aarp.org
Americans for Better Care of the Dying: www.abcd-caring.org
Center to Advance Palliative Care: www.capcmssm.org
Center to Improve Care of the Dying: www.gwu.edu/~cicd
City of Hope Pain/Palliative Care Resource Center: www.cityofhope.org/prc
Community-State Partnerships to Improve End-of-Life Care: www.midbio.org/nPo-about.htm
The Compassionate Friends: www.compassionatefriends.org
End-of-Life Nursing Education Consortium (ELNEC): www.aacn.nche.edu/elnec
The EPEC Project: Education on End-of-Life Care: www.epec.net
Hospice and Palliative Nurses Association: www.hpna.org
Innovations in End-of-Life Care: www.edc.org/lastacts
Last Acts: www.lastacts.org
Mothers Against Drunk Driving: www.madd.org
National Hospice and Palliative Care Organization: www.nhpco.org
Partnership for Caring: www.partnershipforcaring.org
Supportive Care of the Dying: www.careofdying.org

TOOL KIT

Tool Kit for Nurturing Excellence at End-of-Life Transition (TNEEL): www.tneel.uic.edu. Available on CD-ROM, won the 2002 Sigma Theta Tau International, Region 1, Computer-Based Professional Education Award. This tool kit aids nurse educators in developing classes in six areas of end-of-life care.

BOOKS

Byock, I. (1997). *Dying well: The prospect for growth at the end of life.* New York: Riverhead Books.
Callanan, M., & Kelley, P. (1997). *Final gifts: Understanding the special awareness, needs, and communications of the dying.* New York: Bantam Books.

- Set aside time (give your beeper to someone else!).
- Arrange for privacy and quiet.
- Convey empathy ("You must be worried.").
- Ask questions first and listen.
- Explain, using kind words.
- Give information in a graded way.
- Avoid jargon (it confuses).
- Arrange emotional support ("Who will be at home?").
- Offer to meet with family members (a disaster happens to a whole family).
- Offer availability ("Let's meet again next week.").

SUMMARY

Western society's inability to accept and address death and grief can complicate bereavement. Health care professionals are in a unique position to support patients and families through their bereavement journeys. An interactive multidisciplinary approach to care, one that intimately involves the patient and family, can provide a context for anticipatory grief work—a process that can benefit survivors as well

as the person who is dying. Understanding types of grief, typical and atypical responses to loss, and the various impacts that grief has on relationships can equip health care professionals to address the painful realities of loss of patients and their families. Direct and supportive discussions about loss, death, and dying can decrease patient and family fear and help the bereaved adjust to living life without the loved one. Finally, numerous resources exist for providers, patients, and family members who are coping with these serious issues.

Objective Questions

1. The reaction to loss of a loved person is called:

   a. Grief.
   b. Mourning.
   c. Bereavement.
   d. Anticipatory grief.

2. The concept of anticipatory grief was developed by:

   a. Freud, 1917, in *Mourning and Melancholia.*

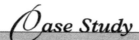

Case Study

Mary, who was 63, had been ill for some time. She suffered from abdominal pain and swelling that got progressively worse. She kept her illness a secret. Pain medication was delivered by a local pharmacy. Her physician, who was known to be generous with his prescriptions, provided it. Mary and her husband James had been married 39 years. They had 10 children, the youngest of whom was away at college and home only on weekends. Mary was able to hide her illness for weeks by staying in bed when anyone was home, with excuses of being tired, having the flu, or just reading. This way no one saw the changes the ovarian cancer was causing to her body. One Friday night, after returning from school, their youngest daughter turned on a light in her mother's room to find her reading a book. She was shocked at what she saw. Mary's face was thin and drawn, and her arms were thin but her abdomen was so bloated that Mary could no longer walk. Mary was taken to the hospital and died

several days later. It took days to reach all the children and get them home. One son arrived just hours before Mary died; another was not able to get home until the funeral. Mary's denial had prevented the family from completing end-of-life tasks. James was shocked and stunned. This 74-year-old gentleman lost his wife of 39 years. Although he had 10 children who loved and supported him, he was unable to talk about his wife's death. For several weeks he was not even able to say her name. A month later he shared, "I dream about her but I don't see her face." He was distraught but unable to share his pain. About a month later he described flu-like symptoms. James was taken to his physician and was diagnosed with Guillain-Barré syndrome. He avoided his painful grief but became physically ill. Guillain-Barré, which is an autoimmune disease, left his feet and legs numb and unstable. This lasted until he died 13 years later.

b. Lindemann, 1944, in *Symptomatology and Management of Acute Grief.*

c. Kübler-Ross, 1969, in *On Death and Dying.*

d. Byock, 1997, in *Dying Well, the Prospect for Growth at the End of Life.*

3. Which of the following feelings would you *not* expect as a result of the anticipatory grief experience?

   a. They permit a healthy reaction to loss.

   b. They can make the actual death less traumatic.

   c. They can cause pain as intense as that felt after the death.

   d. They often cause the terminally ill patient to have an exacerbation of illness.

4. The amount of time a spouse usually experiences grief:

   a. Is not affected by age or coping capability.

   b. Will not usually last longer than 6 to 9 months.

   c. May be related to the value he or she places on the lost person.

   d. Can usually be controlled by the time of year the death occurs.

5. Grief stage theories provide professionals with:

   a. An understanding of the grief process.

   b. A five-step plan for all grieving patients.

   c. Detailed instructions for caring for bereaved individuals.

   d. A clear understanding of how long each patient will grieve.

6. Jack's primary physician has just told him that the pathology from his testicular lump is malignant. He sets aside time each day for prayer where he promises God he will be more devoted to his family if He will allow the treatment to cure him. What stage of anticipatory grief is Jack in?

   a. Denial.

   b. Anger.

   c. Bargaining.

   d. Depression.

7. To adjust well to grief and travel smoothly through bereavement, individuals should:

   a. Realize that painful grief is completely unnatural.

   b. Understand that symptoms wax and wane over time.

   c. Learn to eliminate painful memories rather than live with them.

   d. Believe comfort from a close friend will relieve all of their pain from grief.

8. Successful grief work and recovery from the loss may depend on:

   a. Never becoming angry with God.

   b. The patient's ability to limit the amount of pain medication used.

   c. Allowing the physician providing care the choice of death rituals.

   d. Being allowed to cry and wail loudly at the time of death.

9. The hospice psychosocial director has been following Mrs. Ford in bereavement. During the visits, Mrs. Ford spends most of the time crying. At what point should the psychosocial director consider that this reaction is complicated grief?

   a. 1 week after the funeral.

   b. 1 month after the death.

   c. 2 to 3 months after the death.

   d. 6 to 12 months after the death.

10. The following symptoms are considered an abnormal grief reaction:

    a. Difficulty breathing or swallowing.

    b. Waves of distress lasting up to an hour.

    c. Feelings of extreme guilt and self-reproach.

    d. An intense preoccupation with an image of the deceased.

11. Joan has been divorced for 2 years, but during the 7 years she was married to Ralph he was abusive to her. Joan moved and has started a new life. She is not close to any of Ralph's family and won't attend his funeral. What type of complicated grief is Joan at risk for?

a. Masked grief.
b. Delayed grief.
c. Chronic grief.
d. Disenfranchised grief.

12. Adults in our society generally do *not*:

a. Withdraw from individuals in mourning.
b. Have difficulty discussing death and grief.
c. Prefer medical treatment as a means for hope.
d. Prefer to plan for end-of-life events with family participation.

13. Palliative care professionals recognize that:

a. Pain and symptoms are always controlled at the end-of-life.
b. Family members' concerns do not affect the dying patient.
c. Patients fear the dying process more than they fear death.
d. Once the deceased's funeral is over, pain they experienced at death is forgotten.

14. Johnny is 7 years old. His grandmother is seriously ill and in the hospital. When Johnny visits his grandmother, his parents can expect him to:

a. Act the same way the other 7-year-old boys from their church would act.
b. Not understand anything about his grandmother's illness or potential death.
c. Understand everything his parents explained as long as they did so slowly.
d. Have an ability to understand illness and death that corresponds to his own developmental stage.

15. Laura, a nurse on the oncology floor, has been caring for a gentleman who is of the Muslim faith. She was told he died just a few minutes ago. As Laura goes to be with the family and prepare the body, she knows that:

a. His family will want him cremated immediately.
b. His family will tightly wrap his body with pieces of pure cotton.

c. His family may want his head turned toward his right shoulder.
d. His family will want an autopsy performed.

16. Health care professionals who care for terminally ill patients understand that:

a. Euphemisms are helpful and encourage further communication.
b. Honest communication has detrimental effects.
c. They will gain patient and family trust by withholding the truth and protecting them.
d. Other professionals might fear that providing frank information would lead to blame.

REFERENCES

Bales, D. (Ed.). (1997). More calls for improved end of life care. *Hospice News Network, July 8*, 2.

Blank, H.R. (1969). Mourning. In A.H. Kutscher (Ed.), *Death and bereavement* (pp. 204-206). Springfield, Ill.: Charles C. Thomas.

Buckman, R. (1993). Commnication in palliative care: A practical guide. In D. Doyle, G.W.C. Hanks, & N. MacDonald (Eds.), *Oxford textbook of palliative medicine.* (pp. 47-61). New York: Oxford University Press.

Burge, F. (1999). Grief and bereavement. In N. MacDonald (Ed.), *Palliative medicine: A case-based manual* (pp. 278-284). New York: Oxford University Press.

Byock, I. (1997). Dying well, the prospect for growth at the end of life. New York: Riverhead Books.

Cameron, J., & Parkes, C.M. (1983). Terminal care: Evaluation of effects on surviving family of care before and after bereavement. *Postgrad Med J, 59*, 73-78.

Chesson, R., & Todd, C. (1996). Bereaved carers: Recognizing their needs. *Elder Care, 8*(6), 16-18.

Como, N.D. (Ed.). (1990). *Mosby's pocket dictionary of medicine, nursing, & allied health.* St. Louis: Mosby.

Corr, C.A. (1993). Death in modern society. In D. Doyle, G.W.C. Hanks, & N. MacDonald (Eds.), *Oxford textbook of palliative medicine* (pp. 28-36). New York: Oxford University Press.

Costello, J. (1996). The emotional cost of palliative care. *European J Palliat Care, 3*(4), 171-174.

Couldrick, A. (1992). Optimizing bereavement outcome: Reading the road ahead. *Soc Sci Med, 35*(12), 1521-1523.

Cronin, Y., & Ladd, L.A. (1997). Utilizing the clinical nurse specialist to promote interdisciplinary pain management. *J Fla Med Assoc, 84*(1), 46-48.

Davies, B., & Eng, B.W.S. (1993). Special issues in bereavement and staff support. In D. Doyle, G.W.C. Hanks, & N. MacDonald (Eds.), *Oxford textbook of palliative medicine* (pp. 725-733). New York: Oxford University Press.

Davis-Berman, J., Berman, D., & Faris, R. (1995). Lifestories: Discussions on death using adventure-based activities. *Activities, Adaptation & Aging, 19*(3), 55-63.

deVeber, L L., Jacobson, S.J., Koren, G., et al. (1993). Symptom management. In D. Doyle, G.W.C. Hanks, & N. MacDonald (Eds.), *Oxford textbook of palliative medicine* (pp. 691-699). New York: Oxford University Press.

Doka, K.J. (2000a). I will never get over this. *Hospice Foundation of America: Journeys, Oct.,* 1-2.

Doka, K.J. (2000b). The individuality of grief. *Hospice Foundation of America: Journeys, Nov.,* 1-2.

Doyle, D. (1993). Domiciliary palliative care. In D. Doyle, G.W.C. Hanks, & N. MacDonald (Eds.), *Oxford textbook of palliative medicine* (pp. 629-647). New York: Oxford University Press.

Egan K.A., & Arnold, R.L. (2003). Grief and bereavement care. *Am J Nurs, 103*(9), 42-53.

Engel, G.L. (1961). Is grief a disease? A challenge for medical research. *Psychosom Med, 13*(1), 18-22.

Ferrell, B.R. (1999a). Caring at the end of life. *Reflections, 25*(4), 31-37.

Ferrell, B.R. (1999b). Strengthening nursing education to improve end of life care. *Kans Nurs Newsl, 12*(4), 11.

Gabany, J.M. (2000). Factors contributing to the quality of end-of-life care. *J Am Acad Nurs Pract, 12*(11), 472-474.

Griffie, J., Nelson-Martin, P., & Muchka, S. (2004). Acknowledging the "elephant": Communication in palliative care. *Am J Nurs, 104*(1), 49-50.

Goldberg, S.B. (1973). Family tasks and reactions in the crisis of death. *Social Casework, July,* 398-405.

Greifzu, S. (1996). Grieving families need your help. *RN, 59*(9), 22-27.

Grollman, E.A. (2000a). I thought I knew him. *Hospice Foundation of America: Journeys, Oct.,* 3.

Grollman, E.A. (2000b). Yelling at God. *Hospice Foundation of America: Journeys, Nov.,* 3.

Habel, M. (2001). Caring for people of many cultures. *NurseWeek, Jan.,* 29-30.

Harper, B.C. (2000). Hospice and palliative care: A vision for the new millennium. *J Hospice Palliat Nurs, 2*(1), 21-27.

Hasler, K. (1996). Understanding and managing bereavement. *Nurs Stand, 10*(24), 51-56.

Horowitz, M.J., Siegel, B., Holen, A., et al. (1997). Criteria for complicated grief disorder. *Am J Psychiatry, 154,* 905-910.

House, F. (Jan. 6, 2004). Personal communication.

Huber, R., & Gibson, J.W. (1990). New evidence for anticipatory grief. *Hosp J, 6*(1), 49-67.

Jacob, S.R. (1996). The grief experience of older women whose husbands had hospice care. *J Adv Nurs, 24,* 280-286.

Jacobs, S. (1999). *Traumatic grief: Diagnosis, treatment, and prevention.* Caselton, N.Y.: Brunner/Mazel.

Jalowiec, A., Murphy, S.P., & Powers, M.J. (1984). Psychometric assessment of the Jalowiec Coping Scale. *Nurs Res, 33*(3), 157-161.

Karrer, R. (1996). The Macmillan touch. *Practice Nurse, 9 April,* 377-378, 381-382.

Kaye, P. (1999). *Notes on symptom control in hospice & palliative care.* Essex, Conn.: Hospice Education Institute.

Kleyman, P. (1996). The aging spirit: Living with loss, healing with hope. *Aging Today, Jan./Feb.,* 7-8.

Kristjanson, L.J., Sloan, J.A., Dudgeon, D., et al. 1996). Family members' perceptions of palliative cancer care: Predictors of

family functioning and family members' health. *J Palliat Care, 12*(4), 10-20.

Kübler-Ross, E. (1969). *On death and dying.* New York: Macmillan.

Kurtz, M.E., Kurtz, J.C., Given, C.W., et al. (1997). Predictors of post-bereavement depressive symptomatology among family caregivers of cancer patients. *Support Care Cancer, 5,* 53-60.

Levy, L.H. (1991). Anticipatory grief: Its measurement and proposed reconceptualization. *Hosp J, 7*(4), 1-28.

Lindemann, E. (1944/1994). Symptomatology and management of acute grief. *Am J Psychiatry, 151*(6), 155-160. (Original work published 1944.)

Lloyd-Richards, C., & Rees, C. (1996). Hospital nurses' bereavement support for relatives: Study report. *Int J Palliat Nurs, 2*(2), 106-110.

Maddox, M. (2001). Teaching spirituality to nurse practitioner students: The importance of the interconnection of mind, body, and spirit. *J Am Acad Nurs Pract, 13*(3), 134-139.

Mazanec, P., & Tyler, M.K. (2003). Cultural considerations in end-of-life care. *Am J Nurs, 103*(3), 50-59.

McHale, H.K. (1998). The role of the advanced practice nurse in hospice care. *Kans Nurse, 73*(3), 1-2.

McHale, H.K. (2001). *A study of survivor's progress in bereavement through pre-death work.* Unpublished master's thesis, Pittsburg State University, Pittsburg, Kan.

McHale, H.K. (2002). Palliative care. In K. Kuebler & P. Esper (Eds.), *Palliative care practices from a to z for the bedside clinician* (pp. 193-197). Pittsburgh: Oncology Nursing Press.

McKechnie, J.L. (Ed.). (1973). *Webster's new twentieth century dictionary of the English language* (Unabridged, 2nd ed.). Cleveland: World.

McKissock, M.A., & McKissock, D.R. (1996). The nurses' role in caring for the newly bereaved. *Lamp, 53*(5), 30-32.

Meleski, D.D. (2002). Families with chronically ill children. *Am J Nurs, 102*(5), 47-54.

Monroe, B. (1993). Social work in palliative care. In D. Doyle, G.W.C. Hanks, & N. MacDonald (Eds.), *Oxford textbook of palliative medicine* (pp. 556-574). New York: Oxford University Press.

National Hospice Foundation (NHF). (1999a, June 6). *Baby boomers fear talking to parents about death.* (p. 1) Arlington, Va.

National Hospice Foundation (NHF). (1999b, Oct. 14). NHO board member testifies before congress on pain and end-of-life care. Arlington, Va.

Neuberger, J. (1993). Cultural issues in palliative care. In D. Doyle, G.W.C. Hanks, & N. MacDonald (Eds.), *Oxford textbook of palliative medicine* (pp. 507-513). New York: Oxford University Press.

Norris, F.H., & Murrell, S.A. (1987). Older adult family stress and adaptation before and after bereavement. *J Gerontol, 42*(6), 606-612.

Ott, C.H. (2003). The impact of complicated grief on mental and physical health at various points in the bereavement process. *Death Stud, 27,* 249-272.

Parkes, C.M. (1988). Research: Bereavement. *Omega, 18*(4), 365-373.

Pitorak, E.F. (2003). Care at the time of death. *Am J Nurs, 103*(7), 42-53.

Potocky, M. (1993). Effective services for bereaved spouses: A content analysis of the empirical literature. *Health Soc Work, 18*(4), 288-301.

Prigerson, H.G., Bierhals, A.J., Kasl, S.V., et al. (1997). Traumatic grief as a risk factor for mental and physical morbidity. *Am J Psychiatry, 54,* 617-623.

Quigley, D.G., & Schatz, M.S. (1999). Men and women and their responses in spousal bereavement. *Hosp J, 14*(2), 65-78.

Ransford, H.E., & Smith, M.L. (1991). Grief resolution among the bereaved in hospice and hospital wards. *Soc Sci Med, 32*(3), 295-304.

Rognlie, C. (1989). Perceived short- and long-term effects of bereavement support group participation at the Hospice of Petaluma. *Hosp J, 5*(2), 39-53.

Saunders, J.M. (1981). A process of bereavement resolution: Uncoupled identity. *West J Nurs Res, 3*(4), 319-334.

Sheehan, D.K., & Schirm, V. (2003). End-of-life care of older adults. *Am J Nurs, 103*(11), 48-59.

Shapiro, E.R. (1996). Family bereavement and cultural diversity: A social developmental perspective. *Fam Process, 35*(Sept.), 313-332.

Shuler, P.A., Huebscher, R., & Hallock, J. (2001). Providing wholistic health care for the elderly: Utilization of the Shuler nurse practitioner model. *J Am Acad Nurs Pract, 13*(7), 297-303.

Silverman, P.R. (1974). Anticipatory grief from the perspective of widowhood. In B. Schoenberg (Ed.), *Anticipatory grief* (pp. 320-330). New York: Columbia University.

Speck, P.W. (1978). *Loss and grief in medicine.* London: Bailliere Tindall.

Steele, L.L. (1990). The death surround: Factors influencing the grief experience of survivors. *Oncol Nurs Forum, 17*(2), 235-241.

Stevens, M.M. (1993). Psychological adaptation of the dying child. In D. Doyle, G.W.C. Hanks, & N. MacDonald (Eds.), *Oxford textbook of palliative medicine* (pp. 699-707). New York: Oxford University Press.

Stoudemire, A., & Blazer, D.G. (1985). Depression in the elderly: Normal and pathological grief. In E.E. Beckham & W.R. Leber (Eds.), *Handbook of depression: Treatment, assessment, and research* (pp. 574-575). Homewood, Ill.: Dorsey Press.

SUPPORT Principal Investigators. (1995). A controlled trial to improve care for seriously ill hospitalized patients: The Study to Understand Prognoses and Preferences for Outcomes and Risks of Treatments (SUPPORT). *J Amer Med Assoc, 274,* 1591-1598.

Travelbee, J. (1966). *Interpersonal aspects of nursing.* Philadelphia: F.A. Davis.

Urquhart, P. (1999). Issues of suffering in palliative care. *Int J Palliat Nurs, 5*(1), 35-39.

Valente, S.M., & McIntyre, L.G. (1996). Responding therapeutically to bereavement and grief. *NurseWeek, April*(15), 10-12.

Wheeler, S.R. (1996). Helping families cope with death and dying. *Nursing, 26*(7), 25-30.

Wolfelt, A. (1992). *Understanding grief: Helping yourself heal.* Bristol, Pa.: Accelerated Development.

Wright, L.M., & Leahey, M. (1994). *Nurses and families: A guide to family assessment and intervention.* Philadelphia: F.A. Davis.

Youll, J., & Wilson, K. (1996). A therapeutic approach to bereavement counseling. *Nurs Times, 92*(16), 40-42.

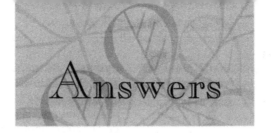
Answers

CHAPTER 1

1. b

The word *palliate* comes from the Latin word *palliare* meaning "to cloak," and according to the Oxford English Dictionary (1975), *palliate* in the context of health care means "to alleviate the symptoms of a disease without curing it." Choices *a, c,* and *d* all are related to but are not part of the strict definition of palliative care. Providing care by an interdisciplinary team (choice *d*) is the means by which palliative care is provided, while quality of life (choice *a*) and hope (choice *c*) are the desired outcomes of providing palliative care.

2. d

The Medicare Hospice Benefit has been instrumental in determining which patients receive hospice services by defining patient eligibility for hospice services based on the certification of two physicians that a patient should have "a medical prognosis that his or her life expectancy is 6 months or less if the illness runs its normal course" (42 Code of Federal Regulations, 1993). It is this requirement (choice *d*), that patients who receive hospice care should have a prognosis of 6 months or less, more than any other, that has defined hospice in the United States and has limited the utilization of hospice services due to difficulties in predicting prognosis. The establishment of the RN as the interdisciplinary team leader, the professional make-up of the team, and the mandate for bereavement services are all important aspects of the Medicare Hospice Benefit but are seldom cited as reasons why hospice services are or are not utilized.

3. d

Palliative care should be provided to patients as part of traditional routine health care (choice *d*). Whether the patient is suffering from cancer or a non-malignant acute or chronic illness and whether the patient is being evaluated, receiving disease-directed therapy for cure or remission, or receiving only symptom-directed therapy (palliative care only), part of the responsibility of the physician and other professionals who care for the patient is to palliate any symptoms the patient is experiencing. Choices *a, b,* and *c* all would limit the population of patients who should receive palliative care, either by diagnosis, by prognosis, or both.

4. a

Under the Medicare Hospice Benefit, professional services of the attending physician (visits and care plan oversight) are the only services that remain reimbursable under Medicare Part B (choice *a*). All other services related to the terminal illness, including diagnostic studies (i.e., laboratory studies, x-rays [choices *b* and *c*]) and treatments that are administered in the attending physician's office are covered under the per diem reimbursement and are the responsibility of the hospice.

5. c

The SUPPORT study Phase II nursing intervention was designed to enhance communication between the patients/families and the physicians and staff caring for them. Unfortunately, the intervention was unsuccessful, and despite the addition of a nurse to facilitate communication, there was no improvement either in the control of pain or in advance care planning among study patients when compared with controls. The authors concluded: "to improve the experience of seriously ill and dying patients, greater individual and societal commitment and more proactive and forceful measures may be needed" (SUPPORT Principal Investigators, 1995).

6. a

The ICU has become an ever-increasing source for patients who require palliative care services, either for symptom management or, in some cases, for end-of-life decision making. According to a 2003 Health Care Advisory Board Report, about one third (33%, choice a) of patients referred to palliative care services come from the ICU setting.

7. b

For a patient living in a long-term care facility to receive care under the Medicare Hospice Benefit, the nursing facility and the hospice must have a contractual relationship. In addition, because the Medicare Hospice Benefit and the Medicare Skilled Nursing Benefit are both Part A and mutually exclusive, a patient may not access the hospice benefit if he or she is receiving care under the skilled nursing benefit (choice b).

8. b

In a study by Casarett and Abrahm published in 2001, a comparison was made between cancer patients cared for by a hospice program and by a pre-hospice bridge program, the latter admitting patients with a prognosis of 1 year or less and/or receiving "life-prolonging" therapies. Comparing patient symptoms between the two groups suggested that the needs of bridge program patients were just as great as those of more traditional hospice patients. Unfortunately, although median survival increased (52 days vs. 20 days), the overwhelming majority of patients still succumbed to their diseases within 6 months (87% bridge vs. 94% hospice) (choice b).

9. d

A preliminary study was conducted that evaluated the role of a palliative care coordinator (PCC) in adding to the management of a group of cancer patients receiving antineoplastic therapy in an academic comprehensive cancer center. The role of the PCC was to facilitate patient/family education regarding the patient's condition as well as to improve patient/family communication with the treating physicians and other health care staff. The study demonstrated neither a survival advantage nor a symptom control benefit for the patients who had the added benefit of the PCC (choices a and b). There was less reduction in quality-of-life measures in the intervention group (choice c). Although the investigators did report a cost advantage in favor of the intervention group, they admitted the results were too preliminary and incomplete to truly conclude that there was a true cost advantage (choice d) (Beresford et al, 2002; Finn et al, 2002; Schapiro et al, 2003).

10. c

As we move into the twenty-first century, with the inevitable aging of our population, it is crucial that we improve patient access to appropriate care at the end of life. One option is an innovative proposal that health care services be tailored to disease trajectory and services would be offered based on the needs of the individual patients and their projected trajectory of decline (choice d). Although this proposal seems worthwhile, it would require a major overhaul of the current health care system, making it an impractical near-term and mid-term solution. Likewise, continuing as we are (confining hospice care to the last days and weeks of life while working to expand palliative care programs) seems impractical, because serious gaps remain in care under the present model of care (choice a). Taking the hospice benefit and eliminating it in favor of a more comprehensive palliative care benefit, although attractive to some, may do more to simply change the descriptor of what is currently available without really changing what we do (choice b).

It is recommended that the approach is to better use what we already have available, namely, to maximize the integration of palliative care and, when appropriate, referral to hospice. This would involve physicians getting more comfortable with referral by adapting a standard based on answering the question "would you be surprised if this patient were to die of his or her illness in the next 12 months?" Hospices should be more willing to admit patients receiving disease-modifying therapies when therapy has potential symptom management benefits and to admit patients participating in investigational studies (especially Phase I trials). For patients who do not desire hospice services, palliative care alternatives should continue to develop, evolve, and remain available (choice c).

CHAPTER 2

1. a
Rapport is necessary for relationship development, is facilitated by provider empathy, is contingent upon verbal and nonverbal behavior, and has not been demonstrated to be related to symptom management.

2. c
Patient reaction to bad news is multifaceted and not determined by one factor alone.

3. b
SOLVER: **S**quarely face the patient, maintain **O**pen posture, **L**ean forward, **V**erbally follow, appropriate **E**ye contact, **R**elax.

4. a
Empathy is not sympathy. Empathy is important in developing patient rapport and empathy is not demonstrated by merely parroting the patient's words.

5. c
Research indicates providers are uncomfortable discussing patient prognosis and that patients generally want the truth about their diagnosis and prognosis.

6. a
Discussing fears with patients is good clinical practice that can help reduce fears and increase efficacy and a sense of personal control

7. b
Countertransference should be examined because it can affect patient care by leading providers to become over-involved or under-involved with patients.

8. b
Wakefield suggests the following to facilitate working through the grief process: saying goodbye to patients, asking questions about the patient's dying trajectory, expressing feelings through stories, and reflecting on grief.

9. b
Novack suggests the following steps to minimize the impact of provider emotional reactions on patient care: (1) name the feeling; (2) accept the normalcy of the feeling; (3) reflect on the emotion and its possible consequences; and (4) consult a trusted colleague.

10. a
Advance care planning should involve family members and the provider, continue even after the completion of advance directives, and be founded on an exploration of the patient's goals and values.

CHAPTER 3

1. a
Choice *a* is correct—scientific basis for practice, which maximizes the chance that the effects of practice will be specific outcomes, as documented in the literature. Choice *b* is wrong because expert opinion presumes desired effects of an intervention but does not support this with research findings. Choices *c* and *d* do not ensure that use of the practice will lead to desired outcomes, only that the practice is being used by others.

2. c
Choice *c* is correct—a treatment that has been tested in randomized controlled trials. Research results from studies with controlled environments with optimal personnel and ideal measures (randomized control trials [RCTs]) give a nonbiased determination of a treatment's effects. Choices *a, b,* and *d* all reflect *efficaciousness*, which refers to results in the real world, in routine clinical practice.

3. a
Choice *a* is correct because conflicting evidence in a body of literature, particularly between RCT and observational data, may not be resolved using levels or hierarchies of evidence. Choice *b* is incorrect; levels of evidence aim to assist in the appraisal of methodologic rigor. Choice *c* is incorrect, because levels of evidence are useful in determining the strength of specific evidence. Choice *d* is not correct. Research based on

homogeneous populations may be very easily evaluated using levels of evidence.

4. d

Choice *d* is correct because it includes "systematically," which alludes to the rigor with which the guideline was developed. This rigor is essential to production of evidence-based guidelines. Choice *a*, standards of care, is incorrect because guidelines are not standards but are recommendations. Choices *b* and *c* are incorrect because these reflect local standards and may not be systematically developed.

5. d

Choice *d* describes the essential elements that make a literature review systematic, both the literature selection and the evaluation process. Choices *a* and *b* are incorrect. These do not play a role in judging a review to be systematic. Choice *c* is incorrect because this defines the single element in most *non*-systematic literature reviews and does not include how the literature was selected or evaluated.

6. d

Choice *d* is correct because the theory of diffusion of innovation considers that new practices are disseminated or spread according to the influence of the perceptions of the innovation, characteristics of those considering the innovation and contextual factors. Choice *a* is incorrect because passive dissemination methods have been ineffective in leading to practice changes. Choice *b* implies a top-down change strategy, which goes against findings about facilitation. Choice *c* is incorrect because most successful facilitation uses multiple strategies.

7. c

Choice *c* is correct because palliative care research often fails to address important outcomes, such as quality of death or best resolution of bereavement, and methodologic limitations, such as high attrition rates. Choice *a* does not describe evidence in palliative care. Choice *b* is incorrect because it is not generally true. There is minimal research in *certain areas* of palliative care. Choice *d* does not pertain to palliative care.

8. d

Choice *d* is correct because this completes the evidence-based practice process by determining whether desired outcomes occurred and by "institutionalizing" the change. Choices *a*, *b*, and *c* are incorrect because these processes should already have occurred when the team has implemented the evidence-based change.

9. d

Choice *d* (National Guidelines Clearinghouse) is correct because this is the repository of guidelines that is monitored and maintained by the Agency for Health Care Quality & Research. Choices *a* and *b* are incorrect because these are computerized databases, which may index clinical practice guidelines that are within other resources but not their sole focus. Choice *c* is not correct because Cochrane Library contains a regularly updated collection of evidence-based medicine databases, including The Cochrane Database of Systematic Reviews, but not specifically CPGs.

10. c

Choice *c* is correct because an aim of the Cochrane Collaboration is to synthesize randomized controlled trials in all aspects of health care. Systematic reviews aim to address a focused area of literature by bringing together results of studies on a topic. Choices *a* and *b* would also give the team a place to look for systematic reviews, but search limits would have to be used to limit types of evidence to reviews. Choice *d* is incorrect because systematic reviews are not indexed at this site.

CHAPTER 4

1. d

Drug half-life ($T_{1/2}$) depends on the volume of distribution (vd) and clearance rate (CL):

$$T_{1/2} = 0.693 \text{ vd} \div CL$$

Half-life is not dependent upon the route of administration. Dosing interval should not change when converting from oral to parenteral route for morphine. Steady state does not depend on drug half-life and is not dependent upon route.

2. d

The semi-log dose efficacy curves for pharma-codynamic responses are linear between EC-20 and EC-80. Toxicity becomes more prevalent and response improvement diminishes with further dose increases thereafter. Opioid conversion or rotation should be done only if there is uncontrolled pain and opioid toxicity. The purpose of pain management is to control pain to the point of improved daily function and patient satisfaction and not necessarily to erad-icate pain. Patients are generally satisfied with an 80% response, and this degree of relief is usually associated with improved daily func-tion. If further analgesia is necessary, an opioid-sparing adjuvant would be reasonable rather than further dose escalation, rotation, or conver-sion. The choice is d.

3. a

Phenytoin does not cause radiation recall, although it is often associated with rash when given during radiation. Phenytoin has been asso-ciated with reduced folate absorption but does not alter dexamethasone absorption. Progressive tumor growth is possible. However, phenytoin does increase dexamethasone clearance, and as a result, doses may need to be doubled.

4. d

Though not covered in this chapter, this is important to know. Diazepam, valproic acid, and carbamazepine are well absorbed per rectum. Gabapentin requires a transport carrier in the small bowel and is not absorbed by the rectum. Phenytoin is not well absorbed by rectum. Another alternative is sublingual lorazepam.

5. b

Both tramadol and codeine require conversion to O-desmethyl tramadol and morphine, respec-tively, to become an analgesic; morphine phar-macokinetics (and metabolism) is not influenced by CYP2D6.

6. c

As a general principle, most drugs can be used in organ failure if low doses and slow titration are utilized. Carbamazepine, valproic acid, and methadone kinetics are relatively uninfluenced by renal failure compared with morphine.

Morphine's active metabolite, morphine-6-glucuronide, is highly dependent upon renal function for clearance and is only partially cleared by hemodialysis. Eventually this patient will be taken off dialysis as she becomes termi-nally ill, which will further alter morphine and morphine-6-glucorinide clearance.

Carbamazepine, but not valproic acid, increases methadone clearance through induc-tion of CYP3A4. There are wide interindividual differences in CYP3A4 induction, leading to significant individual differences in drug inter-actions between carbamazepine and methadone.

The combination with the least risk of drug interactions and the best safety profile in renal failure is methadone and valproic acid.

However alternative dosing strategies such as as-needed or patient-controlled analgesic (PCA) using morphine may be reasonable in renal failure rather than continuous dosing. Because the half-life of morphine and particu-larly morphine-6-glucuronide is increased, a dosing strategy similar to that for methadone (in which q3hr PRN is used) could be adopted.

7. c

The constellation of symptoms she is experienc-ing is most consistent with amitriptyline toxicity. Confusion, drowsiness, and urinary tract symp-toms may be mistaken for urosepsis.

The addition of methylphenidate or haloperi-dol to treat drug toxicity would be inappropri-ate. Removal of the offending drug and in this case ordering amitriptyline drug levels may be helpful.

The Asian population has a significant frequency of CYP2D6#10. This isoenzyme metab-olizes amitriptyline slowly. Therapeutic levels may be reached at less than usual doses. If blood levels are above therapeutic, then amitriptyline should be held and restarted at a lower dose once toxicity resolves. If the response is poor, alternative agents such as carbamazepine, gabapentin, or low doses of opioid may be tried.

8. d

Only about one third of morphine is bound to albumin. Displacement from binding sites and low albumin levels do not significantly alter morphine kinetics. Absorption is not reduced.

Morphine does go through hepatic circulation. Morphine-6-glucuronide is excreted into bile and metabolized to morphine in the gut by bacteria and reabsorbed. However morphine-6-glucuronide elimination is ultimately dependent upon renal function and not bile excretion.

Morphine bioavailability increases as cirrhosis increases, since morphine is a highly extracted drug, subject to first-pass clearance. However, at steady state, morphine clearance is dependent upon UGT activity, which is relatively spared in hepatic failure. As a result, morphine pharmacokinetics is relatively uninfluenced by hepatic failure.

9. c
The volume of distribution is a theoretic volume, which is influenced by peripheral tissue binding as well as plasma and extracellular and intracellular distribution. Avid protein binding may result in volume of distribution larger than body volume. It directly relates to drug half-life but not drug clearance, which is influenced by hepatic and renal function. A large volume of distribution can occur and not increase drug at receptor sites due to avid peripheral tissue binding.

10. c
Morphine kinetics are influenced by hepatic blood flow. Reduced hepatic blood flow increases the oral bioavailability of morphine. Overall clearance is modestly if affected at all due to renal clearance of metabolites and the sparing of hepatic glucuronidation as well as extrahepatic glucuronidation.

11. d
CYP2D6 has a wide range of different isomers, which are unique in frequency among the various ethnicities. CYP2D6 does not metabolize morphine but does metabolize hydrocodone, tramadol, codeine, dextromethorphan, and methadone. CYP2D6 is inhibited by selective serotonin reuptake inhibitors and quinine.

12. d
There are multiple reasons for a drug regimen to fail, and these include under-dosing and failure to dose to symptom pattern. Patients frequently minimize treatments as a means of avoiding side effects or addiction in the case of opioids. Patients on a fixed income may not fill prescriptions (primary pharmaceutical failure) because of cost.

CHAPTER 5

1. b
Sleep is defined according to behavioral, physiologic, and subjective criteria. Behavioral criteria include closed eyes, decreased response to external stimuli, recumbent position, and reversible unconsciousness. The physiologic criteria are based on polysomnographic recordings that include electroencephalography (EEG), electro-oculography (EOG), and electromyography (EMG). Although these definitions and criteria certainly address the phenomenon, they fail to capture the meaning and significance that sleep has within the context of life. Thus subjective measures of or descriptions of a person's experience with sleep are also recognized as important in defining the state.

2. e
Major controversy still exists over the exact function of sleep, and it is not well understood. Some suggest that it is important for mental and physical restoration, energy conservation, memory reinforcement and consolidation, and/or the maintenance of synaptic and neuronal network function. Others propose that during waking, humoral factors accumulate in the blood, which induce tiredness and then are removed by sleep, or that sleep is a state of decreased activity and protein conservation caused by the lack of food intake during the night. Most would agree that although the function of sleep is not well understood, it likely serves multiple purposes (Bonnet, 2000, p. 67).

3. c
Daytime sleepiness refers to the tendency to fall asleep during the day. Under normal circumstances, sleepiness has a biphasic pattern, with an increased sleep tendency in the mid-afternoon and early morning hours. Sleepiness often goes unnoticed if masked by stimulating factors such as excitement or movement. However, it can be unmasked during quiet periods such as watching television, reading a book, or driving a car.

4. a

Decreased concentration, motivation, and memory are often associated with daytime sleepiness. When severe, daytime sleepiness can be debilitating, causing a broad range of neuropsychologic deficits affecting both daytime functioning and quality of life. Sleepiness can even be life-threatening because of associated alterations in alertness and reactivity.

5. e

Sleep usually progresses through repetitive cycles beginning with NREM stages 1 though 4, back again to stage 2, and subsequently into REM. These cycles occur approximately every 70 to 120 minutes in the adult, with four to five cycles normally completed during a sleep period. NREM sleep occupies approximately 75% to 80% of sleep, and REM occupies 20% to 25% of sleep.

6. d

Sleep hygiene refers to practices of daily living that promote good sleep. These behaviors reinforce the time and place for sleep and control factors that interfere with sleep. Individuals should go to bed and get up at approximately the same times each day, carry out a regular bedtime routine, and limit napping. The place for sleep should be physically comfortable and psychologically conducive to sleep. To keep the bed associated with sleep, it should be reserved for that purpose rather than serving as a hub for other activities. Avoiding work or other stimulating activities right before bedtime is also important.

7. c

Insomnia is defined as difficulty falling asleep and staying asleep, waking up too early in the morning, and having unrefreshing sleep.

8. d

Although primarily related to decreased total sleep time and very common in healthy adults, sleep deprivation may compound other types of sleep problems in terminally ill patients. General lifestyle and lifestyle/environment interactions typically underlie sleep deprivation.

9. c

Improvement in or maintenance of quality of life is the primary goal of palliative care. Although numerous studies have examined factors associated with terminal illness and life quality, the role that impaired sleep plays remains to be well characterized. In the general population, nocturnal and daytime sleep abnormalities adversely affect quality-of-life–related measures such as general health status, satisfaction with life, family relationships, mood, and work performance. Good sleep is equally important for those providing the care to patients, because family members have less depression and improved daytime function when adhering to a program of good sleep hygiene (McCurry, Gibbons, Logsdon, et al., 2003).

10. c

Excessive daytime sedation from anxiolytics or pain medications can seriously impair a patient's ability to stay awake during the day, lead to excessive napping, and interfere with sleep onset at night. Thus medications with activating properties may be used to increase daytime alertness. Several antidepressants, such as fluoxetine and bupropion, have both activating and antidepressant effects. Methylphenidate has also been used effectively in cancer patients to decrease daytime sedation and fatigue. Modafinil is increasingly being used to treat daytime sleepiness and fatigue in patients with sleep apnea, narcolepsy, and depression and has recently been shown to reduce opioid-induced sedation in patients treated for nonmalignant pain.

CHAPTER 6

1. c

Choice *a* refers to acute HF, not chronic HF; choices *b* and *d* refer to diastolic dysfunction.

2. a

Choice *b* is incorrect since cardiomyocytes elongate, not shorten; choice *c* is incorrect since there are many causes, not just MI; choice *d* is incorrect since the SNS is activated, not deactivated.

3. d

Sympathetic nervous and renin-angiotensin systems' activation is an adaptive response to stress and injury. Both lead to vasoconstriction, which promotes increased peripheral vascular resistance and ultimately improves cardiac output. Over time, however, continual activation of these systems promotes ventricular remodeling and ultimately worsens heart function.

4. b

Choice *b* occurs in 59% of cases; choice *a* in 24%; the rest occur less than 15% of time.

5. b

Choice *b* occurs in 67% of cases, choice *c* in 28%, and choice *d* in 5% of cases.

6. c

This patient has typical fluid overload (warm and wet); diuresis is the goal of treatment. NOTE: Rales are found in 33% of congested patients. Choice *b* is wrong since this patient does not have signs of severe hypoperfusion; inotropic agents do not confer a benefit to this patient group.

7. d

This patient profile is cold and wet; vasodilation and diuresis are the immediate goals. Choice *b* is wrong since this patient does not have signs of severe hypoperfusion; in fact, his blood pressure is high (for HF standards).

8. a

A low serum sodium after diuresis and stabilization is the only prognosticator in the list that reflects a poor outcome; BNP is a very low value and signifies HF stability; EF improvement after CRT is a positive prognostic sign; and choice *d* is incorrect since patient needs compliance with HF therapies before determining prognostic indicators.

9. d

Before consultation for palliative therapies as the focus of care, it is important for patients to have been optimized on core heart failure therapies (the right drugs at the right doses; other therapies that apply), unless contraindicated. Time must be allowed (i.e., 3 months on core therapies) to determine if the patient is medically refractory to these evidence-based practices. Note: By decreasing the dose of digitalis, increasing the dose of ACE-I, and starting an aldosterone inhibitor, the patient may be able to be weaned from IV inotropic agent.

10. c

Choice *a* is low in fat but deli meats are very high in sodium (used as preservative); pancakes from box mix and packaged bacon are both high in sodium; fat-free foods generally contain significant sodium (for taste).

CHAPTER 7

1. d

Dyspnea is a subjective sensation with multiple causes. Choice *a* is incorrect. Although a subjective sensation, dyspnea, especially on exertion, is a common complaint of patients regardless of their disease severity. Choice *b* is incorrect. Dyspnea is generally episodic in patients with asthma and generally not episodic in patients with COPD. Choice *c* is incorrect. Dyspnea may be defined as the awareness of shortness of breath.

2. c

A diagnosis of COPD is confirmed by spirometry. Choice *a* is incorrect. An EEG is not diagnostic in COPD. Choice *b* is incorrect. A chest x-ray is not diagnostic in COPD. Choice *d* is incorrect. A physical examination alone is rarely diagnostic in COPD.

3. b

Pharmacologic therapy is used to prevent and control the symptoms of COPD. Choice *a* is incorrect. There is currently no cure for COPD. Choice *c* is incorrect. Although it is true that pharmacologic therapy does not modify the disease process in the long run, drug therapy is beneficial in preventing and controlling symptoms. Choice *d* is incorrect. Non-drug interventions are useful as adjunctive therapy to patients with COPD.

4. c

Oxidative stress, chronic airway inflammation, and proteolytic enzymes all contribute to the pathogenesis of COPD. Choice *a* is incorrect.

COPD is not an autoimmune disease. Choice *b* is incorrect. Inflammation mediated by eosinophils and allergens is found with asthma. Choice *d* is incorrect. Many of the factors that contribute to the pathologic changes eventually seen in COPD have been determined.

5. b
Per current guidelines, the use of bronchodilators is recommended as principal pharmacologic treatment. Choice *a* is incorrect. Current guidelines recommend the use of inhaled corticosteroids in those with advanced disease and repeated exacerbations. It is important to note that the evidence that supports steroid use is as an adjunct to bronchodilator therapy, not as replacement. Choice *c* is incorrect. The prophylactic use of antibiotic therapy to prevent exacerbations is not recommended. Choice *d* is incorrect. The effectiveness of antitussives and antioxidants as adjuvant therapy in COPD has not been proven.

6. b
The prevalence of COPD is likely underestimated because of misdiagnosis and under-diagnosis. Choice *a* is incorrect. The prevalence of COPD in the U.S. population is increasing and is expected to be the third leading cause of death by year 2020. Choice *c* is incorrect. The economic burden of COPD is large and estimated to be over 34 billion dollars. Choice *d* is incorrect. The rate of mortality from COPD is increasing. Current available treatment options are palliative.

7. a
Current recommendations for both assessment and management of COPD are based on severity of airflow obstruction. Choice *b* is incorrect. Patient age and smoking history both positively correlate with disease severity. However, these factors do not influence treatment. Choice *c* is incorrect. Patient age and smoking history both positively correlate to disease frequency and severity. However, they are not used to define treatment algorithm. Choice *d* is incorrect. Each drug regimen should be individualized, the choices of which are influenced by many factors, including severity of airflow

obstruction, frequency and severity of exacerbations, and the presence of complications.

8. d
Pulmonary rehabilitation improves exercise tolerance and the patient's sense of well-being. Choice *a* is incorrect. All patients, regardless of disease severity, may benefit from an individualized pulmonary rehabilitation program. Choice *b* is incorrect. All patients, regardless of disease severity, may benefit from an individualized pulmonary rehabilitation program. Choice *c* is incorrect. Pulmonary rehabilitation is psychologically and physiologically helpful to all COPD patients. The net effect is a decrease in overall health care utilization.

CHAPTER 8

1. b
The life expectancy of many dialysis patients is worse than that of patients with AIDS and most cancers.

2. a
In a prospective study of dialysis discontinuation, the mean time to death after discontinuation was 8 days.

3. d
USRDS data based on the CMS death forms filled out on all dialysis patients has consistently reported 20% of all deaths in dialysis patients are preceded by discontinuation. For the past 15 years, the death forms have a specific box that asks if dialysis was discontinued. The other statements, although often assumed, are incorrect.

4. a
Meperidine is metabolized to normeperidine, a metabolite with neurotoxicity. Normeperidine is renally excreted and therefore builds up in renal failure patients.

5. b
Although itching is a common uremic symptom that continues to trouble many dialysis patients, fatigue is more common (40%).

6. a

Most patients prefer to die at home but because of reasons just mentioned, this does not occur in most cases.

7. b

Unfortunately, because of the "medicalization" of death and the lack of adequate home services, most patients die in the hospital.

8. c

Unfortunately, the way the hospice Medicare benefit is written, all medical costs including dialysis must be paid out of the hospice allowance unless there is a separate diagnosis other than renal failure for the terminal illness. This prevents many patients who want to continue dialysis but have a prognosis of less than 6 months from benefiting from hospice.

9. d

Although all these are strong prognostic factors, malnutrition has the worst prognosis.

10. d

In a recent study, patients indicated that they were most comfortable discussing ACP and AD with their family. This might best be accomplished by briefly discussing the issue, explaining the AD form, and emphasizing the importance with the patient/family and asking for the patient to discuss with the family at home and to return the completed form.

CHAPTER 9

1. b

Malignant spreading to other sites in the body not only contributes to the progressive nature of the disease but also influences the concomitant symptoms that contribute to patient discomfort. Depending on a specific diagnosis, metastatic spread to vital organs can be life threatening (e.g., lung cancer that is metastasized to liver).

2. c

Prognostic indicators can be used to discern the goal of therapy. Employing curative or aggressive interventions for a patient who has extensive and progressive disease may be futile and costly. The use of prognostic indicators can help clinicians alter the plan of care and provide a comfort-oriented versus a cure-oriented approach to treatment.

3. a

The correct choice is *a*. The cost associated with end-of-life treatment continues to escalate for both Medicare and non-Medicare expenditures, with 51% of terminal year inpatient care expenses occurring during the final month of life.

4. a

The IOM 2000 report identified that minorities and the poor are often underrepresented in NCI-funded clinical trials. This is often the result of a lack of access to care, initial presentation with advanced or extensive disease, and the lack of enrolling these patients in clinical trials.

5. d

The over-expression in some breast cancers of the glycoproteins' epidermal growth factor receptor (EGF) and HER-2/neu present on normal breast epithelial cells has given them a role in predicting treatment response to chemotherapy.

6. c

While these other mechanisms do contribute to the cancer cachexia syndrome, Omega-3 fatty acids appear to inhibit tumor necrosis factor.

7. d

The other medications may be used for appetite stimulation, but metoclopramide is considered first-line treatment.

8. d

Fatigue is recognized as a syndrome with its own complex pathology and, although anemia is one potential cause of fatigue, it is not the most common cause. Exercise in appropriately selected patients has been shown to increase energy levels and decrease the perception of fatigue.

9. a

Metoclopramide is a dopamine antagonist and GI cholinergic; it is often more effective than other antiemetics alone and is generally well tolerated.

10. d

Bowel obstruction is the correct choice and should always be ruled out. The other choices are appropriate in the management of constipation. Prompt assessment and evaluation are paramount in this situation.

11. c

The correct choice is c. Although the other medications are effective antidepressants, they take days to weeks to reach peak. Methylphenidate is a psychostimulant and is energizing.

12. c

Choice c is correct. Patients with SCC will need to be immobilized to prevent further damage. Bedrest and logrolling are vital. Identifying the cause of the compression is important; however, this will not decrease neurologic damage. Pain management may be accomplished with NSAIDS, opioids, antidepressants, steroids, or anticonvulsants. However, this too, will not decrease neurologic damage.

13. c

Choice c is correct. The mainstay of treatment of SIADH is placement of the patient on strict I&O with a limitation of free water intake to <800-1000 ml/day for 2-3 days. Patients will complain of thirst. Frequent oral hygiene may alleviate some of the discomfort. Thiazide diuretics are contraindicated in SIADH because they are associated with the development of SIADH. Administration of narcotics for pain management is part of the standard of care of patients with SIADH.

14. a

Choice a is correct. Glucocorticoid administration will decrease the inflammatory response to tumor invasion and the edema surrounding the tumor. Chemotherapy is the treatment of choice if the tumor is chemosensitive. Radiation therapy may be given if the underlying tumor is not chemosensitive. Thrombolytic therapy must be initiated within a few days of onset of symptoms to be effective.

15. d

Choice d is correct. Interventions must be implemented to avoid increases in ICP. Such activities to avoid include isometric muscle contractions, head rotation and neck flexion, and sneezing. Patient activities should allow for frequent rest periods. However, activities should not be clustered.

CHAPTER 10

1. d

Cancer pain and chronic nonmalignant pain have the same pathophysiology and neurotransmitter substrate. Cancer pain has been managed in a biomedical model and chronic nonmalignant pain in a biopsychosocial model. This division in models of care may be fundamentally wrong. Cancer patients experience fatigue to a greater degree than pain. Prognosis has no bearing on choice of analgesics—only pain severity. Eighty percent or more of patients will respond to morphine.

2. a

Cancer pain most commonly arises from bone metastases. It is not unusual to have several different distinctive cancer pains and mixed nociceptive and neuropathic pain. Most metastases, even bone metastases, are not painful. Radiographic findings without history and physical findings correlate poorly with cancer pain severity.

3. c

The T12–L1 syndrome produces radiating pain to the sacroiliac crest, and plain radiographs of the lumbrosacral spine may be normal. Bone pain is frequently worse at night in cancer patients. Cough increases pressure on vertebral metastases and unstable spine, causing worsening pain. Physicians may mistake this pain for arthritis or sacroiliac strain. A magnetic resonance image of the lumbar spine may be necessary if standard radiographs are normal.

4. c

Back pain radiating to the groin with leg swelling may be vertebral involvement (L1–L2) and an associated lower extremity venous thrombosis, but lumbar plexopathy and retroperitoneal adenopathy with leg lymphedema are likely. Most lumbar plexopathy arises from intraabdominal cancers.

5. d

Pain interference with activities of daily living correlates with pain severity and does not require the use of a multidimensional pain assessment.

6. c

Pain diaries have been useful in analgesic trials. Patient-derived scaling of pain severity and relief are well-served by home diaries. Pain diaries for the most part improve coping skills and reveal pain patterns for optimal opioid dosing strategies.

7. d

Changes in opioids should be by route, dose, or drug but not simultaneously. Opioids, unlike adjuvant analgesics, do not have a ceiling dose. Tolerance to opioid analgesics does develop but is rarely dose-limiting. Most patients will have continuous and breakthrough pain requiring ATC plus rescue dosing.

8. c

Rate-limiting opioid toxicity is nausea, vomiting, hallucinations, and symptomatic myoclonus. If no pain is present, ATC opioid doses are reduced and rescue doses maintained. If pain is persistent, then changing route, drug, or reducing dose and adding an adjuvant analgesic is likely to work. Patients do not experience toxicity at the same dose, and in fact there can be 100-fold or greater difference among individuals.

9. d

Adjuvant analgesics are opioid-sparing if patients are experiencing opioid-limiting toxicity. The choice depends on the type of pain. Antiseizure medications are for neuropathic pain, and nonsteroidal antiinflammatory drugs are for nociceptive pain. Adjuvants may be primary analgesics for mild pain but are particularly helpful if patients are experiencing severe pain.

10. c

This patient has an abnormal pain behavior manifested as pseudo-addiction. His opioid should be titrated in the hospital and behavior reassessed at the time his pain is relieved. Pseudo-addictive behavior resolves with the relief of pain. These patients become functional with their opioid therapy. However, patients with psychologic addiction will become dysfunctional with opioids. The choice is *c*.

CHAPTER 11

1. c

The El Escorial criteria grade the physical findings as to the likelihood of diagnoses. The patient has fasciculation and weakness in two separate areas and thus has clinically probable ALS.

2. c

ALS was reported to be relatively common in Guam after World War II. The incidence in Guam is now about the same as in the rest of the world. ALS is progressive in course and does not wax and wane nor remit as a general rule. Familial ALS is rare, and most patients have "sporadic" forms of ALS (unless advancement in molecular genetics reveals genetic mutations with variable clinical penetrance).

3. b

The El Escorial criteria were formulated for research purposes as inclusion criteria. They are inaccurate as an exclusion tool. They are valid universally and include familial forms of ALS.

4. c

The clinical course of ALS is measured by serial FVCs, which are performed at 3-month intervals. The FVC can be relatively normal or at least >50% yet hypoventilation may be present. MEP, MIP, and nocturnal oximetry are helpful ancillary tests. Random pulse oximetry is not usually adequate since hypoxemia first occurs at night. An FEV_1 is helpful in chronic obstructive lung disease but is useless in ALS.

5. c

Rehabilitation is important in ALS. Patients need to be taught to be "dependently" (on walking aids) "independent." Early use will allow patients to get to know their equipment, and if it is not met with unusual psychologic resistance, it will be better handled (physically) by patients. Passive range of motion and massage may both reduce pain and provide the comfort of human touch in those with advanced ALS. The choice is *c*.

6. d

Spasticity and fasciculation were previously mentioned in the patient history. Patients need some spasticity to remain mobile. Dantrolene worsens the weakness of ALS. Baclofen is a popular medication and should be used when spasticity or fasciculations are symptomatic. Alternatives are quinine sulfate, carbamazepine, phenytoin, magnesium, and verapamil.

7. c

Nutritional deficiency in ALS increases mortality sevenfold. A PEG tube should be placed before 10% weight loss and/or a FVC <50%. In the actively dying ALS patient, nutrition is not important. The PEG tube may be used to give palliative medications. Some family members may be reluctant to forego or withdraw enteral nutrition in their dying loved one. Sensitivity, compassion, and individualization should rule the day. An open discussion of the pros and cons of continued nutrition may allow for a reasonable compromise.

8. e

All of the first three modalities may be used at one time or another to manage secretions in ALS; diuretics are not useful in the management of respiratory secretions.

9. d

NIPPV is a general term and includes CPAP and BIPAP. The difference between the two is that BIPAP has adjusted pressures between inspiration and expiration and is better able to support ALS patients during inspiration. Mechanical insufflation/exsufflation can be used with BIPAP to help facilitate cough and remove secretions or in lieu of NIPPV. Oxygen therapy in a hypercapnic ALS patient worsens respiratory drive and may lead to further CO_2 retention.

10. c

Morphine can effectively relieve dyspnea and pain in ALS. It is also a cough suppressant. Morphine should not be held in reserve and utilized only with intractable symptoms. It has been shown to be safe in ALS when appropriately titrated to response. Morphine should not be used for anxiety or limited to patients on NIPPV.

CHAPTER 12

1. c

The correct choice is c, based on the study by Kish, Martin, and Price (2000). The others are either much too high or too low.

2. d

The correct choice is d. The SUPPORT study demonstrated that choices b and c are false; but other studies discussed (e.g., Lilly et al. [2000]) show that d is true (and hence, a is false).

3. d

Of the choices presented, d is the one most likely to lead to a decision that both protects the patient's need for pain relief while honoring his or her attitudes toward drugs. Choices a and c would simply ignore his previous wishes; b does not acknowledge the necessity for interpreting advance directives in light of the patient's best interest.

4. c

Choice c is one of the deleterious effects discussed in the text. The other choices are criticized as less likely to occur when information is withheld.

5. b

The evidence for choice b and against the other choices is discussed and referenced in the text (Tomlinson et al., 1990).

6. a

The correct choice is a. Most close family members would have such a conflict, and it is not in itself evidence that a person is not able to fairly represent the patient's wishes. The remaining choices are included among the positive guidelines discussed in the text.

7. c

Choice c is supported by the referenced study (Curtis et al., 2000b). If c is true, the others are false.

8. a

The correct choice is a. As discussed in the text, the DDE would condemn decisions to limit treatment when the patient's earlier death is among the goals. The other choices are either assumptions or implications of the DDE (also discussed).

9. d

Choice *d* is among the primary concerns of Gilligan and Raffin (1996), discussed in the text. Choice *a* is an effect of extubation, but the text explains why this is not a telling ethical objection against it. Choice *b* is false because extubation makes this less likely to happen. Choice *c* refers to a characteristic of terminal weaning, not extubation.

10. b

Choice *b* is the distinction discussed explicitly in the text. Choice *a* is false, since there is nothing in the nature of TS that limits its use to the dying. Choice *c* is false since any withdrawal of treatment could have this objective. Choice *d* is false by definition of VAE.

11. c

The correct choice is *c*. The frequency with which patients and families may desire a quicker death makes it difficult to deny that death may not be among the intentions at work in the use of narcotics. Choice *a* is acceptable under the DDE. Choice *b* is irrelevant for the use of the DDE (and is not in itself a good reason not to use pain medications in the terminally ill, as discussed). Choice *d* is a false statement about the DDE, which does not assume that death is always the greatest evil.

CHAPTER 13

1. c

Choices *a, b,* and *d* (ethnic cultural influences, Western medicine's culture, and the dominant U.S. culture) are among the numerous factors that influence an individual patient's end-of-life decision making.

2. b

Longstanding experiences with oppression and discrimination, including abuses in medical research, institutional racism, and slavery, are possible contributors to African-Americans' distrust of the American health care system.

3. b

Blackhall et al., 1999, studied Mexican-Americans', Korean-Americans', African-Americans', and European-Americans' attitudes toward truth telling. Out of the groups listed in the question (African-Americans, Korean-Americans, Cuban Americans, European-Americans), 53% of Korean-Americans believed that patients should not be told of such a diagnosis, the highest reported percentage as compared with the other groups.

4. b

Familismo is an emphasis on the welfare of the family over the individual, jerarquismo refers to respect for hierarchy, and respectismo is not a Pan-Hispanic value.

5. a

As a group, Native Americans do not share a fear of dead bodies, although this belief has been documented among the Navajos. Generally, many Native Americans are not outspoken about their needs and will avoid confrontation. Some Native Americans are traditional Christians.

6. d

The Koran loosely defines death, prohibits suicide, and views death as a transition from one part of life to another.

7. c

Many researchers have used numerous definitions of spiritual needs, conceptualizing them as complex and multidimensional. Spiritual needs are directly related to spiritual well-being.

8. a

In Yates et al. (1981) early research, higher levels of spiritual well-being were associated with lower pain levels, but those patients who reported spiritual well-being did not live longer than those who did not experience spiritual well-being. Other research done with AIDS and cancer patients indicates that those who scored lower on meaning/peace were more likely to be depressed and that patients with lower spiritual well-being were more likely to experience hopelessness.

9. b

Many spiritual assessments, in their totality, can be lengthy and burdensome to patients who are dying. Spiritual assessments usually measure many dimensions, incorporate issues around religion, and can be administered by other members of the health care team in additions to chaplains.

10. a

Victor Frankl (1962) stated that "to live is to suffer, to suffer is to find meaning in the suffering." Growth is possible as a result of suffering, and some cultures see value in it (e.g., redemptive suffering). Good symptom control can alleviate physical suffering, but emotional, spiritual, and existential suffering are often not alleviated by physical symptom control.

CHAPTER 14

1. a
Criticism about the stage-based theory, which was postulated by Kübler-Ross, is that it is prescriptive in nature and does not allow for individualized reactions to the experience of loss.

2. b
Death with dignity is also identified as physician-assisted suicide and most notably in Oregon, as the Death with Dignity Act supports active physician participation in assisting patients to die.

3. d
Fear of using medications and associated addiction is most likely caused from a lack of patient/family knowledge and should be recognized as a barrier to adequate symptom management that requires additional education.

4. c
Dehydration is not a universal benefit in all patients. It is used to reduce symptoms such as myoclonus, delirium, and agitation.

5. d
Hypoactive delirium is progressive in nature and reveals itself through gradual changes in cognition and without an intervention to sleepiness and lethargy.

6. b
Sedation is not synonymous with physician-assisted suicide. Sedation is a palliative intervention that is used to reduce intractable symptoms.

7. d
Sedation is titrated by the clinician in the same fashion that opioids are titrated to reduce the pain experience.

8. c
Palliative practices promote symptom management and are not intended to hasten the death event.

9. d
For Medicare recipients, 47% of deaths were characterized by the frailty trajectory.

10. c
Prognostic models are based on group data and do not accurately by reflect individual variation.

11. b
Heart failure patients are unlike cancer patients, who have an obvious decline in function. Heart failure is a very unpredictable illness.

12. d
Determining a poor prognosis in dementia patients is not unlike in heart failure patients. The data identify that 30% of patients with dementia thought to be terminal and decease within 6 months remain alive almost 3 years later.

13. c
Hospitalized care focuses primarily on the disease, its management, and providing curative efforts. Symptom management is often not a priority.

CHAPTER 15

1. c
Bereavement is the reaction to the loss of a loved person. Choice a is incorrect because grief can also be felt over the loss of an object. Mourning, choice b, includes actions or feelings of sorrowing, expressing grief; lamentation; specifically, a verbal expression of grief over a death. And choice d, anticipatory grief, is grief experienced before the actual loss.

2. b
Although Freud, Kübler-Ross, and Byock all wrote about death, dying, and grief, the concept of anticipatory grief was developed by Eric

Lindemann in 1944 in his work *Symptomatology and Management of Acute Grief.*

3. d

Anticipatory grief work has proven to be helpful, not harmful, to the patient. It often relieves anxiety and depression and allows him or her to enjoy the short time left. The other choices are incorrect because anticipatory grief does permit a healthy reaction to loss, can make the actual death less traumatic, and can cause pain as intense as that felt after the death.

4. c

The amount of time an individual experiences grief may be related to the value he or she places on the lost person. Choice *a* is wrong because the length of time a spouse grieves is affected by age and coping capability. Choice *b* is incorrect because 1 year or more is usually needed for a spouse to grieve. Choice *d* is incorrect because time of year a spouse dies has nothing to do with the length of time the survivor will grieve.

5. a

Grief stage theories provide professionals with an understanding of the grief process. Choice *b* is incorrect because all patients do not follow a five-step grieving plan. Choice *c* is wrong because the stages are not instructions for caring for the bereaved. Choice *d* is incorrect because stage theories do not address the length of grief.

6. c

During bargaining, a patient may try to bargain with God, hoping this will change the disease status. He is not ready to accept the diagnosis as terminal. Choice *a*, denial, is incorrect because Jack acknowledges that he has the illness. Choice *b* is incorrect because at this time Jack does not appear angry. Choice *d* is incorrect because Jack does not show any sign of depression.

7. b

Symptoms of grief can appear unexpectedly or can be triggered by anniversaries such as the loved one's birthday, holidays, or other special events. Choice *a* is incorrect because painful grief is very natural. Individuals must suffer

from the pain of grief to recover from it. Choice *c* is incorrect because facing and sorting through painful memories help the bereaved face their own realities and heal from the grief. Choice *d* is incorrect because comfort alone cannot heal. The bereaved must face issues and memories and feel their own pain before they can really heal.

8. d

Successful grief work and recovery from the loss may depend on being allowed to cry and wail loudly at the time of death. Being allowed to grieve in a way that comes natural to the individual allows that individual to heal. Choice *a* is incorrect because some individuals might need to get angry with God in order to heal. Choice *b* is wrong because limiting the amount of pain medicine may increase the patient's suffering. This memory of suffering can inhibit grief work and recovery. Choice *c* is incorrect because death rituals should be based on the patient's and family's beliefs and wishes.

9. d

The psychosocial director should consider that crying during most of a bereavement visit when 6 to 12 months has passed since the death is complicated grief. Choices *a, b,* and *c* are incorrect because this type of crying may be normal in these earlier times of bereavement.

10. c

Although some bereaved may feel guilt, feelings of extreme guilt and self-reproach are considered a complicated reaction. The key here is the use of the word *extreme*. Bereaved can feel a variety of normal feelings such as those in choices *a, b,* and *d,* but they are experienced in moderation.

11. d

Joan is at risk for disenfranchised grief because she may not be able to attend Ralph's funeral and may not be able to openly express her grief because she may feel it is culturally unacceptable. In masked grief (choice *a*), the survivor does not know his grief is interfering with his life. Delayed grief (choice *b*) is the repression of feelings to prevent pain. Chronic grief (choice *c*) began as normal grief but lasted an extended amount of time.

12. d

Adults in our society generally do not prefer to plan for end-of-life events with family participation. Choices *a, b,* and *c* are incorrect because adults in our society generally do withdraw from individuals in mourning, have difficulty discussing death and grief, and may prefer medical treatment as a means for hope.

13. c

Palliative care professionals recognize that patients fear the dying process more than they fear death. Choices *a, b,* and *c* are incorrect. Pain and symptoms are not always controlled at the end of life, family members' concerns do affect the dying patient, and pain the patient experienced at death is not forgotten after the funeral but lives on in the memories of the bereaved.

14. d

A child's ability to understand death, even his or her own, parallels the series of developmental stages described by Piaget (Stevens, 1993). Choice *a* is incorrect because although children may be the same age, they develop at different paces and will not act the same about illness and death. Choice *b* is incorrect because children usually understand more about illness and death than adults are aware of or care to admit. Choice *c* is incorrect because a child does not understand everything his parents tell him despite how slowly things are explained. He can understand only what he is developmentally ready to.

15. c

Limbs are straightened and the head turned toward the right shoulder, because the face must be turned toward Mecca when buried. Choice *a* is incorrect because "Muslims are always buried, never cremated, and this is carried out as soon as possible" (Neuberger, 1993, p. 509). Choice *b* is incorrect because the unwashed body is wrapped in a plain sheet. Choice *d* is incorrect. Autopsies are rarely performed because an autopsy can cause significant distress for a Muslim.

16. d

Health care professionals who care for terminally ill patients understand that other professionals might fear that providing frank information would lead to blame. They could be blamed "...when the patient's clinical condition begins to deteriorate" (Buckman, 1993, p. 49). Choice *a* is incorrect because euphemisms, by their very nature, deter further communication and prevent open, honest discussion. Choice *b* is incorrect because "There is, in fact, no reliable evidence that honest communication has detrimental effects, at least not when such communication is responsive to the needs of the dying person and is carried out in a thoughtful and caring way" (Corr, 1993, p. 33). Choice *c* is incorrect because the reticent professional may lose patient and family trust by withholding information, especially when the dying person recognizes the terminal changes in his or her body.

Medications by Disorder

Kim Kuebler
James Varga
Mellar P. Davis

CONTENTS

ABBREVIATIONS

ac	before meals
BID	twice daily
cap	capsule
g	gram
hr	hour
HS	hour of sleep
IM	intramuscular
IV	intravenous
liq	liquid
mcg	microgram
mg	milligram
ml	milliliter
PO	by mouth
PR	per rectum
PRN	as needed
q	every
qd	once daily
QID	four times a day
SL	sublingual
tab	tablet
TID	three times a day
tsp	teaspoon

ANXIETY

Benzodiazepines

Drug/Class	Initial Dosing	Routes	Availability	Comments
Alprazolam (Xanax)	Individualize 0.25-1 mg TID, QID Maximum 8 mg/day	PO, SL, PR, Liq	Scored, multi-scored tabs: 0.25 mg, 0.5 mg, 1 mg, 2 mg.	Useful in depression-associated anxiety. The only benzodiazepine with antidepressant activity. The benzodiazepine most likely to cause withdrawal symptoms if abruptly stopped. Do not consider in patients with

ANXIETY—cont'd

Benzodiazepines—cont'd

Drug/Class	Initial Dosing	Routes	Availability	Comments
Diazepam (Valium)	Individualize 2-5 mg BID, TID Maximum 60 mg/day	PO, SL, PR, IM, IV, Liq	Scored tabs: 2 mg, 5 mg, 10 mg. Injection: 5 mg/ml. Suppository: 10 mg.	positive substance history. Use cautiously in elderly patients. Do not use in acute narrow-angle glaucoma. Interfaces with medications that inhibit CYP34 (cimetidine, fluoxetine, paroxetine, propxyphene, grapefruit juice among others). Diazepam has a long plasma half-life with active metabolites. One metabolite specifically has a half-life up to 200 hr in the elderly patient. Use cautiously in the patient with a positive substance history. Metoclopramide increases absorption. Omeprazole prolongs elimination.
Lorazepam (Ativan)	Individualize 0.5-1 mg TID, QID Maximum 10 mg/day	PO, SL, subcuta-neous, IM, IV	Scored, multi-scored tabs: 0.5 mg, 1 mg, 2 mg.	Benzodiazepine of choice for elderly and hepatic dysfunction due to short half-life. Use cautiously in patients with a positive substance history. May exacerbate agitated delirium. Metabolism impeded by valproic acid. May increase digoxin levels. Metabolized through the same glucuronidase system that metabolizes morphine.

Miscellaneous

Drug/Class	Initial Dosing	Routes	Availability	Comments
Amitriptyline (Elavil) Tricyclic anti-depressant	10-25 mg q HS Maximum 150 mg/day	PO, PR, IM	Tabs. 10 mg, 25 mg, 50 mg, 75 mg, 100 mg, 150 mg. Injection: 10 mg/ml.	Do not use in patients with a history of seizures, urinary retention, glaucoma, or heart block (recent myocardial infarction, dysrhythmias). Good for anxiety, depression, and insomnia. High anticholin-ergic profile may be helpful with tenesmus. Potentiates opioids. Can cause hypotension in dehydrated elderly patients.

Continued

ANXIETY—cont'd

Miscellaneous—cont'd

Drug/Class	Initial Dosing	Routes	Availability	Comments
Citalopram (Celexa) (serotonin selective reuptake inhibitor [SSRI] anti-depressant)	10-20 mg qd Maximum 60 mg/day	PO, Liq	Scored, multi-scored tabs: 10 mg, 20 mg, 40 mg.	Use cautiously in patients with history of seizure disorders or hepatic or renal dysfunction. Few drug interactions. May be potentiated by cimetidine and antagonized by carbamazepine. Do not use with tricyclics. An alternative to citalopram is the active metabolite escitalopram (Lexapro).
Chlorpro-mazine (Thorazine)	10-25 mg TID, QID Maximum 600 mg/day	PO, SL, PR, IM, IV, Liq		Antipsychotic, neuroleptic, useful for nausea and vomiting and dyspnea. Palliative sedation for mild agitated delirium. Anticholinergic properties. May cause hypotension if rapidly titrated. Lower incidence of extrapyramidal effects vs. haloperidol.
Haloperidol (Haldol)	0.5-2 mg BID or q4hr PRN Maximum 20 mg/day	PO, SL, subcuta-neous, IM, IV, Liq	Tabs: 0.5 mg, 1 mg, 2 mg, 5 mg, 10 mg, 20 mg. Elixir: 2 mg/ml. Injection: 5 mg/ml.	Antipsychotic, neuroleptic that is useful for the management of agitated delirium, intractable hiccups, and nausea and vomiting. Low incidence of sedation, anticholingeric effects, and cardiovascular toxicity. Greater incidence of extrapyramidal effects. Can potentiate other CNS depressants (opioids, benzodiazepines) and anticholinergics. Interferes with phenytoin metabolism. There is competitive inhibition between tricyclics and haloperidol through CYP2D6.
Mirtazapine (Remeron) (tetracyclic anti-depressant)	7.5-15 mg q HS Maximum 45 mg/day	PO, SL	Scored tabs: 15 mg, 30 mg, 45 mg.	Rapid onset of action. Good choice for patients with marked anxiety/agitation. Combination of mirtazapine and an SSRI are often effective in refractory depression. 50% reduction in dose with severe hepatic and renal dysfunction. Wide therapeutic index. Do not use in patients with a history of seizure disorders. This anti-depressant enhances both norepinephrine and serotonin

ANXIETY—cont'd

Miscellaneous—cont'd

Drug/Class	Initial Dosing	Routes	Availability	Comments
				neurotransmission. Cimetidine reduces clearance, and carbamazepine increases clearance. Few drug interactions. Induces physiologic sleep.
Olanzapine (Zyprexa) (thiobenzo-diazepine atypical anti-psychotic)	2.5-10 mg BID Maximum 20 mg/day	PO	Tabs: 2.5 mg, 5 mg, 7.5 mg, 10 mg, 15 mg, 20 mg.	Use as an alternative to haloperidol for agitation or delirium. Less extrapyramidal effects than haloperidol. Potent antiemetic. Do not use in Parkinson's disease. Use cautiously in elderly patients or those with renal and hepatic dysfunction. Can produce hypotension with antihypertensives, hypovolemia, dehydration. Omeprazole, rifampin, and carbamazepine increases its clearance. Male smokers have greater drug clearance.

References:

Davis, M., Dickerson, D., Pappagallo, M., et al. (2001). Mirtazepine: Heir apparent to amitriptyline? *Am J Hosp Palliat Care*, *18*(1), 42-46.

Davis, M., Khawam, E., Pozueb, L., et al. (2002). Management of symptoms associated with advanced cancer: Olanzapine and mirtazapine. *Expert Rev Anticancer Ther*, *2*(4), 89-100.

Keltner, N., & Folks, D. (2001). *Psychotropic drugs* (3rd ed.). St. Louis: Mosby.

Lipman, A., Jackson, K., & Tyler, L. (2000). *Evidence based symptom control in palliative care*. Binghamton, N.Y.: Pharmaceutical Products Press.

Twycross, R., Wilcock, A., Charlesworth, S., et al. (2002). *Palliative care formulary* (2nd ed.). Oxon, U.K.: Radcliff Medical Press.

Waller, A., & Caroline, N. (2000). *Handbook of palliative care in cancer* (2nd ed.). Woburn, Mass.: Butterworth-Heinemann.

ANOREXIA/CACHEXIA

Corticosteroids

Drug/Class	Initial Dosing	Routes	Availability	Comments
Dexametha-sone (Decadron)	4-10 mg qd BID	PO, SL, subcuta-neous, IM, IV, Liq	Scored tabs: 0.5 mg, 0.75 mg, 4 mg.	Corticosteroid with high gluco-corticoid activity and limited mineralocorticoid effects. 6-12 times more potent than prednisolone. Has a long duration of action and can reduce plasma phenytoin levels. Highly effective in improving short-term appetite

Continued

ANOREXIA/CACHEXIA—cont'd
Corticosteroids—cont'd

Drug/Class	Initial Dosing	Routes	Availability	Comments
				loss. Dosage efficacy is reduced after a few weeks. Not recommended for use in patients with infection or high glucose levels. Useful for nausea and vomiting, bone pain, neuropathic pain, and headaches from central nervous system (CNS) metastasis. Analgesic action is in part related to down-modulation of nitric oxide synthesis and reduction of secondary mediators of N-methyl-D-aspartate (NMDA) receptor activity.
Prednisolone (Prednisone)	10-30 mg qd Maximum 800 mg/day	PO, IM, IV, Liq	Scored tabs: 2.5 mg, 5 mg, 10 mg, 20 mg, 50 mg.	Most frequently prescribed corticosteroid. See "Dexamethasone" comments. Effects lessen after a few weeks. Less muscle wasting than with dexamethasone.

Miscellaneous

Drug/Class	Initial Dosing	Routes	Availability	Comments
Dronabinol (Marinol)	2.5 mg ac, BID, TID Maximum 20 mg/day	PO	Caps (contain sesame oil): 2.5 mg, 5 mg, 10 mg.	Cannabinoid that may be an effective appetite stimulant—better tolerated in younger vs. elderly patients. Should avoid using with other CNS depressant medications. Can potentiate tricyclic antidepressants, anticholinergics, and phenothiazines. Useful in the treatment of nausea/vomiting. Acts on CB1 receptors centrally for appetite. Reduces gastrointestinal motility through peripheral CB2 receptors.
Megestrol acetate (Megace)	40-120 mg QID, 160 mg TID (induces weight gain) Maximum 800 mg/day	PO, Liq	Scored tabs: 20 mg, 40 mg. Suspension: 40 mg/ml.	Progestational agent that stimulates appetite through potentiation of neuro peptide Y, and with higher doses induces weight gain by exerting an anabolic effect. Not recommended for use in patients with history of thrombophlebitis or severe cardiac disease or dyspnea.

References:

Dixon, S., & Esper, P. (2002). Anorexia, cachexia and nutritional support. In K. Kuebler & P. Esper (Eds.), *Palliative practices from A-Z for the bedside clinician* (pp. 13-22). Pittsburgh, Pa.: Oncology Nursing Society.

Driver, L., & Bruera, E. (2000). *The M.D. Anderson palliative care handbook.* Department of Symptom Control and Palliative Care. The University of Texas M.D. Anderson Cancer Center. Houston: The University of Texas—Houston Health Services Center.

Lipman, A., Jackson, K., & Tyler, L. (2000). *Evidence based symptom control in palliative care.* Binghamton, N.Y.: Pharmaceutical Products Press.

Twycross, R., Wilcock, A., Charlesworth, S., et al. (2002). *Palliative care formulary* (2nd ed.). Oxon, U.K.: Radcliff Medical Press.

Waller, A., & Caroline, N. (2000). *Handbook of palliative care in cancer* (2nd ed.). Woburn, Mass.: Butterworth-Heinemann.

ASCITES

Diuretics

Drug/Class	Initial Dosing	Routes	Availability	Comments
Furosemide (Lasix)	20 mg qd initially, followed by 20-80 mg qd. May increase after 6-8 hours Maximum 600 mg/day	PO, IM, IV, Liq	Scored tabs: 20 mg, 40 mg, 80 mg.	Loop diuretic that may be necessary to add to spironolactone to initiate diuresis. Ascites is usually refractory to loop diuretics alone due to increased aldosterone levels. Persistent diuresis may contribute to electrolyte imbalance. Metabolized through the renal glomerulus.

References:

Heidrich, D. (2002). Ascites. In K. Kuebler & P. Esper (Eds.), *Palliative practices from A-Z for the bedside clinician* (pp. 27-33). Pittsburgh, Pa.: Oncology Nursing Society.

Heidrich, D. (2002). Ascites. In K. Kuebler, P. Berry, & D. Heidrich (Eds.), *End-of-life care clinical practice guidelines* (pp. 189-198). Philadelphia: Saunders.

NPPR, *Nurse practitioners' prescribing reference.* (Spring 2003). New York, N.Y.: Prescribing References Inc.

CONSTIPATION

Stimulants

Drug/Class	Initial Dosing	Routes	Availability	Comments
Bisacodyl	5-20 mg qd, BID Maximum 30 mg/day	PO, PR, Liq	Tabs: 10 mg. Suppository: 10 mg.	Acts on both the small and large bowel. When given rectally induces propulsive motor activity through reflex action. Used for first line may cause rectal inflammation.
Senna	8.6 mg BID, TID Maximum 12 tabs/day	PO, Liq	Tabs: 8.6 mg. Granules: 15 mg/tsp. Syrup: 8.8 mg/5 ml.	Stimulant of choice. Dosages vary among patients, may increase 2-4 tabs or use in combination with docusate sodium. Action is on longitudinal smooth muscles, increasing peristalsis.

Continued

CONSTIPATION—cont'd

Miscellaneous

Drug/Class	Initial Dosing	Routes	Availability	Comments
Docusate (Colace)	100 mg BID, TID Maximum 500 mg/day	PO, PR, Liq	Caps: 50 mg, 100 mg. Liq: 10 mg/ml. Syrup: 20 mg/ 5 ml. Micro-enema (glycerin): 200 mg/5 ml.	Stool softener that usually requires combining a stimulant in palliative care. May induce peristalsis at higher doses. Can be given orally in bowel obstruction, whereas stimulating laxatives should be avoided.
Lactulose (Kristalose)	10 g, 20 g dissolved in 4 oz of water qd, BID Maximum 40 g/day	PO	Singe-dose packets: 10 g, 20 g.	An osmotic that helps retain water in the large bowel. Not systemically absorbed. Safe to use in diabetic patients. Slow onset of action up to 48 hours.
Magnesium salts (Citrate of Magnesium)	120 ml qd, BID Maximum 240 ml/day	PO	120 ml. Magnesium salts: 1-2 tsp in at least ½ cup of water in the AM.	Second-line agent—harsh laxative that produces evacuation in 3-6 hours. Should be considered for use in constipation resistant to other laxatives. Is contraindicated in patients with congestive heart failure or renal dysfunction.
Milk of magnesium	15 ml qd, BID Maximum 60 ml/day	PO	120-ml bottle.	Use with caution in patients with congestive heart failure and renal failure.

References:

Driver, L., & Bruera, E. (2000). *The M.D. Anderson palliative care handbook.* Department of Symptom Control and Palliative Care. The University of Texas M.D. Anderson Cancer Center. Houston: The University of Texas—Houston Health Services Center.

NPPR, *Nurse practitioners' prescribing reference.* (Spring 2003). New York, N.Y.: Prescribing References Inc.

Twycross, R., Wilcock, A., Charlesworth, S., et al. (2002). *Palliative care formulary.* Oxon, U.K.: Radcliff Medical Press.

Waller, A., & Caroline, N. (2000). *Palliative care in cancer* (2nd ed.). Woburn, Mass.: Butterworth-Heinmann.

Zielke, K. (2002). Constipation. In K. Kuebler & P. Esper (Eds.), *Palliative practice from A-Z for the bedside clinician* (pp. 59-62). Pittsburgh, Pa.: Oncology Nursing Society.

COUGH

Drug/Class	Initial Dosing	Routes	Availability	Comments
Benzonatate (Tessalon Perles)	100-200 mg TID Maximum 600 mg/day	PO	Caps: 100 mg, 200 mg.	Antitussive properties; suppresses cough by blocking peripheral lung J receptors. Can cause drowsiness, dizziness. Encourage patients to swallow whole and not to chew or suck caps due to local anesthetic.
Dextromethor-phan/ guaifenesin	100 mg QID Maximum 1200 mg/day	PO	Dextromethor-phan 10 mg + guaifenesin	Antitussive and expectorant. Useful for nonproductive cough or cough due to acute throat irritation.

COUGH—cont'd

Drug/Class	Initial Dosing	Routes	Availability	Comments
(Robitussin DM)			100 mg per 5 ml syrup: available in 4 oz, 8 oz, 12 oz, or pint.	Not useful for chronic cough.
Morphine immediate release (Roxanol, MSIR)	In the opioid-naïve patient 2.5-5 mg q3-4hr No maximum dose	PO, SL, PR, subcuta-neous, Liq	Soluble tabs: 10 mg. Solution: 10 mg/5 ml, 20 mg/5 ml. Tabs: 15 mg, 30 mg.	Opioids suppress the cough reflex in the brain. Morphine is particularly beneficial for those with pain and dyspnea. Small doses at bedtime for opioid-naïve patients. May be useful if all other options have failed.
Nebulized bupivacaine (Marcaine)	0.25% 5 ml up to q8hr	Nebuli-zed		See comments above.
Nebulized xylocaine (Lidocaine)	2% 5 ml PRN up to q6hr	Nebuli-zed	5 ml PRN	Nebulized anesthetics are useful in the management of cough but not breathlessness. There is conflicting evidence for the usefulness of local anesthetics for breathlessness. Beneficial for lymphangitis carcinomatosa. Avoid eating and drinking for 2 hours after use—may reduce the gag reflex. Risk for bronchospasm.

References:
Cohen, B. (2002). Cough. In K. Kuebler & P. Esper (Eds.), *Palliative practices from A-Z for the bedside clinician.* Pittsburgh, Pa.: Oncology Nursing Society.
Lacy, C., Armstrong, L., Goldman, M., et al. (2001-2002). *Drug information handbook.* Hudson, Ohio: Lexi-Comp Inc.
Twycross, R., Wilcock, A. Charlesworth, S., et al. (2002). *Palliative care formulary* (2nd ed.). Oxon, U.K.: Radcliff Medical Press.

DELIRIUM

Benzodiazepines

Drug/Class	Initial Dosing	Routes	Availability	Comments
Lorazepam (Ativan)	0.5-2 mg q1-4hr continuous or intermittent PRN dosing	PO, SL, subcuta-neous, IM, IV	Scored tabs: 0.5 mg, 1 mg, 2 mg.	Generally not effective when used as a single-agent therapy. Consider combination with haloperidol for refractory hyperalert delirium.
Midazolam (Versed)	1-5 mg loading dose Continuous or intermittent PRN dosing	subcuta-neous, IM, IV, Liq	Injection: 1 mg/ ml, (50 ml vial); 5 mg/ml, (2 ml, 5 ml, 10 ml, 18 ml vials).	Very short half-life and best reserved if using for terminal sedation in the last days and hours of life due to tolerance. Can be given subcutaneously.

Continued

DELIRIUM—cont'd

Benzodiazepines—cont'd

Drug/Class	Initial Dosing	Routes	Availability	Comments
			Injection: 2 mg/5 ml (5 ml ampule).	Useful agent for palliative sedation if patients are unresponsive to other agents. Short half-life allows for safer titration to effect. Limited versatility (parenteral only). Cost may limit use in hospice. Like lorazepam, consider adding haloperidol before increasing dose. Anecdotally useful for intractable hiccups.

Miscellaneous

Drug/Class	Initial Dosing	Routes	Availability	Comments
Chlorpromazine (Thorazine)	12.5-50 mg q4-12hr Maximum 600 mg/day	PO, SL, PR, IM, IV, Liq	Tabs: 10 mg, 25 mg, 50 mg, 100 mg, 200 mg. Sustained-release spansules: 30 mg, 75 mg, 150 mg. Suppositories: 25 mg, 100 mg.	Anticholinergic, antihistamine, antidopaminergic properties may be useful to manage respiratory distress and secretions. Monitor for cardiovascular effects, can cause hypotension. Can increase morphine if used in combination. Alternative for palliative sedation. Increased CNS depression, hypotension, respiratory depression. Caution in titrating upward too rapidly.
Haloperidol (Haldol)	0.5-5 mg q1-4hr Maximum 20 mg/day	PO, SL, subcutaneous, IM, IV, Liq	Tabs: 2 mg, 5 mg, 10 mg, 20 mg. Oral solution: 1 mg/ml, 2 mg/ml. Injection: 5 mg/ml (1 ml amp).	First-line agent for restlessness/agitation and delirium. Do not use in combination with metoclopramide; can increase likelihood of extrapyramidal effects/tardive dyskinesia. An excellent antiemetic. Start with high doses for paranoia.
Phenobarbital (Phenobarb)	1-3 mg/kg loading dose continuous or intermittent dosing Maximum 600 mg/day	PO, subcutaneous, IM, IV, Liq	Tabs: 8 mg, 16 mg, 32 mg, 100 mg. Elixir: 15 mg/5 ml, 20 mg/5 ml. Injection: 30 mg/ml, 60 mg/ml, 65 mg/ml, 130 mg/ml.	Long half-life makes titration difficult. Excellent and inexpensive. Useful in terminal sedation and refractory seizures. Paradoxical improvement in cognition and resolution of delirium can occur if delirium is due to subclinical seizure. Use only if familiar with dosing schedules and concomitant medications. Can be given SQ.

References:

Driver, L., & Bruera, E. (2000). *The M.D. Anderson palliative care handbook*. Department of Symptom Control and Palliative Care. The University of Texas M.D. Anderson Cancer Center. Houston: The University of Texas—Houston Health Services Center.

Keltner, N., & Folks, D. (2001). *Psychotropic drugs* (3rd ed.). St. Louis: Mosby.

Smith, H. (2002). Delirium. In K. Kuebler & P. Esper (Eds.), *Palliative practices from A-Z for the bedside clinician*. Pittsburgh, Pa.: Oncology Nursing Society.

Twycross, R., Wilcock, A., Charlesworth, S., et al. (2002). *Palliative care formulary* (2nd ed.). Oxon, U.K.: Radcliff Medical Press.

DEPRESSION

Tricyclic Antidepressants (TCAs)

Drug/Class	Initial Dosing	Routes	Availability	Comments
Amitriptyline (Elavil)	10-25 mg HS Maximum 150 mg/day	PO, PR, IM, Liq	Tabs: 10 mg, 25 mg, 50 mg. Oral solution: 25 mg/5 ml, 50 mg/5 ml.	Antidepressant effects may take up to 2 weeks or more; whereas if using to adjuvantly manage neuropathic pain, the response may be effective in 3-7 days. Titrate dosage slowly— especially in the elderly. Anticholinergic effects may be problematic and can cause urinary retention. Avoid abrupt withdrawal if using for prolonged periods. Has the potential of inducing dysrhythmias.
Desipramine (Norpramin)	10-25 mg HS Maximum 300 mg/day	PO	Tabs: 10 mg, 25 mg, 50 mg, 75 mg, 100 mg, 150 mg.	Tricyclic of choice in the elderly, less anticholinergic activity than amitriptyline. Potentiates CNS depressants (benzodiazepines, alcohol). Can cause urinary retention.

Selective Serotonin Reuptake Inhibitors (SSRIs)

Drug/Class	Initial Dosing	Routes	Availability	Comments
Citalopram (Celexa)	20 mg qd Maximum 40 mg/day	PO, Liq	Scored tabs: 10 mg, 20 mg, 40 mg. Oral solution (peppermint flavor): 2 mg/ml.	SSRI with fewer drug interactions. Steady state is achieved in 1 week. Avoid use with other CNS depressants (benzodiazepines, alcohol).
Sertraline (Zoloft)	25-50 mg qd Maximum 200 mg/day	PO, Liq	Scored tabs: 25 mg, 50 mg, 100 mg. Oral concentrate: 20 mg/ml, dilute just before administration in 4 oz water, ginger ale, orange juice.	Useful for depression-associated panic attacks. May potentiate cimetidine, warfarin, and digitoxin. Do not discontinue abruptly. Steady-state plasma concentrations are achieved after 1 week. Can also be useful in the management of diabetic neuropathic pain.

Continued

DEPRESSION—cont'd

Miscellaneous

Drug/Class	Initial Dosing	Routes	Availability	Comments
Methylphenidate (Ritalin)	5 mg qd, BID Maximum 40 mg/day	PO	Scored tabs: 5 mg, 10 mg, 20 mg. Sustained-release: 20 mg, 30 mg, 40 mg.	Psychostimulant that increases alertness, motivation, and mood. Antidepressant of choice in treating depression in patients with a prognosis of less than 3 months. Can reduce opioid-related drowsiness. Quick onset. Avoid with angina, and use cautiously with dysrhythmias. Addiction is low.
Mirtazapine (Remeron)	15 mg HS Maximum 45 mg/day	PO, SL	Scored tabs: 15 mg, 30 mg, 45 mg. Soluble tabs (orange-flavored, orally disintegrating): 15 mg, 30 mg, 45 mg.	A tetracycline antidepressant that also reduces anxiety associated with depression. Also provides antiemetic and appetite stimulant properties. Has a rapid onset of action and better tolerated than SSRIs and TCAs. Now generic and lower priced.

References:

Brietbart, W., Dickerson, D., Shuster, J., et al. (2002). Depression. In K. Kuebler & P. Esper (Eds.), *Palliative practices from A-Z for the bedside clinician* (pp. 85-88). Pittsburgh, Pa.: Oncology Nursing Society.

Davis, M., Dickerson, D., Pappagallo, M., et al. (2001). Mirtazapine: Heir apparent to amitriptyline? *Am J Hosp Palliat Care*, 18(1), 42-46.

Keltner, N., & Folks, D. (2001). *Psychotropic drugs*. (3rd ed.). St. Louis: Mosby.

Kuebler, K. (2002). Depression. In K. Kuebler, P. Berry, & D. Heidrich (Eds.), *End-of-life care clinical practice guidelines* (pp. 269-280). Philadelphia: Saunders.

NPPR, *Nurse practitioners' prescribing reference*. (Spring 2003). New York, N.Y.: Prescribing References Inc.

Twycross, R., Wilcock, A., Charlesworth, S., et al. (2002). *Palliative care formulary*. Oxon, U.K.: Radcliff Medical Press.

DYSPNEA

Drug/Class	Initial Dosing	Routes	Availability	Comments
Albuterol (Proventil, Ventolin)	Proventil 2 inhalations q4-6hr Nebulizer 0.5 ml TID, QID Ventolin same dosing	PO inhalation (mouth), ventilatory mask	Proventil 90 mcg/ inhaler metered-dose. Inhalation solution: 0.5 ml.	Beta-2 agonist first for bronchospasm and chronic obstructive pulmonary disease (COPD). Short acting. May be useful to add to corticosteroid if wheezing is persistent. Avoid excessive use.
Chlorpromazine (Thorazine)	25 mg q4-6hr	PO, SL, PR, IM, IV, Liq	Tabs: 10 mg, 25 mg, 50 mg,	Phenothiazine, which provides antianxiety relief

DYSPNEA—cont'd

Drug/Class	Initial Dosing	Routes	Availability	Comments
	Maximum 600 mg/day		100 mg, 200 mg. Syrup: 10 mg/ml. Suppositories: 25 mg, 100 mg. Injection: 25 mg/ml.	associated with dyspnea, and anticholinergic effects, which reduce respiratory secretion. Less sedating than benzodiazepines.
Dexamethasone (Decadron)	4-8 mg qd May titrate to higher doses	PO, SL, subcuta- neous, IM, IV, Liq	Scored tabs: 0.5 mg, 0.75 mg, 4 mg. 5-12 Pak: package of 12 scored 0.75-mg tabs. Injectable: 24 mg/ml.	Corticosteroid, which provides antiinflammatory effects. Second-line agent for refractory dyspnea. Beneficial for acute exacer- bations of COPD. Use with caution with diabetic and immunosuppressed patients. Useful for dyspnea associated with lymph- angitic carcinoma of the pulmonary parenchyma.
Ipratropium (Atrovent)	2 inhalations QID Maximum 12 inhalations/ day Nebulizer 500 mcg TID, QID	PO inhalation (mouth), ventilatory mask	18 mcg metered- dose inhaler 500 mcg (500 mcg in 2.5 ml).	Anticholinergic used in combination with albuterol. Slow onset of action but long acting. Useful for bron- chospasm associated with chronic bronchitis and COPD. Long-term inhaler of choice.
Morphine	5 mg TID, QID No maximum dosage	PO, SL, subcuta- neous, IM, IV, PR, Liq	Various preparations— should use short- acting morphine for relief of dyspnea. If patient is taking opioids for pain, consider using 5%-10% of total daily dose for dyspnea. No clear evidence to date supports the use of nebulized morphine other than anecdotal reports.	Morphine is the main therapy for managing dyspnea. Opioids decrease the perception of breathlessness and reduce ventilatory drive that is responsive to hypoxia. Lower doses than those required for analgesia.
Oxygen	Continuous or inter- mittent	Nasal cannula Ventilation mask	Canister or room air concentrator.	Often considered standard therapy for dyspnea but may offer only a placebo effect in patients who are not hypoxic. May work through stimulation of trigeminal nerve.

Continued

DYSPNEA—cont'd

Drug/Class	Initial Dosing	Routes	Availability	Comments
Theophylline (Uniphyl)	200 mg BID Maximum 900 mg/day	PO, Liq	Controlled-release scored tabs: 400 mg, 600 mg.	Second-line agent—may serve useful when combined with albuterol and ipratropium. Sustained-release products should not be crushed or chewed. Take with meals. Smokers metabolize quicker. May stimulate diaphragm to decrease dyspnea.
Tiotropium	Daily inhalation Maximum 18 mcg/day	PO inhalation (mouth)	18 mcg/day Handihaler.	Anticholinergic with limited systemic absorption. Prolonged muscarinic receptor 3 affinity. 24-hr sustained release anticholinergic.

References:

Driver, L., & Bruera, E. (2000). *The M.D. Anderson palliative care handbook*. Department of Symptom Control and Palliative Care. The University of Texas M.D. Anderson Cancer Center. Houston: The University of Texas—Houston Health Services Center.

Kuebler, K. (2002). Dyspnea. In K. Kuebler, P. Berry, & D. Heidrich (Eds.), *End-of-life care clinical practice guidelines* (pp. 301-316). Philadelphia: Saunders.

Lipman, A., Jackson, K., & Tyler, L. (2000). *Evidence based symptom control in palliative care*. Binghamton, N.Y.: Pharmaceutical Products Press.

Twycross, R., Wilcock, A., Charlesworth, S., et al. (2002). *Palliative care formulary*. Oxon, U.K.: Radcliff Medical Press.

Van Noord, J., Smeets, J., Custers, F., et al. (2002). Pharmocodynamic steady state of tiotropium in patients with chronic obstructive pulmonary disease. *Europ Resp J* 19(4): 639-644.

NAUSEA AND VOMITING

Histamine Blockers

Drug/Class	Initial Dosing	Routes	Availability	Comments
Meclizine (Antivert)	12.5-25 mg BID, TID Maximum dose may vary on individual patient response	PO	Tabs: 12.5 mg, 25 mg, 50 mg.	Useful for nausea related to motion sickness or vertigo. Ancillary antiemetic in nausea and vomiting caused by mechanical bowel obstruction and raised intracranial pressure.
Prochlorperazine (Compazine)	5-10 mg q6-8hr Maximum 40 mg/day	PO, PR, IM, IV, Liq	Tabs: 5 mg, 10 mg. Fruit-flavored syrup: 5 mg/5ml. Sustained-release spansules: 10 mg, 15 mg. Rectal suppositories: 2.5 mg, 5 mg, 25 mg.	Usually reserved as a second-line therapy for nausea and vomiting unresponsive to narrow-spectrum butyrophe-nones. Moderate dopamine and anticholinergic activity. May worsen gastric stasis and urinary retention. May

NAUSEA AND VOMITING—cont'd

Histamine Blockers—cont'd

Drug/Class	Initial Dosing	Routes	Availability	Comments
Promethazine (Phenergan)	12.5-25 mg q6-8hr Maximum 200 mg/day	PO, PR, IM, IV, Liq	Injection: 5 mg/ml. Scored tabs: 12.5 mg, 25 mg, 50 mg. Rectal suppositories: 12.5 mg, 25 mg, 50 mg.	treat vertigo-related nausea. Useful for motion-related nausea and vomiting. Second-line therapy if butyrophenones fail. Moderate dopamine and antihistaminic activity. Can cause excessive drowsinessand also lower seizure threshold.

5HT$_3$ Blockers

Drug/Class	Initial Dosing	Routes	Availability	Comments
Ondansetron (Zofran)	4-8 mg BID, TID Maximum 32 mg/day	PO, SL, IV, Liq	Tabs: 4 mg, 8 mg, 24 mg. Dissolvable strawberry tabs: 4 mg, 8 mg. Strawberry-flavored solution: 4 mg/5 ml. Premixed IV fluid: 32 mg/50 ml. IV, IM injection: 2 mg/ml.	5HT$_3$ antagonist. Used primarily to prevent chemotherapy-induced nausea and vomiting. Useful for radiation-induced nausea. Nausea from intracranial pressure. May also be useful for patients with bowel obstruction as a third line. Usually given in combination with pheno-thiazines and corticosteroids.

NK1 Inhibitor

Drug/Class	Initial Dosing	Routes	Availability	Comments
Aprepitant (Emend)	125 mg on day 1 of chemotherapy and followed by 80 mg qd on days 2 and 3. No current data on maximum dosage	PO	Tabs: 80 mg, 125 mg.	Usually administered with a corticosteroid and a 5HT$_3$ antagonist for the prevention of acute and delayed nausea and vomiting associated with highly emetogenic chemotherapy. Known for its efficacy in the prevention of delayed nausea and vomiting. Has many drug interactions including warfarin, corticosteroids, azole antifungal, diltiazem, and oral contraceptives.

Continued

NAUSEA AND VOMITING—cont'd

Miscellaneous

Drug/Class	Initial Dosing	Routes	Availability	Comments
Dexamethasone (Decadron)	4-24 mg qd, BID Maximum 96 mg (taper)	PO, SL, subcutaneous, IM, IV, Liq	Scored tabs: 0.5 mg, 0.75 mg, 4 mg. IV injection: 24 mg/ml.	Corticosteroid with low mineral corticoid activity, higher antiinflammatory efficacy, and longer half-life. Useful adjunctive as an antiemetic with metoclopramide. Used as primary antiemetic for raised intracranial pressure.
Haloperidol (Haldol)	0.5-2 mg q4hr or BID Maximum 20 mg/day	PO, SL, subcutaneous, IM, IV, Liq	Tabs: 1.5 mg, 5 mg, 10 mg. Oral solution: 2 mg/ml. Injection: 5 mg/ml (1-ml ampule).	Antiemetic of choice for mechanical bowel obstruction and metabolic causes of nausea and vomiting. Extremely high dopamine (D2) affinity. Less sedation and cardiotoxicity than phenothiazines.
Dronabinol (Marinol)	2.5-5 mg use 1 hour ac or BID-QID Maximum 5 mg/m^2/day	PO	Sesame oil caps: 2.5 mg, 5 mg, 10 mg.	Indicated for refractory or intractable chemotherapy-induced nausea and vomiting.
Metoclopramide (Reglan)	10 mg ac and HS or q6hr or continuous subcutaneous 20-120 mg over 24 hours	PO, PR, IV, subcutaneous	Scored tabs: 5 mg, 10 mg.	Prokinetic through acetylcholine and antiemetic through dopamine antagonism. High doses are associated with $5HT_3$ antagonist. Useful for nausea, gastroparesis, and early satiety.
Olanzapine (Zyprexa)	5 mg qd, BID Maximum 20 mg/day	PO	Tabs: 2.5 mg, 5 mg, 7.5 mg, 10 mg, 15 mg, 20 mg. Oral dissolving tabs: 5 mg, 10 mg, 15 mg, 20 mg.	Very broad receptor blockade (i.e., muscarinic, histamine, $5HT_3$, dopamine) and therefore can be effective as a single agent in refractory nausea and vomiting. Dissolvable disk for patients with dysphagia, mucositis, or nausea who cannot swallow.
Transdermal Scopolamine (Scope Patch)	1.5 mg transdermal patch delivers 1 mg over 3 days	Transdermal	Comes in a box of 4 patches (12 days).	Used for motion sickness or preoperative surgery. Has a slow onset of action up to 12 hours. Each patch is effective up to 72 hours.

References:

Campos, D., Pereira, J., & Reinhardt, R. (2001). Prevention of cisplatin-induced emesis by the oral neurokinin-1 antagonist, MK-869, in combination with granisetron and dexamethasone or with dexamethasone alone. *J Clin Oncol, 19*(6), 1759-1767.

Davis, M. (2002). Nausea and vomiting. In K. Kuebler & P. Esper (Eds.), *Palliative practices from A-Z for the bedside clinician.* Pittsburgh, Pa.: Oncology Nursing Society.

NPPR, *Nurse practitioners' prescribing reference.* (Fall 2003). New York, N.Y.: Prescribing References Inc.

Twycross, R., Wilcock, A., Charlesworth, S., et al. (2002). *Palliative care formulary* (2nd ed.). Oxon, U.K.: Radcliff Medical Press.

www.PDR.net. (2003). *Physicians desk reference.* On-line resource.

NEUROPATHIC PAIN, ADJUVANT ANALGESICS

Tricyclic Antidepressants

Drug/Class	Initial Dosing	Routes	Availability	Comments
Amitriptyline (Elavil)	10-25 mg HS Maximum 150 mg/day	PO, PR, IM	Tabs: 10 mg, 25 mg, 50 mg, 75 mg, 100 mg, 150 mg. Injection: 10 mg/ml.	Provides analgesic for neuropathic pain by blocking the reuptake of serotonin and norepinephrine in descending tracts. Analgesic effects occur sooner (3-7 days) than antidepressant effects (>2 wk). Analgesia can occur at lower doses. Consider useful for patients with neuralgia or diabetic neuropathy. Can produce weight gain from increased appetite. Antimuscarinic effects—use cautiously in elderly patients. Is the most anticholinergic of any of the tricyclics.
Desipramine (Norpramin)	10-25 mg HS Maximum 150 mg/day	PO	Tabs: 10 mg, 25 mg, 50 mg, 75 mg, 100 mg, 150 mg.	Similar to amitriptyline. Has the least anticholinergic effects of any of the tricyclics and is the tricyclic of choice for the elderly.
Nortriptyline (Pamelor)	10-25 mg HS Maximum 150 mg/day	PO	Caps: 10 mg, 25 mg, 50 mg, 75 mg. Oral solution: 10 mg/5 ml.	Is similar to desipramine and has the least cardiovascular side effects.

Anticonvulsants

Drug/Class	Initial Dosing	Routes	Availability	Comments
Carbamazepine (Tegretol)	100-200 mg QID Maximum 1200 mg/day	PO, Liq	Scored and chewable tabs: 100 mg, 200 mg. Extended-release tabs: 100 mg, 200 mg, 400 mg. Citrus vanilla–flavored suspension: 100 mg/5 ml. Rectal suppository: 250 mg.	Do not use in marrow suppression. Can be useful in the treatment of lancinating neuropathic or analgesic-resistant pain. Has multiple drug interactions.
Gabapentin (Neurontin)	100-300 mg qd, TID	PO, Liq	Caps: 100 mg, 300 mg, 400 mg.	Inhibits glutamate release and is a calcium channel blocker.

Continued

NEUROPATHIC PAIN, ADJUVANT ANALGESICS—cont'd
Anticonvulsants—cont'd

Drug/Class	Initial Dosing	Routes	Availability	Comments
	Maximum 3600 mg/day		Strawberry-anise oral solution: 250 mg/ml.	The drug of choice for lancinating neuropathic pain and postherpetic neuralgia. Useful in allodynia and hyperanalgesia. Potentiates the sedation of CNS depressants such as opioids and benzodiazepines. Useful for opioid-related myoclonus.
Valproic acid (Depakene)	250 mg BID-TID Maximum 2500 mg/day	PO, subcutaneous, IV, Liq, PR	Caps: 250 mg. Syrup: 250 mg/ml.	Decreases neuronal sensitization by blocking sodium channels. Gamma-aminobutyric acid (GABA) agonist. Fewer drug interactions compared with classic antiseizure medications. Once or twice daily dosing is an advantage and cost effective compared with gabapentin and carbamazepine (3 times/day). Less costly than the other anticonvulsants. Versatility includes rectal administration.

Miscellaneous

Drug/Class	Initial Dosing	Routes	Availability	Comments
Ketamine	100-200 mg subcutaneously over 24 hr Maximum 600 mg/day	subcutaneous, IM, IV, Liq	Oral solution: 50 mg/5 ml Injection: 10 mg/ml (in 20-ml vial).	NMDA antagonist. May be useful oral or subcutaneous second-line agent. Narrow therapeutic index. High risk for psychomimetic effects.
Lioresal (Baclofen)	5-10 mg TID Maximum 120 mg/day	PO	Scored tabs: 10 mg, 20 mg.	GABA agonist. Useful as an opioid adjuvant for neuropathic pain syndromes. Baclofen doses should be titrated slowly to limit side effects. Taper doses gradually when discontinuing. Reduce doses in the setting of renal dysfunction.
Mexiletine (Mexitil)	150 mg BID Maximum 200 mg TID	PO	Caps: 150 mg, 200 mg, 250 mg.	Sodium channel stabilizer. Consider as a second or third agent for refractory neuropathic pain. May be useful in patients with nerve injury–related pain. Do not use in patients with any cardiac conduction

NEUROPATHIC PAIN, ADJUVANT ANALGESICS—cont'd
Miscellaneous—cont'd

Drug/Class	Initial Dosing	Routes	Availability	Comments
				abnormalities. Discontinue antidepressant adjuvants at least 48 hours before initiating.

References:
American Pain Society. (1999). *Principles of analgesic use in the treatment of acute pain and cancer pain* (4th ed.). Glenview, Ill.: Author.
Pappagallo, M., Dickerson, D., Varga, J., et al. (2002). Management of neuropathic pain. In K. Kuebler & P. Esper (Eds.), *Palliative practices from A-Z for the bedside clinician* (Appendix A). Pittsburgh, Pa.: Oncology Nursing Society.
Twycross, R., Wilcock, A., Charlesworth, S., et al. (2002). *Palliative care formulary* (2nd ed.). Oxon, U.K.: Radcliff Medical Press.

PAIN: NON-OPIOIDS

Drug/Class	Initial Dosing	Routes	Availability	Comments
Acetaminophen (Tylenol)	325-650 mg q4-6hr Maximum 4 g/day	PO, PR, Liq	Scored tabs: 325 mg. Extra-strength tabs, caps, gelcaps: 500 mg. Mint-flavored liq: 500 mg/15 ml.	Useful for pain that is not somatic in nature. Doses in 2 g can show hepato-cellular damage. Excess of 4 g daily is hepatotoxic. May consider in combination with hydrocodone. No studies available to confirm efficacy in cancer pain. Can be effective in neoplastic fever.

Cox-2 Inhibitors*

Drug/Class	Initial Dosing	Routes	Availability	Comments
Celecoxib (Celebrex)	100-200 mg qd, BID Maximum 400 mg/day	PO	Caps: 100 mg, 200 mg, 400 mg.	Cox-2 selective medication. Potential does exist for GI adverse effects when used at higher doses for long durations. Do not use in combination with cortico-steroids, aspirin, or anti-coagulants. Avoid in renal dysfunction or when using with angiotensin-converting enzyme (ACE) inhibitors. Does not inhibit platelets.

*Should be reserved for patients with predisposed risk for developing gastrointestinal (GI) toxicity and ulcer.

Continued

PAIN: NON-OPIOIDS—cont'd

Cox-2 Inhibitors—cont'd

Drug/Class	Initial Dosing	Routes	Availability	Comments
Valdecoxib (Bextra)	10 mg qd Maximum 20 mg/day	PO	Tabs: 10 mg, 20 mg.	Useful in patients with a history of osteoarthritis, rheumatoid arthritis. See comments for all Cox-2 inhibitors. Works peripherally and centrally through Cox-1 and Cox-2 to reduce cancer pain.

Combination Cox-1 and Cox-2 Inhibitors*

Drug/Class	Initial Dosing	Routes	Availability	Comments
Diclofenac (Arthrotec)	25-50 mg TID Maximum 225 mg/day	PO	Tabs: 50 mg, 75 mg.	Traditional mixed Cox-1 and Cox-2 inhibitor. May consider adding an H-2 antagonist or an acid pump inhibitor for patients with a predisposed risk for GI toxicity. Avoid magnesium antacids. Avoid in patients with congestive heart failure (CHF) and uncontrolled hypertension.
Etodolac (Lodine)	300-500 mg BID, TID Maximum 1.2 g/day	PO	Caps: 200 mg, 300 mg. Tabs: 400 mg, 500 mg.	Same comments as above. Antacids reduce efficacy. May antagonize ACE inhibitors.
Naproxen (Aleve)	250-500 mg BID Maximum 1.5 g/day	PO, Liq	Tabs: 250 mg, 375 mg, 500 mg. Pineapple-orange suspension: 125 mg/5 ml.	See comments as above. Difference is in cost-effective dose when given BID for compliance.

Nonsteroidal Antiinflammatory Drugs (NSAIDs)

Drug/Class	Initial Dosing	Routes	Availability	Comments
Ibuprofen (Motrin, Advil)	200-400 mg q4-6hr Maximum 3.2 g/day	PO, Liq	Gelcaps, caplets, tabs: 200 mg. Tabs: 400 mg, 600 mg, 800 mg. Chewable citrus-flavored tabs: 50 mg, 100 mg. Berry-flavored suspension: 100 mg/5 ml.	Cost-effective medication of choice for patients with a low risk of GI toxicity. Easy to obtain over the counter. May potentiate anticoagulants, methotrexate. May decrease the effects of thiazide diuretics and furosemide.

*GI toxicity is generally associated with Cox-1 enzyme affinity. Therapeutic effectiveness is related to Cox-2 affinity.

PAIN: NON-OPIOIDS—cont'd
Nonsteroidal Antiinflammatory Drugs (NSAIDs)—cont'd

Drug/Class	Initial Dosing	Routes	Availability	Comments
Ketorolac (Toradol)	15-60 mg q6hr	PO, subcutaneous, IV, IM	Tabs: 10 mg. Injection: 15 mg/ml, 30 mg/ml.	Use for 4-5 days to control severe pain. High risk for GI toxicity and renal dysfunction. Is opioid-sparing in the presence of opioid toxicity or impending bowel obstruction.

References:
NPPR, *Nurse practitioners' prescribing reference.* (Fall 2003). New York, N.Y.: Prescribing References Inc.
www.PDR.net. (2003). *Physicians desk reference.* On-line reference.
Twycross, R., Wilcock, A., Charlesworth, S., et al. (2002). *Palliative care formulary* (2nd ed.). Oxon, U.K.: Radcliff Medical Press.

PAIN: OPIOIDS

Drug/Class	Initial Dosing	Routes	Availability	Comments
Fentanyl IR (Actiq)	0.5-2 ml of 50 mcg/ml lozenge on a stick	PO (buccal)	Lozenge: 200, 400, 600, 800, 1600 mcg.	50% of dose absorbed buccally. Remove lozenge from mouth with pain relief. Not more than 2 lozenges should be used concomitantly.
Hydromorphone (Dilaudid)	2-4 mg q4-6hr continuous or intermittent. No ceiling to dose escalation	PO, subcutaneous, IM, IV, PR, Liq	Tabs: 2 mg, 4 mg, 8 mg. Elixir: 5 mg/5 ml. Rectal suppository: 3 mg. Injections: 1 mg/ml, 2 mg/ml, 4 mg/ml, 10 mg/ml.	Similar properties of morphine both pharmacokinetic and pharmacodynamic. Almost 5-7.5 times more potent than morphine. Duration of action is approximately 4 hours of analgesia. Use cautiously in severe renal failure.
Methadone	2.5-10 mg. Follow dosing guidelines. No ceiling to dose escalation— titrate slowly	PO, subcutaneous, IV, IM, Liq	Tabs: 5 mg, 30 mg. Elixir: 1 mg/ml, 10 mg/ml, 20 mg/ml. Injection: 10 mg/ml (1 ml, 2 ml, 3.5 ml, 5 ml ampules).	Broader-spectrum opioid, with benefit against neuropathic pain. Drug accumulation can occur due to unique kinetics. Absorbed well from all routes. Extensive half-life. Hepatic and/or renal impairment do not affect clearance. Use cautiously with carbamazepine, phenytoin, or phenobarbital as they increase clearance. Azole antifungal, fluvoxamine, macrolide, and cimetidine decrease metabolism.

Continued

PAIN: OPIOIDS—cont'd

Drug/Class	Initial Dosing	Routes	Availability	Comments
Morphine sulfate (immediate release) IR (Roxinol, MSIR)	5-10 mg q3-4hr PRN for breakthrough pain. No ceiling to dose escalation	PO, SL, IV, IM, subcutaneous, PR, Liq	Soluble tabs (Lilly): 10 mg. Scored tabs: 15 mg, 30 mg. Caps: 15 mg, 30 mg. Elixir: 10 mg, 20 mg/5 ml. Concentrated oral solution: 20 mg/ml.	If rotating from morphine, the usual initial dose is 1/10 of the 24-hour oral morphine dose. See specific dosing parameters. Morphine is the first-line agent among strong opioids. Active opioid from opium. Liver primary site of metabolism. Analgesic properties of the metabolites (morphine-6-glucronide) are increased in renal failure. Always treat for constipation, as with other opioids, along with analgesia. Also useful for cough, dyspnea, diarrhea. Immediate-release preparation used in combination with sustained-release and dosed at 5%-15% of total daily sustained-release dose.
Morphine sulfate (sustained release) SR (Oramorph, MS Contin, Avinza)	15-30 mg BID No ceiling to dose escalation	PO, PR	Extended-release (24 hr) (Avinza): 30 mg, 60 mg, 90 mg, 120 mg. Sustained-release (12 hr) (MS Contin, Oramorph): 15 mg, 30 mg, 60 mg, 100 mg, 200 mg.	Long-acting preparation requires titration from immediate-release dosing to determine individual dose.
Oxycodone IR (Oxy IR, Oxyfast)	5 mg q3-4hr PRN for breakthrough pain. No ceiling to dose escalation	PO, SL, PR, Liq	Caps: 5 mg. Elixir: 20 mg/ml.	Broader-spectrum agent, usually reserved for patients who have adverse reactions or become physically tolerant to morphine preparations. Metabolized to oxymorphone and 10 times stronger than parenteral morphine—but plays little role in analgesia. Use cautiously with hepatic and renal failure, both of which significantly prolong half-life. PO dose is 1.5 to 2 times more potent than morphine. Immediate-release dose for breakthrough pain and dosed at 5%-15% of total daily sustained-release dose.

PAIN: OPIOIDS—cont'd

Drug/Class	Initial Dosing	Routes	Availability	Comments
Oxycodone SR (Oxycontin)	10 mg BID. No ceiling to dose escalation	PO, PR	Sustained-release caps: 10 mg, 20 mg, 40 mg, 80 mg.	Long-acting preparation requires individual titration.
Transdermal fentanyl (Duragesic)	2 mcg q48-72hr	Trans-dermal	25 mcg, 50 mcg, 75 mcg, 100 mcg.	Reserve for patients who are unable to tolerate oral opioids. Difficult to titrate in patients who have poorly managed pain. Steady-state plasma levels are achieved in 36-48 hours—due to pharmaceutical preparation. After patch removal, opioid elimination can take from 13-22 hours. Morphine to fentanyl is 100/70:1. The rate of absorption is affected by heat (i.e., febrile, heating pad, body positioning [bed-bound patient with patch placed on back and increased body heat, increases absorption]). Useful in patients with dysphagia and relatively safe in renal dysfunction. Prolonged half-life in severe renal failure.

References:

Davis, D. (2003). Equianalgesia: Paradox and pitfalls. *J Terminal Oncol, 2(?),* 89-91.

Davis, M. (in press). *Acute pain in advanced cancer: An opioid dosing strategy and illustration.* (manuscript).

Davis, M., Weissman, D., & Arnold, R. (in press). *Opioid dose titration for severe cancer pain: A systemic evidence based review.* (manuscript).

Davis, M., Varga, J., Dickerson, D., et al. (2003). Normal-release and controlled-release oxycodone: Pharmacokinetics, pharmacodynamics, and controversy. *Support Care Cancer, 11,* 84-92.

NPPR, *Nurse practitioners' prescribing reference.* (Fall 2003). New York, N.Y.: Prescribing References Inc.

Twycross, R., Wilcock, A., Charlesworth, S., et al. (2002). *Palliative care formulary* (2nd ed.). Oxon, U.K.: Radcliff Medical Press.

Walsh, D., Rivera, N., Davis, M., et al. (2003). *Opioid dosing in cancer pain: 40 strategies for 10 clinical problems: The Cleveland Clinic Foundation Guidelines.*

PRURITUS

Drug/Class	Initial Dosing	Routes	Availability	Comments
Cimetidine (Tagamet)	300 mg q6hr Maximum 1200 mg/day	PO, IM, IV, Liq	Tabs: 300 mg, 400 mg, 800 mg. 2.8% alcohol-based mint-peach flavored liquid: 300 mg/5 ml. Phenol-based	Can be considered if patient is not taking other medications. Should be avoided due to the multiple drug interactions. H2-blocker (in skin) is useful in pruritus but has multiple drug interactions. Best used in

Continued

PRURITUS—cont'd

Drug/Class	Initial Dosing	Routes	Availability	Comments
			injection: 300 mg/2 ml. Premixed IV infusion (preservative free): 300 mg/50 ml in 0.9% NaCl.	patients with active benign duodenal or gastric ulcers. Prevention of upper GI bleeding in critical care patients. May potentiate anticoagulants, phenytoin, theophylline. May also alter absorption of medications that require gastric pH.
Cyproheptadine HCl (Periactin)	2-4 mg TID Maximum 20 mg/day	PO, Liq	Scored tabs: 4 mg.	Antihistamine/H1-blocker used for urticaria. Can cause drowsiness. Use cautiously in patients with history of hyperthyroidism, cardiovascular disease, hypertension, asthma, or glaucoma. Can be used as a premedication when giving blood/blood products. Has a minimal role in palliative care.
Diphenhydramine (Benadryl)	25 mg q6hr Maximum 200 mg/day	PO, Topical, IM, IV, Liq	Capsules, tabs: 25 mg. Gel-filled caps: 25 mg. Chewable tabs: 12.5 mg. Alcohol-free cherry-flavored liquid: 12.5 mg/5 ml. Injection: 50 mg/ml (10-ml vial, 1-ml ampule, 1-ml pre-filled syringe).	Antihistamine/H1-blocker (in skin). Can potentiate CNS depression with other CNS depressants (benzodiazepines, alcohol). Is anticholinergic; use caution if using other anticholinergic medications. Use cautiously in patients with a history of cardiovascular disease, hypertension, hyperthyroidism, and glaucoma. Can induce congestive heart failure and has multiple drug interactions through CPP2D6.
Dexamethasone (Decadron) (corticosteroid)	0.75-2 mg qd, BID Maximum 8 mg/day	PO, SL, subcutaneous, IM, IV, Liq	Tabs: 0.5 mg, 0.75 mg, 4 mg. 5-12 Pak: package of 12 scored 0.75-mg tabs. Multi-dose vial: 24 mg/ml.	Glucocorticoid serves as an antiinflammatory. May be used short term due to multiple side effects in long-term therapy. Do not use if patient has chickenpox, measles, or shingles. Can escalate blood glucose and not recommended in brittle diabetics.
Doxepin (Sinequan)	5 mg q HS Maximum 150 mg/day	PO	Caps: 10 mg, 25 mg, 50 mg, 75 mg, 100 mg, 150 mg. Liquid concentrate:	Tricyclic with antihistamine properties. Anticholinergic. Is potentiated with other CNS depressant medications and alcohol. Can cause drowsiness.

PRURITUS—cont'd

Drug/Class	Initial Dosing	Routes	Availability	Comments
			10 mg/ml, dilute in 4 oz fluid.	Highest potent H1-blocker.
Methyltestos-terone (Android)	10-25 mg BID Maximum 50 mg/day	PO, SL	Caps: 10 mg.	Androgenic steroid may be useful in cholestatic pruritus. Do not consider if patient is jaundiced or has abnormal liver functions. Can potentiate oral anticoagulants. Use cautiously in patients who are insulin-dependent diabetics.
Mirtazapine (Remeron)	7.5-15 mg q HS Maximum 45 mg/day	PO, SL	Scored tabs: 15 mg, 30 mg, 45 mg. Chewable tabs (orange-flavored): 15 mg, 30 mg, 45 mg.	Tetracyclic antidepressant. Blocks H1, $5HT_2$ and $5HT_3$ receptors in the skin. Has a high affinity for H1 histaminic receptors.
Ondansetron (Zofran)	4 mg qd, BID Maximum 8 mg/day	PO, SL, IM, IV, Liq	Tabs: 4 mg, 8 mg, 24 mg. Chewable strawberry-flavored tabs: 4 mg, 8 mg. Oral solution: 4 mg/5 ml. IV prefilled bags: 32 mg/50 ml. Ampules: 2 mg/ml. Multi-dose vial: 2 mg/ml (20-ml vial).	Selective $5HT_3$ blocker (located in the skin). Used predominately in the setting of chemotherapy for the management of nausea and vomiting. Particularly in platinum-based agents. May be useful in patients with severe pruritus with obstructive jaundice and renal failure. Useful in radiation-induced nausea.
Paroxetine (Paxil)	10 mg qd Maximum 40 mg/day	PO, Liq	Controlled-release tabs: 12.5 mg, 25 mg, 37.5 mg. Orange-flavored suspension: 10 mg/5 ml.	SSRI down-modulates serotonin dermal receptors. Has many drug interactions. Potentiated by cimetidine. Use cautiously with warfarin.

References:
Davis, M., Dickerson, D., Pappagallo, M., et al. (2001). Mirtazapine: Heir apparent to amitriptyline? *Am J Hosp Palliat Care,* *18*(1), 42-46.
Davis, M., Khawam, E., Pozueb, L., et al. (2002). Management of symptoms associated with cancer: Olanzapine and mirtazapine. *Expert Rev Anticancer Ther,* *2*(4), 89-99.
Lipman, A., Jackson, K., & Tyler, L. (2000). *Evidenced based symptom control in palliative care.* Binghamton, N.Y.: Pharmaceutical Products Press.
NPPR, *Nurse practitioners' prescribing reference.* (Fall 2003). New York, N.Y.: Prescribing References Inc.
Twycross, R., Wilcock, A., Charlesworth, S., et al. (2002). *Palliative care formulary* (2nd ed.). Oxon, U.K.: Radcliff Medical Press.
Waller, A., & Caroline, N. (2000). *Handbook of palliative care in cancer* (2nd ed.). Woburn, Mass.: Butterworth-Heinemann.

APPENDIX B

Medication Routes and Metabolism

Kim Kuebler

James Varga

Mellar P. Davis

NOTE: The cytochrome P-450 enzyme system is identified as a general system for metabolism. It is the clinician's responsibility to have a working knowledge of individual drug metabolism that can contribute to adverse drug interactions. The P-450 enzymes metabolize medications as either substrates, inhibitors, and/or inducers and determine the efficacy of individual medications.

Medication	PO	SL	PR	Subcutaneous	IM	IV	Liq	Metabolism
Acetaminophen (Tylenol)	•		•				•	Hepatic, glucuronidated, and 10% by cytochrome P-450 (CYP2E1, CYP1A2)
Alprazolam (Xanax)	•	•	•				•	Hepatic, cytochrome P-450(CYP3A4/5)
Amitriptyline (Elavil)	•		•		•			Hepatic, cytochrome P-450 (CYP2D6, CYP2C9, CYP2C19, CYP3A4)
Benzonatate (Tessalon)	•							Local anesthetic effects on cough
Bisacodyl (Dulcolax)	•						•	Pass unchanged and unabsorbed through the small bowel
Carbamazapine (Tegretol)	•						•	Hepatic, cytochrome P-450 (CYP3A4)
Celecoxib (Celebrex)	•							Hepatic, cytochrome P-450 (CYP2C9)
Chlorpromazine (Thorazine)	•	•	•		•	•	•	Hepatic, cytochrome P-450 (CYP2D6)
Cimetidine (Tagamet)	•				•	•	•	Hepatic, cytochrome P-450, many interactions (CYP3A4/5, CYP1A2, CYP2C9/10, CYP2C18/19, CYP2D6)
Citalopram (Celexa)	•						•	Hepatic, cytochrome P-450 (CYP2C19)

Above columns headed: **Route**

Route

Medication	PO	SL	PR	Subcutaneous	IM	IV	Liq	Metabolism
Clonazepam (Klonopin)	•							Hepatic, cytochrome P-450 (CYP3A4)
Clonidine (Catapress)	•			•				50% excreted unchanged in the kidney, the remainder by hepatic, cytochrome P-450
Cyproheptadine (Periactin)	•						•	GI tract
Desipramine (Norpramin)	•							Hepatic, cytochrome P-450 (CYP2D6)
Dexamethasone (Decadron)	•	•		•	•	•	•	Hepatic, cytochrome P-450 (CYP3A4)
Diazepam (Valium)	•	•	•		•	•	•	Hepatic, cytochrome P-450 (CYP3A4)
Diclofenac (Arthrotec, Voltran)	•							Hepatic, cytochrome P-450 (CYP2D6)
Diphenhydramine (Benadryl)	•				•	•	•	Hepatic, cytochrome P-450 (CYP2D6)
Diphenoxylate/ Atropine (Lomotil)	•						•	GI tract
Docusate sodium (Colace, Peri-Colace)	•		•				•	GI tract
Dronabinol (Marinol)	•							Hepatic, cytochrome P-450 (CYP2C9)
Etodolac (Lodine)	•							Hepatic, cytochrome P-450
Fentanyl (Duragesic)				Transdermal route				Hepatic, cytochrome P-450 (CYP3A4)
Fluoxetine (Prozac)	•						•	Hepatic, cytochrome P-450 (CYP2D6)
Furosemide (Lasix)	•				•	•	•	Hepatic, glucuronidation
Gabapentin the kidneys (Neurontin)	•							Excreted unchanged by
Glycopyrrolate (Robinul)	•			•	•	•		Dependent upon renal and hepaticfunction
Haloperidol (Haldol)	•	•		•	•	•	•	Hepatic, cytochrome P-450 (CYP2D6)
Hydrochlorothiazide (HCTZ)	•							Renal
Hydrocodone/APAP (Vicodan)	•						•	Hepatic, cytochrome P-450 (CYP2D6)

Continued

Route

Medication	PO	SL	PR	Subcutaneous	IM	IV	Liq	Metabolism
Hydromorphone (Dilaudid)	•		•	•	•	•	•	Hepatic, glucuronidation
Hydroxyzine (Atarax)	•				•		•	GI tract
Hyoscyamine (Levsin, Urised)	•	•		•		•	•	Small bowel
Ibuprofen (Motrin, Advil)	•						•	Hepatic, cytochrome P-450 (CYP2C9)
Ketamine	•	•		•		•	•	Hepatic, cytochrome P-450 (CYP3A4, CYP2B6, CYP2C9)
Lidocaine (Xylocaine)				•		•	•	Hepatic, cytochrome P-450 (CYP2D6, CYP3iA4)
Lioresal (Baclofen)	•							Hepatic, cytochrome P-450
Loperamide (Imodium)	•						•	P glycoprotein efflux
Lorazepam (Ativan)	•	•		•		•	•	Hepatic, glucuronidation
Meclizine (Antivert)	•							GI tract
Megestrol acetate (Megace)	•						•	GI tract
Methadone (Dolophine)	•			•		•	•	Hepatic, cytochrome P-450 (CYP3A4, CYP2D6, CYP1A2, CYP2B6)
Methylphenidate (Ritalin)	•							De-esterfied peripherally
Methyltestosterone (Android)	•	•						Hepatic, cytochrome P-450 (CYP3A4, CYP3A5-7)
Metoclopramide (Reglan)	•			•		•	•	Hepatic, cytochrome P-450 (CYP2D6)
Metolazone (Mykrox)	•							Renal
Mexilitine (Mexitil)	•							Hepatic, cytochrome P-450 (CYP2D6)
Midazolam (Versed)	•			•		•	•	Hepatic, cytochrome P-450 (CYP3A4)
Mirtazapine (Remeron)	•	•						Hepatic, cytochrome P-450 (CYP3A4, CYP2D6, CYP2C9, CYP1A2)
Morphine (MS Contin, MSIR, Oramorph SR, Roxanol)	•	•	•	•		•	•	Hepatic, glucuronidation

Route

Medication	PO	SL	PR	Subcutaneous	IM	IV	Liq	Metabolism
Naproxen (Aleve)	•						•	Hepatic, cytochrome P-450 (CYP1A2, CYP2C9, CYP2C18)
Octreotide (Somatostatin)				•		•		GI tract
Olanzapine (Zyprexia)	•							Hepatic, cytochrome P-450 (CYP1A2, CYP3A4, CYP2D6)
Omperazole (Prilosec)	•							Hepatic, cytochrome P-450 (CYP2C19, CYP2C18, CYP2C8)
Ondansetron (Zofran)	•	•				•	•	Hepatic, cytochrome P-450 (CYP2D6, CYP1A2, CYP2E1, CYP3A4)
Oxycodone (OxyContin, OxyFast, OxyIR)	•	•					•	Hepatic, cytochrome P-450 (CYP2D6)
Pemoline (Cylert)	•							Hepatic, cytochrome P-450
Phenobarbital (Phenobarb)	•				•	•	•	Hepatic, cytochrome P-450 (CYP2C9)
Prednisone (Deltasone)	•				•	•	•	Hepatic, cytochrome P-450 (CYP3A4)
Prochlorperazine (Compazine)	•		•		•	•	•	Hepatic, cytochrome P-450 (CYP2D6)
Promethazine (Phenergan)	•		•		•	•	•	Hepatic, cytochrome P-450 (CYP2D6)
Ranitidine (Zantac)	•				•	•	•	GI tract
Senna (Senekot)	•						•	GI tract
Sertraline (Zoloft)	•							Hepatic, cytochrome P-450 (CYP2D6)
Spironolactone (Aldactone)	•							Renal
Temazepam (Restoril)	•							Hepatic, cytochrome P-450 (CYP2D6)
Theophylline (Theo-24)	•						•	Hepatic, cytochrome P-450 (CYP1A2, CYP2E1, CYP3A4)
Tramadol (Ultracet, Ultram)	•							Hepatic, cytochrome P-450 (CYP2D6)

Continued

Route

Medication	PO	SL	PR	Subcutaneous	IM	IV	Liq	Metabolism
Trazodone (Desyrel)	•							Hepatic, cytochrome P-450 (CYP2D6, CYP3A4)
Valproic acid (Depakene, Depacon)	•			•	•		•	Hepatic, glucuronidation
Zolpidem (Ambien)	•							GI tract

References:

NPPR, *Nurse practitioners' prescribing reference* (Fall 2003). Prescribing References, Inc.

Twycross, R., Wilcock, A., Charlesworth, S., et al. (2002). *Palliative care formulary* (2nd ed.). Oxon, U.K.: Radcliff Medical Press.

www.PDR.net. (2003). *Physicians desk reference.* On-line resource.

www.georgetown.edu/departments/pharmacology/clinlist.html

Varga, J. (in press). *Interactive palliative care center* (website resource under construction).

PO, By mouth; *SL,* sublingual; *PR,* per rectum; *SQ,* subcutaneous; *IM,* intramuscular; *IV,* intravenous; *Liq,* liquid; *GI,* gastrointestinal.

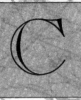

APPENDIX C

Palliative Care Assessment Tools

Marilyn O'Mallon
Kim Kuebler

CONTENTS

By Category:

By Tool:

FAMILY ASSESSMENT TOOLS

Family Pain Questionnaire

The Family Pain Questionnaire (FPQ) is a 16-item ordinal scale that measures the knowledge and experience of a family caregiver in managing chronic cancer pain. This tool can be useful in clinical practice as well as for research. This instrument can be administered by mail or in person.

Directions: The caregiver is asked to read each question thoroughly and decide if he or she agrees with the statement or disagrees. The caregiver is then asked to circle a number to indicate the degree to which he or she agrees or disagrees with the statement according to the word anchors on each end of the scale.

The FPQ includes 9 items that measure knowledge about pain and 7 items that measure the caregiver's experience with pain. All of the items have been formatted such that 0 = the most positive outcome and 10 = the most negative outcome.

This tool is used in conjunction with a version created for use by patients, the Patient Pain Questionnaire (PPQ). The FPQ tool has been tested with established reliability (test-retest, internal consistency) and validity (content, construct, concurrent). A series of psychometric analyses were performed on the instrument including content validity (CVI = .90), construct validity (ANOV A, $p < .05$), concurrent validity ($r = .60$, $p. < .05$), factor analysis and test-retest reliability ($r = .80$), established with a retest of caregivers ($n = 67$).

Below are a number of statements about cancer pain and pain relief. Please circle a number on the line to indicate your response.

Knowledge

1. Cancer pain can be effectively relieved.
   Agree   0   1   2   3   4   5   6   7   8   9   10   Disagree
2. Pain medicines should be given only when pain is severe.
   Agree   0   1   2   3   4   5   6   7   8   9   10   Disagree
3. Most cancer patients on pain medicines will become addicted to the medicines over time.
   Agree   0   1   2   3   4   5   6   7   8   9   10   Disagree
4. It is important to give the lowest amount of medicine possible to save larger doses for later when the pain is worse.
   Agree   0   1   2   3   4   5   6   7   8   9   10   Disagree
5. It is better to give pain medications around the clock (on a schedule) rather than only when needed.
   Agree   0   1   2   3   4   5   6   7   8   9   10   Disagree
6. Treatments other than medications (such as massage, heat, relaxation) can be effective for relieving pain.
   Agree   0   1   2   3   4   5   6   7   8   9   10   Disagree
7. Pain medicine can be dangerous and can often interfere with breathing.
   Agree   0   1   2   3   4   5   6   7   8   9   10   Disagree
8. Patients are often given too much pain medicine.
   Agree   0   1   2   3   4   5   6   7   8   9   10   Disagree
9. If pain is worse, the cancer must be getting worse.
   Agree   0   1   2   3   4   5   6   7   8   9   10   Disagree

Experience

10. Over the past week, how much pain do you feel your family member has had?
    No Pain   0   1   2   3   4   5   6   7   8   9   10   A Great Deal

FAMILY ASSESSMENT TOOLS—cont'd

Family Pain Questionnaire—cont'd

11. How much pain is your family member having now?

    No Pain   0   1   2   3   4   5   6   7   8   9   10   A Great Deal

12. How much pain relief is your family member currently receiving?

    No Pain   0   1   2   3   4   5   6   7   8   9   10   A Great Deal

13. How distressing do you think the pain is to your family member?

    No Pain   0   1   2   3   4   5   6   7   8   9   10   A Great Deal

14. How distressing is your family member's pain to you?

    No Pain   0   1   2   3   4   5   6   7   8   9   10   A Great Deal

15. To what extent do you feel you are able to control the patient's pain?

    No Pain   0   1   2   3   4   5   6   7   8   9   10   A Great Deal

16. What do you expect will happen with your family member's pain in the future?

    No Pain   0   1   2   3   4   5   6   7   8   9   10   A Great Deal

Used with permission from City of Hope National Medical Center.

FAMILY ASSESSMENT TOOLS—cont'd

Home Care Assessment Tool

	Yes	No
1. Does the Patient have Spiritual/Religious Support?		
2. Does the Patient desire a home death?		
3. Does the Primary Caregiver desire a home death?		
4. Does the Primary Physician agree to a home death?		
5. Does the Primary Physician agree to regular home visits?		
6. Are there an adequate number of caregivers (2 or more)?		
7. Are there physical barriers within the home that do not support a home death?		

Reference:

Cantwell, P., Turco, S., Bruera, E., et al. (1998). Home death assessment tool: A prospective study. *J Palliat Care, 14,* 104 (abstract).

Used with permission from Dr. Eduardo Bruera, M.D. Anderson Cancer Center.

NOTE: One or more "yes" answers is an indication that additional resources should be considered because the patient is at risk for a home death.

FAMILY ASSESSMENT TOOLS—cont'd

Quality of Life Family Version

The Quality of Life (Family Version) is a 37-item ordinal instrument that measures the quality of life (QOL) of a family member caring for a patient with cancer. This tool can be useful in clinical practice as well as for research. This instrument can be administered by mail or in person.

The caregiver is asked to read each question thoroughly and decide if he or she agrees with the statement or disagrees. The caregiver is then asked to circle a number to indicate the degree to which he or she agrees or disagrees with the statement according to the word anchors on each end of the scale.

The scoring should be based on a scale of 0 = worst outcome to 10 = best outcome. Several items have reverse anchors, and therefore when you code the items you will need to reverse the scores of those items. For example, if a subject circles "3" on such an item, $(10 - 3 = 7)$, you would record a score of 7. The items to be reversed are 1-4, 6, 13-20, 22, 24-29, and 33. Subscales can be created for analysis purposes by adding all of the items within a subscale and creating a mean score.

The family version of the QOL tool is an adaptation of the patient version QOL tool. The instrument was revised and tested from 1994 to 1998 in a study of 219 family caregivers of cancer patients. The test-retest reliability was $r = .89$ and internal consistency was alpha $r = .69$. Factor analysis confirmed the 4 QOL domains as subscales for the instrument. Psychometric data are provided in the patient version QOL tool (see letter that accompanies patient version QOL Tool).

Directions: We are interested in knowing how your experience of having a loved one with cancer affects *your* quality of life. Please answer all of the following questions based on *your* life at this time.

Please *circle* the number from 0-10 that best describes your experiences:

Physical Well-Being

To what extent are the following a problem for you:

1. Fatigue
   No problem   0   1   2   3   4   5   6   7   8   9   10   Severe problem
2. Appetite changes
   No problem   0   1   2   3   4   5   6   7   8   9   10   Severe problem
3. Pain or aches
   No problem   0   1   2   3   4   5   6   7   8   9   10   Severe problem
4. Sleep changes
   No problem   0   1   2   3   4   5   6   7   8   9   10   Severe problem
5. Rate your overall physical health.
   Extremely poor   0   1   2   3   4   5   6   7   8   9   10   Excellent

Psychological Well-Being Items

6. How difficult is it for you to **cope** as a result of your family member's disease and treatment?
   None at all   0   1   2   3   4   5   6   7   8   9   10   Extremely well
7. How good is your **overall quality of life**?
   Extremely poor   0   1   2   3   4   5   6   7   8   9   10   Excellent
8. How much **happiness** do you feel?
   None at all   0   1   2   3   4   5   6   7   8   9   10   Completely
9. Do you feel like you are in **control** of things in your life?
   Not at all   0   1   2   3   4   5   6   7   8   9   10   Completely
10. How **satisfying** is your life?
    Not at all   0   1   2   3   4   5   6   7   8   9   10   Completely

Continued

FAMILY ASSESSMENT TOOLS—cont'd

Quality of Life Family Version—cont'd

11. How is your present ability to **concentrate or to remember things**?
    Extremely poor   0   1   2   3   4   5   6   7   8   9   10   Excellent
12. How **useful** do you feel?
    Not at all   0   1   2   3   4   5   6   7   8   9   10   Extremely
13. How distressing was your family member's **initial diagnosis** for you?
    Not at all   0   1   2   3   4   5   6   7   8   9   10   Extremely
14. How distressing were your family member's **cancer treatments** (i.e., chemotherapy, radiation, BMT, or surgery) for you?
    Not at all   0   1   2   3   4   5   6   7   8   9   10   Extremely
15. How distressing has the time been **since your family member's treatment ended**?
    Not at all   0   1   2   3   4   5   6   7   8   9   10   Extremely
16. How much **anxiety** do you have?
    None at all   0   1   2   3   4   5   6   7   8   9   10   Severe
17. How much **depression** do you have?
    None at all   0   1   2   3   4   5   6   7   8   9   10   Severe
18. Are you **fearful of a second cancer** for your family member?
    Not at all   0   1   2   3   4   5   6   7   8   9   10   Extremely
19. Are you **fearful of recurrence** of your family member's cancer?
    Not at all   0   1   2   3   4   5   6   7   8   9   10   Extremely
20. Are you **fearful of the spreading** (metastasis) of your family member's cancer?
    Not at all   0   1   2   3   4   5   6   7   8   9   10   Extremely
21. Rate your **overall psychological well being**.
    Extremely poor   0   1   2   3   4   5   6   7   8   9   10   Excellent

Social Concerns

22. How distressing has your family member's illness been for your **family**?
    Not at all   0   1   2   3   4   5   6   7   8   9   10   Extremely
23. Is the amount of **support** you receive from others sufficient to meet your needs?
    Not at all   0   1   2   3   4   5   6   7   8   9   10   Completely
24. To what degree has your family member's illness or treatment interfered with your **personal relationships**?
    Not at all   0   1   2   3   4   5   6   7   8   9   10   Completely
25. To what degree has your family member's illness or treatment interfered with your **sexuality**?
    Not at all   0   1   2   3   4   5   6   7   8   9   10   Completely
26. To what degree has your family member's illness or treatment interfered with your **employment**?
    No problem   0   1   2   3   4   5   6   7   8   9   10   Severe problem
27. To what degree has your family member's illness or treatment interfered with your **activities at home**?
    No problem   0   1   2   3   4   5   6   7   8   9   10   Severe problem
28. How much **isolation** is caused by your family member's illness or treatment?
    None   0   1   2   3   4   5   6   7   8   9   10   Complete
29. How much **financial burden** resulted from your family member's illness or treatment?
    None   0   1   2   3   4   5   6   7   8   9   10   Extreme
30. Rate your **overall social well being**.
    None   0   1   2   3   4   5   6   7   8   9   10   Extreme

FAMILY ASSESSMENT TOOLS—cont'd

Quality of Life Family Version—cont'd

Spiritual Well-Being

31. Is the amount of support you receive from **religious activities** such as going to church or temple sufficient to meet your needs?

    Not at all   0   1   2   3   4   5   6   7   8   9   10   Completely

32. Is the amount of support you receive from **personal spiritual activities** such as prayer or meditation sufficient to meet your needs?

    Not at all   0   1   2   3   4   5   6   7   8   9   10   Completely

33. How much **uncertainty** do you feel about your family member's future?

    None at all   0   1   2   3   4   5   6   7   8   9   10   Extreme

34. Has your family member's illness made **positive changes** in your life?

    None at all   0   1   2   3   4   5   6   7   8   9   10   Extremely

35. Do you have a **purpose/mission** for your life or a reason for being alive?

    Not at all   0   1   2   3   4   5   6   7   8   9   10   Completely

36. How **hopeful** do you feel?

    None at all   0   1   2   3   4   5   6   7   8   9   10   Extremely

37. Rate your **overall spiritual well-being.**

    Extremely poor   0   1   2   3   4   5   6   7   8   9   10   Excellent

Used with permission from City of Hope National Medical Center.

FUNCTIONAL ASSESSMENT TOOLS

Edmonton Functional Assessment Tool (EFAT)

To measure a functional status specifically, oncologists rely on various scales such as the Karnofsky or Eastern Cooperative Oncology Groups (ECOG) Functional Index. These are, however, unreliable in the lower ratings (i.e., in patients with advanced cancer) and are not useful to evaluate rehabilitation measures. Consequently, our unit developed the EFAT, which was specifically designed to evaluate functional performance of patients with advanced cancer over time and to document the degrees of functional performance of patients throughout the terminal phase. It is also useful in the evaluation of the rehabilitation effect. It assesses the status of 10 functions: communication, pain, mental status, dyspnea, sitting or standing balance, mobility, walk or wheelchair locomotion, activities of daily living (ADL), fatigue, and motivation. These are assessed by the physical and occupational therapists and are quick and simple and do not require much training. Each item in the EFAT is evaluated by 4-point rating scale from 0 to 3 (0 = functional independent performance; 3 = total loss of functional performance). A total possible score on the EFAT is 30. In addition to the EFAT, a global performance status (PS) rating asks for an overall judgment of functional performance taking into account the 10 functions assessed by the EFAT.

FUNCTIONAL ASSESSMENT TOOLS—cont'd

New Edmonton Functional Assessment Tool

	0 Functional	1 Min. Dysfunction	2 Mod. Dysfunction	3 Severe Dysfunction	Date
Communication	Independent with all aspects of communication	Requires glasses, hearing aid(s), or communication devices	Communicates effectively <50% of time	Unable to communicate	
Mental Status	Oriented ×3. Memory intact	Impair 2/6 orientation/ memory. Follows simple commands	Impair 3-4/6 orientation/ memory. Responds inconsistently or restless, agitation, anxious	Impair 5-6/6 orientation/ memory or unresponsive to verbal commands	
Pain	None or occ. pain. Pain does not impact function	Pain limits some activity. Inhibits function minimally	Pain present all the time. Inhibits functions mod.	Unable to do any activities because of pain	
Dyspnea*	No dysfunction	Urgency—counting or SOBOE or intermittent	1 extra breath with counting or O_2 at 1-3 litres	$\geq$ 2 breaths with counting or O_2 at $\geq$ 4 litres	
Balance* Sit Stand	Normal balance	↓ balance. Attain/maintain position with equip or 1 person. Min. safety risk	Unsafe balance. Maintain position with mod. assist 1 or more. Risk of fall	Maintain position with max. assist 1-2 person or unable to evaluate	
Mobility*	Controls/moves all limbs at will. Performs safely and independently	Control/move all limbs but degree of limitation. 1 assist to move/safety	Can assist another person who initiates movement. Requires 2 persons assist for safe transfer	Unable to assist with position change. Mechanical lift to transfer	
Locomotion† Walk Wheelchair	Walks unassisted or independently in lead up and propelling	Walks with 1 person assist/± walk aid or supervision with lead up	Walks with 2 person assist short distance or requires assist with lead up/ propel wheelchair	Unable to walk WB for transfer. Dependent W/C management	
Fatigue‡ Motivation‡	Rarely needs to rest Wants to participate despite limitations	Rest <50% of day Active/passive participant >50% of time	Rest >50% of day Active/passive participant <50% of time	Bedridden due to fatigue No desire to participate in activity	
ADL	Independent	Independent using adaptive equipment	Manual assist of 1, verbal cueing/supervision to complete task	Total assist with ADL	
Performance Status	Independent in room or unit	Independent with minimal assist of 1	Mod. assist of 1 person room/unit	Assist of 1-2 persons in room	

Sensation—deleted.
* Reworded to ↑ objectivity.
† Activity/WC mobility collapsed.
‡ New items added.

Educational component supported by the Capital Health Authority. Used with permission from Dr. Eduardo Bruera, M.D. Anderson Cancer Center.

FUNCTIONAL ASSESSMENT TOOLS—cont'd
Palliative Performance Scale (version 2) (PPSv2)

PPS Level	Ambulation	Activity & Evidence of Disease	Self-Care	Intake	Conscious Level
100%	Full	Normal activity & work No evidence of disease	Full	Normal	Full
90%	Full	Normal activity & work Some evidence of disease	Full	Normal	Full
80%	Full	Normal activity with effort Some evidence of disease	Full	Normal or reduced	Full
70%	Reduced	Unable normal job/work Significant disease	Full	Normal or reduced	Full
60%	Reduced	Unable hobby/house work Significant disease	Occasional assistance necessary	Normal or reduced	Full or confusion
50%	Mainly sit/lie	Unable to do any work Extensive disease	Considerable assistance required	Normal or reduced	Full or confusion
40%	Mainly in bed	Unable to do most activity Extensive disease	Mainly assistance	Normal or reduced	Full or drowsy +/− confusion
30%	Totally bed bound	Unable to do any activity Extensive disease	Total care	Normal or reduced	Full or drowsy +/− confusion
20%	Totally bed bound	Unable to do any activity Extensive disease	Total care	Minimal to sips	Full or drowsy +/− confusion
10%	Totally bed bound	Unable to do any activity Extensive disease	Total care	Mouth care only	Drowsy or coma +/− confusion
0%	Death	—	—	—	—

1. PPS scores are determined by reading horizontally at each level to find a "best fit" for the patient, which is then assigned as the PPS % score.
2. Begin at the left column and read downwards until the appropriate ambulation level is reached; then read across to the next column and downward again until the activity/evidence of disease is located. These steps are repeated until all five columns are covered before assigning the actual PPS for that patient. In this way, "leftward" columns (columns to the left of any specific column) are "stronger" determinants and generally take precedence over others.

   Example 1: A patient who spends the majority of the day sitting or lying down due to fatigue from advanced disease and requires considerable assistance to walk even for short distances but who is otherwise fully conscious level with good intake would be scored at PPS 50%.

   Example 2: A patient who has become paralyzed and quadriplegic requiring total care would be PPS 30%. Although this patient may be placed in a wheelchair (and perhaps seem initially to be at 50%), the score is 30% because he or she would be otherwise totally bed bound due to the disease or complication if it were not for caregivers providing total care including lift/transfer. The patient may have normal intake and full conscious level.

FUNCTIONAL ASSESSMENT TOOLS—cont'd

Example 3: However, if the patient in example 2 was paraplegic and bed bound but still able to do some self-care such as feed themselves, then the PPS would be higher at 40% or 50% since he or she is not "total care."

3. PPS scores are in 10% increments only. Sometimes, there are several columns easily placed at one level but one or two which seem better at a higher or lower level. One then needs to make a "best fit" decision. Choosing a "half-fit" value of PPS 45%, for example, is not correct. The combination of clinical judgment and "leftward precedence" is used to determine whether 40% or 50% is the more accurate score for that patient.

4. PPS may be used for several purposes. First, it is an excellent communication tool for quickly describing a patient's current functional level. Second, it may have value in criteria for workload assessment or other measurements and comparisons. Finally, it appears to have prognostic value.

PSYCHOSOCIAL AND SPIRITUAL ASSESSMENT TOOLS

CAGE Questionnaire

Sample Questions:

1. Have you ever felt you should **C**ut down on your drinking? Yes or No
2. Have people **A**nnoyed you by criticizing your drinking? Yes or No
3. Have you ever felt bad or **G**uilty about your drinking? Yes or No
4. Have you ever had a drink first thing in the morning to steady your nerves or to get rid of a hangover (**E**ye opener)? Yes or No
5. Have you ever had any problem with non-prescription or prescriptive medications? Please specify. Yes or No

   Two or more yes responses indicate a positive CAGE (2/5 = a positive CAGE).

Scoring: Item responses on the CAGE are scored 0 or 1, with a higher score an indication of alcohol problems. A total score of 2 or greater is considered clinically significant.

REFERENCES:

Bruera, E., Moyano, J., Seifert, L., et al. (1995). The frequency of alcoholism among patients with pain due to terminal cancer. *J Pain Symptom Manage, 10,* 599-603.

Moore, R., Bone, L., Gellar, G., et al. (1989). Prevalence, detection, and treatment of alcoholism in hospitalized patients. *JAMA, 26,* 403-407.

PSYCHOSOCIAL AND SPIRITUAL ASSESSMENT TOOLS—cont'd

FACIT-Sp-Ex (version 4)

Below is a list of statements that other people with your illness have said are important. *By circling one (1) number per line, please indicate how true each statement has been for you during the past 7 days.*

0 = Not at all
1 = A little bit
2 = Somewhat
3 = Quite a bit
4 = Very much

Sp1	I feel peaceful	0 1 2 3 4
Sp2	I have a reason for living	0 1 2 3 4
Sp3	My life has been productive	0 1 2 3 4
Sp4	I have trouble feeling peace of mind	0 1 2 3 4
Sp5	I feel a sense of purpose in my life	0 1 2 3 4
Sp6	I am able to reach down deep into myself for comfort	0 1 2 3 4
Sp7	I feel a sense of harmony within myself	0 1 2 3 4
Sp8	My life lacks meaning and purpose	0 1 2 3 4
Sp9	I find comfort in my faith or spiritual beliefs	0 1 2 3 4
Sp10	I find strength in my faith or spiritual beliefs	0 1 2 3 4
Sp11	My illness has strengthened my faith or spiritual beliefs	0 1 2 3 4
Sp12	I know that whatever happens with my illness, things will be okay	0 1 2 3 4

REFERENCES:

Bradley, M.J., Peterman, A.H., Fitchett, G., et al. (1999). A case for including spirituality in quality of life instruments in oncology. *Psychooncology, 8,* 417-428.

Peterman, A.H., Fitchett, G., Brady, M.H., et al. (2002). Measuring spiritual well-being in people with cancer: The Functional Assessment of Chronic Illness Therapy-Spiritual Well-Being Scale (FACIT-Sp). *Ann Behav Med, 24*(1), 49-58.

US English 3/19/03, Copyright 1987, 1997. Derived from David Cella, PhD, Professor and Director, CORE, 1001 University Place, Evanston, IL 60201; e-mail d-cellla@northwestern.edu.

FACIT-Sp-Ex (version 4), Functional Assessment of Chronic Illness Therapy—Spiritual Well-Being, Expanded version.

PSYCHOSOCIAL AND SPIRITUAL ASSESSMENT TOOLS—cont'd

Mini-Mental State Examination (MMSE)

The Mini-Mental State Examination (MMSE) is a widely used method for assessing cognitive mental status. The evaluation of cognitive functioning is important in clinical settings because of the recognized high prevalence of cognitive impairment in medical patients. As a clinical instrument, the MMSE has been used to detect impairment, follow the course of an illness, and monitor response to treatment. The MMSE has also been used as a research tool to screen for cognitive disorders in epidemiologic studies and follow cognitive changes in clinical trials.

MMSE Sample Items

1. **Orientation to time**
   "What is the date?"

2. **Registration**
   "Listen carefully; I am going to say three words. You say them back after I stop. Ready? Here they are... HOUSE *(pause)*, CAR *(pause)*, LAKE *(pause)*.
   Now repeat those words back to me." *(Repeat up to 5 times, but score only the first trial.)*

3. **Naming**
   "What is this?" *(Point to a pencil or pen.)*

4. **Reading**
   "Please read this and do what it says." *(Show examinee the words on the stimulus form.)*

Reproduced by special permission of the Publisher, Psychological Assessment Resources, Inc., 16204 North Florida Avenue, Lutz, FL 33549, from the Mini-Mental State Examination, by Marshall Folstein and Susan Folstein, Copyright 1975, 1998, 2001 by Mini Mental LLC, Inc. Published 2001 by Psychological Assessment Resources, Inc. Further reproduction is prohibited without permission of PAR, Inc. The MMSE can be purchased from PAR, Inc. by calling (800) 331-8378 or (813) 968-3003.

PSYCHOSOCIAL AND SPIRITUAL ASSESSMENT TOOLS—cont'd

Pain, Suffering, and Spiritual Assessment

Pain is a complex subjective experience that involves both neurophysiological *and* emotional aspects. Many individual factors can affect a person's experience of pain and subsequent response to treatment including their past experiences with pain, the meaning they assign to their current pain, and underlying mood disorders (e.g., anxiety, depression, anger). At times affective and cognitive dimensions of pain along with psychosocial and spiritual issues can produce an overwhelming amount of suffering. However, pain and suffering are not inextricably linked. That is, some patients with pain report no suffering.

Attending to suffering, by listening, and offering empathy is a critical nonpharmacologic intervention. Obtaining a spiritual history can help patients and their caregivers further understand and attend to the suffering aspects of pain.

Obtaining a Spiritual History

S = Spiritual belief system	Do you have a spiritual life that is important to you? Do you have a formal religious affiliation? What is your clearest sense of the meaning of your life at this time?
P = Personal spirituality	When you are afraid or in pain, how do you find comfort? Describe the beliefs and practices of your religion that you personally accept. In what ways is your spirituality/religion meaningful to you in your daily life?
I = Integration with spiritual community	Do you belong to any religious or spiritual groups? How do you participate in this group? In what ways is this group a source of support to you?
R = Ritualized practices and restrictions	What lifestyle activities or practices does your religion encourage, discourage, or forbid? What meaning do these practices hold for you? To what extent do you follow these practices?
I = Implications for medical care	Would you like to discuss religious/spiritual implications of health care? Are there specific elements of medical care that your beliefs/religion discourage/forbid? Are there any persons you would like us to include in your spiritual care planning?
T = Terminal events planning	Are there any unresolved areas of your life at this point that you would like us to assist you with addressing? Are there practices or rituals you would like available in the hospital or home? For what in your life do you still feel gratitude even though you are in pain?

Hints for conversations about suffering and faith:
- Let the patient set the agenda; you don't need to ask about fear, unless they open the door to it.
- Don't underestimate the power of silence. Sometimes the best support is simply listening.
- A person generally isn't looking for advice, just someone to listen and affirm that fear, anger, sadness, etc. are normal.

REFERENCES:

Ambuel, B., & Weissman, D. (2000). *Fast fact and concept #19: Taking a spiritual history.* EPERC. www.epercmcw.edu.
Byock, L. (1997). *Dying well: The prospect for growth at the end of life.* Putnam, Riverhead.
Cassell, E.J. (1991). Diagnose suffering. *Ann Intern Med, 131*(7), 531-534.
Paice, J.A. Managing psychological conditions in palliative care. *Am J Nurs, 102*(11), 36-43.

PSYCHOSOCIAL AND SPIRITUAL ASSESSMENT TOOLS—cont'd

Psychosocial Pain Assessment Form

Patient: _____ Age: _____ Date: _____

Med. Record #: _____ Significant Other: _____

Diagnosis: _____ Primary Physician: _____

Pain Syndrome: _____

Duration of Pain: _____ Assessed by: _____

Please circle appropriate descriptors.

1. **Build:**   Cachectic   Thin   Medium   Heavy   Obese
2. **Attire:**   Disheveled   Hospitalized   Casual   Professional
3. **Eye Contact:**   Avoided   Appropriate   Stared
4. **Attention:** Distracted <····································|····································> Hypervigilant
   Focused
5. **Manner:**   Flat   Depressed   Distant   Cooperation
   Engaging   Humorous   Dramatic   Agitated
   Anxious   Tearful   Sobbing   Defensive
   Sarcastic   Argumentative   Angry   Hostile
6. **Verbal Expression:**   Terse   Vague   Average   Articulate   Verbose
7. **Reasoning Ability:**   Impaired   Age-Appropriate   Advanced
8. **Overall Perspective:**   Pessimistic <·································> Optimistic
   Unrealistic <·································> Realistic
9. **Impressions:**

   _____

   _____

   _____

10. **Interventions:**

    _____

    _____

    _____

11. **Recommendations:**

    _____

    _____

    _____

<u>Rating (0-10)</u>

(0 = no concern, 10 = greatest concern)

	Interviewer	Patient	Significant Other
Economic			
Social support			
Activities of daily living			
Emotional			
Coping			

PSYCHOSOCIAL AND SPIRITUAL ASSESSMENT TOOLS—cont'd

Psychosocial Pain Assessment Form—cont'd

Introduction

We recognize that people are often concerned about the impact of pain on many areas of their lives. Unrelieved pain can cause economic, emotional, spiritual and social problems in addition to medical and physical ones. We will be looking at the overall impact of pain in your life and asking several questions to help the Pain Team better understand your personal concerns. The first area we will be addressing is the economic impact of your pain.

Economic

1. How are you supporting yourself financially?

   Work_____ Family_____ Disability _____

   Partner_____ Retirement/Pensions_____ Other_____

   Friends_____ Savings _____

2. Some people we see are concerned about meeting their economic needs. Which of these are worrisome to you?

   None _____

   Housing _____ Clothing _____ Prescriptions_____

   Food_____ Childcare_____ Insurance_____

   Transportation_____ Medical bills_____ Other _____

3. How has your economic situation changed? **Better** _____ **Worse** _____
   Describe:

   _____

   _____

   _____

4. How upsetting have these changes been to you?
   Describe:

   _____

   _____

   _____

5. What would be different in your life if you could afford to change it?
   Describe:

   _____

   _____

   _____

6. Please rate your overall level of concern regarding these economic issues.

   Rating (0-10)
   (0 = no concern; 10 = greatest concern)

	Interviewer	Patient	Significant Other
Economic			

Continued

PSYCHOSOCIAL AND SPIRITUAL ASSESSMENT TOOLS—cont'd

Psychosocial Pain Assessment Form—cont'd

Social Support

We believe that pain affects not just you, but your entire family. We'd like to look at ways in which you've noticed this impact.

1. Who do you turn to when you're uncomfortable or in pain?

   Self _____ **Others** _____ **God** _____

   Name: _____ Relationship: _____

   How accessible is this person to you?

   _____

   How helpful is this to you?

   _____

2. How comfortable are you sharing your feelings/fears with your loved ones?
   What makes this difficult for you?
   Describe:

   _____

   _____

   _____

3. How satisfied are you with communication with your doctor/medical team?
   Describe:

   _____

   _____

4. Losing people who are important to us affects us deeply. Have you suffered any recent losses?
   Yes_____ No_____
   Describe:

   _____

   _____

   Breaking up _____ Separation _____
   Divorce _____ Death _____
   Moving away _____ Other _____

5. Please rate your overall level of concern regarding these social support issues.

   #### Rating (0-10)
   (0 = no concern: 10 = greatest concern)

	Interviewer	Patient	Significant Other
Social support			

PSYCHOSOCIAL AND SPIRITUAL ASSESSMENT TOOLS—cont'd

Psychosocial Pain Assessment Form—cont'd

Activities of Daily Living

Physical impact

Often unrelieved pain affects a person's daily routine. How has your pain impacted you in these activities of daily living?

1. Affecting your sleeping patterns? **Yes**_____ **No**_____

Frequent napping	_____	Difficulty going to sleep	_____
Nightmares	_____	Difficulty staying asleep	_____
Drowsiness	_____	Difficulty waking up	_____
Chronic Fatigue	_____	Other	_____

2. Affecting your eating habits? **Yes**_____ **No**_____

Weight loss/gain	_____	Special diet	_____
Loss of appetite	_____	Feeding tube	_____
Nausea/vomiting	_____	Difficulty swallowing	_____
Changes in taste	_____	Other	_____

3. Affecting your hygiene/elimination habits? **Yes**_____ **No**_____

Diarrhea	_____	Constipation	_____
Catheter	_____	Ostomy	_____
Difficulty grooming	_____	Incontinence	_____
Difficulty bathing	_____	Other	_____

4. Affecting your ability to move? **Yes**_____ **No**_____

Generalized weakness	_____	Limited range of motion	_____
Bed bound	_____	Wheel chair	_____
Crutches/walker/cane	_____	Walking/standing	_____
Getting in/out of car	_____	Climbing stairs	_____
Lifting/carrying	_____	Other	_____
No longer athletic	_____	Shortness of breath	_____

5. Affecting your roles in your family? **Yes**_____ **No**_____
   In what ways?

   _____

6. Affecting your sexual functioning? **Yes**_____ **No**_____
   In what ways?

   _____

7. Affecting your physical appearance? **Yes**_____ **No**_____
   In what ways?

   _____

8. How has your energy level changed? Less_____ Same_____ Improved _____
9. Please rate your overall level of concern regarding these physical changes.

Rating (0-10)
(0 = no concern; 10 = greatest concern)

	Interviewer	Patient	Significant Other
Activities of daily living			

Continued

PSYCHOSOCIAL AND SPIRITUAL ASSESSMENT TOOLS—cont'd

Psychosocial Pain Assessment Form—cont'd

Emotional

Pain affects our emotions. These questions will help us better understand your pain's impact upon you emotionally.

1. Have you been troubled by feelings of:
   Depression **Yes**_____ **No**_____ *Describe:* _____
   Frustration/Anger **Yes**_____ **No**_____ *Describe:* _____
   Anxiety **Yes**_____ **No**_____ *Describe:* _____
   Panic Attacks **Yes**_____ **No**_____ *Describe:* _____
   Mood Swings **Yes**_____ **No**_____ *Describe:* _____
   Difficulty Concentrating **Yes**_____ **No**_____ *Describe:* _____
   Loss of Motivation **Yes**_____ **No**_____ *Describe:* _____
2. Do you ever see or hear things that others don't? **Yes**_____ **No**_____
   Describe:
   _____
   _____
3. Are there any medical tests or procedures that frighten you? **Yes**_____ **No**_____
   Describe:
   _____
   _____
4. Have you ever thought about hurting yourself or taking your life? **Yes**_____ **No**_____
   Describe:
   _____
   _____
5. Please rate your overall level of concern regarding these emotional issues.

   #### Rating (0-10)
   (0 = no concern; 10 = greatest concern)

	Interviewer	Patient	Significant Other
Emotional issues			

Coping

People handle pain and distress in many ways. These questions will help us better understand how you cope with upsetting situations.

1. Sometimes, doing things we enjoy distracts us from our pain. What activities are you able to do that you enjoy?
   None _____

Family _____	Friends _____	Hobbies _____	Reading _____
Religion _____	Gardening _____	Traveling _____	Exercise _____
Art/Music _____	TV _____	Pets _____	Other: _____

2. Some people find comfort in spirituality to help them cope with difficult situations. What role does spirituality have in helping you?
   Describe:
   _____
   _____

PSYCHOSOCIAL AND SPIRITUAL ASSESSMENT TOOLS—cont'd

Psychosocial Pain Assessment Form—cont'd

3. Many people in your situation ask "Why did this happen to me?" How have you attempted to "make sense" of your painful experiences?
   Describe:
   _____
   _____

4. Past stressful events can impact us in the present. What kinds of stress have you had to handle before?
   Describe:
   _____
   _____

   Child abuse? **Yes**_____ **No**_____ *Describe:* _____
   Sexual abuse? **Yes**_____ **No**_____ *Describe:* _____
   Family violence? **Yes**_____ **No**_____ *Describe:* _____

5. Some people find that counseling sessions or attending support groups can help them cope with stressful situations.
   Have you ever been in counseling? **Yes**_____ **No**_____
   What was the focus of your therapy? _____
   Have you ever attended a support group? **Yes**_____ **No**_____
   What kind? _____
   How helpful was this?_____
   _____

6. Some people are prescribed medications to help them cope. Which of these have you been prescribed? **None**_____
   Other: _____
   Anti-Anxiety medications? **Yes**_____ **No**_____ *Describe:* _____
   Anti-Depressant medications? **Yes**_____ **No**_____ *Describe:* _____
   Pain Medications? **Yes**_____ **No**_____ *Describe:* _____
   Do you ever take your prescriptions differently than ordered? **Yes**_____ **No**_____
   Describe: _____

7. Some people use chemicals to help them cope. Which of these do you use?
   Tobacco? **Yes**_____ **No**_____ *Describe:* _____
   Alcohol? **Yes**_____ **No**_____ *Describe:*_____
   Recreational drugs? **Yes**_____ **No**_____ *Describe:* _____
   Have you ever tried to stop using these? **Yes**_____ **No**_____ *Describe:* _____
   Do you worry about your usage of these? **Yes**_____ **No**_____ *Describe:* _____
   Has your family worried about your usage of these? **Yes**_____ **No**_____ *Describe:* _____

8. What changes do you expect in your future?
   Describe: _____

9. Overall, how satisfied are you with your present quality of life?
   Describe: _____

10. Please rate your overall level of concern regarding your ability to cope or manage your pain.
    Rating (0-10)
    (0 = no concern: 10 = greatest concern)

	Interviewer	Patient	Significant Other
Coping			

Used with permission from Shirley Otis-Green, City of Hope National Medical Center.

PSYCHOSOCIAL AND SPIRITUAL ASSESSMENT TOOLS—cont'd

Quality Of Life Inventory (QOLI®)

The QOLI assessment, a test from Pearson Assessments, is a brief inventory to help measure life satisfaction that can also be used to help measure outcomes. Brief but comprehensive, the QOLI assessment has an overall measure of life satisfaction and helps assess problems in living in 16 key areas of life including love, work, and recreation.

Applications of the QOLI assessment include:

- Outcome assessment and treatment planning for mental and physical disorders
- Non–health-related personal counseling settings such as organizational development, EAPs and college counseling centers to help people focus on improving their quality of life
- Tracking patient treatment progress and documenting change
- Helping to identify people at risk for developing health problems or disorders
- Assisting in gathering information to help establish the efficacy of different treatments or services
- Substance abuse treatment and assessment
- Behavioral medicine assessment
- Personnel selection to help predict future job performance and satisfaction

The QOLI test is a copyrighted instrument 1996-2004. **DO NOT COPY.** The QOLI test consists of 32 items. Listed below is a sampling of the QOLI test items and condensed test directions.

(*This survey asks how satisfied you are with parts of your life such as your work and your health. For each question, blacken the circle that best describes you.*)

Health is being physically fit, not sick, and without pain or disability.

"How important is HEALTH to your happiness?" (0: Not important; 1: Important; 2: Extremely important)

"How satisfied are you with your HEALTH?" (−3: Very dissatisfied; −2: Somewhat dissatisfied; −1: A little dissatisfied; +1: A little satisfied; +2: Somewhat satisfied; +3: Very satisfied)

"QOLI" is a registered trademark of Michael B. Frisch, PhD. Selected items and test instructions reproduced with permission of Pearson Assessments. 1-(800) 627-7271, ext. 3225. www.pearsonassessments.com/tests/qoli.htm.

PSYCHOSOCIAL AND SPIRITUAL ASSESSMENT TOOLS—cont'd

Spiritual Well-Being Scale

For each of the following statements circle the choice that best indicates the extent of your agreement or disagreement as it describes your personal experience:

SA = Strongly Agree
MA = Moderately Agree
A = Agree
D = Disagree
MD = Moderately Disagree
SD = Strongly Disagree

1. I don't find much satisfaction in private prayer with God.	SA	MA	A	D	MD	SD
2. I don't know who I am, where I came from, or where I am going.	SA	MA	A	D	MD	SD
3. I believe that God loves me and cares about me.	SA	MA	A	D	MD	SD
4. I feel that life is a positive experience.	SA	MA	A	D	MD	SD
5. I believe that God is impersonal and not interested in my daily situations.	SA	MA	A	D	MD	SD
6. I feel unsettled about my future.	SA	MA	A	D	MD	SD
7. I have a personally meaningful relationship with God.	SA	MA	A	D	MD	SD
8. I feel very fulfilled and satisfied with life.	SA	MA	A	D	MD	SD
9. I don't get much personal strength and support from my God.	SA	MA	A	D	MD	SD
10. I feel a sense of well-being about the direction my life is headed in.	SA	MA	A	D	MD	SD
11. I believe that God is concerned about my problems.	SA	MA	A	D	MD	SD
12. I don't enjoy much about life.	SA	MA	A	D	MD	SD
13. I don't have a personally satisfying relationship with God.	SA	MA	A	D	MD	SD
14. I feel good about my future.	SA	MA	A	D	MD	SD
15. My relationship with God helps me not to feel lonely.	SA	MA	A	D	MD	SD
16. I feel that life is full of conflict and unhappiness.	SA	MA	A	D	MD	SD
17. I feel most fulfilled when I'm in close communion with God.	SA	MA	A	D	MD	SD
18. Life doesn't have much meaning.	SA	MA	A	D	MD	SD
19. My relation with God contributes to my sense of well-being.	SA	MA	A	D	MD	SD
20. I believe there is some real purpose for my life.	SA	MA	A	D	MD	SD

SYMPTOM ASSESSMENT TOOL

Edmonton Symptom Assessment Scale

Numerical intensity	1	2	3	4	5	6	7	8	9	10
Pain										
Tiredness										
Nausea										
Depression										
Anxiety										
Drowsiness										
Appetite										
Well-being										
Dyspnea										
Date:										

Reference:
Bruera, E., Kuehn N., Miller, M., et al. (1991) The Edmonton Symptom Assessment System (ESAS): A simple method for the assessment of palliative care patients. *J Palliat Care, 7,* 6-9.

Used with permission from Dr. Eduardo Bruera, M.D. Anderson Cancer Center.

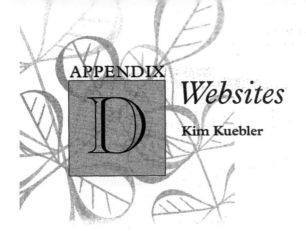

APPENDIX D

Websites

Kim Kuebler

CONTENTS

COMPLEMENTARY AND ALTERNATIVE MEDICINE

American Holistic Nurses Association
www.ahna.org

Cancer Consultants
www.cancerconsultants.com

MD Anderson's Complementary/Integrative
Education Resource
www.mdanderson.org/departments/cimer

Memorial Sloan-Kettering
www.mskcc.org

National Center for Complementary and
Alternative Medicine
www.nccam.nih.gov

NCI's Office of Cancer and Complementary and
Alternative Medicine
www.3cancer.gov/occam

Rosenthal Center for Complementary and
Alternative Medicine
www.rosenthal.hs.columbia.edu

ETHICS

Center for Clinical Ethics and Humanities in
Healthcare
http://wings.buffalo.edu/faculty/research/bioethics/
main.htm

Ethics Committee of the Society of Critical Care
www.sccm.org

Ethics in Medicine—University of Washington
School of Medicine
http://eduserv.hscer.washington.edu/bioethics/

European Association for Palliative Care
www.eapcnet.org

Institutes of Medicine
www.iom.edu

Medical College of Wisconsin Bioethics
www.mcw.edu/bioethics

EVIDENCE-BASED PRACTICE

Agency for Health Care and Research Quality
(AHRQ)
www.ahrq.gov

BioMed Central/Palliative Care
www.biomedcentral.com

Centre for Evidence-Based Medicine
www.cebm.utoronto.ca

Cochrane Library
www.cochrane.org

Critical Care Workgroup
www.mywhatever.com/cifwriter/content/41/
pe1208.html

Evidence-Based Nursing
http://ebn.bmjjournals.com

Federal Government National Guidelines
Clearinghouse
www.guidelines.gov

Graduate Research in Nursing
www.graduateresearch.com

International Medical Volunteers Association
www.imva.org

Oncology Nursing Society Evidence-Based
Practice
www.ons.org/nursingEd/

Online Journal of Clinical Innovations
www.cinahl.com/cexpress/ojcionline3/

Online Journal of Knowledge Synthesis for
Nursing
www.stti.iupui.edu/VirginiaHendersonLibrary/

Quality of Life Care
www.cddc.vt.edu

ONCOLOGY PATIENT INFORMATION

American Cancer Society
www.cancer.org

American Institute for Cancer Research
www.aicr.org

American Lung Association
www.lungusa.org

American Society of Clinical Oncology
www.asco.org

Association of Pediatric Oncology Nurses
www.apon.org

Cancer Care, Inc
www.cancercare.org

Cancer Index
www.cancerindex.org

Intercultural Cancer Control
www.iccnetwork.org

National Cancer Institute
www.nci.nih.gov

Oncolink
www.oncolink.upenn.edu

People Living with Cancer
www.peoplelivingwithcancer.org

PAIN

American Chronic Pain Association
www.theacpa.org

American Pain Foundation
www.painfoundation.org

American Pain Society
www.ampainsoc.org

American Society of Addiction Medicine
www.asam.org

American Society of Pain Management Nurses
www.aspmn.org

Association of American Sickle Cell Disease
www.sicklecelldisease.org

British Medical Journal Pain Articles
www.bmj.com/cgi/collection/pain

City of Hope Pain/Palliative Care Resource Center
http://cityofhope.org/prc/

International Association for the Study of Pain
(IASP)
www.iasp-pain.org

Mayday Pain Project
www.painandhealth.org

MD Anderson Cancer Center Pain Management
www.mdacc.tmc.edu

Pain and Policy Studies Group
www.partnershipforcaring.org

Pain Medicine and Palliative Care
www.stoppain.org

Partners Against Pain
www.partnersagainstpain.com

Wisconsin Cancer Pain Initiative
www.wisc.edu/wcpi

World Institute of Pain
http://wipain.org

PALLIATIVE CARE RESOURCES

Aging with Dignity
www.agingwithdignity.org

American Academy of Hospice and Palliative
Medicine
www.aahpm.org

Americans for Better Care of the Dying
www.abcd-caring.org

Association of Multicultural Counseling and
Development
www.amcd-aca.org

Association of Oncology Social Work
www.aosw.org

Caregiver Survival Resources
www.caregiver911.com

Center for Practical Bioethics
www.midbio.org

Center to Advance Palliative Care
www.capcmssm.org

Center to Improve Care of the Dying
www.medicaring.org

Centre for Grief Education
www.grief.org.au

Cleveland Clinic Palliative Medicine
www.clevelandclinic.org/palliative

Compassion in Dying Federation
www.compassionindying.org

Dying Well
www.dyingwell.com

Edmonton Palliative Care Service
www.palliative.org

Education for Physicians on End-of-Life Care
www.epec.net

End-of-Life Nursing Education Consortium
www.aacn.nche.edu/elnec

Family Caregiver Alliance
www.caregiver.org

Family Care Research Program
www.healthteam.msu.edu

Growth House, Inc
www.growthhouse.org

Hospice Association of America
www.hospice-america.org

Hospice Foundation of America
www.hospicefoundation.org

Hospice and Palliative Nurses Association
www.hpna.org

IAHPC access to palliative care journals
www.palliativecarejournals.com

IAHPC access to palliative care texts
www.pallcarebooks.com;
www.palliativebooks.com

Innovations in End-of-Life Care
www.edc.org/lastacts

International Association for Hospice and
Palliative Care (IAHPC)
www.iahpc.com

International Workgroup Group on Death, Dying
and Bereavement
www.wwdc.com

Last Acts
www.lastacts.org

MD Anderson Cancer Center Palliative Care and
Rehabilitation Medicine
www.mdanderson.org/palliative/clinician

National Association of Social Workers
www.socialworkers.org

National Hospice and Palliative Care
Organization
www.nhpco.org

National Prison Hospice Association
www.npha.org

Oncology Nursing Society
www.ons.org

Partnership for Caring
www.partnershipforcaring.org

Promoting Excellence in End-of-Life Care
www.promotingexcellence.org

San Diego Hospice and Palliative Care
www.grief.org

Shaare Zedek Cancer Pain and Palliative Medicine
Reference Database
www.chernydatabase.org

Social Work Resources
www.clinicalsocialwork.com

Supportive Care of the Dying
www.careofdying.org

PATIENT ADVOCACY

Hospice Network
www.hospicenet.org

Hospice Patients Alliance
www.hospicepatients.org

National Academies, Office of News and Public
Information
www.nationalacademies.org/news.nsf

National Institute on Aging
www.nia.nih.gov

National Public Radio The End of Life
www.npr.org/programs/death

Purdue Pharma LLP
www.patientadvocacy@pharma.com

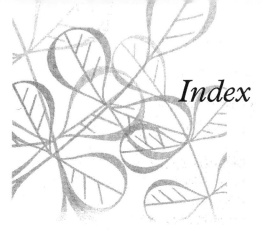

Index

Page numbers followed by f indicate figures; t, tables; b, boxes.

Accurate oncology information...

fast!

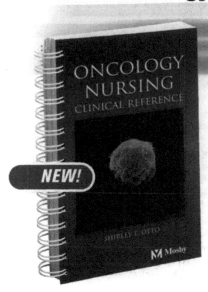

NEW!

Oncology Nursing Clinical Reference

Shirley E. Otto, MSN, CRNI, AOCN
2004 • 528 pp., illustd.
ISBN: 0-323-02517-X • A Mosby title

Written by an experienced practitioner and author, the new **Oncology Nursing Clinical Reference** covers essential information and numerous hot topics in oncology — all in a great rapid-reference, spiral-bound format that's ideal for clinical use in any practice settting.

Its clear, consistent organization and concise outline format provide succinct coverage of common types of cancer — based on a uniquely practical symptom-management approach.

This outstanding clinical tool includes:

- ➡ Details on 12 different **oncologic emergencies**
- ➡ Important **end-of-life and grief/bereavement issues**
- ➡ **Support therapies** such as complementary, alternative, and herbal medicine, hormonal therapy, and nutrition
- ➡ A **symptom management** emphasis that helps you identify and share important comfort strategies with patients
- ➡ Facts on 200 of the most commonly prescribed **chemotherapeutic agents and pain medications** for cancer patients
- ➡ A **pediatric cancers** chapter for adolescent patients seen in adult care areas

Designed to help you retrieve the information you need *fast*, this expert resource lets you focus on giving prompt, informed, compassionate care to cancer patients in any setting — acute, ambulatory, home, or extended care.

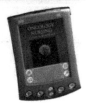

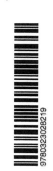